ATLAS *of* COSMETIC SURGERY

ATLAS *of* COSMETIC SURGERY

MICHAEL S. KAMINER, MD
SkinCare Physicians of Chestnut Hill
Chestnut Hill, Massachusetts
Adjunct Assistant Professor of Medicine (Dermatology)
Dartmouth Medical School
Hanover, New Hampshire

JEFFREY S. DOVER, MD, FRCPC
SkinCare Physicians of Chestnut Hill
Chestnut Hill, Massachusetts
Adjunct Professor of Medicine (Dermatology)
Dartmouth Medical School
Hanover, New Hampshire

KENNETH A. ARNDT, MD
SkinCare Physicians of Chestnut Hill
Chestnut Hill, Massachusetts
Clinical Professor of Dermatology
Harvard Medical School
Boston, Massachusetts
Adjunct Professor of Medicine (Dermatology)
Dartmouth Medical School
Hanover, New Hampshire

With 479 illustrations

W.B. SAUNDERS COMPANY
A Division of Harcourt Health Sciences
Philadelphia London New York St. Louis Sydney Toronto

W.B. SAUNDERS COMPANY
A Harcourt Health Sciences Company

The Curtis Center
Independence Square West
Philadelphia, Pennsylvania 19106

Library of Congress Cataloging-in-Publication Data

Atlas of cosmetic surgery / [edited by] Michael S. Kaminer, Jeffrey S. Dover, Kenneth A. Arndt.
p. ; cm.
Includes bibliographical references and index.
ISBN 0-7216-8413-0
1. Surgery, Plastic—Atlases. I. Kaminer, Michael S. II. Dover, Jeffrey S. III. Arndt, Kenneth A., 1936-
[DNLM: 1. Surgery, Plastic—Atlases. WO 517 A87905 2002]
RD119 .A87 2002
617.9′5—dc21
2001042967

Acquisitions Editor: Elizabeth M. Fathman
Developmental Editor: Ellen Baker Geisel
Project Manager: Patricia Tannian
Project Specialist: Anne Salmo
Book Design Manager: Gail Morey Hudson
Cover Designer: Teresa Breckwoldt

ATLAS OF COSMETIC SURGERY ISBN 0-7216-8413-0

Printed in the United States of America

Last digit is the print number: 9 8 7 6 5 4 3 2 1

To my wonderful children

Lexi and Jake

Who keep me honest and motivated,
and whose love and devotion make me smile every day

To my parents

For everything

And to my wife

Heather

For her strength, support, commitment, and love,
which I rely on and cherish more than she can know

MSK

To my daughters

Sophie and Isabel

For their unconditional love

And my wife

Tania

For her never ending encouragement, support,
love, friendship, and patience

JSD

To my colleagues and friends

and as always

to my family

(with a welcome to Alexander)

Who make my life exciting, fulfilling, fun,
productive, and filled with love.

KAA

Contributors

MURAD ALAM, MD
Department of Dermatology
Columbia University, College of Physicians & Surgeons
New York, New York

KENNETH A. ARNDT, MD
SkinCare Physicians of Chestnut Hill
Chestnut Hill, Massachusetts
Clinical Professor of Dermatology
Harvard Medical School, Boston, Massachusetts
Adjunct Professor of Medicine (Dermatology)
Dartmouth Medical School
Hanover, New Hampshire

ERIC F. BERNSTEIN, MD
Director
Laser Surgery and Cosmetic Dermatology Centers
Marlton, New Jersey
Clinical Associate Professor of Dermatology
University of Pennsylvania
Philadelphia, Pennsylvania

BRIAN S. BIESMAN, MD
Associate Clinical Professor of Ophthalmology
The University of Tennessee Health Sciences Center
Memphis, Tennessee
The Center for Eyelid & Aesthetic Surgery
Nashville, Tennessee

JOHN BRAMHALL, PhD, MD
Assistant Professor of Anesthesiology
University of Washington
Attending Physician, Harborview Medical Center
Seattle, Washington

STEVEN H. DAYAN, MD
Clinical Assistant Professor
Division of Facial Plastic Surgery
Department of Otolaryngology, University of Illinois
Chicago, Illinois

ELIZABETH R. DIDIE, MA
Doctoral Candidate in Clinical Psychology
Department of Clinical and Health Psychology
Medical College of Pennsylvania—Hahnemann University
Philadelphia, Pennsylvania

CHRISTINE DIERICKX, MD
Private Practice, Antwerp, Belgium
Visiting Faculty Member, Harvard Medical School
Boston, Massachusetts

JEFFREY S. DOVER, MD, FRCPC
SkinCare Physicians of Chestnut Hill
Chestnut Hill, Massachusetts
Adjunct Professor of Medicine (Dermatology)
Dartmouth Medical School
Hanover, New Hampshire

ZOE DIANA DRAELOS, MD
Clinical Associate Professor
Department of Dermatology
Wake Forest University School of Medicine
Winston-Salem, North Carolina

RICHARD E. FITZPATRICK, MD
Associate Clinical Professor of Medicine/Dermatology
University of California, San Diego
San Diego, California

BARBARA A. GILCHREST, MD
Professor and Chairman, Department of Dermatology
Boston University School of Medicine
Chief of Dermatology, Boston Medical Center
Boston, Massachusetts

RICHARD G. GLOGAU, MD
Clinical Professor of Dermatology
University of California, San Francisco
Professor of Dermatology
University of California, San Francisco Medical Center
San Francisco, California

TED A. GROSSBART, PhD
Assistant Clinical Professor of Psychology
Department of Psychiatry, Harvard Medical School
Senior Supervisor, Department of Psychiatry
Beth Israel-Deaconess Hospital
Boston, Massachusetts

ELIZABETH HAIKEN, PhD
El Cerrito, California

C. WILLIAM HANKE, MD, FACP
Clinical Professor, Indiana University School of Medicine
Indianapolis, Indiana
Medical Director, Laser & Skin Surgery Center of Indiana
Carmel, Indiana

GEORGE J. HRUZA, MD
Clinical Associate Professor of Dermatology and Otolaryngology-Head and Neck Surgery
St. Louis University School of Medicine
Director, Laser & Dermatologic Surgery Center
St. Louis, Missouri

MAMI AIELLO IWAMOTO, MD
Instructor of Ophthalmology
Harvard Medical School
Associate Surgeon, Department of Ophthalmology
Massachusetts Eye & Ear Infirmary
Boston, Massachusetts

DARLENE S. JOHNSON, MD
Clinical Instructor, Department of Dermatology
Harvard University, Boston, Massachusetts
Staff Physician, Department of Medicine
Division of Dermatology, Lahey Clinic
Burlington, Massachusetts

MICHAEL S. KAMINER, MD
SkinCare Physicians of Chestnut Hill
Chestnut Hill, Massachusetts
Adjunct Assistant Professor of Medicine (Dermatology)
Dartmouth Medical School
Hanover, New Hampshire

ARNOLD WILLIAM KLEIN, MD
Professor of Dermatology/Medicine
University of California, Los Angeles School of Medicine
UCLA Center for Health Sciences
Los Angeles, California

MADELINE KRAUSS, MD
Director, Center for Cosmetic Skin Surgery
Department of Dermatology, New England Medical Center
Assistant Professor of Dermatology
Tufts University School of Medicine
Boston, Massachusetts

PATRICK J. LILLIS, MD
Assistant Clinical Professor of Dermatology
University of Colorado Health Sciences Center
Loveland, Colorado

JULIE R. McCOY, PharmD
Adjunct Faculty, College of Pharmacology
Washington State University, Pullman, Washington
Clinical Pharmacist, Sacred Heart Medical Center
Spokane, Washington

RICHARD J. ORT, MD
Clinical Faculty, Department of Dermatology
University of Colorado School of Medicine
Denver, Colorado

STEPHEN W. PERKINS, MD
Clinical Associate Professor
Department of Otolaryngology-Head and Neck Surgery
Indiana University School of Medicine
Meridian Plastic Surgery Center, St. Vincent Hospitals
Indianapolis, Indiana

THOMAS E. ROHRER, MD
Associate Professor of Dermatology
Boston University School of Medicine
Director, Mohs and Dermatologic Surgery
Director
Boston University Center for Cosmetic and Laser Surgery
Boston Medical Center
Boston, Massachusetts

DAVID B. SARWER, PhD
Assistant Professor of Psychology
Departments of Psychiatry and Surgery
University of Pennsylvania School of Medicine
Philadelphia, Pennsylvania

LORI L. SCHOONOVER, PharmD
Scientific Manager, U.S. Medical and Regulatory Affairs
Aventis Pharmaceuticals
Spokane, Washington

ROBIN TRAVERS, MD
SkinCare Physicians of Chestnut Hill
Chestnut Hill, Massachusetts
Adjunct Assistant Professor of Medicine (Dermatology)
Dartmouth Medical School
Hanover, New Hampshire

RODNEY L. TRYTKO, MD, MBA
Anesthesiologist, Deaconess Medical Center
Anesthesia Associates
Spokane, Washington

SANDY S. TSAO, MD
Instructor in Dermatology, Harvard Medical School
Assistant in Dermatology, Massachusetts General Hospital
Boston, Massachusetts

WALTER P. UNGER, MD
Clinical Professor of Dermatology
Co-Director, Division of Cosmetic Dermatologic Surgery
Department of Medicine (Dermatology)
Mt. Sinai Hospital, New York, New York
Associate Professor of Medicine (Dermatology)
University of Toronto
Co-Director, Division of Dermatologic Surgery
St. Michael's Hospital
Toronto, Ontario, Canada

ROBERT A. WEISS, MD
Assistant Professor
Johns Hopkins University School of Medicine
Department of Dermatology
Director, Maryland Laser, Skin & Vein Institute
Baltimore, Maryland

Foreword

Achieving cosmetic perfection has been a human preoccupation since before recorded time. For the ancient Greeks, the ideal body was found in perfect proportion. The second century Greek sculpture *Aphrodite of Cyrene* was crafted with elegant proportions that have been a model for artists ever since. The Greeks were so enamored of ideal human proportions that they used mathematical extrapolations of idealized bodies to design Greek temples and other structures. In fact, the architect of the temple built to Hermes revealed that, unbeknownst to all, the structure was actually the mathematical image of a young woman of Corinth whom he had the good fortune to love.

Our human sense of self, as we chose to express it in art, probably first emerged about 30,000 years ago. Prehistoric statuettes identified in the ancient world were barely larger than the palm of a hand and, sculpted out of stone or other natural materials, took advantage of natural features such as protrusions for breasts and irregularities for hair. They were primitive but reflected an obvious effort to capture human identity. Of course, there were practical purposes to early art: its use in fertility rights and in religious ceremonies reflected a desire to understand the nature of human mortality. These counterpoints of self-image and beauty, fertility, and immortality provide a direct connection between the preoccupations of the prehistoric human and our own today. While it is true that previous generations probably died too young to look old, concern about appearance is universal, transcultural, and ineluctable.

Cosmetic surgery is hardly a new endeavor. History indicates that human beings have always tried to modify their appearance for religious purposes, for reasons of love and sex, or because of personal dissatisfaction. In the final analysis, cosmetic surgery today is intended to enhance our personal beauty. Beauty engenders attractiveness; appeal leads to a sense of youthful exuberance, and youth is the single rigid finger that we can poke in the eye of mortality. We pursue laser treatment to remove blemishes or other marks considered disfiguring to make ourselves more perfect. We undergo liposuction to remodel ourselves into the form that we think we should be, a shape in which we think we would be happier. For those of us who practice cosmetic surgery and intimately touch the lives of our patients it is important to remember that perfection is never wholly obtainable. In fact, as the ancient artists and cultures have taught us, perfection is merely a goal. The Greeks understood quite clearly that Aphrodite, goddess of love, represented an image of absolute beauty rather than the beauty a mortal could achieve.

It is axiomatic that as our population ages, our youth-oriented culture creates greater demands upon those of us who practice cosmetic surgery to help the patient remain youthful in appearance. There is no doubt that great progress is being made in our understanding of aging at the cellular level, but this does not necessarily translate for now into clinical benefits that we can perceive. Claims for the role of antioxidants and other topical compounds have not been scientifically substantiated, and the variety of nonsurgical approaches that do not in any way alter the biology, structure, or anatomy of the skin and its associated tissues cannot be expected to yield significant cosmetic benefits. In a field that is so emotion laden, the physician who establishes his or her credibility with the patient will be the cosmetic surgeon with the greatest success. This *Atlas of Cosmetic Surgery* details not only the scientific basis of cosmetic procedures but also the clinical potential of the expanding realm of legitimate cosmetic surgery. From the explosion of laser technology to advances in liposuction this *Atlas* provides a detailed roadmap to obtaining the highest possible level of cosmetic improvement.

Because of the substantial psychological overlay that inevitably is associated with issues of self-image and cosmesis the reader should take special note of the emphasis on careful evaluation, patient discussion, management of expectation, and skilled execution of the procedures. For the patient who presents in your office wanting to look like the model on the cover of the beauty magazine she is holding, take a hint. To the patient who sits across from you and states, "I don't want to look tired all the time. I just want to look a bit more refreshed," you can likely offer much.

Doctors who perform cosmetic surgery are truly physicians and scientists of the skin. Understanding the interdisciplinary nature of this exciting field is critical to success. The editors, Drs. Kaminer, Dover, and Arndt, whom I know well, are superbly qualified to knit together the diverse strands of a discipline that includes laser surgery, hair restoration, liposuction, and many others. This extremely well-written book reflects the cumulative experience of the authors and editors and focuses on the practical applications designed to help you achieve success with your patients, as well as the science underlying the processes and procedures. Dr. Arndt, editor of the *Archives of Dermatology* for almost twenty years, has a broad perspective on cosmetic surgery that helps shape the heft of the book. Dr. Dover and Dr. Kaminer, through their research, publications, and active clinical practice, have a combined expertise that provides valuable perspective and depth of knowledge. By using this *Atlas,* you will be able to take advantage of their experience and knowledge as you enjoy the challenges of cosmetic surgery.

An atlas is necessarily intended to inform and instruct. Cosmetic surgery is a practical field, and the atlas format provides the most efficient means of disseminating useful information in a lucid and visually comprehensible fashion. In addition to using this atlas it is important for you to be a true expert in any of the procedures that you choose to perform. This expertise can be enhanced further by reading primary articles, visiting with colleagues who are already expert, and by participating in formal didactic and hands-on courses. Another way to become well-known for expertise in particular procedures is to publish articles based on your own experience and to participate in clinical trials that relate to the procedures you are performing.

As you seek to perfect, remember always, as the Greeks believed, that beauty is an elusive goal and that immortality will similarly slip between our fingers. Conversely, be mindful that through the judicious use of the procedures described in this book one can hope to approximate more closely the goal of the appearance of eternal youth, and the attendant happiness that may bring will be a consolation for the immortality that eludes us all.

David J. Leffell, MD

Professor of Dermatology, Plastic Surgery, and Otolaryngology
Yale School of Medicine
Chief, Section of Dermatologic and Laser Surgery
Yale New Haven Hospital, New Haven, Connecticut

Preface

What is cosmetic surgery? This deceptively simple question is in many ways the foundation for how and why the *Atlas of Cosmetic Surgery* came together. At first glance, the simple answer appears to be, procedures that make people look better. But then come the harder questions, such as, Who performs cosmetic surgery? What is a cosmetic surgeon? What is the minimum amount of invasiveness required to make a procedure "surgery"? and finally, Who are the cosmetic surgery patients?

In some ways, the answer to the "what is cosmetic surgery" question depends on whom you ask. Interspecialty and intraspecialty disagreements have often dominated the discussion and unfortunately have made it difficult to accurately assess the current field of cosmetic surgery as a whole. Clearly, cosmetic surgery is a multifaceted specialty practiced by physicians from a variety of disciplines. This diversity of cosmetic surgery practitioners has made it difficult to define the field because by its nature it is broad and evolving. Because of this, a clear definition of cosmetic surgery has until now been lacking. It is our intent with this book to give cosmetic surgery a name, a face, an identity, and in so doing help to answer the question, What is cosmetic surgery?

The concept of appearance enhancement has been with us for centuries, but over the latter part of the twentieth century, surgical procedures to improve the way we look became not only commonplace but also, and even more importantly, socially acceptable. The media and our patients began to talk about surgery to improve appearance in an open and accepting format that previously was unthinkable. Unfortunately the medical community has in many ways lagged behind the popular press in bringing accurate and ethically sound information about cosmetic surgery not only to the public but also to our colleagues.

Specialties such as dermatology, plastic surgery, facial plastic surgery, anesthesiology, oral and maxillofacial surgery, and oculoplastic surgery have all participated in the academic process of improving surgery to enhance appearance. Yet the fact that so many diverse groups are involved has made it difficult to provide consistent information to the public and the medical community about cosmetic surgery. Cosmetic surgery procedures are now safer, more effective, and less invasive than at any time in history, and the reason for this is directly linked to the contributions of numerous doctors from a variety of specialties. The *Atlas of Cosmetic Surgery* is a comprehensive, interdisciplinary textbook that is intended to provide physicians with the information and tools necessary to understand cosmetic surgery patients, evaluate them, learn about the field of cosmetic surgery as a whole, and perform the procedures central to helping patients improve their appearance.

So how did the *Atlas of Cosmetic Surgery* come to be? Every once in a while, something happens that can have a significant impact on your life. It was toward the end of 1997 that one of those moments happened to the three of us. We were sitting in Ken Arndt's office at Beth Israel Deaconess Medical Center. There were diplomas and honorary degrees on the wall too numerous to count, photographs, the buzz of a busy office outside the door. We were discussing several issues, including our philosophies on patient care, the future of dermatology and dermatologic surgery, and the daunting amount of work we were facing as we prepared to open a new cosmetic surgery and laser facility.

At the time the new facility was one of the first of its kind in the world, and it was the first and only comprehensive cosmetic surgery facility at Harvard Medical School. It was state-of-the-art, with thirteen lasers, two full operating rooms, and a physician staff that could perform virtually all of the laser and cosmetic surgery procedures available in cutaneous cosmetic surgery. The space was designed to accommodate physicians from all over the world who might come to learn some of the techniques we were using. As we went over the architect's drawings and started to bring the abstract thought of an academic, world-class cosmetic surgery facility into a reality, one of us (K.A.A.) made a simple statement. In effect, he said that the only way to really disseminate information about the techniques we were going to use in the new office was to write a textbook. Not just any textbook, but a comprehensive textbook of cosmetic surgery that encompassed virtually the entire field. It *sounded* so simple and straightforward, only to be followed by one of the biggest understatements of all time, "It will take a little bit of work, but it will be worth it in the end."

Now nearly four years later, that comment was essentially right on target, except for the minor detail that it took an enormous amount of work with the help of dozens of people. In many ways the experiences and challenges we had editing this textbook are similar to the task ahead of any physician who seeks to expand his or her cosmetic surgery skills.

It is not easy to learn new procedures, especially when they are elective and cosmetic. Some are complicated and require a great deal of time, effort, and skill to learn and master. Others are not technically difficult to learn, but they can be intimidating, and many of us have spent sleepless nights thinking about the patient we treated for the first time with a new procedure.

Even though this book was a challenge to write and edit, it is no different from the task ahead of all of us when we seek to learn something new. Fortunately, there is a wealth of knowledge and experience available for physicians to learn from in cosmetic surgery. What we have done in the *Atlas of Cosmetic Surgery* is bring together many of the greatest minds in cosmetic surgery in one text and ask them to share not only their knowledge but also their skill and expertise to help others learn about and how to perform cosmetic procedures. They have written comprehensive literature reviews of the procedures and have gone the extra length to provide detailed information on how to actually perform the procedures. This book provides a unique opportunity to learn from many of the world's leaders in cosmetic surgery from a diverse group of specialties.

In the end, the only way to create something of value that will endure is through hard work. This book has been an enormous amount of hard work for many people, and we thank everyone who has helped us along the way. In the same way, hard work will usually pay off when learning a new procedure, in particular the cosmetic procedures discussed in this text. If only it were as simple as reading a book and becoming proficient at a surgical procedure. Rather, this book will serve as the foundation on which to build a skill-set in cosmetic surgery. It was intended to be useful for physicians and surgeons from all specialties and all skill levels. Each and every chapter was written in a way that gives an enormous amount of information in a well-designed, user-friendly format, with an emphasis on the how-to atlas section of each chapter. We also went to great lengths to have authors from multiple specialties (dermatology, dermatologic surgery, facial plastic surgery, oculoplastic surgery, psychology, history, and anesthesiology), and it is our hope that this has made the *Atlas of Cosmetic Surgery* a unique text that bridges the interdisciplinary field of cosmetic surgery.

It has been a pleasure working on this book together, and we are delighted that it has finally become a reality.

Michael S. Kaminer, MD
Jeffrey S. Dover, MD, FRCPC
Kenneth A. Arndt, MD

Contents

PART I

EVALUATION OF THE COSMETIC SURGERY PATIENT

CHAPTER 1

The History of Cosmetic Surgery

ELIZABETH HAIKEN

Aesthetic surgery is one of the fastest-growing medical practices in the world. The American Society for Aesthetic Plastic Surgery recently reported that more than 2 million Americans elected to undergo cosmetic procedures (surgical and nonsurgical) in 1998—an increase of 4% over the previous year. Because this organization's statistics cover only activities reported by three specialty boards (plastic surgery, dermatology, and otolaryngology), the number of procedures performed in North America alone is clearly higher. Worldwide, from China to Peru, the number of people who are convinced that anatomy does not equal destiny increases each year.[1]

The history of aesthetic surgery both parallels and diverges from the history of medicine more generally. In the early twentieth century, like most would-be specialists, those physicians interested in pursuing aesthetic surgery (which was then as often called featural surgery, cosmetic surgery, or even—derisively—beauty surgery) forged their own paths through medical school, individually sought out apprenticeships with experienced physicians in North America or in Europe, and struggled to make a place for themselves in medical practice. After the First World War, which drew physicians of all backgrounds into wartime medical service, aspiring aesthetic surgeons (again, like their colleagues in other specialties) organized professional societies and negotiated and established the boundaries of their specialty. They took up these activities with renewed vigor after World War II, which like the first interrupted personal career paths and at the same time provided unparalleled opportunities for professional training and experience. Today, aesthetic surgeons attend medical school, complete internships and residencies, work in medical offices, surgical suites, and hospitals, and define their work in medical terms. Like other physicians, they see patients who come to them seeking help and who judge them according to their ability to effect cure. As the World Health Organization now defines health as "complete physical, mental, and social well-being, and not merely the absence of disease or infirmity," so aesthetic surgeons have come to see their work not simply as removing a distressing flaw but rather as facilitating patients' total mental and physical health.[2]

Just as all physicians share certain formative experiences, aesthetic surgery shares a common history with other medical practices. Like all medical practices, it was built on a foundation of basic anatomy, informed by developments such as asepsis, antisepsis, and anesthesia, and supported by an institutional framework of schools, hospitals, and professional associations; like all medical practices, it both drove and was driven by technological innovation, from the stethoscope to the dermabrader to the laser.[3]

These commonalities are important; they remind us that aesthetic surgery has always been and remains firmly grounded in medicine. Yet what is most interesting about aesthetic surgery, and crucial to an understanding not only of its past but of its present and future, is how, where, and why it has diverged from other medical practices.[4]

As a medical practice, aesthetic surgery differs from other practices in significant ways. While many medical specialties developed around a particular part of the body—ophthalmology, gynecology, and cardiology are among the obvious examples—aesthetic surgery took instead a less definable center. In claiming as its purview the aesthetics of the human body, from eyelids to abdomen to calves, aesthetic surgery at once confuses, challenges, and bridges professional divisions. In the 1920s and 1930s, those who believed that the specialty of plastic surgery should be grounded primarily in reconstructive surgery argued vociferously against the pursuit of cosmetic or aesthetic work. After the Second World War, the discovery and widespread use of antibiotics generated tension between otolaryngologists, who began to do more aesthetic work as infections became easier to treat, and plastic surgeons, who saw rhinoplasty as their "turf." In the 1960s, some plastic surgeons believed that the founding of a new society dedicated solely to aesthetic work threatened to split, and weaken, the specialty of plastic surgery. Claiming a philosophy (or perhaps orientation) rather than a specific part of the body has made aesthetic surgery controversial at times. But while anxiety over professional boundaries has sometimes led to tension between various groups, the specialty of aesthetic surgery—precisely *because* it draws practitioners from a range of specialties, from plastic surgery to dermatology to general surgery, and brings them together based on common interests to pursue a common goal—also has greater potential than many specialties to bridge the professional divisions that so characterize modern medicine.

Perhaps the most significant factor that differentiates aesthetic surgery from other medical practices is the extent to which it is grounded in culture as well as in medicine, and specifically in the increasingly visual, psychologized culture of contemporary North America. Early in the twentieth century, the intertwined processes of industrialization, urbanization, and immigration and migration transformed the United States. From a predominantly rural nation, in which identity was firmly grounded in family and region and wrinkles and sagging breasts were simply facts of life, the United States became an increasingly urban nation, in which identity derived from self-presentation—and in which wrinkles were no longer facts to be accepted but "problems" to be conquered. Proponents of aesthetic surgery, who began to discuss and emphasize the social and economic importance of external appearance, were inspired by this new culture even as they themselves helped to shape it. In more recent years, the extension of a Western (and by nature Westernizing) visual culture around the globe has influenced both the desire for aesthetic surgery and its practice. Just as in the 1920s movies and fan magazines showed young American women what beauty looked like, today young Asians and Africans cannot help but come in contact with American fashion magazines and American movies, which familiarize them with Western ideals of beauty.[5]

The "public" nature of aesthetic surgery has also influenced its development to a significant degree. Human growth hormone and Prozac offer comparatively recent examples of cases in which popularity and public enthusiasm have driven medical developments and shaped the response to them, but aesthetic surgery was the first, and it is the longest-lived. Largely in response to market demand for aesthetic surgery, plastic surgeons moved to incorporate cosmetic surgical techniques and concerns into the specialty of plastic surgery, and dermatologists, otolaryngologists, rhinologists, and a host of other specialists likewise claimed it for their own. By doing so these practitioners created an entirely new range of optional medical treatments that was available for purchase.

Aesthetic surgery's public nature has shaped the physician-patient relationship in important ways. As in other medical specialties, education, training, and credentials comprise one set of variables that create the surgeon's professional authority. In the case of aesthetic surgery, however, authority derives as much from the patient (and, more broadly, from the realm of the consumer culture the patient both inhabits and embodies) as from the surgeon. Patients who seek aesthetic surgery are physically healthy. The diseases they want cured—aging, ugliness, poor self-esteem—are many, but they share the characteristic of being difficult to diagnose in the precise terms medicine normally employs. Etiology, nosology, and symptomology are individualized: they are defined by the patient before they are diagnosed by the physician, and they are impossible to quantify.

Because it took shape in the public realm, plastic surgery represents a revealing and ambiguous case of medical economics, as well as negotiation of professional authority. The economics of aesthetic surgery has always been distinctive. In the early twentieth century, medicine was a cash business, and family funds were carefully husbanded to cover the necessities of childbirth and contagious illness; in this context, aesthetic surgery was a luxury of the few. Over the course of the twentieth century, an increasing proportion of Americans were covered either by a proprietary medical plan or by the federal government, but with the exception of some Public Health Service hospitals and military medical centers, whose coverage was generous enough to spark a minor scandal in the early 1960s ("Facelifts on the Taxpayer!" the *San Francisco Chronicle* cried),[6] procedures defined as aesthetic or cosmetic were generally not covered. As a specialty defined by elective medical procedures that were paid for in advance, aesthetic surgery remained distinctive. Today, that distinctiveness remains, although the reasons for it have changed. Aesthetic surgery has begun to seem like a refuge for physicians abandoning the trenches of managed care in favor of the freedom and independence they once enjoyed (or hoped to enjoy) in the medical free market. As a result, its economics is changing rapidly, as physicians, finance companies, and credit bureaus collaborate to extend their services to a wider sector of the population.

A TWENTIETH-CENTURY PHENOMENON

Precursors

Because its development was powered as much by consumer dream and desire as by perceived medical necessity, plastic surgery constitutes a peculiar historical puzzle. But because plastic surgeons proudly proclaim themselves practitioners of both an ancient art and an ancient medical practice, the history of medicine provides one of the essential contexts. Modern surgeons trace their history to India, where as early as 600 B.C. the

Hindu surgeon Sushruta described a method of reconstructing a nose from a patient's cheek: "A careful physician having taken a plant leaf of the size of the nose of that person, and having cut adjoining cheek according to that measurement, and having scarified the nose tip should attach it to the nose tip and quickly join it with perfect sutures." The first written account of the Indian (or forehead) reconstruction rhinoplasty was not published until 1794, but the operation was performed as early as 1000 A.D. Modern plastic surgeons also claim kinship with Gasparo Tagliocozzi of Bologna, Italy, often called the "father of modern plastic surgery." In the mid-sixteenth century, inspired by "the great need for plastic operations . . . due to the frequent duels, street brawls, and other clashes of armed men," Tagliocozzi pioneered the Italian method of nasal reconstruction, in which a flap from the upper arm is gradually transferred to the nose.[7]

Around the world, isolated practitioners continued to pursue effects that today we would categorize as aesthetic surgery. Around the turn of the twentieth century, interest coalesced around a few practitioners at a few "hot spots." Suzanne Noël, the pioneering Paris surgeon who concentrated on face lifts, and Berlin's Jacques Joseph, one of the inventors of the modern nose job, were deservedly famous. (Infamous, perhaps, more appropriately characterizes Chicago surgeon Charles C. Miller, who claimed to have invented a number of innovative procedures, including an original method for creating dimples.) Not until the twentieth century was well under way, however, did technological innovation and medical advancement combine with a critical mass of interest among practitioners and potential patients.

Beginnings

Pioneers in nasal reduction like Jacques Joseph and John Orlando Roe are better remembered today, but most of the earliest nasal operations were undertaken to build up the nose rather than reduce it. Of greatest concern was the condition, much more common then than now, called "saddle nose." A saddle nose can be inherited or caused by trauma, an abscess, or infection, but scrofula, lupus, and especially syphilis—scourge of the American landscape—were the more common causes. Americans knew that one of the most common results of untreated syphilis was a depressed nose, and surgeons who attempted to correct depressed noses knew the challenge they faced was cultural as well as medical. As New York surgeon Joseph Safian observed in 1926, "Many persons with a saddle nose . . . are suspected of having inherited disease and are greatly handicapped, both in their social and business relations."[8]

The "saddle nose deformity" was particularly difficult to treat because it is easier to subtract from the human body than to add to it. Practitioners had recorded a variety of attempts to build up noses using internal prostheses or bone and cartilage grafts, but these techniques were time consuming and often unsuccessful. In contrast, paraffin—which was relatively easy to inject, did not require any troublesome incisions, and, at least initially, appeared to remain inert once introduced into the body—seemed ideal.

Toward the end of the nineteenth century, New York City neurologist J. Leanard Corning and Viennese physician Robert Gersuny began to experiment with paraffin, and news of this apparently ideal substance began to spread through the medical community. By September 1903, it had reached Leadville, Colorado, where physician F. Gregory Connell cautiously characterized the surgical use of paraffin as "more or less" experimental, but noted hopefully that its potential was rapidly increasing: "prosthetic operations, undertaken solely for cosmetic effect," he forecast, "should be absolutely harmless." Apparently successful in treating saddle noses, paraffin quickly came to be seen, by some practitioners, as an instant panacea for soft-tissue defects: it was used to fill out facial wrinkles, in one case to create a testicle, and was rumored to have been injected into breasts.[9]

But paraffin proved not to be the miracle cure originally described (and because of this casts a long shadow over the history of aesthetic surgery). Physicians soon began to observe that it had an unfortunate tendency to migrate (particularly if recipients spent time in the sun); more serious was the proliferation of "wax cancers" called paraffinomas. Removing paraffin proved to be much more difficult than injecting it; the process often left the patient severely scarred. Physicians were loath to abandon a practice that had seemed to hold such promise, but experiments with different mixtures of substances (including petroleum jelly, wax, white oak bark, glycerine, olive oil, and goose grease, with or without carbolic acid for antisepsis) produced no better results, and by 1920, most reputable physicians had abandoned the practice of injecting paraffin.[10]

That year, New York physician Seymour Oppenheimer chronicled paraffin's rise and fall; the lessons he drew from the episode are still valuable. He attributed paraffin's meteoric rise in popularity to the belief, common among even "skilled and well-recognized surgeons and rhinologists," that "the operation was practically without pain, caused no scars . . . and corrected nasal deformities that could not well be overcome otherwise." The more significant problem, however, was the widespread awareness and fear of the moral implications of such deformities, which drove public demand and made patients particularly vulnerable: "the charlatans, the advertising 'beauty doctor' and others of that ilk were quick to see the possibilities in a financial sense in its appeal to the popular imagination, and seized upon the method with avidity, and with this added to their armentarium reaped, and still reap, a harvest from the willing victims among the laity." He called on his colleagues to participate in an educational campaign to inform the public that paraffin injections, while "dangerous even in the hands of the well-equipped surgeon" were "doubly more dangerous . . . at the hands of the ignorant, unscrupulous and uneducated 'beauty doctor.' "[11]

World War I

Injuries to the mouth and jaws were not unknown before the war, but in general, as one surgeon recalled, "prior to 1915, the treatment of maxillofacial injuries was not one of the major preoccupations of surgery." Trench warfare meant that heads and necks were particularly vulnerable; steel helmets saved lives but contributed to facial injury, as fragments of helmets (and the projectiles that shattered on them) hit soldiers' unprotected faces. Facial injuries and resulting deformities received great attention not just because they were visible and often horrifying, but because these particular types of injuries were among the most numerous. Dentist Varaztad Kazanjian's skill and inventiveness earned him the name "the miracle man of the Western Front," and the *New York Times* proudly reported, "the skill of American dentistry holds undisputed first place, and is particularly highly esteemed in France." England's Sir Arbuthnot Lane, New Zealand's Harold Delf Gillies, and France's Hypolyte Morestin were also highly regarded.[12]

Reflecting the concerns of soldiers and surgeons alike, almost everything the American public learned about plastic surgery during the war years concerned reconstructive rather than aesthetic efforts. Early in 1916, for example, Mrs. William K. Vanderbilt excitedly told readers of the *New York Times* about her visit to the American Ambulance Hospital in France. Many of the men looked "frightful" when they came in, she conceded, but the "big thing" at the hospital was "re-making": "The Ambulance takes these torn, mutilated beings, without any faces, who would otherwise be unbearably repulsive and almost certainly economically dependent, and makes them over. It turns them into normal men again, so that they can live normal lives, as individuals, and be of service to their country as well." In 1919, Dr. William Seaman Bainbridge of the Navy medical corps told *Current Opinion* readers that the surgical work being done was "little short of miraculous . . . one of the greatest triumphs ever achieved by the beneficent art of surgery."[13]

In many cases, however, surgeons' and patients' best efforts fell short of the challenges the trenches posed. Both the British and the French medical services employed artists to construct full or partial facial masks for those whom surgery could not help further. Captain Derwent Wood, an artist attached to Britain's Third London General Hospital, stated, "My work begins when the work of the surgeon is completed. When the surgeon has done all he can to restore function, to heal wounds, to support fleshy tissues by bone grafting, to cover areas by skin grafting, I endeavor by means of the skill I happen to possess as a sculptor to make a man's face as near as possible to what it looked like before he was wounded." Years later, Ernest Hemingway wrote of *"les geules cassées,"* who still bore visible signs of their war experience: "There was always an almost iridescent shiny cast about the considerably reconstructed face, rather like that of a well packed ski run, and we respected these clients more than we did the *savants* or the professors."[14]

Coming Home

American surgeons returned from the war eager to build the specialty (and by the beginning of the Second World War would claim about 60 practicing plastic surgeons—more than 10 times as many as Britain, and almost twice as many as the rest of the world combined). Kazanjian, who returned to Harvard in 1919 to finish medical school, later recalled that although previously plastic surgery was "never looked upon too favorably by the medical profession at large," the war "created an interest and demand for reconstructive surgery." Vilray P. Blair returned from Sidcup to found the plastic surgery department at Washington University School of Medicine and Barnes Hospital in St. Louis. At Johns Hopkins University, John Staige Davis became the first titled professor of plastic surgery in the United States, following the publication in 1919 of his textbook *Plastic Surgery,* which plastic surgeon Frank McDowell later called "perhaps the first respected book with that title in the English language."[15]

Wartime reconstructive surgery had enabled surgeons to gain experience and confidence, but the end of the war seemed to signal a contraction. Physicians and surgeons who wished to practice plastic surgery when they returned home were thus aware that they were in a transitional position. Unlike the well-established fields of general or abdominal surgery, plastic surgery was in its infancy, and while reconstructive surgery had achieved some status, aesthetic surgery was still regarded with suspicion. At the same time, however, surgeons saw that aesthetic surgery offered great potential for growth. New York surgeon Seymour Oppenheimer, for example, noted that although "the world war, with its pressing demands for the practice of reconstructive surgery . . . has not alone brought cosmetic rhinoplasty into its own, ethically speaking," it has "created a great demand for surgical workers." He continued optimistically, "the time seems auspicious . . .

for all cosmetic surgery and cosmetic rhinoplasty in particular, to be elevated to its proper dignity in the profession, to be popularized and made available for the large number of individuals in civil life who could be benefited in mind no less than in feature."[16]

As they turned their sights toward the civilian practice of plastic surgery, American surgeons began to address questions that would occupy their profession for years to come: Who should do plastic surgery? How and by whom should they be trained? But it was the realization that beauty, as a business, offered seemingly limitless potential—and that American women would spend as much time and effort (and significantly more money) in the quest for beauty than even the most severely injured soldiers—that drove surgeons to confront the most important question that emerged from the war: Was there a difference between reconstructive plastic surgery and aesthetic or cosmetic plastic surgery, and if so, where was the dividing line? Surgeons did not immediately resolve this question (and have not resolved it yet). But as they attempted to define the parameters that would enable them to feel comfortable and confident about their status as medical specialists, while still acknowledging and responding to patients' needs and demands, the basic lines along which aesthetic surgery would develop emerged.[17]

The writings of Portland, Oregon, surgeon Adalbert G. Bettman, whose practice bridged the two world wars, are instructive here. "Whenever I see a group of people," Bettman noted in 1920, "I am struck with the fact that there is offered a great field for practising the beautifying and practical, I might say grateful art of plastic surgery." He asserted that "removing wrinkles of the face and neck, double chins and such like deformities" is "probably the most interesting work in plastic surgery" and urged his colleagues to accept such patients. "Persons with these cruel deformities (for they certainly are more cruel than the loss of a leg, for instance)," Bettman wrote, "can and should be relieved."[18]

Bettman was an innovative, as well as enthusiastic, proponent of aesthetic surgery. In a 1919 presentation to the Alumni Association of the University of Oregon Medical School in Portland, he introduced the extensive face lift incision that, with modifications, is still used today (and he may have been the first to demonstrate such an operation using before and after pictures). He made extravagant claims for his work. It was practically painless: "One woman after having this operation done proceeded immediately to a local department store, where she purchased a new hat suitable to her now youthful appearance, certainly an amusement not indulged in when one is in pain." It could be kept secret, even from close relatives: "Another woman," he reported, went home to her husband, mother and grown daughter and "not one of these noticed the dressings." But perhaps most significant was the new terminology Bettman employed. In specifically referring to wrinkles and double chins as deformities, Bettman broke new ground in what critics have termed the medicalization of nonmedical conditions, and over the course of the twentieth century practitioners have moved toward, rather than away from, his generous definition.[19]

A small group of self-defined "reputable surgeons" met initially at the Chicago Athletic Club on August 8, 1921, to found the first plastic surgical organization in North America and would eventually found and organize the specialty of plastic surgery in the United States. They agreed that because few surgeons on either side of the Atlantic followed the path Tagliocozzi had forged, not until World War I was plastic surgery "reborn," as an art and a profession; even then, they said, it was a medical response to the medical emergency of modern warfare. The language they used to describe their work evokes the classical context in which they preferred to place themselves; the term *plastic surgery* derives from the Greek *plastikos,* to shape or mold. They chose the term *plastic surgeon* to distinguish themselves from the practitioners they called "beauty doctors" and claimed the inclusive term plastic surgery to differentiate their work from what they variously called "featural," "beauty," "cosmetic," or "aesthetic" surgery.[20]

But just two short years later, comedienne and Ziegfield Follies star Fanny Brice had her nose bobbed, and aesthetic surgery, practically overnight, became a cultural phenomenon.

Consolidating: 1923-1972

During the 1920s and 1930s, as the physicians who aspired to become known as the "first generation" of plastic surgeons struggled to organize their specialty, the most divisive question they faced was whether or not to define surgery undertaken specifically to improve appearance as a legitimate medical practice. The more demanding standards of appearance that the nation's burgeoning consumer culture seemed to impose provided one compelling justification for the practice of cosmetic surgery. As a 1927 advice book for teenagers called *Any Girl Can Be Good-Looking* put it, "Being good looking is no longer optional. . . . There is no place in the world for women who are not." The danger posed by "quacks and charlatans" who preyed on human insecurity provided a second: the sad case of aspiring actress Sadye Holland, who developed gangrene and lost both legs at the knee following an adventurous surgeon's attempt to reshape her calves, provided ample warning. The third revealed itself in the form of the inferiority complex, a concept originally formulated by Viennese psychologist Alfred Adler that became a major fad in America between the two world wars. By medicalizing cosmetic surgery—defining it not as vanity surgery but as psychiatry with a scalpel—it encouraged the organizing profession to expand its boundaries to incorporate surgery with a purely cosmetic goal. By 1941, when the American Board of Plastic Surgery achieved full specialty status, it was clear that most practitioners would do both reconstructive and cosmetic work.[21]

World War II and After. When the Second World War ended, the United States—its physical plant untouched and its economy intact—emerged as the world's major economic and military power. In addition to producing a larger share of manufactured goods than ever before, the United States produced an increasingly large share of the world's science and medicine. New medical technologies and the expansion of scientific information accelerated the evolutionary process that had begun before the war; they were cause and consequence of an increase in both relative and absolute numbers of specialists. These changes were compounded by overall growth in the profession: in the years after World War II, the number of medical schools in the United States almost doubled, and the number of doctors more than doubled.[22]

Even against this backdrop, the growth in the field of plastic surgery was significant. In 1960, for example, the American Board of Plastic Surgery reported that the specialty had certified 462 surgeons: it had tripled in size since its founding two decades earlier. Plastic surgeons were not only more numerous, they were distributed more widely around the country. Starting from the east and west coasts where they had initially congregated, they were spreading out: by 1965 only five states—Idaho, Montana, Alaska, South Dakota, and Wyoming—had no plastic surgeons. Reliable statistics are difficult to come by, but it was generally agreed that the number of surgeries performed had also increased. According to one report, more than 130,000 Americans had plastic surgery in 1958, compared with just 15,000 a decade earlier, and the numbers were increasing annually.[23]

The postwar surge of interest in aesthetic surgery was sparked, in part, by the enthusiastic coverage wartime plastic surgery had received in the popular press. Throughout the war surgeons warned the press and the public about plastic surgery's limitations: as Lieutenant Colonel James Barrett Brown put it, "We are giving the injured the best modern surgery can provide . . . [but] we cannot duplicate what God has made." But the awe-struck tone of articles such as "New Faces for New Men" shaped popular perceptions about plastic surgery. Films like Bela Lugosi's *The Raven* (1935), *A Woman's Face* (with Joan Crawford, 1941), and particularly *Dark Passage* (1947), which starred Humphrey Bogart as an escaped prisoner and Lauren Bacall as the angel who takes care of him after plastic surgery, helped to buttress plastic surgery's magic aura.[24]

By increasing their numbers, making their services more widely available, and pricing aesthetic surgery with an eye on the expanding middle class (New York surgeon E. Hoyt de Kleine, in 1955, asserted that "the total cost of standard cosmetic procedures must be brought down to prices not exceeding what the average man pays for his television"), practitioners of aesthetic surgery expanded their market in the postwar years, but as the following anecdote suggests, this is only part of the story. In June 1944, the *New York Times* reprinted a letter that had been sent anonymously to Senator Ralph O. Brewster of Maine proposing a novel morale booster: a federal lend-lease program to provide cosmetic surgery for wives and families of men in the armed services as a morale booster. "What woman, wife or mother, among us wants that man to return to a wrinkled face, dried up, flabby neck; knowing men do not age as quickly as women?" the writer had asked. "We've suffered at home—many of us are still in our 30s, but our necks and eyes, faces, do not respond to cream and exercises. We need these skins made youthful again. That would help the morale of returning fighting men." The *Times* treated the suggestion as a joke, but the letter Senator Brewster had received was a harbinger of things to come.[25]

Beauty remained important for women in the postwar world, and was increasingly equated with youth. As Lily Daché put it in her 1956 *Glamour Book,* "If you want to keep up with this modern, wonderful world, you must be young in thought, feeling and appearance . . . and all you have to do is stretch out your hand to receive the magic bounty of glamour that modern science has prepared for you." Increasingly, American women did just that. As writer Olga Kahler commented in a 1948 article about face lifting, "Some think it's wonderful; some think it's silly; and a few think it's horrible. But all, including the horrified, are extremely interested and listen eagerly to the smallest detail." Kahler's article generated so much interest that it was reprinted verbatim a few months after its initial appearance with an explanatory note citing the "unusual number of requests for information about this particular branch of plastic surgery" that the magazine had received.[26]

Real Men Get Face Lifts. As middle-class Americans became increasingly convinced that an aging face exacted significant social, economic, and psychological costs, men also began to see their wrinkles in this new light. Face lifts had been rare among men for several reasons: the popular belief that where age made women ugly, it made men mature and distinguished, and the fact that until after the war, surgical techniques were less effective on male patients. (In the standard

Today, when mass-market magazines and newspapers routinely run cleverly designed advertisements enticing readers to change their lives by changing their faces and bodies, mid-twentieth-century marketing efforts look pretty tame. As the following two stories suggest, however, even when they tried to be cautionary, advocates of aesthetic surgery often encouraged their patients to think in terms of sweeping transformation. The first ran in *American Weekly*, a widely distributed Sunday newspaper supplement, in 1946. The caption reads, "To the homely girl, life may seem an endless succession of embarrassments, frustrations and anguish until she decides, one day, to . . . have a plastic surgery operation. Then a remodeled nose, a rounded chin, may alter her personality—and her whole life." The accompanying illustration, which depicts, first, a disconsolate secretary doodling caricatures of large noses as her boss ignores her, and second, the same secretary with a smaller nose basking in the welcome attentions of said boss, underscores the idea of unlimited possibility.[46]

The idea of transformation is equally—if perhaps unintentionally—replicated in an *Esquire* article from 1965. "Sometimes it's very hard to decide about the patient," a surgeon told his interviewer. "I had a woman patient recently; a very smart, chic, well dressed woman . . . she wanted a facelift . . . she was married to a very responsible man in an upper income bracket, and she wanted to look better for her husband. It sounded okay. . . . Later on I heard she absolutely ran amok—divorced her husband, ran off to Mexico, took a 25-year-old boy as a lover—the whole route. It was dreadful." Dreadful, perhaps, for the surgeon; probably dreadful for the unsuspecting husband, but dreadful is probably not the word that leaped to the mind of the middle-aged woman sidelined by the youth culture of the 1960s who stumbled across this article as she waited her turn in the beauty shop.[47]

Throughout the 1960s, when plastic surgeons meditated on the question of aging and its effects on identity, they were clearly concerned only with women. When they did mention men, it was only in the context of comparison (where aging was widely perceived to alter female identity in a negative way, it brought benefits to men, who were perceived to become more powerful as they aged). In the context of the economic retrenchment of the 1970s, however, surgeons and cultural commentators begin to reexamine men through the same lens they had applied to women. Today, stories of downsized, middle-aged men who resort to eye lifts, face lifts, liposuction, and hair transplants to reconstruct a more masculine, more youthful, more powerful identity have become so common in publications ranging from *Esquire* to the *Wall Street Journal* they seem like tropes.[48]

For practitioners of aesthetic surgery, the question of what it means to do aesthetic surgery has always been and continues to be central. It is also something of a catch-22: If cosmetic surgery is not about culture and identity—if, in other words, it's only about changing external appearance—then it's not deep and meaningful, it's superficial (and it may not even be medicine).

This is a stance that most practitioners have rejected. Just as the first generation of surgeons struggled to distance themselves from what they perceived as the less than honorable history of the "barber-surgeon," the first generation of aesthetic surgeons fought long and hard to shed the pejorative label of "beauty doctor." They did this, in part, by organizing themselves into associations (and, a bit later, into specialty boards), by prescribing standards in education, training, and professional behavior, and by enforcing these standards (granted, with varying degrees of success) through examinations, licensing requirements, and self-policing.[49]

As important was that they formulated a philosophical foundation for the practice of altering appearance through surgery. Medicine, they say, has evolved from a preoccupation with curing disease to a concern with the wellness of the whole person. Individual well-being depends on mental as well as physical health, and a mentally healthy person is one who feels comfortable functioning in the society in which she or he lives. Medical practitioners have accepted, even embraced, the conviction that their mission is to repair the disjunction that can develop between the internal and the external—to facilitate "wellness" by facilitating the development of an identity that feels authentic. Thus, they argue, aesthetic surgery is very much about culture and identity, about feeling good in society as well as looking good.

Granted, if medical practitioners are to maintain their status and their self-image as responsible professionals, they simply cannot say, "Let's face it, it's all about what sells in the market." Yet to acknowledge that aesthetic surgery is about identity is to raise some troubling questions. Within the context of the medical profession, acknowledging this connection naturally invites the question of whether plastic surgeons, dermatologists, ear, nose, and throat specialists, general surgeons, and others who routinely perform surgical procedures that we would define as aesthetic are the appropriate professionals to deal with this issue. The first generation of plastic surgeons argued that a mark of "progress" in twentieth-century medicine was the recognition that psychological functioning is just as important as physical functioning. In the 1920s and 1930s they congratulated themselves for recognizing this and for providing the services their patients needed (smaller noses, smoother brows) to function effectively in consumer society. But the relationship between those who practice "physical medicine" and those who practice "mental medicine" (psychiatrists, psychologists, psychotherapists) has not been smooth. Currently, it ranges from respectful (we can cooperate and learn from each other) to dismissive (make sure you send the prospective patient to a psychiatrist to find out if she's the litigious type) to competitive (we can fix this problem faster and better than you can).

Perhaps more importantly, the fact that surgeons prescribe aesthetic surgery as the solution for complex problems involving individual, social, and cultural identity reflects not only their grounding in medical culture but the limitations of that culture. For much of the past century, medicine has encouraged practitioners to search for "magic bullets" (as well as to protect and when possible expand their specialty turf). A face lift may indeed be a "magic bullet"—i.e., the quickest, even the most effective, solution for an individual patient who is convinced that her sagging chinline is making her life miserable—but by giving and receiving the lift, the surgeon and the patient affirm the culture that created the disjunction in the first place.

Medical practitioners naturally tend to situate themselves within medical culture. From this point of view, it seems that aesthetic surgery emerged from plastic surgery, which evolved out of general surgery, which is a branch of medicine, and the drive toward technical and technological advancement comes out of the recognition that functional defects ought to be repaired. Thus efforts to repair cleft palates and war injuries inspire surgeons to experiment and to take risks that lead to the development of other facial surgeries; efforts to reconstruct breasts after mastectomy lead to breast augmentation; the two world wars are major turning points, in facial reconstruction and in burn technique, respectively.[50]

There is, however, another way to view the history of the phenomenon we call aesthetic surgery. As a practice, aesthetic surgery is contemporaneous with reconstructive surgery, which means that it emerged out of culture, as well as medicine. The drive toward technical and technological advancement is given impetus by consumer conviction that certain features are not advantageous and thus should be improved, and by the whiff of money. Thus anti-Semitism and anti-immigrant sentiment inspire prospective patients to request, and surgeons to perform, nasal surgery beginning in the late nineteenth century and the vogue for sweater girls after World War II inspires a clamor for breast augmentation to which surgeons respond by inventing breast implants. From this point of view, the two world wars may be turning points in terms of technique and in terms of the supply of surgeons, but the real turning point—the acceptance of and accommodation to a media-driven, urban, consumer culture—comes in between.

In a broader sense, to acknowledge that aesthetic surgery is about identity is to open up a discussion about how identities have been constructed in the modern world in the twentieth century, and whether this will change in the twenty-first. In the United States, attitudes toward aesthetic surgery have been based on a series of assumptions: that inside every person who looks "other" is an "American" struggling to get out; that from every homely girl a confident girl is trying to emerge; that inside every middle-aged woman the "essential (read: 25-year-old) self" remains intact; that inside every balding, middle-aged former executive lurks a virile power broker at the top of his game.

These assumptions rest on a complex web of beliefs about what is good, desirable, and aesthetically pleasing. Methods for measuring and calculating objective standards of beauty have gone in and out of style (the science of anthropometry having replaced the "profilometer," an early twentieth century invention) but the rhetoric in which many practitioners of aesthetic surgery indulge has not. Those who devote themselves to altering the human face and body are artists, sculptors whose medium is human flesh; it is not insignificant that one mid-century surgeon chose *Dr. Pygmalion* as the title for his autobiography. The standards of beauty that shape their work (and their patients' faces and bodies) are informed, they say, by objective measurement and educated, professional judgment of what is aesthetically most pleasing to the human eye.[51]

But if the phenomenon of aesthetic surgery is shaped by culture as well as by medicine, it seems logical that its practitioners would be as well. The vision of artistic inspiration described above is problematic because it obscures, even denies, the extent to which physicians shape and are shaped by the specific culture they inhabit, in this case, the visual culture (movies, magazines, models) of the contemporary United States. Surgeons who in the 1920s and 1930s described Semitic noses as "too large" were clearly operating within the realm of a culture that defined certain looks as beautiful and others as less so, an orientation suggested by their choice (in the 1930s) of the Venus di Milo as the central icon of their first official societal logo and today by their frequent use of the adjective *sleepy* to describe the way Asian eyelids look before they are Westernized.[52]

Surgeons have long acknowledged the effect of "culture." In defense of aesthetic surgery, they say (and have said since the 1920s) that consumer demand exists and is increasing because we live in a culture that pays big benefits (and extracts significant costs) for certain kinds of looks, and that therefore it is important that reputable, responsible practitioners be available to meet that demand safely and effectively. They have, in short, been quick to acknowledge "culture" as something that has driven them. They have been less forthright about—or perhaps simply less aware of—the extent to which they themselves shape culture. There can be no question that surgeons have played a reactive role, flooded with requests for Jane Russell breasts in one decade and for Sandra Dee noses in the next. Yet to think of surgeons merely as hapless carpenters buffeted by the capricious demands of generations of fashion conscious women is to do them a grave disservice. That complex web of beliefs, desires, and dreams we call culture is no solid thing. It is created each day in each practitioner's office during the series of exchanges in which a patient's requests are found to fit, or not, with what a physician believes to be appropriate and desirable. Individual identity evolves through a complex social and cultural process of perception and reflection. Surgeons who over the course of the century have agreed with their patients that Jewish noses should be made smaller, that Asian eyes should be made to open wider, that wrinkles and small breasts and chubby thighs are ugly and have then acted on those convictions have played a role commensurate with the flood of perfect images that inspired the initial inquiries. From the beginning, aesthetic surgery has been shaped by pressures and priorities within American culture as well as within the profession of medicine. Its history illuminates the complex interplay between medical and cultural imperatives; for better or worse, appearance and identity are tightly intertwined. As writer Lucy Grealey has so cogently observed, "It is no mistake that in movies and literature the dead sometimes know they are dead only after they can no longer see themselves in mirrors."[53]

NOTES

1. The most recent statistics are tracked and posted periodically by the American Association for Aesthetic Plastic Surgery at www.surgery.org and by the American Society of Plastic and Reconstructive Surgeons at www.plasticsurgery.org.
2. The WHO definition is quoted in Thomasma DC. The goals of medicine and society. In: Brock DH, ed. The Culture of Biomedicine. Newark: University of Delaware Press, 1984:51.
3. See Reiser SJ. Medicine and the Reign of Technology. Cambridge: Cambridge University Press, 1978.
4. Historians, of course, do not necessarily agree. See Haiken E. Venus Envy: A History of Cosmetic Surgery. Baltimore: Johns Hopkins University Press, 1997, on which this introduction is based, and Gilman S. Making the Body Beautiful: A Cultural History of Aesthetic Surgery. Princeton, NJ: Princeton University Press, 1999.
5. NY Times, December 12, 1978:C10:1. This phenomenon is unique to the United States. British, French, and American surgeons participated equally in World War I, but at the onset of World War II, Britain claimed only four plastic surgeons, and France, two. The United States, in contrast, had almost fifty. This pattern continued in subsequent decades. Brazil is usually recognized as the first country to develop a comparable interest and industry. Today aesthetic surgery is less American than ever as the practice is growing, and thriving, in countries as diverse as Argentina and China.
6. San Francisco Chronicle, July 20, 1971:33; San Francisco Examiner and Chronicle, November 24, 1974:A18; San Francisco Examiner, March 23, 1979:7; March 25, 1979:A2.
7. Both quoted in Stark RB. The history of plastic surgery in wartime. Clin Plast Surg 1975; 2:509-510.
8. Brandt AM. No Magic Bullet: A Social History of Venereal Disease in the United States since 1880. New York: Oxford University Press, 1987:10, 40, 161. Safian J. Ethical plastic surgery vs. the quack beauty doctor. Radio lecture, Station WEAF, New York City, June 30, 1926, given under the auspices of the Gorgas Memorial Institute. National Archives of Plastic Surgery, Countway Library, Harvard University (hereafter cited as NAPS); Safian Correspondence. Campbell JT. The subcutaneous injection of paraffin more particularly for the correction of nasal deformities. Ill Med J 1904; 6:381.
9. Perhaps because paraffin reached its zenith as a solution to cosmetic problems, Gersuny, who pioneered its use in this arena, is generally remembered as having popularized its use. Goldwyn RM. The paraffin story. Plast Reconstr Surg 1980; 65:517-524. Connell FG. The subcutaneous injection of paraffin for the correction of deformities of the nose. JAMA 1903; 41:697-699 and JAMA 1903; 41:781. San Francisco County Medical Society. Society proceedings. Occidental Med Times 1903; 17:393. See also Smith H. Paraffin injected subcutaneously for the correction of nasal and other deformities. JAMA 1903; 41:773-776.
10. Goldwyn RM. The paraffin story. Plast Reconstr Surg 1980; 65: 517-524. DeVries JC. The surgical correction of featural deformities. Am J Dermatol Genito-Urinary Dis 1909; 13:427-428. Chicago Laryngological and Otological Society Meeting of October 13, 1908. Ill Med J 1909; 15:104. Rogers BO. A chronologic history of cosmetic surgery. Bull NY Acad Med 1971; 47:269.
11. Oppenheimer S. A condemnatory note on the use of paraffin in cosmetic rhinoplasty. Laryngoscope 1920; 30:595. For examples of reports of negative results, see Davis BF. Coal and petroleum products as causes of chronic irritation and cancer. JAMA 1914; 62:1716-1720. Paraffinoma and wax cancer. JAMA 1920; 75:1709-1711.
12. NY Times, August 4, 1916:4:4; Rank BK. The story of plastic surgery, 1868-1968. Practitioner 1968; 201:115. Wallace AF. The development of plastic surgery for war. J R Army Med Corps 1985; 131:29. Converse JM. The extraordinary career of Doctor Varaztad Hovhannes Kazanjian. Plast Reconstr Surg 1983; 71:140. Kazanjian V. Remembrance of things past. Plast Reconstr Surg 1965; 35:5-13. Jennings HB. Plastic surgery in the army: A short historical account. Plast Reconstr Surg 1971; 48:413-418.
13. Vanderbilt (Mrs.) WK. Miracles of surgery on men mutilated in war. NY Times Magazine, January 16, 1916:6:1. Bainbridge WS. Restoration of the warrior's lost face. Current Opinion, September 1919:169.
14. Vanderbilt (Mrs.) WK. Miracles of surgery on men mutilated in war. NY Times Magazine, January 16, 1916:6:1. NY Times, July 27, 1919:12:1. Hemingway E. A moveable feast. New York: Scribner, 1964:82.
15. Converse JM. The extraordinary career of Doctor Varaztad Hovhannes Kazanjian. Plast Reconstr Surg 1983; 71:140. Kazanjian V. Remembrance of things past. Plast Reconstr Surg 1965; 35:5-13. Barsky AJ. A personal memoir: Plastic surgery in the twentieth century. Surg Clin N Am 1978; 58:1019.
16. Oppenheimer S. The surgical correction of the aquiline or hump nose. Am J Surg 1920; 34:121. Smith F. Plastic surgery: Its interest to otolaryngologists. JAMA 1920; 75:1556.
17. Webb MS. Beyond Beauty: Philosophy, Ethics and Plastic Surgery. Ph.D. dissertation, Yale University, 1985 offers a cogent discussion of how the developing specialty dealt with these values. Anyone who thinks this discussion is no longer current should see Ringel E. The morality of cosmetic surgery for aging. Arch Dermatol 1998; 134:427-431 and the responses to it in Arch Dermatol 1998; 1204-1206, 1293-1297.
18. Bettman AG. Plastic and cosmetic surgery of the face. Northwest Med 1920; 19:205-209 reprinted in Aesthetic Plast Surg 1988; 12:5-7.
19. Bettman AG. Plastic and cosmetic surgery of the face. Northwest Med 1920; 19:205-209 reprinted in Aesthetic Plast Surg 1988; 12: 5-7. Rogers BO. A chronologic history of cosmetic surgery. Bull NY Acad Med 1971; 47:280-281.

20. Stark RB. History of plastic surgery in wartime. Clin Plast Surg 1975; 2:511. Wallace AF. The early development of pedicle flaps. J R Soc Med 1978; 71:834-835. Barsky AJ. A personal memoir: Plastic surgery in the twentieth century. Surg Clin North Am 1978; 58:1019.
21. Cades HR. Any Girl Can Be Good-Looking. New York: D. Appleton-Century, 1927:3. Editorial. Schireson—The disgrace of Illinois. JAMA 1928; 90:387-388. Haiken E. Venus Envy: A History of Cosmetic Surgery. Baltimore: Johns Hopkins University Press, 1997:44-130.
22. Starr P. The Social Transformation of American Medicine. New York: Basic Books, 1982:335-337. Relman AS. The future of medical practice. In: Bulger RJ, ed. In Search of the Modern Hippocrates. Iowa City: University of Iowa Press, 1987:199-205 .
23. Greeley PW. Progress. Plast Reconstr Surg 1952; 9:89. Secretary-Treasurer's Report, May 1960. NAPS, American Board of Plastic Surgery (hereinafter cited as ABPS) #406. Figi FA. Presidential address. Plast Reconstr Surg 1957; 10:2. McCoy TR. Beauty can be bought. American Weekly, April 26, 1959:8-9. NY Times, July 14, 1959:30:1. Conway H. Distribution of plastic surgeons in the United States. Plast Reconstr Surg 1965; 35:183. See also Aufricht G. The development of plastic surgery in the United States. Transactions of the American Society of Plastic and Reconstructive Surgeons 13th Annual Meeting 1944:9-32.
24. NY Times, December 8, 1944:14:6. See also July 2, 1944:IV 9:6; October 1, 1944:IV 11:6.

Examples of popular coverage include: Maisel AQ. New faces for new men. Sci Digest, April 1943:28-32. Ray MB. Saving his face. Woman's Home Companion, September 1944:25, 56, 58. Schacht B. Giving the boy a new face. St. Louis Globe-Democrat, March 10, 1946:E1.

Writer Geri Trotta called *Dark Passage* "near witchery . . . absurd," but Americans loved it. The face plastic surgery can build you, Look, April 3, 1948:78.
25. de Kleine EH. The crossroads of cosmetic surgery. Plast Reconstr Surg 1955; 16:145-149. NY Times, June 24, 1944:17:2.
26. Daché L. Lily Daché's Glamour Book. Lewis DR, ed. Philadelphia: J.B. Lippincott, 1956:30-31. Kahler O. I'm glad I had my face lifted. Your Life, December 1948:80-84.
27. Davis I, Davis S. The great male face race. LA Magazine, February 1975:63, 103-104. Alvarez W. Face-lifting: For what . . . Good Housekeeping, September 1957:86-87, 186-189. NY Times, November 9, 1967:51:1. San Francisco Examiner, August 4, 1972:26. New wrinkles. Newsweek, April 28, 1969:70. See also NY Times, April 8, 1969:49:7.
28. Mercer M. Plastic surgery for men. Coronet, May 1961:100-104.
29. Maltz M. New Faces, New Futures: Rebuilding Character with Plastic Surgery. New York: Richard R. Smith, 1936. Davis M. Does plastic surgery work? Pictorial Review, December 1937:18. Breast reduction: Is it for you? Women's Sports and Fitness, July 1986: 56. Now I can be free. People, April 26, 1993:83. For the big picture see Yalom M. A History of the Breast. New York: Knopf, 1997.
30. For a fascinating take on this part of the story see Jacobson N. Cleavage: Technology, Controversy, and the Ironies of the Man-Made Breast. New Brunswick, NJ: Rutgers University Press, 1999.

Some surgeons, most neither members of the plastic surgical societies nor certified by the American Board of Plastic Surgery, did claim early successes in surgically treating small breasts. Henry Junius Schireson was one of these; in his 1938 book As Others See You: The Story of Plastic Surgery (New York: Macaulay, 1938:218-226) he reported successful breast augmentation using a "pedical flap/fat-fascia graft."
31. Franklyn RA. Beauty Surgeon. Long Beach, Calif: Whitehorn, 1960: 15-22. Honor E. Cosmetic surgery. Cosmopolitan, August 1956:28-31. Wade C. Instant beauty through plastic surgery. Lady's Circle, April 1965:19 (In: NAPS, HMS C87 #403).
32. Abreast of the times. JAMA 1966;195:863. Ashley FL, Braley S, Rees TD, Goulian D, Ballantyne DL. Present status of silicone fluid in soft tissue augmentation. Plast Reconstr Surg 1967; 39: 411-415. Boo-Chai K. The complications of augmentation mammaplasty by silicone injection. Br J Plast Surg 1969; 22:281. Chaplin CH. Loss of both breasts from injections of silicone (with additive). Plast Reconstr Surg 1969; 44:447. No national statistics on complications are available but one San Diego physician told a reporter that 20% of the approximately 400 complications he saw between 1967 and 1974 required amputation. See Larned D. A shot—or two, or three—in the breast. Ms., September 1977:55.
33. Schalk D. History of augmentation mammaplasty. Plast Surg Nurs 1988; 8:89. Braley S. Use of silicones in plastic surgery: A retrospective view. Plast Reconstr Surg 1973; 51:285-286. NY Times, November 13, 1988:IV 9:1.
34. Time, March 27, 1964:48. Broadbent TR, Woolf RM. Augmentation mammaplasty. Plast Reconstr Surg 1964; 40:517-523. Perras C. Plastic reconstruction of the small breast. J Am Med Womens Assoc 1965; 20:951-952. Schalk D. History of augmentation mammaplasty. Plast Surg Nurs 1988; 8:89. Braley S. Use of silicones in plastic surgery: A retrospective view. Plast Reconstr Surg 1973; 51: 285-286. See also Blocksma R, Braley S. Implantation materials. In: Grabb W, Smith J, eds. Plastic Surgery. Boston: Little, Brown, 1965:3-148.
35. Time, March 27, 1964:48. Yes, you can have a bigger bosom! Cosmopolitan, January 1970:66. Over the years, popular magazines have presented a range of opinions on cosmetic breast augmentation, often offering alternative viewpoints in back-to-back issues (for example, an article one month touting the benefits and an article the next month profiling a case that went wrong). In general, coverage was positive until the late 1980s and in some cases the early 1990s, when stories about risks and problems, often sparked by one of the widely publicized court cases or by FDA action, began to appear.
36. Hoge W. Doctor vanity: The jet set's man in Rio. NY Times Magazine, June 8, 1980:42-46, 52-62, 66-70. Stanley A. Lifting the spirit (and face) in Russia. NY Times, June 6, 1995:A6. Koop D. Bogus plastic surgeons prey on Peru's poor and desperate. Associated Press, February 13, 1998. Pomfret J. China syndrome: "True happiness" is no more than a nose job away. Washington Post, January 10, 1999:A1.
37. Articles on these topics are innumerable; a good starting point is Rosenthal E. Cosmetic surgeons seek new frontiers. NY Times, September 24, 1991:B5:1. For a regional take: Kramer J. Sharper images. Pacific Sun, March 31-April 6, 1999:11. On penile enhancement see Haiken E. Virtual virility or, does medicine make the man? Men & Masculinity (2000). On labioplasty see Kamps L. Labia envy. Salon Magazine, February 1, 1999; www.salonmagazine.com/mwt/feature/1998/03/16feature.html
38. On the FTC episode, see McCoy FJ. Report on the activities of the ASPRS. Plast Reconstr Surg 1977; 59:315-317. Randall P. Federal Trade Commission vs. reliance upon board certification in a specialty. Plast Reconstr Surg 1979; 63:453-456. Gorney M. F.T.C., Woodstock, and plastic surgery. Plast Reconstr Surg 1980; 65:245. Gorney M. The morning after. Plast Reconstr Surg 1980; 66:751-752. Ship AG. To advertise or not to advertise. Plast Reconstr Surg 1984; 74:123.

The debate on advertising dominates the letters pages of most specialty journals in these months.
39. Regush N. Toxic breasts. Mother Jones, January/February 1992: 25-31. See also Goldrich SN. Restoration drama. Ms., June 1988, which played a significant role in sparking the recent controversy, and Blakeslee S. The true story, Glamour, August 1991:186, which details the early history of the polyurethane covered implant. For an example of how the Même was discussed in the popular press, see Lippert JL. A better breast implant. Health, April 1983:21-22. Also Angell M. Science on Trial: The Clash of

Medical Evidence and the Law in the Breast Implant Case. New York: Norton, 1996.

40. Goldrich SN. Restoration drama. Ms., June 1988:20. Press coverage was extensive.
41. Goldrich SN. Restoration drama. Ms., June 1988:20. NY Times, November 10, 1988:I 18:1; November 24, 1988:II 16:5. Silicone breast implants on trial. Science News, December 10, 1988:380.
42. Marks C. The new breast implant scare. Mademoiselle, February 1989:124-125. FDA to require safety data on breast implants. FDA Consumer, March 1989:2.
43. NY Times, June 14, 1918:6:2. Ryan L. Plastic surgery. Ill Med J 1918; 34:69.
44. Roberts JB. The cosmetic surgery of the nose. JAMA 1892; 19:231-233. On immigration see Higham J. Strangers in the Land: Patterns of American Nativism, 1860-1925. New York: Atheneum, 1963, 1973; also Kraut A. Silent Travelers: Germs, Genes, and the Immigrant Menace. New York: Basic Books, 1994. NY Times, August 15, 1923:10:3 and August 16, 1923:14:4. Katkov N. The Fabulous Fanny. New York: Knopf, 1953:141.
45. Harris H. 9 Myths about face-lifting. McCall's, June 1961:78-79, 182.
46. Potter R. Farewell to ugliness. American Weekly, April 14, 1946.
47. Harris DD. Now you can have. . . . Esquire, November 1965:134-136, 189-192.
48. A few examples: Kelly J. Cosmetic lib for men. NY Times Magazine, September 25, 1977:119. What cosmetic surgery can and can't do. Business Week, January 21, 1980:104-105, 108. Put on a successful face. Psychology Today, December 1983:70.
49. See, for example, Davis JS. The art and science of plastic surgery. Ann Surg 1926; 84:203-210.
50. There are many examples of this version; one is Rank BK. The story of plastic surgery, 1868-1968. Practitioner 1968:201.
51. For early and late attempts at quantification, see Straith CL. Reconstructions about the nasal tip. Am J Surg 1939; 43:223-236, and Farkas LG, Kolar JC. Anthropometrics and art in the aesthetics of women's faces. Clin Plast Surg 1987; 14:599-616. Maltz M. Dr. Pygmalion: The Autobiography of a Plastic Surgeon. New York: Thomas Y. Crowell, 1953. For a more modern example: www.bodybybloch.com
52. On Asian eyes, see Kaw E. Medicalization of racial features: Asian American women and cosmetic surgery. Med Anthropol Q 1993; 7:74-89.
53. Grealey L. Autobiography of a Face. Boston: Houghton-Mifflin, 1994:222.

CHAPTER 2

The History of Cosmetic Dermatologic Surgery

C. WILLIAM HANKE

BACKGROUND AND HISTORY

Dermatology is a mature medical-surgical specialty with a distinguished history of innovation. Although this historical perspective will emphasize surgical dermatology (dermatologic surgery), the history of medical dermatology has been just as impressive. Furthermore, this chapter will focus on cosmetic dermatologic surgery as opposed to general dermatologic surgery and skin cancer surgery. Similarly, the evolution of skin cancer surgery, particularly Mohs micrographic surgery and reconstruction, has been remarkable.

Training in Dermatologic Surgery

Unlike some other surgical specialties, dermatologists receive nearly all of their surgical training during dermatology residency and surgical fellowships. The 3-year residency is preceded by a Graduate Level I year, which may be spent in internal medicine, pediatrics, surgery, or rotating. Each dermatology residency program is required to have a full-time surgical program director who is responsible for resident training in surgery.

Dermatologic surgery is required to be given special emphasis during residency training, and includes anesthesia, cryosurgery, nail surgery, biopsy techniques, electrosurgery, laser surgery, excisional surgery, and reconstructive surgery including flaps and grafts. Residents are also expected to be familiar with Mohs micrographic surgery, hair transplantation, sclerotherapy, dermabrasion, liposuction, laser resurfacing, tissue augmentation, and chemical peels. Resident experience in dermatologic surgery can be continued in one of more than 60 dermatologic surgery fellowships, which are 1 or 2 years in duration. Residents, fellows, and practitioners can also register for postgraduate courses in various aspects of dermatologic surgery that are sponsored by the American Academy of Dermatology, the American Society for Dermatologic Surgery, and other organizations that will be mentioned later. Many of these postgraduate courses involve didactic lectures, hands-on laboratories, and live surgery sessions.

Dermatologic Surgery Organizations

Four professional dermatologic surgery organizations have been established to fulfill various educational missions.

1. The American College of Mohs Micrographic Surgery and Cutaneous Oncology (ACMMSCO) was founded in 1967 as the American College of Chemosurgery. The College held annual meetings to share experience in Mohs surgery and cutaneous oncology. Early "chemosurgeons" learned Mohs surgery via short preceptorships with Frederic Mohs. In 1967, Tromovitch and Stegman began performing Mohs surgery without zinc chloride fixative paste and the "fresh tissue technique" was born. Immediate reconstruction of wounds, previously impossible because of devitalized zinc chloride fixed tissue, was now possible. Perry Robins established the first 1-year Mohs Surgery Fellowship at New York University in 1970. Henry Menn, who later established his own Mohs Surgery Fellowship at the University of Miami, was the first fellow. There are presently over 60, 1- to 2-year Mohs Surgery/Dermatologic Surgery Fellowships available. All fellowships are accredited by the College. The American College of Chemosurgery changed its name to the American College of Mohs Micrographic Surgery and Cutaneous Oncology in 1986, to reflect the changes in the scope of practice that had occurred. The reconstructive skills that are presently taught during fellowship have direct application to larger excisional procedures.
2. The American Society for Dermatologic Surgery (ASDS) was founded in 1970 by Leonard Lewis, Sorrel Resnik, and 27 other founding members. Norman Orentreich was the first president. The ASDS annual meetings have evolved into a showcase of procedural learning for all aspects of dermatologic surgery including skin cancer surgery, laser surgery, and cosmetic surgery. The Society, currently the second largest in dermatology, has more than 2400 members. The ASDS became a member of the AMA House of Delegates in 1987. In 1993, the Society elected to join

the Accreditation Association for Ambulatory Health Care (AAAHC) as one of 13 sponsoring health care organizations. C. William Hanke and Roy C. Grekin were appointed to represent ASDS on the AAAHC Board of Directors. In 2000, the American Academy of Dermatology (AAD) also joined AAAHC as a sponsoring organization. C. William Hanke was elected to a 2-year term as president of AAAHC beginning in 2001. In 1995, the ASDS acquired the publishing rights to *Dermatologic Surgery* from Elsevier Science Publishers. New, focused ASDS-sponsored postgraduate courses for dermatologic surgeons on tumescent liposuction, laser, and phlebology were held in the year 2000.

3. The International Society for Dermatologic Surgery (ISDS) was founded by Perry Robins in 1979 to promote and teach dermatologic surgery worldwide. The ISDS became the first sponsoring society for the *Journal of Dermatologic Surgery and Oncology* in 1986. ISDS world congresses have been held in the following cities: Lisbon, Portugal (1979); Paris, France (1980); Vienna, Austria (1981); Granada, Spain (1983); Jerusalem, Israel (1984); Rome, Italy (1985); London, England (1986); Barcelona, Spain (1987); Edinburgh, Scotland (1988); Brussels, Belgium (1989); Florence, Italy (1990); Munich, Germany (1991); Paris, France (1992); Seville, Spain (1993); Toronto, Canada (1994); Tel Aviv, Israel (1995); Budapest, Hungary (1996); Amsterdam, Netherlands (1997); Salvador, Brazil (1998); Athens, Greece (1999); and Madrid, Spain (2000).

   The ISDS congresses provide an opportunity for dermatologic surgeons from around the world to share experiences. Live surgery workshops have become a highlight of recent Congresses. The ISDS formed the Council of National Dermatologic Surgery Societies (CNDSS) in 1992 to include representatives from all of the national dermatologic surgery societies from around the world. The CNDSS meets each fall during the ISDS congress.
4. The Association of Academic Dermatologic Surgeons (AADS) was founded in 1988 by Ed Krull. The purpose of the organization is the promotion of dermatologic surgery education, research, and patient care. The membership is composed of the surgical training directors from all of the dermatology residency programs. The annual meetings provide an opportunity for academic surgical faculty to interact and solve common problems.

Allied Surgical Societies

Six additional surgical societies provide postgraduate education in various aspects of cosmetic surgery and dermatologic surgery. All of these societies have large numbers of dermatologic surgeons as members. These societies include the American Society for Lasers in Medicine and Surgery (ASLMS), the International Society of Cosmetic Laser Surgeons (ISCLS), the American Academy of Cosmetic Surgery (AACS), the American College of Phlebology (formerly the North American College of Phlebology), and the International Society of Hair Restoration Surgeons (ISHRS). In addition to comprising large percentages of the membership, dermatologic surgeons have served as officers and directors of these organizations.

1. The American Society for Lasers in Medicine and Surgery (ASLMS) was founded by Goldman and Drake in 1981. ASLMS is a multidisciplinary organization that holds a comprehensive educational and research meeting each spring. The organization currently has 3000 members from all areas of medicine and dentistry.
2. The International Society of Cosmetic Laser Surgeons (ISCLS) was founded as a multidisciplinary organization by David in 1990 and focuses on education in cosmetic laser surgery. Members from around the world gather at the Annual ISCLS Symposium each spring to assess the latest advances in cosmetic laser surgery. A live surgery observational session has always been part of the annual symposium. The Society has 461 members.
3. The American Academy of Cosmetic Surgery (AACS) was founded in 1985 as a multidisciplinary society for the advancement of education in cosmetic surgery. The annual meeting each January brings together cosmetic surgeons from around the world. Each year, the AACS also sponsors a World Congress and multiple smaller workshops on various aspects of cosmetic surgery. AACS currently has 1349 members. Dermatologic surgeons comprise 25% of the membership.
4. The North American College of Phlebology (NACP) was founded in 1985. The College selected *Dermatologic Surgery* as its official journal in 1990. *Dermatologic Surgery* has devoted special issues to sclerotherapy (1989), phlebology (1995), and ambulatory phlebectomy (1998). In 1998, the College changed its name to the American College of Phlebology. The College has 600 members.
5. The International Society for Hair Restoration Surgeons (ISHRS) was founded by Norwood and Stough in 1987. The multidisciplinary membership currently numbers 825. A world symposium is held each year to share experience and assess advancements in technique.

Journal of Dermatologic Surgery

The Journal of Dermatologic Surgery was founded by Perry Robins and George Popkin in 1975, in spite of critics who felt the *Journal* was unnecessary and would fail. The *Journal* grew in size and stature and was selected by six societies as their official publication: International Society for Dermatologic Surgery (ISDS), American Society for Dermatologic Surgery (ASDS), American College of Mohs Micrographic Surgery and Cutaneous Oncology (ACMMSCO), American College of Phlebology (ACP), International Society of Cosmetic Laser Surgeons (ISCLS), and International Society of Hair Restoration Surgeons (ISHRS). A number of editors-in-chief have served with distinction: Perry Robins (1975-1977), Morris Leider (1978-1981), George L. Popkin (1982-1985), C. William Hanke (1986-1990), Leonard M. Dzubow (1991-1996), and Ronald Moy (1997-2001). In 1977 the *Journal*'s name was changed to the *Journal of Dermatologic Surgery and Oncology.* In 1995 the name was shortened to *Dermatologic Surgery.* In 1990, Elsevier Science Publishers purchased the *Journal* from Perry Robins. In 1995, C. William Hanke, then president of the ASDS, negotiated the ASDS purchase of the *Journal* from Elsevier. In 1999 Blackwell Science Publishers began publishing the *Journal* under ASDS ownership. The *Journal* thus became a business as well as a professional asset for ASDS. The *Journal* continues to grow and publishes state-of-the-art manuscripts on all aspects of dermatologic surgery. In recent years, an increasing number of manuscripts on laser and cosmetic surgery have been published. Other dermatology journals such as the *Archives of Dermatology* and the *Journal of the American Academy of Dermatology* have added special sections on dermatologic surgery.

HISTORY OF ADVANCES IN COSMETIC DERMATOLOGIC SURGERY

Dermatologic surgeons have either developed or refined the surgical procedures that are part of the specialty of dermatology. Dermatologic surgeons have also been generous teachers of dermatologic surgical procedures to other specialties. Many of the procedures have been assimilated by other specialties without mention of where they originated. This series of procedural timelines and commentary will document the origins and advances in dermatologic cosmetic surgery. The first timeline, Milestones in Cosmetic Dermatologic Surgery (Box 2-1), presents some of the highlights. Many of the procedures will have a separate timeline.

Dermabrasion (Box 2-2)

Dermabrasion has a long history in dermatology. In 1905, Kromayer[1] used rotating burrs for dermabrasion. He also used carbon dioxide snow to firm the skin. The real breakthrough came in 1953 when Kurtin[2] and Robbins collaborated to develop motorized dermabrasion apparatus, wire brushes, and the diamond fraise. Also in 1953, Lowenthal[3] described punch transplants for scars. Blau and Rein[4] coined the term *dermabrasion* in 1954. In 1955, Burks[5] published his book *Wire Brush Surgery,* which described his extensive experience with dermabrasion. Wilson et al[6] developed new skin refrigerants for dermabrasion. Burks[7,8] later published studies on wound healing following dermabrasion and also dermabrasion for severe actinic damage. In 1969, Orentreich[9] reviewed the many cosmetic and therapeutic indications for dermabrasion. In 1977, Stagnone[10] published his experiences with "chemabrasion," which was dermabrasion following a chemical peel. In 1983, Mandy[11] described more rapid healing when polyethylene oxide gel was used following dermabrasion. Various skin refrigerants were being used for dermabrasion. In 1985, Hanke and co-workers[12] reported a laboratory analysis of all skin refrigerants currently in use. Rubenstein[13] et al provided evidence that abnormal healing can occur if dermabrasion is performed too soon after isotretinoin treatment. In 1986, Mandy[14] reported more rapid reepithelialization if tretinoin was used preoperatively for dermabrasion. Also in 1986, Johnson's[15] publication popularized punch transplants for scars. Yarborough[16] demonstrated that early dermabrasion of scars can enhance results. In 1992, Klein and Coleman[17] described dermabrasion under tumescent anesthesia. The American Academy of Dermatology published "Guidelines of care for dermabrasion" in 1994.[18] Also in 1994, Harris and Noodleman[19] revived manual dermasanding for sun-damaged skin. Microdermabrasion with aluminum oxide crystals has recently come into common use in the United States as a minimally invasive procedure.

Chemical Peeling (Box 2-3)

In 1882, Unna described salicylic acid, trichloroacetic acid, phenol, and resorcinol for chemical peeling. In 1941, Eller and Wolff[20] reported their work with salicylic acid, phenol, and carbon dioxide snow. Monash[21] described low-strength trichloroacetic acid peels in 1945. Urkov[22] described peeling with phenol under occlusion in 1946. In 1950, Winter[23] used phenol to permanently remove freckles. A landmark article appeared in 1952 when Mackee[24] reported his 50-year experience with phenol face peels. Ayres[25] popularized trichloroacetic acid and phenol peels in the early 1960s. Resnik and co-workers[26] refined trichloroacetic acid peeling in the 1970s. Stagnone[10] utilized chemical peel followed by dermabrasion and coined the term *chemabrasion.* In the early 1980s, Stegman[27,28] studied the effects of dermabrasion and chemical peeling agents in animal and human skin. In 1984, Van Scott and co-workers[29] reported the effectiveness of α-hydroxy acids for superficial peeling. In 1986, Brody and Hailey[30] utilized solid carbon dioxide and 35% trichloroacetic acid for medium-depth peeling. Monheit[31] popularized a simplified medium-depth peel using Jessner's solution and 35% trichloroacetic acid in 1989. Coleman and Futrell[32] later de-

BOX 2-1 Timeline: Milestones in Dermatologic Cosmetic Surgery

1905 Kromayer develops early dermabrasion techniques in Germany
1952 Mackee reports his 50-year experience with phenol peels
1953 Kurtin develops modern dermabrasion techniques
1955 Burks publishes book on *Wire Brush Surgery*
1956 Epstein publishes first of six editions of *Skin Surgery*
1957 Spangler describes fibrin foam for depressed scars
1959 Orentreich reports on hair transplantation
1960 Ayres reports on phenol and TCA for aging skin
1961 Goldman is first physician to treat patients with laser
1966 Zacarian reports on cryosurgery with liquid nitrogen
1970 The American Society for Dermatologic Surgery (ASDS) is founded
1972 ASDS sponsors first surgical postgraduate course at the University of Miami
1974 ASDS sponsors first dermabrasion–chemical peel seminar
1974 ASDS sponsors first hair transplant workshop
1975 Robins and Popkin found the *Journal of Dermatologic Surgery*
1977 Field learns early liposuction techniques in Paris
1978 Unger and Unger describe scalp reduction
1979 Robins founds International Society for Dermatologic Surgery (ISDS)
1980 Stegman describes chemical peel and dermabrasion in an animal model
1980 Stegman and Tromovitch consult with Collagen Corp. for Zyderm development
1982 Florida Society of Dermatologic Surgeons is founded
1986 Johnson popularizes treatment of pitted scars with punch transplants
1987 Klein publishes his first report on tumescent liposuction
1987 Carruthers begins cosmetic surgical use of BOTOX
1988 FDA approves pulsed-dye laser for cutaneous vascular lesions
1988 The *Journal of Dermatologic Surgery and Oncology* publishes first special issue devoted to liposuction
1988 Association of Academic Dermatologic Surgeons is founded
1989 Monheit reports his experiences with Jessner's–35% TCA peel
1990 Alt is first dermatologic surgeon elected president of American Academy of Cosmetic Surgery
1990 AAD publishes first guidelines of care for liposuction
1992 Carruthers reports experience with cosmetic use of BOTOX
1992 ISDS founds Council of National Dermatologic Surgery Societies
1993 ASDS becomes thirteenth sponsoring organization for AAAHC
1995 Hanke et al report on "Safety of tumescent liposuction in 15,336 patients"
1996 Grossman et al report on laser hair removal

BOX 2-2 Timeline: Milestones in Dermabrasion by Dermatologic Surgeons

1905 Kromayer describes motorized dermabrasion with metal burrs in Germany
1953 Kurtin and Robbins develop ethyl chloride spray and rotary brushes
1953 Lowenthal describes punch grafting for scars
1954 Blau and Rein coin the term *dermabrasion*
1956 Wilson et al publish research on skin refrigerants
1956 Burks publishes book on *Wire Brush Surgery*
1957 Burks publishes studies on wound healing following dermabrasion
1963 Burks et al recommend dermabrasion for actinic damage
1969 Orentreich reviews dermabrasion treatment for multiple conditions
1977 Stagnone presents his experience with "chemabrasion"
1983 Mandy uses polyethylene oxide gel to speed healing after dermabrasion
1985 Hanke et al perform laboratory evaluation of skin refrigerants
1986 Rubenstein et al recommend delayed dermabrasion after isotretinoin treatment
1986 Mandy uses pre-op tretinoin cream to speed healing after dermabrasion
1986 Johnson popularizes punch transplants for scars
1988 Yarborough describes use of early dermabrasion for scars
1992 Klein and Coleman describe dermabrasion by tumescent anesthesia
1994 AAD publishes "Guidelines of care for dermabrasion"
1994 Harris and Noodleman describe manual dermasanding for sun-damaged skin

BOX 2-3 Timeline: Milestones in Chemical Peeling by Dermatologic Surgeons

1882 Unna describes salicylic acid, resorcinol, phenol, and TCA for peeling

1941 Eller and Wolff describe peeling with phenol, salicylic acid, and CO_2 snow

1945 Monash describes low-strength salicylic peels in dermatology

1946 Urkov describes occluded phenol peels

1950 Winter removes lentigines with phenol

1952 Mackee reports his 50-year experience with phenol peels

1960 Ayres describes TCA and phenol peeling for actinic damage

1976 Resnik et al popularize peeling with TCA

1977 Stagnone describes chemical peel followed by dermabrasion ("chemabrasion")

1980 Stegman compares chemical peeling agents and dermabrasion in animal model

1982 Stegman reports histology of dermabrasion and chemical peel in human skin

1984 Van Scott describes α-hydroxy acids for superficial peels

1986 Brody and Hailey develop medium-depth peeling with solid CO_2 and TCA

1989 Monheit reports his experience with Jessner's–35% TCA peel

1992 Brody publishes first edition of *Chemical Peeling*

1994 Coleman and Futrell describe 70% glycolic acid–35% TCA peel

1995 Rubin publishes *Manual of Chemical Peels*

1997 Brody publishes second edition of *Chemical Peeling*

scribed a medium-depth peel with 70% glycolic acid followed by 35% trichloroacetic acid. Chemical peeling techniques utilized by modern dermatologists were detailed by Brody[33] and Rubin[34] in books in the 1990s.

Dermatologic Laser Surgery (Box 2-4)

The theoretical concepts of laser were discussed by Einstein[35] in 1917 as part of quantum theory. In 1955, Townes and Gordon[36] worked with a laser precursor dubbed MASER. The first operational ruby laser was developed by Maimon in 1960.[37] Goldman, a dermatologist at the University of Cincinnati, was the first physician to treat patients with ruby laser in 1961. The Helium-Neon and Nd:YAG lasers were developed in 1961. The argon laser followed in 1962, and the carbon dioxide laser in 1964. Goldman[38] described his experience treating nevi and melanomas with ruby laser in 1964, and vascular lesions with argon laser in 1968. In 1981, Anderson and Parrish[39] reported that yellow laser light of 577 nm would be ideal for vascular lesions. Goldman and Drake founded the American Society for Lasers in Medicine and Surgery in 1981. Gilchrest[40] reported on the protective effects of chilling of the skin for argon laser treatment of vascular lesions. A major breakthrough occurred in 1983, when Anderson and Parrish[41] published their "theory of selective thermolysis," which has enhanced understanding of laser effects on the skin. Goldman[42] reported his experience with copper vapor laser for vascular lesions in 1987. Kaufman and Hibst[43] published the first report on laser resurfacing with Er:YAG laser in 1989. Tan and coworkers[44] reported on pulsed-dye laser treatment for portwine stains in children in 1989. The International Society of Cosmetic Laser Surgeons was founded in 1990 with David as the first president. Taylor and Dover[45] reported on treatment of tattoos with the Q-switched ruby laser in 1990. Garden[46] described pulsed-dye laser treatment of capillary hemangiomas in 1992. Fitzpatrick and David were the first to use the Ultrapulse carbon dioxide laser for skin resurfacing in 1992. Koop developed the Computerized Pattern Generator (CPG) for the Ultrapulse in 1995. Grossman[47,48] and co-workers reported on various lasers for hair removal in the late 1990s. Arndt et al,[49] Ratz,[50] and Dover et al[51] published books on cutaneous laser surgery between 1983 and 1990.

Liposuction (Boxes 2-5 and 2-6)

Fischer[52] published the first description of hollow cannula liposuction in 1976. Field,[53] an American dermatologist, first learned about liposuction in Paris that same year. The period from 1977 to 1981 was essentially the French period. Illouz introduced the "wet technique," which utilized hypotonic saline and hyaluronic acid. Fournier developed the "crisscross" technique and syringe liposuction. Martin, an otolaryngologist in Los Angeles, was the first to perform liposuction in the United States in 1981.[54] Newman and Dolsky taught the first liposuction course in the United States in 1982. The first live surgery workshop on liposuction was held in Hollywood, California, in 1983.

The American period for dermatologic liposuction surgery begins with the first published articles on liposuction by Field and Chrisman[55,56] in 1984 in the *Journal of Dermatologic Surgery and Oncology.* Klein performed his first prototype liposuction procedure under local anesthesia in 1985. In 1986, Asken[57] published his first book, *Manual of Liposuction Surgery.* The breakthrough

BOX 2-4 Timeline: Milestones in Dermatologic Laser Surgery

1917	Einstein publishes theoretical concepts of laser as part of quantum theory
1955	Townes and Gordon develop MASER
1960	First laser (ruby) is developed by Maimon
1961	Goldman is first physician to treat patients with ruby laser
1961	Helium-neon, Nd:YAG lasers developed
1962	Argon laser is developed
1964	Carbon dioxide laser is developed
1964	Goldman publishes on ruby lasers for nevi and melanomas
1968	Goldman treats vascular lesions with argon laser
1981	Anderson and Parrish propose yellow laser (577 nm) for vascular lesions
1981	Goldman and Drake found ASLMS
1982	Gilchrest proposes chilling of skin for argon laser treatment
1983	Anderson and Parrish publish theory of selective photothermolysis
1987	Goldman uses copper vapor laser for vascular lesions
1988	Anderson publishes on Q-switched Nd:YAG laser for pigmented lesions
1988	Wheeland publishes book on *Lasers in Skin Disease*
1989	Tan, Sherwood, and Gilchrest report on PDL for portwine stains in children
1989	Kaufman and Hibst report on Er:YAG laser resurfacing
1990	ISCLS is formed with David as first president
1990	Taylor and Dover publish on Q-switched ruby laser for tattoos
1992	Garden treats capillary hemangiomas with PDL
1992	Fitzpatrick and David use Ultrapulse CO_2 laser for resurfacing
1995	Koop develops CPG for Ultrapulse
1997	Grossman, Dierickx, Anderson use long-pulse ruby laser for hair removal
1998	Grossman and Dierickx use 800 nm diode laser for hair removal

BOX 2-5 Timeline: Early Liposuction Pioneers

1976	Fischers publish first description of blunt hollow cannula liposuction
1977-1981	Illouz introduces "wet technique" with hypotonic saline and hyaluronic acid
1977-1981	Fournier advocates "crisscross technique" and syringe liposuction
1981	Martin (an otolaryngologist) performs first liposuction in Los Angeles, California
1982	Newman and Dolsky teach first American course in liposuction
1983	First live surgery workshop on liposuction is held in Hollywood, California

report occurred in 1987 when Klein[58] published his early results with the tumescent technique. In 1988, Bernstein and Hanke[59] reported on the safety of liposuction performed by dermatologists on 9478 patients. Also, in 1988, the *Journal of Dermatologic Surgery and Oncology* devoted an entire issue to liposuction by dermatologists. The first guidelines of care for liposuction were approved by the AAD in 1989.[60] Klein[61] reported in 1990 that safe liposuction could be performed with tumescent lidocaine 35 mg/kg. In 1995, Hanke and coworkers[62] reported on "Safety of tumescent liposuction in 15,336 patients." Ostad et al[63] reported on safe liposuction using tumescent lidocaine 55 mg/kg in 1996.

BOX 2-6 Timeline: Milestones in Liposuction by Dermatologic Surgeons

1977	Field first learns about liposuction in Paris
1984	Field and Chrisman publish first liposuction articles in *Journal of Dermatologic Surgery and Oncology*
1985	Klein performs his first liposuction procedure under local anesthesia
1986	Asken publishes *Manual of Liposuction Surgery*
1987	Klein publishes his landmark article on tumescent liposuction
1988	Bernstein and Hanke report on safety of liposuction by dermatologists in 9478 patients
1988	*Journal of Dermatologic Surgery and Oncology* devotes an entire issue to liposuction
1989	First "Guidelines of care for liposuction" are approved by AAD
1990	Klein reports safe liposuction with tumescent lidocaine 35 mg/kg
1995	Hanke et al report on "Safety of tumescent liposuction in 15,336 patients"
1996	Ostad et al report safe liposuction with tumescent lidocaine 55 mg/kg
1998	Sommer, Sattler, and Hanke publish first book on *Tumescent Local Anesthesia* in German
2000	Klein publishes his comprehensive book on *Tumescent Technique*

BOX 2-7 Timeline: Milestones in Phlebology/Phlebologic Surgery by Dermatologic Surgeons

1966 Muller's first article on ambulatory phlebectomy

1982 Chrisman publishes on hypertonic saline injections for leg veins

1982 Shields and Jansen publish on sodium tetradecyl sulfate for leg veins

1985 Bodian's publication in *Journal of Dermatologic Surgery and Oncology* popularizes sclerotherapy

1985 Butie founds North American Society of Phlebology (NASP)

1986 First lectures on phlebology are given at AAD annual meeting

1987 American Board of Dermatology develops first board questions on phlebology

1988 Duffy advocates sclerotherapy with hypertonic saline and polidocanol

1988 First Congress of North American Society of Phlebology is held in San Diego

1988 *Journal of Dermatologic Surgery and Oncology* devotes an entire issue to sclerotherapy

1990 *Journal of Dermatologic Surgery and Oncology* is selected as official publication of NASP

1991 Goldman publishes comprehensive book on sclerotherapy

1993 AAD publishes "Guidelines of care for sclerotherapy"

1994 Sattler publishes on endoscopic vein surgery

1995 *Dermatologic Surgery* devotes a second special issue to phlebology

1996 Muller publishes his 40-year experience with ambulatory phlebectomy

1998 NASP is renamed the American College of Phlebology

1998 *Dermatologic Surgery* devotes a special issue to ambulatory phlebectomy

Sommer et al[64] published the first book on *Tumescent Local Anesthesia* in German in 1998. In 2000, Klein[65] published a comprehensive book, *Tumescent Technique.*

Phlebology/Phlebologic Surgery (Box 2-7)

Phlebology began in Europe and has been transplanted to the United States. An article by Chrisman[66] in 1982 advocated hypertonic saline for spider veins. Shields and Jansen[67] described the use of sodium tetradecyl sulfate for spider veins, also in 1982. Bodian's[68] publication in 1985 served to popularize sclerotherapy in dermatology. The North American Society of Phlebology (NASP) was founded by Butie in 1985 with many American dermatologists as founding members. In 1986, the first lectures on phlebology were given at the annual meeting of the American Academy of Dermatology (AAD). The American Board of Dermatology developed its first test questions on phlebology in 1987. In 1988, Duffy[69] advocated sclerotherapy with hypertonic saline and polidocanol. Also in 1988, the First Congress of the NASP was held in San Diego. The *Journal of Dermatologic Surgery and Oncology* published an entire issue on sclerotherapy in 1989, and the NASP selected the *Journal* as its official publication in 1990. Goldman and Fitzpatrick[70] published on pulsed-dye laser for leg telangiectasia in 1990. Goldman[71] completed a book on *Treatment of Varicose and Telangiectatic Leg Veins* in 1991. Guidelines of care for sclerotherapy were published by the AAD in 1993. A special issue of *Dermatologic Surgery* was devoted to phlebology in 1995. In 1998, the NASP was renamed the American College of Phlebology. Also in 1998, *Dermatologic Surgery* devoted an entire issue to ambulatory phlebectomy. Muller[72,73] described ambulatory phlebectomy in 1966, and provided a long-term follow-up report in 1996. Sattler and co-workers[74] reported on endoscopic vein surgery and endoscopic perforating vein ligation in 1994.

Hair Transplantation (Box 2-8)

Okuda[75] initially described punch grafting in the *Japanese Journal of Dermatology* in 1939. There was very little activity in hair transplantation in the United States until Orentreich began performing transplants in New York in 1952. He published his results and "theory of donor dominance" in 1959.[76] Ayres and Arouet began transplant practices in California and Paris, respectively, in 1961. Rabineau began a hair transplant practice in Paris in 1963 following instruction from Orentreich in New York. Ayres used skill and innovation to develop a high-profile practice in Beverly Hills. An article by Ayres[77] in 1964 contained the first description of micrografts and minigrafts. Alt performed his first hair transplant in 1972 and became one of the greatest innovators and teachers. Norwood[78] published the first edition of his book on *Hair Transplant Surgery* in 1973. Unger and Unger described scalp reduction in 1978.[79] Unger[80] published the first edition of his book on *Hair Transplantation* in 1979. Norwood and Shiel[81] produced the second edition of *Hair Transplant Surgery* in 1984. Also in 1984, Norwood[81] described his classification of androgenetic alopecia. Unger and Nordstrom[82] co-edited the second edition of *Hair Transplantation* in 1991. The International Society for Hair Restoration Surgery (ISHRS) was founded by Nor-

BOX 2-8 Timeline: Milestones in Hair Transplantation by Dermatologic Surgeons

1939 Okuda describes punch grafting in *Japanese Journal of Dermatology*

1952 Orentreich performs his first hair transplant in New York

1959 Orentreich publishes early results with hair transplantation

1959 Orentreich publishes research supporting his "theory of donor dominance"

1961 Ayres begins "celebrity" hair transplant practice in California

1961 Arouet performs his first hair transplant in Paris after instruction from Orentreich

1963 Rabineau begins hair transplants in Paris after instruction from Orentreich

1964 Ayres describes micrografts and minigrafts in *Archives of Dermatology*

1972 Alt performs his first hair transplant after instruction from Stough, Orentreich, and Burks

1973 Norwood publishes his first book on *Hair Transplant Surgery*

1978 Unger and Unger publish on scalp reduction

1979 Unger publishes first edition of his book on *Hair Transplantation*

1984 Norwood and Shiel publish second edition of *Hair Transplant Surgery*

1984 Norwood publishes his classification for androgenetic alopecia

1989 Norwood and Stough found ISHRS

1989 Arouet publishes textbook on hair transplantation

1991 Limmer reports on follicular unit transplants in *Hair Transplant Forum International*

1995 Norwood founds *Hair Transplant Forum*

wood and Stough in 1987. A book on hair transplantation was published by Arouet in 1989. In 1995, Norwood founded the *Hair Transplant Forum.*

Filler Materials and Botulinum Toxin (Box 2-9)

Spangler[83] reported on fibrin foam (porcine collagen) for scars initially in 1957. A long-term follow-up study was published in 1975.[84] Gottlieb[85] refined and popularized the technique. This new porcine collagen filler, called Fibrel, was approved by the FDA for scars in 1988 and for wrinkles in 1990. Long-term follow-up studies demonstrated long-lasting effects.[86] Regrettably, the production of Fibrel has been discontinued and it is no longer available for use.

In the late 1970s, Stegman and Tromovitch began working with the Collagen Corporation on the development of bovine collagen for clinical use. Zyderm I was approved by the FDA for soft-tissue defects in 1981, Zyderm II in 1983, and Zyplast in 1985. Stegman and Tromovitch taught others including Klein[87] and Elson,[88] who did much to advance the technique.

In 1992, Carruthers and Carruthers[89] published on botulinum toxin type A (BOTOX) for glabellar frown lines and a new revolution in minimally invasive cosmetic surgery began. Dermatologists outside the United States began to use injectable hyaluronic acid with success for wrinkles and scars. Elson[90] and Klein[91] published comprehensive books on soft-tissue augmentation in 1995, and 1998, respectively. Carruthers and Carruthers[92] published the first book on botulinum toxin in cosmetic surgery in 2001.

BOX 2-9 Timeline: Filler Materials and Botulinum Toxin

1957 Spangler uses fibrin foam for acne scars

1975 Spangler reports on long-term follow-up with fibrin foam

1980 Stegman and Tromovitch report on bovine collagen for scars

1992 Carruthers and Carruthers describe therapeutic and cosmetic use of botulinum toxin

1995 Elson publishes book on *Treatment of the Aging Face*

1995 Hyaluronic acid is used as an injectable dermal implant

1998 Klein publishes book on *Tissue Augmentation*

2001 Carruthers and Carruthers publish comprehensive book on cosmetic use of botulinum toxin

Many dermatologic surgeons believe that autologous fat is the most natural appearing filler material. Asken[93,94] wrote books on the subject in the 1980s. Skouge and co-workers[95] have studied autologous fat in animal models.

Blepharoplasty and Facelift

Dermatologic surgeons such as Noel[96] were leaders in blepharoplasty and face lift techniques in the 1920s. Interest by dermatologists in these techniques was rekindled by Webster, who taught cosmetic surgery to all specialties. Dermatologists Asken and Alt were two of

Webster's pupils. Asken[97-100] wrote early books on liposuction and also refined blepharoplasty and face lift techniques. Alt[101,102] became a great teacher-practitioner of blepharoplasty, face lift, dermabrasion, chemical peel, and hair transplantation. Chrisman refined Asian blepharoplasty and browlift.[103] Chrisman and Field[104] utilized liposuction for face lift surgery. David[105] began performing carbon dioxide laser transconjunctival lower lid blepharoplasty in 1985, and published his initial results in 1987. Current renewed interest in face lift by dermatologic surgeons is a direct result of advances in tumescent liposuction of the neck. Klein's initial report[58] on tumescent liposuction in 1987 provided the technical advance for dermatologic surgeons to perform safe liposuction of the neck totally under local anesthesia. The publications of Cook[106] have documented the excellent results that can be achieved. Weinstein[107,108] has reported her results for laser resurfacing done in conjunction with laser blepharoplasty, brow lift, and endoscopic forehead lift.

SUMMARY

Dermatologists have been pioneers in dermatologic and skin surgery for decades. The latter half of the twentieth century has seen an unprecedented rise in the popularity of cosmetic surgery, and dermatologists have been central in the development of new, improved, and safer techniques. However, it is fascinating that this interest in surgical improvement of the skin dates back to the late nineteenth and early twentieth century in dermatology. Dermatologists are in a unique professional position to see and evaluate changes of the skin, and the development of the field of cosmetic dermatologic surgery has been a natural extension of the surgical aspect of dermatology.

In addition to creating the field of microscopically controlled skin cancer removal (Mohs micrographic surgery), dermatologists have been at the forefront of skin surgery for decades. Recent advances including tumescent liposuction, micro and mini grafting for hair transplantation, soft tissue augmentation, botulinum A exotoxin injection, and laser surgery confirm the importance and relevance of the dermatologic surgeon's role in cosmetic surgery. Many of the most exciting advances in cosmetic surgery in the twentieth century have come from the collegial and academic field of dermatology.

It is interesting to note the role that intra- and interspecialty education and cooperation has played in the developments in cosmetic dermatologic surgery. Dermatology has a long history as a specialty with a solid academic foundation, and it is this fundamental interest in education and learning that has propelled many of the techniques in use today. Educational and hands-on courses abound, as do didactic and academic meetings on a national level. It has become clear to dermatologic surgeons that it is through the shared knowledge of experiences that true innovations and progress evolve. This forward-thinking cooperative approach has enabled many new techniques to flourish and enjoy widespread use and acceptance, and it is clear that dermatologic cosmetic surgery is a field with a rich history and bright future.

REFERENCES

Dermabrasion

1. Kromayer E. Rotation Instrumente: ein neues Techisches verfahren in der Dermatologischen. Kleinchirurgie Dermatol Z 1905; 12:26.
2. Kurtin A. Corrective surgical planing of skin. Arch Dermatol Syphilol 1953; 68:389-397.
3. Lowenthal L. Punch biopsy with autograft. Arch Dermatol Syphilol 1953; 67:629-631.
4. Blau S, Rein CR. Dermabrasion of the acne pit. Arch Dermatol Syphilol 1954; 70:754-766.
5. Burks JW. Wirebrush Surgery. Springfield, Ill: Charles C Thomas, 1955.
6. Wilson J, Ayres S, Luikart R. Mixtures of fluorinated hydrocarbons as refrigerated anesthetic. Arch Dermatol 1956; 74:310-311.
7. Burks JW, Marascalco J, Clark WH. Half-face planing of precancerous skin after five years. Arch Dermatol 1963; 88:572-585.
8. Burks JW, Brewer JM. Surgical planing for the prevention of cancer of the skin. South Med J 1966; 53:86-91.
9. Orentreich N. Dermabrasion. J Am Med Womens Assoc 1969; 24:331-336.
10. Stagnone JJ. Chemabrasion, a combined technique of chemical peeling and dermabrasion. J Dermatol Surg Oncol 1977; 3:217-219.
11. Mandy SH. A new primary wound dressing made of polyethylene oxide gel. J Dermatol Surg Oncol 1983; 9:153-155.
12. Hanke CW, O'Brian JJ, Solow EB. Laboratory evaluation of skin refrigerants used in dermabrasion. J Dermatol Surg Oncol 1985; 11:45-49.
13. Rubenstein R, Roenigk HH Jr,. Stegman SJ, Hanke CW. Atypical keloids after dermabrasion of patients taking isotretinoin. J Am Acad Dermatol 1986; 15:280-285.
14. Mandy SH. Tretinoin in the preoperative and postoperative management of dermabrasion. J Am Acad Dermatol 1986; 15: 878-879, 888-889.
15. Johnson W. Treatment of pitted scars: punch transplant techniques. J Dermatol Surg Oncol 1986; 12:260-265.
16. Yarborough JM Jr. Ablation of facial scars by programmed dermabrasion. J Dermatol Surg Oncol 1988; 14:292-294.
17. Coleman WP, Klein JA. Use of the tumescent technique for scalp surgery, dermabrasion, and soft-tissue augmentation. J Dermatol Surg Oncol 1992; 18:130-135.
18. Mandy SH, Gross KKG, Yarborough JM. Guidelines of care for dermabrasion. J Am Acad Dermatol 1994; 31:654-657.
19. Harris DR, Noodleman FR. Combining manual dermasanding with low strength trichloroacetic acid to improve actinically injured skin. J Dermatol Surg Oncol 1994; 20:436-442.

Chemical Peeling

20. Eller JJ, Wolff S. Skin peeling and scarification. JAMA 1941; 116:934-938.
21. Monash S. The uses of diluted trichloroacetic acid in dermatology. Urol Cut Rev 1945; 49:119-120.
22. Urkov JC. Surface defects of skin: treatment by controlled exfoliation. Ill Med J 1946; 89:75.
23. Winter L. Method of permanent removal of freckles. Br J Dermatol Syph 1950; 62:83.

24. Mackee GM, Karp FL. The treatment of post-acne scars with phenol. Br J Dermatol 1952; 64:456-9.
25. Ayres S. Dermal changes following application of chemical cauterants to aging skin. Arch Dermatol 1960; 82:578-585.
26. Resnik SS, Lewis LA, Cohen BH. Trichloroacetic acid peeling. Cutis 1976; 17:127-129.
27. Stegman SJ. A study of dermabrasion and chemical peels in an animal model. J Dermatol Surg Oncol 1980; 6:490-497.
28. Stegman SJ. A comparative histological study of the effects of three peeling agents and dermabrasion on normal and sun-damaged skin. Aesthet Plast Surg 1982; 6:123-135.
29. Van Scott EJ, Yu RJ. Hyperkeratinization, corneocyte cohesion and alpha hydroxy acids. J Am Acad Dermatol 1984; 11:867-879.
30. Brody HJ, Hailey CW. Medium-depth chemical peeling of the skin: a variation of superficial chemosurgery. J Dermatol Surg Oncol 1989; 15:945-950.
31. Monheit G. The Jessner's + TCA peel: a medium depth chemical peel. J Dermatol Surg Oncol 1989; 15:945-950.
32. Coleman WP, Futrell JM. The glycolic acid and trichloroacetic acid peel. J Dermatol Surg Oncol 1994; 20:76-80.
33. Brody HJ. Chemical Peeling. St. Louis: Mosby–Year Book, 1992.
34. Rubin MG. Manual of Chemical Peels. Philadelphia: JB Lippincott, 1995.

Dermatologic Laser Surgery

35. Einstein A. Zar Quantentheorie der Stahlung. Physical Z 1917; 18:121-128.
36. Gordon JP, Zeigler HJ, Townes CH. The MASER—New type of amplifier, frequency standard and spectrometer. Physiol Rev 1955; 99:1264-1274.
37. Maimon TH. Stimulated optical radiation in ruby. Nature 1960; 187: 493-494.
38. Goldman L, Igelman JM, Richfield DF. Impact of the laser on nevi and melanomas. Arch Dermatol 1964; 90:71-75.
39. Anderson RR, Parrish JA. Microvasculature can be selectively damaged using dye lasers: a basic theory and experimental evidence in human skin. Lasers Surg Med 1981; 1:263-276.
40. Gilchrest BA, Rosen S, Noe JM. Chilling portwine stains improves the response to argon laser therapy. Plast Reconstr Surg 1982; 69:278-283.
41. Anderson RR, Parrish JA. Selective photothermolysis: precise microsurgery by selective absorption of pulsed radiation. Science 1983; 220:524-527.
42. Goldman L, Taylor A, Putnam T. New developments with heavy metal vapor lasers for the dermatologist. J Dermatol Surg Oncol 1987; 13:163-165.
43. Kaufman R, Hibst R. Pulsed Er:YAG and 308 NM UV-eximer laser: in vitro and in vivo study of skin ablative effects. Lasers Surg Med 1989; 9:132-140.
44. Tan OT, Sherwood K, Gilchrest BA. Treatment of children with portwine stains using the flashlamp-pulsed tunable dye laser. N Engl J Med 1989; 320:416-421.
45. Taylor CR, Grange RW, Dover JS et al. Treatment of tattoos by Q-switched ruby laser. Arch Dermatol 1990; 126:893-899.
46. Garden JM, Bakus AD, Paller AS. Treatment of cutaneous hemangiomas by the flashlamp-pumped pulse dye laser: prospective analysis. J Pediatr 1992; 120:555-560.
47. Grossman MC, Dierickx CC, Farinelli WA et al. Damage to hair follicles by normal-mode ruby laser pulses. J Am Acad Dermatol 1997; 35:889-894.
48. Grossman MC, Dierickx CC, Quintana A et al. Removal of excess body hair with an 800 NM pulsed diode laser. Lasers Surg Med 1998; 108:42.
49. Arndt KA, Noe JM, Rosen S. Cutaneous Laser Therapy: Principles and Methods. New York: Wiley, 1983.
50. Ratz JL. Lasers in Cutaneous Medicine and Surgery. Chicago: Year Book, 1986.
51. Dover JS, Arndt KA, Geronemus R et al. Illustrated Cutaneous Laser Surgery. Norwalk, Conn: Appleton & Lange, 1990.

Liposuction

52. Fischer A, Fischer G. First-surgical treatment for molding body's cellulite with three 5 mm incisions. Bull Int Acad Cosmet Surg 1976; 3:35-36.
53. Field LM. The dermatologist and liposuction—a history. J Dermatol Surg Oncol 1987; 13:1040-1041.
54. Hetter CP. The history of LSNA. Lipoplasty 1999; 16:9.
55. Field LM. Lipo-suction surgery: a review. J Dermatol Surg Oncol 1984; 10:530-538.
56. Chrisman BB, Field LM. Facelift surgery update: suction assisted rhytidectomy and other improvements. J Dermatol Surg Oncol 1984; 10:544-548.
57. Asken S. Manual of Liposuction Surgery and Autologous Fat Transplantation Under Local Anesthesia. Irvine, Calif: Terry and Associates, 1986.
58. Klein JA. The tumescent technique for liposuction surgery. Am J Cosm Surg 1987; 4:263-267.
59. Bernstein G, Hanke CW. Safety of liposuction: a review of 9478 cases performed by dermatologists. J Dermatol Surg Oncol 1988; 14:1112-1114.
60. Liposuction practice guidelines. American Academy of Dermatology, 1989.
61. Klein JA. Tumescent technique for regional anesthesia permits lidocaine doses of 35 mg/kg for liposuction; peak plasma lidocaine levels are diminished and delayed for 12 hours. J Dermatol Surg Oncol 1990; 16:240-263.
62. Hanke CW, Bernstein G et al. Safety of liposuction in 15,336 patients. Dermatol Surg 1995; 21:459-462.
63. Ostad A, Kageyama N, Moy RL. Tumescent anesthesia with a lidocaine dose of 55 mg/kg is safe for liposuction. Dermatol Surg 1996; 22:921-927.
64. Sommer B, Sattler G, Hanke CW, eds. Tumescenz Lokalanasthesie. Berlin: Springer, 1998.
65. Klein JA. Tumescent technique: tumescent anesthesia and microcannular liposuction. St Louis: Mosby, 2000.

Phlebology/Phlebologic Surgery

66. Chrisman BB. Treatment of venous ectasias with hypertonic saline. Hawaii Med J 1982; 41:406.
67. Shields JL, Jansen GT. Techniques of sclerotherapy for superficial telangiectasias of the lower extremities. J Dermatol Surg Oncol 1982; 8:857-860.
68. Bodian EL. Techniques of sclerotherapy for sunburst venous blemishes. J Dermatol Surg Oncol 1985; 11:696-704.
69. Duffy D. Small vessel sclerotherapy: an overview. In: Callen et al., eds. Advances in Dermatology, Vol 3. St Louis: Mosby, 1988.
70. Goldman MP, Fitzpatrick RE. Pulsed-dye laser treatment of leg telangiectasia with and without simultaneous sclerotherapy. J Dermatol Surg Oncol 1990; 16:338-344.
71. Goldman MP. Sclerotherapy Treatment of Varicose and Telangiectatic Leg Veins. St Louis: Mosby–Year Book, 1991.
72. Muller R. Traitement des varices par la phlebectomie ambulatoire. Phlebologie 1966; 19:227-229.
73. Muller R. Misse au point sur la phlebectomie ambulatoire selon Muller (PAM). Phlebologie 1996; 49:335-344.
74. Sattler G, Mossler K, Hagedorn M. Prophylaxe und therapie des ulcer cranis: endoskopische perforansuenendiszision und antegrade paratibiale fasziotomie. In: Wundheilung-Wundverschluss Theorie und Praxis, Chirurgische und Kunservative Massnahmen. Berlin: Springer-Verlag, 1994:225-229.

Hair Transplantation

75. Okuda S. Clinical and experimental studies on transplanting of living hair. Jpn J Dermatol Urol 1939; 46:135-138.

76. Orentreich N. Autografts in alopecias and other selected dermatologic conditions. Ann NY Acad Sci 1959; 83:465.
77. Ayres S III. Conservative surgical management of male pattern baldness. Arch Derm 1964; 90:492-499.
78. Norwood O. Hair Transplant Surgery. Springfield, Ill: Charles C Thomas, 1973.
79. Unger MG, Unger WP. Management of alopecia of the scalp by a combination of excisions and transplantations. J Dermatol Surg Oncol 1978; 4:670-672.
80. Unger W. Hair Transplantation. New York: Marcel Dekker, 1979.
81. Norwood O, Shiel R. Hair Transplant Surgery. 2nd ed. Springfield, Ill: Charles C Thomas, 1984.
82. Unger WP, Nordstrom REA. Hair Transplantation. 2nd ed. New York: Marcel Dekker, 1988.

Filler Materials and Botulinum Toxin

83. Spangler AS. New treatment for pitted scars. Arch Dermatol 1957; 76:708.
84. Spangler AS. Treatment of depressed scars with fibrin foam—seventeen years of experience. J Dermatol Surg Oncol 1975; 1:65.
85. Gottlieb S. GAP repair techniques. Poster exhibit. American Academy of Dermatology Annual Meeting. Dallas, Texas, 1977.
86. Millikan LE et al. A 5-year safety and efficacy evaluation with Fibrel in correction of cutaneous scars following one or two treatments. J Dermatol Surg Oncol 1991; 17:223-229.
87. Elson EL. The role of skin testing in the use of collagen injectable materials. J Dermatol Surg Oncol 1989; 15:301-303.
88. Klein AW. In favor of double skin testing. J Dermatol Surg Oncol 1989; 15:263.
89. Carruthers JDA, Carruthers JA. Treatment of glabellar frown lines with *C. botulinum*-A exotoxin. J Dermatol Surg Oncol 1992; 18:17-21.
90. Elson ML. Evaluation and Treatment of the Aging Face. New York: Springer-Verlag, 1995.
91. Klein AW. Tissue Augmentation in Clinical Practice. New York: Marcel Dekker, 1998.
92. Carruthers A, Carruthers J. The Cosmetic Use of Botulinum Neurotoxin. New York: Marcel Dekker, 2001.
93. Asken S. A Manual of Liposuction Surgery and Autologous Fat Transplantation Under Local Anesthesia. Irvine, Calif: Terry and Associates, 1986.
94. Asken S. Liposuction Surgery and Autologous Fat Transplantation. East Norwalk, Conn: Appleton & Lange, 1988.
95. Skouge JW, Canning DA, Jefs RD. Long-term survival of perivascular fat harvested and injected by microlipo injection techniques in a rabbit model. Presented at 16th Annual Meeting of American Society for Dermatologic Surgery, Fort Lauderdale, Fla, 1989.

Blepharoplasty and Face Lift

96. Noel AS. La chirurgie esthetique. In: Masson et al. Son Role Sociale. Paris, 1926.
97. Asken S. Cosmetic eyelid surgery—blepharoplasty. In: Coleman WP, Hanke CW, Alt TH, Asken S, eds. Cosmetic Surgery of the Skin. Philadelphia: BC Decker, 1991.
98. Asken S. Blepharoplast. In: Coleman WP, Hanke CW, Alt TH, Asken S, eds. Cosmetic Surgery of the Skin. 2nd ed. St Louis: Mosby–Year Book, 1997.
99. Asken S. The facelift-cervicofacial rhytidectomy. In: Coleman WP, Hanke CW, Alt TH, Asken S, eds. Cosmetic Surgery of the Skin. Philadelphia: BC Decker, 1991.
100. Asken S. Cervicofacial rhytidectomy. In: Coleman WP, Hanke CW, Alt TH, Asken S, eds. Cosmetic Surgery of the Skin. 2nd ed. St Louis: Mosby–Year Book, 1997.
101. Alt TH. Chemical peeling, alopecia surgery, dermabrasion. In: Coleman WP, Hanke CW, Alt TH, Asken S, eds. Cosmetic Surgery of the Skin. Philadelphia: BC Decker, 1991.
102. Alt TH. Chemical peeling, dermabrasion, hair transplantation, scalp reduction. In: Coleman WP, Hanke CW, Alt TH, Asken S, eds. Cosmetic Surgery of the Skin. 2nd ed. St Louis: Mosby–Year Book, 1997.
103. Chrisman B. Blepharoplasty and browlift with surgical variations in non-white patients. J Dermatol Surg Oncol 1986; 12:58-66.
104. Chrisman B, Field L. Facelift surgery 1984—suction assisted rhytidectomy and other improvements. J Dermatol Surg Oncol 1984; 10:544-548.
105. David LM, Sanders GH. Carbon dioxide laser blepharoplasty: a comparison to cold steel knife methods. J Dermatol Surg Oncol 1987; 13:110-114.
106. Cook W. Laser neck and jowl liposculpting including platysmal laser resurfacing, dermal laser resurfacing, and vaporization of subcutaneous fat. Dermatol Surg 1997; 23:1143-1148.
107. Weinstein C. Ultrapulse carbon dioxide laser removal of periocular wrinkles in association with laser blepharoplasty. J Clin Lasers Med Surg 1994; 12:205-209.
108. Weinstein C. Endoscopic forehead lifts. In: Coleman WP, Hanke CW, Alt TH, Asken S, eds. Cosmetic Surgery of the Skin. 2nd ed. St Louis: Mosby–Year Book, 1997:379-385.

CHAPTER 3

Evaluation of the Aging Face

RICHARD G. GLOGAU

Wrinkles should merely indicate where smiles have been.

MARK TWAIN (1897)

With advancing years, the aging appearance has taken center stage as a presenting complaint for many patients. The reasons for their unhappiness with their appearance may include

- Job pressures in a highly competitive and increasingly technical job market
- A high rate of divorce and successive remarriage
- The incessant advertising media reflecting the icons of beauty and appearance
- Awareness of the wider availability of cosmetic services
- An unsurpassed decade of economic growth, with higher discretionary income
- A wider social tolerance of cosmetic rejuvenation procedures
- An explosion of medical and surgical technology

Liposuction surgery was literally unheard of only two decades ago and now is one of the most commonly performed cosmetic surgical procedure in the United States. Cosmetic lasers, which didn't exist two decades ago, have surpassed liposuction in sheer number of cases performed and patients treated. Use of injectable soft-tissue fillers and the hottest current aesthetic agent, botulinum toxin, may surpass lasers and liposuction in the next few years in sheer numbers of patients treated.

ANATOMIC BASIS FOR AGING APPEARANCE

The physician should approach an analysis of the aging face using an anatomic model to provide a systematic framework to counsel patients and rationally select among a wide variety of therapeutic options. Too often, patients encounter physicians who have developed a preference for one therapeutic "hammer," and all the patients become "nails." Failure to match a given therapeutic technique to the anatomic basis for the cosmetic problem leads to mediocre results at best and disasters at worst.

The human face ages in response to a number of factors that appear in varying degrees in different individuals:

1. Chronic ultraviolet light damage to the skin
2. Loss of subcutaneous fat
3. Changes in the intrinsic muscles of facial expression
4. Gravitational changes from loss of elasticity of the tissue
5. Remodeling of the underlying bony and cartilaginous structures

Identifying the relative mix and proportion of these factors in the patient often points the way to selecting the most appropriate procedure. By knowing the risk/benefit ratio for the procedure and communicating this information to the patient, the physician can successfully complete the cosmetic consultation visit.

Clearly there is a great deal of confusion among medical professionals since we still see patients with distinct cosmetic defects being mismatched with the wrong therapeutic procedure on a regular basis:

- Patients with severe chronic sun damage having face lifts without consideration of resurfacing
- Patients with jowls and platysmal banding of the neck undergoing liposuction without redraping the superficial musculoaponeurotic system (SMAS) and skin
- Patients already gaunt from the lipoatrophy associated with aging getting laser resurfacing and rhytidectomy, producing a skeletonized appearance
- Patients with deep glabellar furrows treated with injectable fillers without botulinum toxin to paralyze the intrinsic muscles producing the frown

Mismatching the procedure to the patient results from failing to appreciate the underlying anatomic defect causing the undesired aesthetic appearance. Considered in turn, each one lends itself to some aspect of therapy that may be used individually or combined with other therapies aimed at a different component of the anatomy to give the desired aesthetic effect.

PHOTOAGING

With the increase in leisure time, air travel, and outdoor activity, the boomers spent their formative years out in the sun, without the benefit of currently available sunscreens. Years of "baby oil and iodine," more revealing clothing, and the desire of the physically fit to acquire the oxymoronic "healthy tan" have produced high rates of skin cancer and prematurely aging skin. Cumulative exposure to sun remains the largest factor in aging skin and is responsible for a large portion of the unwanted aesthetic effects. Clinical signs of photoaging of the skin include rhytides, lentigines, keratoses, telangiectasia, loss of translucency, loss of elasticity, and sallow color.[1,2]

I have developed a simple systematic classification of patient photoaging types, Type I through Type IV (Box 3-1 and Fig. 3-1).[3] Younger patients, usually in their 20s or 30s, show only the earliest signs of photoaging, usually as a change in homogeneity of color, but generally have no rhytides at all, even when the face is animated by talking or expression. They are categorized as Type I: No Wrinkles. They generally wear no makeup foundation at all, because they do not require it for either color or lines.

As the patient ages, the ultraviolet damage to the elastic fibers becomes chronic and the inherent "snap back" quality of the skin becomes impaired. Wrinkles begin to appear, at first only when the face is in motion, usually as expression lines parallel to the meilolabial fold, the corners of the mouth, and the lateral canthal areas and over the zygomatic arch and malar eminences. These patients frequently utilize makeup foundation to conceal the irregularity in color or the sallow tones that result from the chronic sun exposure. These patients are commonly in their 30s or 40s and look unlined when their faces are at rest. However, as soon as they begin to talk, the lines appear. They are classified as Type II: Wrinkles on Motion.

As the photoaging proceeds, the damage to the elastic fibers becomes more severe. Eventually the wrinkles

BOX 3-1 Glogau Photoaging Classification

Type 1: No Wrinkles
Early photoaging
- Mild pigmentary changes
- No keratoses
- Minimal wrinkles

Patient age: 20s or 30s
Minimal or no makeup

Type II: Wrinkles in Motion
Early to moderate photoaging
- Early senile lentigines visible
- Keratoses palpable but not visible
- Parallel smile lines beginning to appear

Patient age: late 30s or 40s
Usually wears some foundation

Type III: Wrinkles at Rest
Advanced photoaging
- Obvious dyschromia, telangiectasia
- Visible keratoses
- Wrinkles even when not moving

Patient age: 50s or older
Always wears heavy foundation

Type IV: Only Wrinkles
Severe photoaging
- Yellow-gray color of skin
- Prior skin malignancies
- Wrinkled throughout, no normal skin

Patient age: 60s or 70s
Cannot wear makeup—"cakes and cracks"

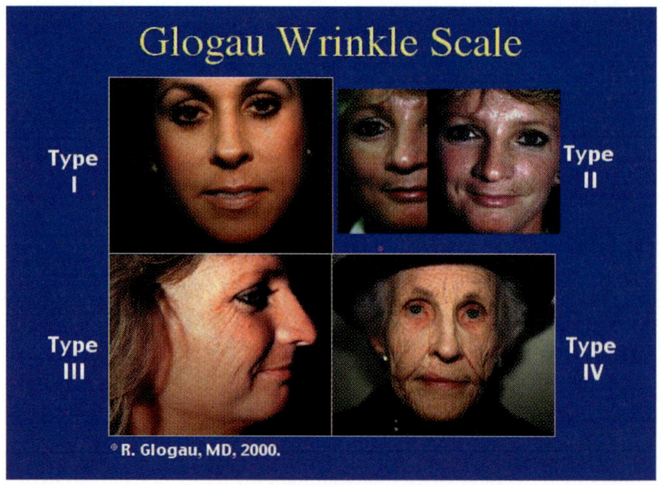

FIG. 3-1 Glogau Wrinkle Scale
Type I: No Wrinkles. Skin is uniform in color. There is an absence of lines even at the corners of the eyes and mouth. *Type II: Wrinkles in Motion.* When the face is at rest (IIa), the patient appears similar to Type I. But when the face is animated by expression (IIb), there are many parallel lines that appear, first at the corners of the mouth, then parallel to the nasolabial folds, then at the corners of the eyes, and finally over the malar cheeks. *Type III: Wrinkles at Rest.* This patient clearly shows the parallel lines seen with animation in Type II except they are now present with the face at complete rest. *Type IV: Only Wrinkles.* The perioral skin in particular is likely to demonstrate the total replacement of normal skin with minute, rhomboid, and geometric rhytides, clearly seen in this patient. The entire face shows similar rhytides on close inspection.

produced by dynamic movement of the face persist even when the face is at rest. Generally by the 50s there are visible parallel lines at the crow's feet, parallel to the corners of the mouth, radiating down from the lower eyelids onto the malar cheeks, and across the upper lip and lower lip. Makeup foundation still helps with the color problem in these patients but tends to accentuate the appearance of the lines. These patients appear lined even when their faces are at rest and are classified as Type III: Wrinkles at Rest.

With continued photoaging, the wrinkles gradually spread to cover the majority of the facial skin, while the dermis becomes totally engorged with thick debris of poorly staining ground substance, giving a thickened, coarse quality to the skin. Usually this occurs by the 60s or 70s, but earlier in the severest cases. Many of these patients have already had one or more skin cancers. Makeup is completely impractical because it gives the appearance of cracked mud when applied to such an uneven surface. These patients really have no unlined skin anywhere on their faces and are classified as Type IV: Only Wrinkles.

PIGMENTARY SYSTEM

Patients must also be categorized according to their Fitzpatrick Sun-Reactive Skin Type.[4] This classification (Table 3-1) is based on the skin's response to erythema-producing doses of ultraviolet light. Patients differ in their sun reactivity, and the scale gives a good indication of the potential for dyschromia following epidermal or papillary dermal injury and the likelihood that postinflammatory hyperpigmentation will develop during the short-term postoperative period and of the potential for permanent hypopigmentation resulting from destruction of melanocytes.

Evaluating the degree of photodamage present and the pigmentary ultraviolet response can be expressed as shorthand to classify the patient's degree of damage.

Table 3-1 Fitzpatrick's Sun-Reactive Skin Types

Skin Type	Skin Color	Tanning Response
Type I	White	Always burns, never tans
Type II	White	Usually burns, tans with difficulty
Type III	White	Sometimes mild burn, tans average
Type IV	Brown	Rarely burns, tans with ease
Type V	Dark brown	Very rarely burns, tans very easily
Type VI	Black	No burn, tans very easily

A patient who is a Fitzpatrick III, Glogau Photoaging III is a very different candidate for resurfacing than a Fitzpatrick I, Glogau Photoaging II. The risk/benefit ratios are entirely different in these two patients. The presence of lines and wrinkles alone is not sufficient indication for resurfacing.

As a general rule, patients with Fitzpatrick Skin Types I to III will tolerate resurfacing without significant risk of color change. Although resurfacing may be undertaken in Fitzpatrick Skin Types IV to VI, the risk of pigmentary change is certainly high enough that the patient should be warned that there can be color change in the treated skin.

LOSS OF SUBCUTANEOUS FAT

An aspect of the aging face that is a major component of aesthetic disharmony is the redistribution and loss of subcutaneous fat. While some compartments such as the submental fat may lend themselves to removal via liposuction, in general there is a growing appreciation that removal of fat should be done with caution because of the flattening or hollowing of contours that may occur. Aging produces a profound loss of subcutaneous fat in the peri-oral area, the temporal fossae, the premalar areas, chin, and forehead. The older face has a flattened quality to the cheekbones, a sunken appearance to the lips, a bulging of the inferior fat pads of the eye, and in general a loss of the fullness and roundness of youth. Experienced plastic surgeons have recognized this and are moving away from excessive fat removal to fat repositioning or augmentation. Dr. Steven Hoefflin has written, "in the aging face it is not the tightness of the SMA (platysma aponeurosis) or skin that makes the difference, but the quantity and position of subcutaneous fat."[5]

For example, the routine removal of the infraorbital fat as a part of blepharoplasty, which often accentuated the deep grooves between the lower eyelid and the cheek, has become outdated. Now the surgeons prefer to utilize an arcus marginalis release and mobilize the fat medially and anteriorly to fill in that groove and return a more youthful appearance to the lower eyelids through restoration of fullness. Similarly, repositioning of the pre-malar fat has become an important part of routine face lifting, reversing the aged appearance that comes from flattening of the cheekbone contours.

The ultimate recognition of the importance of the subcutaneous volume of the face comes from the work of surgeons like Fournier and Coleman and others who have evolved techniques of fat transfer to restore the volume contours of the aged face. Microlipoinjection in small and larger volumes, placed subcutaneously and intramuscularly, has been used with great success to reshape the aging face. While difficulties remain in the predictability and longevity of fat transfers, the aesthetic effects are often impressively natural in the resulting appearance.

Restoration of loss of volume lies behind the appeal of injectable fillers such as collagen, hyaluronic acid gel, and microdroplet silicone. Lip augmentation with injectables remains one of the most frequently sought after cosmetic procedures performed in aesthetic medicine today. The market is literally overflowing with new injectable agents and alloplastic implants of expanded polytetrafluoroethylene (SoftForm, Gore-Tex).

Analysis of the aging face must include an assessment of the quality and position of the subcutaneous fat. Are the lips thin? Have they lost their shape? Are the cheekbones flattened? Is there wasting in the temporal fossae, above the eyebrows, in the buccal pads? Resurfacing or face lifting or both will not address these problems and may make them stand out even more.

CHANGES IN FACIAL MUSCULATURE

Perhaps nothing else has driven home the impact of facial musculature on facial aging like the introduction of botulinum toxin for selective chemical denervation of selected muscles of the face. Paralysis or partial weakening of the glabellar corrugator/procerus complex, the forehead frontalis, and the lateral orbicularis muscles has simply revolutionized the management of the upper third of the aging face. Deep glabellar lines, which could be only briefly improved with injectable fillers, now melt away with the placement of botulinum toxin in the corrugator/procerus complex. Crow's feet lines, which routinely reappeared after deep resurfacing, now vanish in a few days. Even the troublesome horizontal lines and creases of the lower eyelid, which persisted after blepharoplasty or resurfacing or both, now can be treated with botulinum toxin. The toxin is both safe and temporary. It has now become a mainstream tool in cosmetic surgery.

The interesting thing about the use of botulinum toxin is that it allows us to see precisely what the components of the various anatomic compartments may be in the aging face. For example, the patient who has deep photoaging lines may not get complete resolution of the glabellar furrows with initial treatment with botulinum toxin. Because the sun-damaged skin has been repeatedly folded, a line may still be visible for several months after botulinum toxin has completely paralyzed the corrugators. These patients require either resurfacing or a dermal filler such as Zyderm collagen to address the remaining component of the glabellar line. Similarly the occasional male patient will have such hypertrophy of the glabellar muscle complex that with botulinum-induced paralysis and atrophy of the muscles, the underlying contour of the bone becomes more prominent, and the patient perceives a "bump" appearing in the brow. Volume in the face can be at least partly related to musculature as well as subcutaneous fat.

INHERENT LOSS OF ELASTICITY

As the facial soft tissue ages, the skin and underlying supporting structures, while sagging under the effects of gravity, lose their inherent resiliency or ability to resist stretching. The most striking example of this is the development of brow ptosis with age. The most common problem in patients' own analysis of the aging face is their inability to relate the hooding of the upper eyelid skin to malposition of the brows and forehead. How many patients ask for (and receive) upper lid blepharoplasty when the source of their problem is ptosis of the upper brow and forehead? In a similar vein, inappropriate and overzealous use of botulinum toxin in the upper third of the face routinely produces brow ptosis, a feeling of "heaviness" and a slightly Neanderthal appearance because the older forehead does not have the inherent resiliency to maintain any brow position without the support of the underlying frontalis.

In contrast, the surgeon who inappropriately elevates the brow to a position that would be mismatched to the patient's gender or age does the patient no aesthetic favor. Careful consideration of the quality of elasticity of the skin and soft tissue must be taken into account before attempting to address the position of the brow either surgically or with botulinum toxin.

In the lower third of the face, the face lift is the sine qua non of the successful aesthetic outcome. Redraping, repositioning, and judicious removal of skin and soft tissue that has lost elasticity achieves a restoration of youthful appearance that cannot be achieved with resurfacing, fillers, fat transfer, or botulinum toxin. While in truth many of these other techniques properly applied have made it possible for patients to delay and defray, virtually no one escapes the effects of gravity and the loss of intrinsic elasticity. The face lift procedure is not in danger of extinction, though it now requires more selective application and execution that is mindful of the other components of aging discussed previously.

CHANGES IN UNDERLYING CARTILAGE AND BONE

The aging nose elongates and the tip droops. The aging mouth is affected by bony remodeling of the maxilla. The chin sharpens and protrudes. The ears appear to lengthen as the lobes droop. The tarsal plate softens and no longer holds the lower lid margin in proper curve or position. Various surgical procedures address these problems: tip rhinoplasty, tarsal lid tightening, canthoplasty, etc. Newer dental implant procedures and maxillofacial surgery can address intrinsic changes affecting the lower face.

But the practiced diagnostic eye of the cosmetic surgeon should not overlook the contribution of the underlying hard structures of the face—particularly when assessing presence (or more commonly absence) of facial symmetry. Patients often present with requests for treatment of facial problems without appreciating the contribution of underlying structures to their facial asymmetry. Although subtle, the asymmetry is not due to the soft tissue. No amount of collagen is going to correct an underlying difference in maxillary structure of the cheekbones, for example.

These preexisting differences in facial asymmetry need to be identified so they can be pointed out to the patient and discussed. We have seen too many patients who are unhappy with their face lift results who rail against the surgeon when it is their underlying facial structures that are the root cause of the difference in the appearance of their lifts. Recognizing preexisting facial asymmetry due to underlying bony or cartilaginous structural differences is an important part of setting realistic patient expectations.

The most common example of preexisting asymmetry is in cosmetic ear piercing. Patients recognize that their earlobes differ in size, volume, position, and orientation. They know how difficult it is to pierce earlobes so that their jewelry will hang at the proper angle. The surgeon can often use this example to point out other asymmetries and put them in terms the patients can recognize.

COMBINATION THERAPIES

Optimal improvement in appearance can more often be obtained by combining procedures. At one end of the therapeutic spectrum, topical medical therapy utilizing agents like tretinoin, α-hydroxy acids, hydroquinones, and 5-fluorouracil can inhibit or reverse ultraviolet-associated changes in aging skin. At the other end of the therapeutic spectrum, rhytidectomy, blepharoplasty, brow lift, and suction-assisted lipectomy often provide dramatic results in facial rejuvenation. The choice of therapy rests on the ability of the surgeon to look at the face, analyze the anatomic components of the aging appearance, and then prioritize them, matching procedure risk/benefit ratio to each element. Is the predominant problem sun damage, sagging, or loss of volume? Often there are overriding constraints; e.g., the "down time," surgical risk, cost, and likelihood of benefit all weigh in the selection of the appropriate therapy. But underlying all of these choices must be a rational analysis of the various elements that go into making up the aging face.

REFERENCES

1. Balin A, Pratt L. Physiological consequences of human skin aging. Cutis 1989; 43:431-436.
2. Montagna W, Carlisle K, Kirchner S. Epidermal and Dermal Histological Markers of Photodamaged Human Facial Skin. Shelton, Conn: Richardson-Vicks, 1988.
3. Glogau RG. Chemical peeling and aging skin. J Geriatr Dermatol 1994; 2(1):30-35.
4. Fitzpatrick T. The validity and practicality of sun-reactive skin types I through VI. Arch Dermatol 1988; 124:869-871.
5. Hoefflin SM. The youthful face: tight is not right, repositioning is right [letter]. Plast Reconstr Surg 1998; 101(5):417.

CHAPTER 4

Photoaging: Mechanisms, Consequences, and Prevention

THOMAS ROHRER
MURAD ALAM
ROBIN TRAVERS
BARBARA A. GILCHREST

BACKGROUND AND HISTORY

Aging is a process that leads to progressive reduction in organ function and increased vulnerability to disease. As a highly visible organ at the environmental interface, the skin is subjected to both intrinsic and extrinsic factors that combine to produce an aged appearance as well as compromised function.[1-3] Intrinsic aging, also called chronologic aging, occurs at a genetically determined rate throughout the body, and its skin manifestations can be observed in sun-protected areas of older people. Extrinsic aging is primarily the superposition of chronic sun damage on intrinsic aging and is therefore also called photoaging.

Chronologic aging primarily causes physiologic changes in the skin. Epidermal turnover, barrier function, sensory perception, vitamin D production, immunosurveillance, thermoregulation, DNA repair capacity, and mechanical protection are all reduced during the intrinsic aging process. Consequences of these changes include poor wound healing, increased risk of irritant dermatitis, skin cancer, and easy tearing or blistering of skin. Morphologic changes of intrinsic aging are relatively subtle and consist of laxity, fine wrinkling, and a variety of benign neoplasms such as seborrheic keratoses and cherry angiomata.

Photoaging refers to essentially permanent changes in skin that are largely the result of ultraviolet (UV) radiation, almost always received from the sun. Other possible sources of UV exposure include phototherapy, arc welding, fluorescent light, and tanning beds. Photoaging has unique features but also exaggerates many of the changes seen in chronologic aging (Box 4-1). Of great importance to patients, photoaged skin has prominent morphologic changes in addition to functional decrements.

Clinically, photoaged skin is characterized by irregular pigmentation, roughness, variable atrophy and hyperplasia, a pebbly quality termed elastosis, fine and coarse wrinkling, telangiectases, and a variety of benign neoplasms (Fig. 4-1). Skin cancers occur almost exclusively on habitually sun exposed skin, and the risk correlates closely with severity of photoaging. Both severity of photoaging and risk of skin cancer generally increase with an individual's lifelong insolation (intensity, frequency, and duration of sun exposure). The character of photoaging is also determined by phototype, with fair-skinned individuals (skin types I and II) tending to have generally atrophic and dysplastic changes (Fig. 4-2), and darker-skinned individuals (skin types III through VI) tending to have hyperplastic changes, with prominent coarse wrinkling and elastosis.

The common unwanted changes in the skin that occur with aging are largely preventable by avoiding photoinjury. However, in our society, many younger people enjoy the appearance of a dark tan and ignore the inevitable delayed effects of sun exposure on their skin. Hence, our society will have to deal with the unwanted effects of too much sun exposure over at least the next several decades and perhaps indefinitely despite the availability of excellent sunscreens. Beyond the burden of skin cancer, demand for treatment of wrinkling, mottled, and coarse skin will surely increase. The following sections focus on action spectra and molecular mechanisms of photoaging.

BOX 4-1 Clinical Features of Photoaging

Irregular pigmentation	Purpura
Roughness	Laxity
Diffuse erythema	Sagging
Telangiectasia	Fine wrinkles
Lentigines	Coarse wrinkles

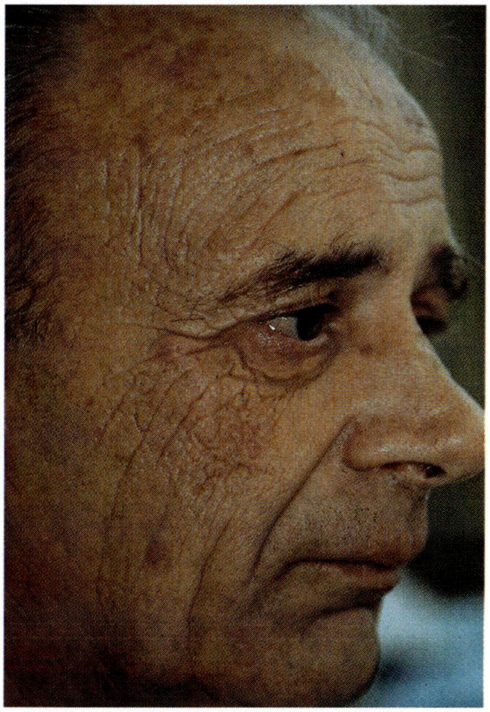

FIG. 4-1
This man, skin type III, has had ample lifelong sun exposure. There is coarse wrinkling and distinct elastosis affecting the lateral cheek and forehead. Solar lentigines are also apparent.

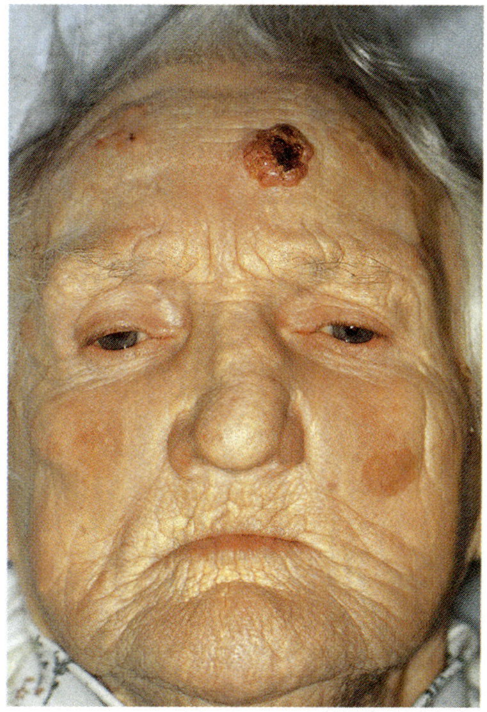

FIG. 4-2
This elderly woman, skin type II, has coarse wrinkling and solar lentigines as signs of photoaging. In addition, there is a large basal cell carcinoma on the forehead, in an area of habitual sun exposure.

BASIC SCIENCE

Action Spectrum

Terrestrial sunlight contains UV radiation (290 to 400 nm), visible light (400 to 700 nm), and infrared radiation (>700 nm). While visible light and infrared radiation have negligible effects on skin, UV radiation has significant deleterious effects. Ultraviolet radiation is divided into UVC (200 to 290 nm), the most energetic UV wavelengths; UVB (290 to 320 nm), also called the sunburn spectrum; and UVA (320 to 400 nm), also called black (invisible) light or near-UV. UVC is filtered efficiently by the ozone layer and hence is virtually absent from terrestrial sunlight, so that UVB, which constitutes less than 0.5% of terrestrial sunlight, is responsible for most of the acute and chronic photoinjury to normal skin.

Ultraviolet rays are reflected, scattered, or absorbed during their passage through the epidermis and upper dermis. The depth of penetration of UV is directly related to wavelength. The most energetic photons of shortest wavelength are absorbed more superficially, many in the stratum corneum. Longer UVB wavelengths tend to penetrate into the epidermis where they may be absorbed by nucleic acids. Photon absorption by nucleic acids rapidly declines with increasing wavelength. Therefore, UVA rays tend to penetrate into the dermis where they are scattered and absorbed by cellular chromophores such as NADH and riboflavin. On average, approximately 10% of UVB photons and 50% of UVA photons reach the dermis, a depth of 0.1 to 0.2 mm. The corollary is that UVB photons preferentially affect the epidermis, whereas UVA photons are equally likely to affect molecular targets in the papillary dermis.

Action spectra for acute effects of sun exposure, such as sunburn and tanning, have been determined experimentally in humans. The action spectra for these two consequences of sun exposure are virtually identical and peak sharply in the UVB portion of the spectrum, at approximately 300 nm, falling off exponentially with increasing wavelength through approximately 3 to 4 orders of magnitude over the UVA range. The curves also closely conform to the action spectrum for formation of DNA photoproducts such as thymine dimers, strongly implicating UV-induced DNA damage as a primary etiology. Similarly, photocarcinogenesis has been determined in animal models to be caused most efficiently by UVB wavelengths, in accord with the major recognized role for UV-induced mutations in DNA, the consequence of incorrectly repaired DNA photoproducts. Indeed, more than 90% of human squamous cell carcinomas contain mutations in the p53 tumor suppressor protein and transcription factor, with many of these qualifying as UVB "signature mutations," characteristic base substitutions in the DNA strand that can result only from incorrect repair of UV-induced pyrimidine dimers. Further support for UVB's major role in photocarcinogenesis derives from the human disease xeroderma pigmentosum (XP), in which inherited mutations in one of several loci required for repair of DNA photoproducts results in a greater than thousandfold increase in skin cancer incidence, with many patients succumbing to metastatic squamous cell carcinoma or melanoma in the first decades of life. Note, however, that pure UVA irradiation is also capable of causing skin cancers in experimental animals, and a contribution of lifelong UVA irradiation to human photocarcinogenesis cannot be excluded. Whether the UVA contribution to photocarcinogenesis is proportionate to the UVA contribution to sunburn and suntanning is a subject of current debate.

The action spectrum for human photoaging is least well studied and remains controversial. Indeed, it is possible and perhaps likely that different components of the photoaged phenotype (e.g., dyspigmentation versus wrinkling versus elastosis) have different action spectra. For example, the epidermal changes of "dryness" or surface roughness and irregular pigmentation that often characterize photoaged skin appear at a very early age in patients with XP and are indeed the features for which the condition was named, strongly suggesting a relationship to UVB-induced DNA damage. In contrast, patients with XP do not have prominent wrinkling or elastosis, changes presumed to result from UV damage to dermal targets. In considering the likely action spectrum for dermal photoaging, much is made of the fact that UVA is far more abundant in terrestrial sunlight than UVB (on average, tenfold more) and penetrates on average more deeply into the dermis. However, it remains unclear whether it is the occasional UVB photon or the more numerous UVA photons reaching the dermis that account for the cumulative and long-lasting effects on collagen, elastin, and the vasculature. Studies in the hairless mouse model of photoaging have established that UVB is quite capable of producing elastosis and wrinkling, but data vary regarding the relative efficacy of UVA wavelengths. One carefully performed study suggests that the action spectrum for elastosis closely parallels that for erythema and tanning, while other publications suggest that UVA wavelengths are nearly as effective as UVB photons in altering the dermis. Studies in human subjects have determined that repeated suberythemal exposures to pure UVA causes lysozyme deposition on dermal elastin fibers, interpreted by the authors as predictive of long-term photodamage (elastosis), although this interpretation remains speculative. It must be noted that the alteration of dermal collagen and elastin that is so characteristic of photodamaged dermis may not reflect direct effects of UV on the extracellular matrix, known to turn over slowly in adult skin, but may instead be due to permanent DNA-based changes in the fibroblasts responsible for matrix production.

Molecular Mechanisms

The precise molecular mechanisms of photoaging are unknown. However, recent studies have provided new insights into likely molecular mechanisms of intrinsic cellular aging that by definition contribute to the photoaging process.

Progressive changes in individual cells within tissues and organs presumably lead ultimately to aging of the organism. Three interactive components of this process have been studied at the molecular level: proliferative senescence (the Hayflick phenomenon), dysfunctional differentiation, and isolation from environmental stimuli.

Hayflick first demonstrated that the lifespan of cells in vitro is inversely related to the chronologic age of the donor and that normal human cells have a finite lifespan or ability to divide, after which they remain viable but can no longer undergo mitosis, a state termed senescence. For newborn human fibroblasts, the number of serial divisions prior to senescence is approximately 60, while fibroblasts from adult donors divide approximately 20 times prior to senescence. In general, cells from short-lived organisms senesce after fewer doublings than do cells derived from organisms with longer lifespans, and cells derived from individuals with premature aging syndromes generally undergo senescence far sooner than cells from normal age-matched controls. Together these observations suggest that the lifespan of the individual and senescence of its cultured cells are under similar genetic control.

Several studies suggest the "biologic clock" that determines replicative senescence and aging is telomere length. Telomeres are the terminal portion of eukaryotic chromosomes and in mammals consist of tandem repeats up to several kilobases in length of the sequence TTAGGG. During proliferation, DNA polymerase cannot replicate the final base pairs at the chromosome end, resulting in progressive shortening with each round of cell division. A reverse transcriptase, telomerase, can replicate the chromosomal ends, but with very few exceptions is expressed only in germline and malignant cells. Telomere length is known to decrease with advancing donor age both in cultured cells and in cells harvested directly from tissue. Adequate telomere length is believed critical to DNA stability, and sufficient telomere shortening triggers cell growth arrest or apoptosis (programmed cell death), depending on the cell type. Transfecting telomerase into cultured human cells greatly extends their culture lifespan, although in some cell types additional manipulation is needed for immortalization.

Proliferative senescence of entire populations of dividing cells presumably does not occur during the lifetime of the organism, although loss of melanocytes from the hair bulb, leading to graying, may be such an example. It is postulated, however, that with increasing age tissues contain a growing portion of senescent cells. Such cells would no longer be able to respond to proliferative signals, for example during wound healing, and would continue to accumulate damage, impairing their differentiated function. Evidence for the accumulation of cells in skin with a dysfunctional differentiated phenotype includes the increased expression of collagenase in fibroblasts from old donor dermis, presumably contributing to loss of collagen and dermal thinning with age. Keratinocytes also overexpress a variety of differentiation-associated genes in old donor versus young donor cultures, although the functional consequence for older skin is largely unknown.

Another well-documented feature of cells from old adult donors is their decreased responsiveness to physiologic stimuli in the cell environment. Impaired mitogen responsiveness is best documented, and old donor cells routinely proliferate far less extensively than do newborn or young adult cells. In the well-studied example of responsiveness to epidermal growth factor (EGF), with increasing donor age there are fewer receptors per cell, decreased EGF binding affinity for these receptors, and decreased activation of post-receptor-signal transduction pathways even in the presence of saturating EGF concentrations. This is consistent with the finding in lymphocytes that mitogen responsiveness is impaired in old cells even if the receptor/ligand interaction can be bypassed by directly stimulating the postreceptor signaling molecules. Overall, the consequence in tissues is less cellular response to critical environmental signals intended to modify growth or differentiated function.

All these factors impact photoaged skin as well as intrinsically aged skin. Skin that is habitually sun exposed, however, also manifests the effects of UV-induced damage. DNA, both nuclear and mitochondrial, appears to be the major target. Mutations in genomic DNA presumably compromise a variety of protein functions, of which the best studied is cell growth regulation, and damage to mitochondrial DNA impairs cellular respiration and presumably therefore a wide variety of metabolic functions.

Photoaging is a common problem in older fair skinned individuals, responsible for the majority of unwanted age-associated changes in skin appearance. The central role of UV damage is unquestioned, although the specific wavelengths responsible for the roughness, dyspigmentation, wrinkling, and coarseness of photoaged skin have not been determined. Present evidence suggests a major role for UVB, largely through DNA damage, but a substantial contribution from UVA wavelengths cannot be excluded. These uncertainties dictate that general sun avoidance and broad spectrum sunscreens are prudent preventive measures. Molecular mechanisms responsible for photoaging are those of intrinsic aging, with the superposition of UV-induced cell damage. Proliferative senescence alternating with inappropriate unregulated cell division, dysfunctional differentiation, and inability to respond appropriately to environmental signals are all contributing factors.

CLINICAL STUDIES

Epidemiology of Skin Cancer

Population studies have confirmed that prolonged sun exposure over a span of years can lead to a prematurely aged appearance. The degree of clinically apparent photodamage is related to skin type, with increased susceptibility in fair-skinned people. Undesired features include fine and coarse wrinkles, skin laxity, textural irregularity, mottled pigmentation, lentigines, telangiectases, and diffuse erythema[4] (see Box 4-1). While some of these manifestations are related to intrinsic aging and would accrue regardless of the extent of photoinjury, they are at the least significantly exacerbated by sunlight.

Squamous Cell Carcinoma. Incidence of skin cancers also appears to be related to photodamage (Table 4-1). The relationship is clearest for squamous cell carcinomas.[5] Both recent and lifetime sun exposure have been shown to be risk factors for squamous cell carci-

Table 4-1 Association of Common Skin Cancers with Solar Radiation

Cancer Type	Associated Solar Radiation Pattern
Squamous cell carcinoma	Recent and lifetime sun exposure. Cumulative ultraviolet exposure is a risk factor, with highest risk on anatomic sites receiving heavy sun. Same pattern of solar radiation is associated with the incidence of actinic keratoses, which can also develop into squamous cell carcinomas.
Basal cell carcinoma	Relatively small amounts of sun at an early age. Lesions frequently occur on sites of only moderate cumulative sun exposure.
Melanoma	Childhood sun exposure and recreational (intermittent) exposure. As with basal cell carcinoma, the timing of exposure appears more important than the cumulative dose. Lentigo maligna type frequently does occur on anatomic sites of maximal cumulative sun exposure.

noma in humans.[6,7] Actinic keratoses, which may develop into invasive squamous cell carcinomas, as well as squamous cell carcinomas themselves are reduced by the use of sunscreen.[8-10] An Australian study that entailed application of SPF 17 sunscreen or vehicle to experimental and control subjects, respectively, confirmed the protective effect of the active substance.[9] After one summer, patients in the sunscreen group had on average 0.6 fewer actinic keratoses than when they had begun, and patients in the control group, 1 additional such lesion. Squamous cell carcinoma of the lip is, similarly, less common in women who use lip protection than women who do not, or in men.[11]

Given that squamous cell carcinoma is most frequently seen on sites of heavy sun exposure, it is interesting and disturbing that the world incidence appears to be rising in recent decades. Population-based studies have corroborated anecdotal reports. The Rochester Epidemiology Project, a registry that captures virtually all the inhabitants of Olmsted County, Minnesota, noted a marked rise in the rate of new squamous cell carcinomas between 1984 and 1986 (incidence: 46.5/100,000, female; 71.2/100,000, male) and 1990 to 1992 (incidence: 125.9/100,000, female; 155.5/100,000, male).[12] The magnitude of the difference was significantly greater than could be explained by demographic shifts or other incidental factors.

Basal Cell Carcinoma. Basal cell carcinoma, the other primary nonmelanoma skin cancer, accounts for most of the estimated 1.2 million annual cases of nonmelanoma skin cancer in the United States.[13] While most of the 2100 annual deaths from nonmelanoma skin cancer are attributable to squamous cell carcinoma,[13] basal cell carcinomas generate a relatively greater proportion of patient inconvenience and medical visits. Surprisingly, there is relatively little evidence to support the efficacy of sunscreen in the prevention of basal cell carcinoma.[5] Unlike squamous cell carcinoma, basal cell carcinomas often arise on areas, such as the upper trunk in men and women and the lower leg in women, receiving only moderate sun exposure.[14] Retrospective data indicate that basal cell carcinoma genesis may be linked to relatively small amounts of ultraviolet light exposure at an early age.[6,7]

Melanoma. Melanoma may be partly caused by sun exposure but the relationship is complex. As in the case of basal cell carcinoma, and in contrast to squamous cell carcinoma, the timing of solar exposure may be more important than the cumulative dose.[5] The exception is lentigo maligna melanoma, a type that typically evolves on areas of maximum sun exposure.[5]

In general, the action spectrum for melanoma is not known.[15] Risk does increase with significant childhood exposure to sunlight,[5] and a history of sunburns during childhood is positively correlated with the likelihood of eventual melanoma.[16-19] In a study conducted within the Nurse's Health Study, blistering sunburns at ages 15 to 20, but not after age 30, were associated with a significantly increased risk (relative risk of 2.2 for greater than five sunburns).[20] Migration studies have also verified that long periods of sun exposure in childhood are correlated with heightened melanoma risk in adulthood.[21] Outdoor activity and sun during the early years of life is also associated with development of greater numbers of melanocytic nevi, a known risk factor for melanoma.[22-24] The elements involved in the promotion of melanoma rates via childhood exposure are not well understood. There may be an age-specific constitutional sensitivity to sunlight, or perhaps exposure is more pervasive because there is more leisure time and less clothing worn.[14] Nonetheless, exposure during childhood to light sufficient to induce burns is a consistent finding in case-control studies of melanoma.[25]

Likelihood of melanoma is actually decreased in persons with occupational exposure to ultraviolet light as adults.[26,27] Recreational exposure to sun, conversely, adds to the baseline risk of melanoma.[5,15,28] Since vacationers and outdoor enthusiasts are only intermittently exposed to sunlight whereas outdoor workers undergo more constant exposure, intermittent exposure may be the relevant risk factor. On the other hand, history of actinic keratoses and nonmelanoma skin cancer, which are more obviously related to cumulative sun exposure, is a risk factor for melanoma.[29] So, at least indirectly, and maybe to a lesser extent, the total amount of sun exposure also appears to influence the likelihood of melanoma.[30]

Limited evidence exists that sunscreen use prevents melanoma.[5] Intuitively obvious, the proof of a beneficial effect is difficult to establish due to methodological constraints.[31-34] Study participants have difficulty precisely recalling details, such as degree of sun exposure and number of burns, from the distant past. Moreover, since the widespread use of sunscreens, people may be staying out in the sun for longer periods and consequently accumulating greater ultraviolet light exposure because they are not deterred by sunburns. In view of these and other confounders, it is understandable that studies of sunscreen use have indicated increased risk of melanoma,[35-39] decreased risk,[19,40] or no change in risk.[34,41] Reliable meta-analyses of the available studies are precluded by irreconcilable differences in methodology.[42]

Interestingly, worldwide incidence of melanoma has been rising for decades, and this trend precedes the ubiquity of sunscreen.[43] It has been postulated that the cause may be increased sun-related leisure activities made possible by growing affluence in industrialized nations. Certainly, the increase in incidence of melanoma is both indisputable and alarming. Annual incidence rates among fair-skinned populations have increased 3% to 7% per year during the last three decades.[14] An examination of population-based incidence rates for the period 1973 to 1994 using the US Surveillance, Epidemiology, and End Results tumor registries indicated an annual increase in incidence of 3.6 %.[44] Rates rose for melanomas less than 1 mm in thickness, 1 to 3 mm, and greater than 3 mm, as well as for 2-year mortality from melanoma.[44,45] Absolute annual mortality rates range from 1 to 3/100,000 for fair-skinned people in the northern hemisphere to 5 to 10/100,000 in Australia and New Zealand.[46-48] In the United States, the American Cancer Society[49] estimates that there will be 51,400 new cases of melanoma in 2001, with melanoma (excluding basal and squamous cell carcinoma) being the sixth most common cancer in men (5% of all new cancer cases) and seventh most common cancer in women (4% of new cancer cases). Five thousand American men and 2800 American women will die of melanoma in 2001, and the lifetime risks for melanoma are 1 in 60 and 1 in 80, respectively, for men and women.

Skeptics have wondered to what extent the growing frequency of melanoma is medically significant.[43] More frequent registration of newly found lesions, vigilant monitoring of melanocytic lesions by patients and physicians, and submission of numerous nevi for pathologic diagnosis may contribute to the apparent increased incidence. Early and aggressive detection may also result in increasing diagnosis of a low-risk, nonmetastasizing form of melanoma. Overall, however, the magnitude of the increase suggests that at least part of the growing number of melanomas are clinically important. And rates of melanoma remain higher in those who burn only and never tan,[50] thus providing credence to the view that sun exposure is likely a major causative factor.

Environmental Influences

In addition to recreational and leisure sun exposure, environmental changes may be contributing to higher rates of photodamage. Impairment of the ozone layer, a natural shield in the stratosphere that absorbs much of the biologically damaging ultraviolet radiation emanating from the sun, may be resulting in more potentially harmful light reaching the earth's surface.[51] When present in adequate quantities, ozone blocks all incident UVC, 90% of UVB, especially wavelengths from 290 to 300 nm, and a small amount of UVA.[4,52] Unfortunately, in the early 1980s, scientists amassed evidence that chlorofluorocarbons (CFCs) and other synthetic agents were depleting the ozone layer.[51] Especially in Antarctica, the destruction of ozone is exceeding its natural replenishment. It has been shown that heavily populated areas are now absorbing more ultraviolet radiation than two decades ago.[53]

Several measures have been devised to quantify the extent and significance of the ultraviolet light hitting the planet. The radiation amplification factor (RAF) is the percentage increase in biologically active ultraviolet light seen by individuals that results from a 1% decrease in the ozone layer at a particular location.[54] Values vary, with the RAF of 0.7 to 1.2 for the erythema action spectrum; 1.1 to 1.6 for the skin cancer action spectrum; and 1.5 to 2.3 for the DNA damage action spectrum. While these numbers are highly speculative estimates, the observed ozone layer decrease of 4.8% to 7.4% over the United States during the period 1979 to 1992 clearly indicates a substantially increased risk of photo-induced skin aging and skin cancer. A similar statistic is the amplification factor (AF), the percentage rise in nonmelanoma skin cancer attributable to a 1% decrease in ozone.[55] Estimated AF values of 1.7 for basal cell carcinoma and 3.0 for squamous cell carcinoma, respectively, point to a substantial growth in incidence of these lesions if there is a sustained decrease in the thickness of the ozone layer.

Variables other than the ozone layer can affect the amount of sunlight impinging on the earth.[51] Ultraviolet light intensity is maximal at high altitudes, where there is less atmosphere to absorb incoming radiation. Equatorial latitudes are high radiation areas as well, since the sun there is directly overhead. A contributing effect is the relative attenuation of the ozone layer at the equator. Seasonal influences can similarly result in differential sun exposure, with ultraviolet intensity in the northern hemisphere greatest in the summer months, when the incident angle of sunlight is approximately 90 degrees. Thin cloud cover typically blocks 20% to 40% of sun-related ultraviolet radiation, and window glass, virtually 100% of UVB but only 50% of UVA.[4,56] Sand, snow, concrete, and water can reflect up to 85% of sunlight, thus nearly doubling the ambient ultraviolet exposure. Beachgoers ostensibly protected by an umbrella may therefore be subject to the equivalent of direct sunlight due to the proximity of numerous reflective surfaces. About 50% of ultraviolet radiation can reach skin submerged in shallow water.[4]

Sunscreens

Mitigation of sun-induced photoaging is possible with the appropriate use of sunscreens. During the past several decades, these substances have become easily available and moderately priced. Use of sunscreen, however, continues to lag behind the public's perception of its importance. In a survey of beachgoers, 70% indicated that they were there to get or maintain a tan, and during the average stay of 4 hours, only half applied sunscreen.[57] In the United States, as few as 25% of sunbathers routinely used a sunscreen product with sun protection factor (SPF) of 15 or greater.[58] The National Canadian Survey of Sun Exposure and Protective Behaviors revealed that 62% of respondents did not wear sunscreen on the face, and 68% did not use sunscreen on the rest of their bodies.[59] Young adolescents,[60] male college students,[61] and skiers with past experience of sunburns[62] have been shown to utilize sunscreen at low rates. Childhood exposure continues to be significant, but although past burn history is a determinant of future sunscreen application,[60] as few as one third of parents adequately protect their children.[63] Sunscreen use is most prevalent in Australia, where three quarters of adults visiting a family physician reported frequent sun protection behaviors.[64]

Definition and Rationale for Use. Sunscreens are topical preparations designed to reduce actinic damage.[32] Initially, these substances were created to prevent sunburn. Active ingredients within sunscreens diminish the amount of ultraviolet radiation penetrating the skin (Table 4-2). Most commercially distributed products contain a number of active compounds that collectively impart broad spectrum protection. Animal evidence indicates that sunscreens, especially those with high SPF, can reduce the visible and microscopic stigmata of photoaging.[5] Sunlight-induced skin sagging has been demonstrably reduced in experimental animals after sunscreen application. Reduction of risk of certain skin cancers (see previous section) may also accrue from regular use of sunscreens. Since UVA penetrates more deeply than UVB, a significant proportion of chronic photodamage may be secondary to UVA effects,[65] and optimal sunscreens therefore must be able to efficiently block both UVB and UVA.

A grading system has been devised to measure sunscreen-derived protection against erythema, primarily UVB induced (given that UVB is 1000 times as erythemogenic as UVA).[32] SPF is a ratio of the amount of ultraviolet radiation required to generate a minimal erythema response, 24 hours after exposure, in a sunscreen-protected area of the skin to the amount required to induce the same degree of erythema in unprotected skin. Government agencies responsible for sunscreen regulation include the US Food and Drug Administration, the Standards Association of Australia, and Comite de Liaison des Associations Europeenes de l'Industrie de la Parfumerie, des Produits Cosmetiques et de Toilette (COLIPA). SPF values computed from outdoor testing tend to be lower than those obtained from indoor use of a solar simulator. Importantly, measurement of sunscreen's exclusion of UVA is less standardized than that of UVB, and there is concern that biologically significant amounts of UVA are able to pierce even so-called broad-spectrum preparations. UVA blockers such as Parsol 1789 are less common in US sunscreens due to the labyrinthine FDA approval process, which has recently been streamlined.[5]

Historically, sunscreens were classified as *physical* or *chemical* types.[32] In view of the active chemical properties of the sunblocks previously referred to as physical (e.g., titanium dioxide, zinc oxide), the preferred terms are now *inorganic* and *organic* compounds.[32] The former are particulate in sunscreen preparations due to their low solubility, and the latter are soluble. Organic compounds in sunscreens may be primarily useful against UVA or UVB. The major classes of these organics currently available are PABA and its esters (UVB; e.g., octyl dimethyl PABA), salicylates (UVB; e.g., octyl salicylate), cinnamates (UVB; e.g., 2-ethylhexyl p-methoxycinnamate; UVB/UVA; e.g., octocrylene), anthranilates (UVA; e.g., methyl anthranilate), benzophenones (UVA; e.g., oxybenzone), dibenzoylmethanes (UVA; e.g., avobenzone, or Parsol 1789), and benzylidene camphors (UVA; e.g., terephthalylidene dicamphor sulfonic acid, or Mexoryl SX). Users of sunscreen should be aware that the polarity and pH of a particular combination of sol-

Table 4-2 Active Ingredients of Sunscreens

Organic Sunscreens		
Class	Examples	Inorganic Sunscreens
PABA and its esters	Octyl dimethyl PABA (UVB)	Zinc oxide
Salicylates	Octyl salicylate (UVB)	Titanium dioxide
Cinnamates	2-ethylhexyl p-methoxycinnamate (UVB) Octocrylene (2-ethylhexyl-2-cyano-3,3-diphenyl-acrylate) (UVB/UVA)	
Anthranlinates	Methyl anthranilate (UVA)	
Benzophenones	Oxybenzone (UVA)	
Dibenzoylmethanes	Avobenzone (butyl methoxydibenzoylmethane [Parsol 1789]) (UVA)	
Benzylidene camphors	Terephthalylidene dicamphor sulfonic acid (Mexoryl SX) (UVA)	

vents and active compounds can influence the absorption maxima of a given sunscreen[66]; in other words, not all sunscreens with similar compositions are equally protective. The ability of a sunscreen product to maintain its effectiveness, especially when exposed to water, is a desirable feature.

Method of Application. To benefit from sunscreens to the extent of their SPF labeling, users must apply them in a prescribed manner.[5] In the United States, SPF values are determined on the basis of testing at 2 mg/cm^2, and in Europe the hypothetical delivery is defined as 1.5 mg/cm^2. If less than these amounts is used, the corresponding sun protection will be diminished.[67,68] Survey data suggests that actual usage of sunscreen is far below recommended amounts, with layering usually in the range 0.5 to 1 mg/cm^2.[69] This concentration effectively reduces an SPF 15 sunscreen to one providing SPF protection of 3 to 7. Inorganic sunscreens are similarly vulnerable to underuse, and if an SPF 25 titanium dioxide sunscreen that should be applied as 2 mg/cm^2 is used at only 1.3 mg/cm^2, the resulting SPF may be below 10.[70,71] While the evidence indicates that few people use sunscreen correctly, regulatory authorities have not required manufacturers to correct displayed SPF values to reflect this reality. Public health messages impressing the need for adequate thickness layering of sunscreen also remain rare. Producers of sunscreen have been more successful in formulating cosmetically acceptable sunscreen preparations, which consumers are more likely to wear.[32]

Beyond application of sufficient amounts, it is unclear how sunscreen use may influence efficacy. The recommendation that frequent application provides better protection does not appear to be borne out by the evidence.[5] In a study of children subject to 6 hours of sun exposure equivalent to 13 times their minimum erythema doses, one body side received one application of sunscreen and the other side received four applications, but both schedules of sunscreen application were equally protective.[10] The exhortation, often included in public service announcements, that sunscreen should be applied 30 to 60 minutes prior to exposure is also unsupported.[5] Sunscreen appears to work immediately upon application. Despite the absence of convincing evidence, it appears intuitive that some activities may limit the protection afforded by sunscreens. After swimming, or heavy exertion with sweating, reapplication may be warranted.[32]

Use in Vulnerable Populations. Sunscreen use in special populations has been investigated. Among the elderly, few are likely to develop skin cancers or visible photodamage from current sun exposure, yet sunscreen may be useful to prevent acute burns.[5] The active elderly, who engage in outdoor sports and have a significant life expectancy, may benefit from more deliberate sunscreen use comparable to that in younger adults. Older patients treated for actinic keratoses or nonmelanoma skin cancers can become exceedingly anxious about future sun exposure. Such patients should be reassured that major lifestyle changes are not required for health maintenance.

It has been recommended that sunscreen should not be applied to children younger than 6 months.[32] The theoretical concern is that infants may be unable to metabolize the chemicals within these preparations.[72] No confirmatory evidence exists, but in any event, sunscreen may not be necessary to ensure adequate sun protection in the very young. Until babies are able to move independently, they may be best sheltered from the sun by strict sun avoidance and clothing. The Australian Cancer Society, in concert with the Australasian College of Dermatologists, has recommended that sunscreen be used on babies when physical protection, such as apparel, is inadequate.[73] In its policy statement regarding ultraviolet light–related hazards to children, the American Academy of Pediatrics[74] suggests that physicians share with parents the inconclusive information regarding sunscreen use in the very young. The Academy concludes by noting that, even in infants, it may be reasonable to apply sunscreen to small, otherwise poorly protected areas, such as the face and the back of the hands.

Microbiologic and Histologic Benefits. Suberythemal doses of UVB can induce immunosuppression, and sunlight has been observed to suppress resistance to infection.[75] In a study in Italy, 100 minutes of solar exposure at midday resulted in clinically notable reduction in resistance to infection with *Listeria monocytogenes*.[76] Use of sunscreens may decrease ultraviolet light–induced immunosuppression.[77-80] In general, sunscreens reduce but do not eliminate immunosuppression, and the precise extent of protection is not known.[81] Occurrence of ultraviolet-induced herpes labialis has been shown to be prevented by judicious use of lip balm containing sunscreen.[82]

Sunscreens also reduce histologic signs of photodamage. Skin biopsies have verified that regular application of an SPF 30 sunscreen over a period of 24 months results in a significant decrease in solar elastosis compared with control sites.[83] Combined UVA- and UVB-blocking preparations are believed to be most effective in minimizing histologic photoeffects.

Safety. Habitual use of sunscreens appears to be safe. Repeated applications by millions in the United States alone has not resulted in reports of serious ill effects. Photoallergic contact dermatitis has been seen with sunscreen use, but allergy to the active ingredients is rare.[5,32] Irritant reactions are far more likely than allergy.[84] Copious application of sunscreen to the forehead is potentially troublesome, as it can migrate downward and stimulate irritation, redness, and tearing of the eyes. Rubbing the eyes with fingers covered in sunscreen can cause a similar reaction.[5]

Concern that UVB-absorbing sunscreens may interfere with vitamin D synthesis in human skin appears to be unfounded. SPF 17 sunscreen, applied continuously during one summer, did not markedly alter vitamin D levels in subjects over age 40.[85] A double-blind, randomized, placebo-controlled trial that lasted 7 months also did not detect any decrease in mean levels of vitamin D and its precursors in the sunscreen group.[85] Even intensive sun protection practiced by xeroderma pigmentosum patients over a 6-year period was not associated with abnormal vitamin D levels.[86] Long-term treatment of patients with PABA resulted in slightly lower vitamin levels, which were still within the range of normal.[87]

The photochemistry of sunscreens has been partially elucidated. Simply, the protective process entails the absorption of ultraviolet radiation by sunscreen molecules that must then reenter a ground state by dissipating this energy.[32] Stored energy is likely dissipated via fluorescence, phosphorescence, self-quenching, and heat generation.[88] It has been speculated by some that the associated photochemical reactions may create reactive oxygen species and other photoproducts that may subsequently react with cellular proteins, RNA, or DNA. While this has never been shown to occur in a medically significant manner, additional research may help confirm the long-term safety of sunscreens.[88,89]

Other Photoprotective Strategies

Clothing and Apparel. Occasionally, patients in whom sunscreen use is indicated may be reluctant users. Sunscreens may be avoided because they are perceived as unattractive, uncomfortable, messy, or expensive.[90] Alternatively, for some extremely fair-skinned individuals, even diligent sunscreen use may not provide sufficient protection. Both these groups may benefit from wearing clothing that filters sunlight effectively. Transmission of ultraviolet radiation through fabric is quantitated by the ultraviolet protection factor (UPF), which can be determined experimentally for any piece of cloth.[91] Weave, weight, color, and stretch contribute to the UPF.[92,93] Materials with higher UPF are to be preferred for sun protection, and standards have already been established in Australia. According to one study, white-colored cotton, acetate, and rayon samples typically have SPF ratings of less than 15, with polyester fabrics being more protective.[90] SPF rises with mass and weight, yet the relationship is not linear. Closely knit fabrics are associated with higher SPF, and while weight is desirable, even lightweight fabrics that are densely woven can be highly effective at excluding ultraviolet light.[94] Dyeing fabrics tends to greatly enhance their sun-blocking properties.[90] Moisture can diminish the SPF of clothing. For instance, the average T-shirt has an SPF of 15 when dry, but merely SPF 5 when wet.[95] Maximally protective clothing has been measured to have SPFs as high as 36.

In addition to clothing, other devices may be used to reduce sun exposure, particularly to the upper body. A hat with a 10-cm brim can reduce head and neck ultraviolet exposure by as much as 70%, equivalent to an SPF of 3 to 4.[94] Hats and caps with partial or less wide brims are less effective at sun protection and may provide adequate coverage for only part of the face.[96] Eye protection has recently been recognized as a vital component of a complete sun protection regimen. Melanoma of the uveal tract, the most common primary intraocular neoplasm in adults, is associated with a tendency to sunburn and with intense exposure to ultraviolet radiation.[97] The American Academy of Ophthalmology has averred that excess exposure of the eyes to ultraviolet radiation can cause painful burns of the cornea and that long-term exposure to ultraviolet radiation may increase the incidence of cataracts, pterygium, and possibly macular degeneration.[98] Optimally protective sunglasses would block 99% to 100% of UVA and UVB. Filtering of blue light may be helpful provided that colors are not distorted. Sunglasses also effectively protect the eyelids, with larger, curved glasses extending this coverage to the lateral periocular area. Since no uniform labeling system currently exists for the protective efficacy of sunglasses, patients should read package descriptions carefully before purchase. Although well-designed sunglasses afford excellent ocular and periocular sun protection, some wearers may be misled into believing that they are receiving less sun than they really are.[99]

Behavioral Change. Various other protective behaviors can further reduce photodamage sustained from sunlight and artificial sources of ultraviolet radiation. Avoiding the sun during the midday hours, when incident solar radiation is at its peak, can greatly reduce cumulative exposure.[32] Outdoor workers may find this prohibition impractical. Similarly, parents of schoolchildren may be unable to modify the scheduling of team sports or school functions.

Eschewing use of tanning booths is another highly effective means of minimizing ultraviolet damage. Longer-term effects of tanning booth exposure are not yet manifest, and the exact emission spectra of machines in current use are not well described, but there is already substantial information corroborating the hazards of artificial tanning.[15] Atypical melanocytic proliferations, lentigines, phototoxic and photoallergic reactions, and immunosuppression have been attributed to frequent use of tanning beds.[15] Several studies have, furthermore, documented a significant elevation in melanoma risk among those who tan with ultraviolet lamps.[100-106] The UVA radiation sources employed in electronic tanning devices produce a tan not as protective against subsequent sunburn as a UVB-generated tan,[107,108] and tanning with UVA may be more hazardous than with UVB.[109] Prima facie, the configuration of a tanning bed is antithetical to the principles of photoprotection enumerated above: customers lie horizontally, unclad and without sunscreen, receiving maximal exposure to ultraviolet light that is magnified by surrounding reflective surfaces.

At the urging of professional medical organizations, media outlets have in recent decades begun to broadcast messages encouraging photoprotection. Soundbites that have been loudly propagated include the observation that a tan is a response to injury rather than a healthy change in appearance[32]; that people obtain up to 80% of their lifetime sun exposure before age 18[98]; that skin cancer can be prevented by sun avoidance, and is curable if detected early[16]; and that cosmetically undesirable photoaging can result from unprotected tanning.

Public Policy. Public policy makers have also become more animated in addressing issues related to photodamage. Thus, the American Academy of Dermatology and the Centers for Disease Control and Prevention Consensus Conference have adopted a set of guidelines for appropriate sun protection[110] (Box 4-2). Recommendations include limiting exposure to ultraviolet light, especially between 10 AM and 4 PM; wearing protective clothing and sunglasses; using sunscreen with SPF of at least 15 in combination with SPF lip balms; avoiding artificial tanning devices; and encouraging children to practice the shadow rule, which notes the importance of seeking shade at times when ultraviolet exposure is high, as indicated by one's shadow being shorter than oneself.

Longer-term strategies for human photoprotection may require cooperation among large groups. For example, provision of shady areas requires redesign of public spaces to include permanent shade structures.[32] At present, shade is often difficult to find in schoolyards, where the competing need to construct sports fields results in areas bereft of trees. Shady areas may also be built adjacent to children's wading pools and at beaches. Wide umbrellas can provide personal shade, but their use is often impractical, particularly for active children.[98] In April 1999, the American Academy of Dermatology, with the help of the National Dermatology Awareness Program and KaBOOM!, a nonprofit organization that builds safe playgrounds, constructed the first sun-safe playground in the United States in Staten Island, New York. Sun-safe elements included shade structures for caregivers, trees and landscaping that provided shade, and a shade structure covering the entire playground area.[111]

Slowing and eventually correcting the loss of ozone in the stratosphere is an even greater public policy challenge. Until this is accomplished, it may be necessary to rely on public service announcements to warn people of impending increases in solar radiation. In 1994, the National Weather Service, in cooperation with the US Environmental Protection Agency and the Centers for Disease Control and Prevention, initiated the "UV index" for 58 cities[112] (Table 4-3). This index informs the public of the intensity of ultraviolet light reaching the surface at a particular location and time. Satellite measurements of total ozone are used in the computation of the UV indices. Ratings range from very high (10+: fair-skinned persons may burn in less

BOX 4-2 Guidelines for Appropriate Sun Protection

Behavior

- Limit exposure to ultraviolet radiation, especially between 10 AM and 4 PM.
- Seek shelter in shaded areas if outdoors for a prolonged period.
- Avoid artificial tanning devices.
- Modify daily sun protection measures based on the local UV index reading.
- Conduct self-examinations for melanoma based on the ABCD rule.

Apparel

- Wear protective clothing that is colored, closely knit, and dry.
- Use hats with 10-cm brims.
- Cover the eyes with wrap-around sunglasses that completely block ultraviolet light.

Sunscreen

- Apply sunscreen with SPF of at least 15 to all exposed body surfaces every day.
- Substitute more protective sunscreen when in bright light or during long exposures.
- Include the daily application of lip balm with SPF protection.
- Select broad-spectrum sunscreen products including UVB and UVA blocking agents.

Children

- Protect infants from sun exposure, and use protective garments when outdoors.
- If necessary for adequate protection, apply sunscreen to infants younger than 6 months.
- Encourage children to follow the "shadow rule."
- Provide children with sun-safe play areas.
- Model appropriate behaviors for children to imitate.

Table 4-3 UV Index Exposure Categories

Numerical Index	Word Index	Recommendations
10+	Very high	Very high risk of harm from unprotected sun exposure. Fair-skinned persons may burn in less than 5 minutes. Outdoor workers and vacationers at especially high risk.
7-9	High	High risk of harm from unprotected sun exposure. Fair-skinned persons may burn in less than 10 minutes.
5-6	Moderate	Moderate risk of harm from unprotected sun exposure. Fair-skinned persons may burn in less than 15 minutes.
3-4	Low	Low risk of harm from unprotected sun exposure. Fair-skinned persons may burn in less than 20 minutes.
0-2	Minimal	Minimal danger from the sun's ultraviolet radiation for the average person. Most people can stay in the sun for up to 1 hour during the hours of peak sun strength, 10 AM to 4 PM, without burning. People with very sensitive skin and infants should always be protected from prolonged sun exposure.

than 5 minutes), to high (7 to 9: burn in 10 minutes), moderate (5 to 6: burn in 15 minutes), low (3 to 4: burn in 20 minutes), and very low (0 to 2: burn in greater than 1 hour). Because indices are location specific, they may be different for nearby locations. Similarly, ultraviolet light reflected from water or snow may raise ultraviolet exposure above predicted levels.

More effective patient education may result in reduced rates of photodamage in the future. It has been suggested that inculcation regarding the harmful effects of sunlight should begin as early as age 3.[16] Messages should be tailored to children's ages and levels of sophistication, and authorities agree that parents can contribute by modeling responsible photoprotective behaviors.

DISCUSSION

All persons who are exposed to sufficient sun will develop photoaging. For fair-skinned people, the extent of this damage will be proportionately greater, as will the likelihood of sun-induced skin cancer. Unfortunately, even the most strident public declarations by dermatologists may have limited impact on changing behaviors. While the attractiveness of a "healthy tan" is quickly apparent, the adverse effects are delayed and often perceived as hypothetical. Changes in behavior may thus be more effectively induced by itemizing not the horrors of cancer but rather the deleterious cosmetic effects of premature photoaging. Physical beauty is associated with high self-esteem, social success, and career advancement. If people are convinced that any short-term gains from sun exposure will be vastly outweighed by a protracted period of impaired physical appearance, they may be reluctant to sit outside in the summer.

REFERENCES

1. Gilchrest BA, ed. Photodamage. Cambridge, Mass: Blackwell Science, 1995.
2. Gilchrest BA, Bohr VA, eds. The Role of DNA Damage and Repair in Cell Aging. New York: Elsevier Scientific, 2001:255.
3. Yaar M, Gilchrest BA. Aging of the skin. In: Freedberg IM, Eisen AZ, Wolff K, et al, eds. Fitzpatrick's Dermatology in General Medicine, 5th ed. New York: McGraw-Hill, 1999:1697-1706.
4. Kaminer MS. Photodamage: magnitude of the problem. In: Gilchrest BA, ed. Photodamage. Cambridge, Mass: Blackwell Science, 1995.
5. McLean DI, Gallagher R. Sunscreens: use and misuse. Dermatol Clin 1998; 16:219-226.
6. Gallagher RP, Hill GB, Badjik CD. Sunlight exposure, pigmentary factors, and risks of nonmelanoma skin cancer, part I: basal cell carcinoma. Arch Dermatol 1995; 131:164-169.
7. Rosso S, Zanetti R, Martinez C. The multicentre south European study "Hellos," part II: different sun exposure patterns in the etiology of basal cell and squamous cell carcinomas of the skin. Br J Cancer 1996; 73:1447-1454.
8. Naylor MF, Boyd A, Smith DW. High sun protection factor sunscreens in the suppression of actinic neoplasia. Arch Dermatol 1995; 131:170-175.
9. Thompson SC, Jolley D, Marks R. Reduction of solar keratoses by regular sunscreen use. N Engl J Med 1993; 329:1147-1151.
10. Miyagi T, Bhutto AM, Nonaka S. The effects of sunscreens in UVB erythema and Langerhans' cell depression. J Dermatol 1994; 21:645-651.
11. Pogoda JM, Preston MS. Solar radiation, lip protection, and lip cancer risk in Los Angeles County women. Cancer Causes Control 1996; 7:458-463.
12. Gray DT, Suman VJ, Su WPD, Clay RP. Trends in the population-based incidence of squamous cell carcinoma of the skin first diagnosed between 1984 and 1992. Arch Dermatol 1997; 133:735-740.
13. Chuang T-Y, Reizner GT, Elpem DJ, et al. Squamous cell carcinoma in Kauai, Hawaii. Int J Dermatol 1995; 34:393-397.
14. Marks R. Epidemiology of melanoma. Clin Exp Dermatol 2000; 25:459-463.
15. Weinstock MA, Lim HW, DeLeo V, et al. Tanning, tanning booths, and melanoma: risky or protective? J Am Acad Dermatol 1999; 41:84-87.

16. Lim HW, Bergfeld W. Prevention strategies. J Am Acad Dermatol 1999; 41:95-96.
17. Zanetti R, Franceschi S, Rosso S, et al. Cutaneous melanoma and sunburns in childhood in a southern European population. Eur J Cancer 1992; 28A:1172-1176.
18. Cress RD, Holly EA, Ahn DK. Cutaneous melanoma in women, part V: characteristics of those who tan and those who burn when exposed to summer sun. Epidemiology 1995; 6:538-543.
19. Holly EA, Aston DA, Cross RD, et al. Cutaneous melanoma in women, part I: exposure to sunlight, ability to tan, and other risk factors related to ultraviolet light. Am J Epidemiol 1995; 141:923-933.
20. Weinstock MA, Colditz GA, Willett WC. Nonfamilial cutaneous melanoma incidence in women associated with sun exposure before 20 years of age. Pediatrics 1989; 84:199-204.
21. Khlat M, Vail A, Parkin M, Green A. Mortality from melanoma in migrants to Australia: variation by age at arrival and duration of stay. Am J Epidemiol 1992; 135:1103-1113.
22. Harrison SL, MacLennan R, Speare R, Wronski I. Sun exposure and melanocytic nevi in young Australian children. Lancet 1994; 344:1529-1532.
23. Green A, Siskind V, Hansen ME, et al. Melanocytic nevi in schoolchildren in Queensland. J Am Acad Dermatol 1989; 20: 1054-1060.
24. Fritschi L, McHenry P, Green A, et al. Nevi in schoolchildren in Scotland and Australia. Br J Dermatol 1994; 130:599-603.
25. Autier P, Dore JF. Influence of sun exposures during childhood and during adulthood in melanoma risk. Int J Cancer 1998; 77:533-537.
26. Elwood JM, Gallagher RP, Hill GB. Cutaneous melanoma in relation to intermittent and constant sun exposure—the Western Canada Melanoma Study. Int J Cancer 1985; 35:427-433.
27. Gallagher RP, Elwood JM, Yang CP. Is chronic sunlight important in accounting for increases in melanoma incidence? Int J Cancer 1989; 44:813-815.
28. Elwood JM. Melanoma and sun exposure: contrasts between intermittent and constant exposure. World J Surg 1992; 16:157-166.
29. Green AC, O'Rourke MG. Cutaneous malignant melanoma in association with other skin cancers. J Nat Cancer Inst 1985; 74: 977-980.
30. Armstrong BK. Epidemiology of malignant melanoma: intermittent or total accumulated exposure to the sun? J Dermatol Surg Oncol 1988; 14:835-846.
31. Holly EA, Kelly JW, Ahn DK. Risk of cutaneous melanoma by number of melanocytic nevi and correlation of nevi by anatomic site. In: Gallagher RP, Elwood JM, eds. Epidemiological Aspects of Cutaneous Malignant Melanoma. Boston: Kluwer Academic Publishers, 1994:159-172.
32. Rosen CF. Photoprotection. Semin Cutan Med Surg 1999; 18: 307-314.
33. Rosen CF. Unanswered questions on the use of sunscreens. J Am Acad Dermatol 1999; 41:87-93.
34. Osterlind A, Tucker MA, Stone BJ. The Danish case-control study of cutaneous malignant melanoma, part II: importance of UV-light exposure. Int J Cancer 1988; 42:319-324.
35. Westerdahl J, Olsson H, Masback A. Is the use of sunscreens a risk factor for malignant melanoma? Melanoma Res 1995; 5: 59-65.
36. Beitner H, Norell SE, Ringborg U. Malignant melanoma: Aetiological importance of individual pigmentation and sun exposure. Br J Dermatol 1990; 122:43-51.
37. Klepp O, Magnus K. Some environmental and bodily characteristics of melanoma patients: a case-control study. Int J Cancer 1979; 23:482-486.
38. Autier P, Dore J-F, Schifflers E. Melanoma and use of sunscreens: an EORTC case-control study in Germany, Belgium and France. Int J Cancer 1995; 61:749-755.
39. Graham S, Marshall J, Haughey B. An inquiry into the epidemiology of melanoma. Am J Epidemiol 1985; 122:606-619.
40. Rodenas JM, Delgado-Rodriguez M, Herranz M. Sun exposure, pigmentary traits, and risk of cutaneous malignant melanoma: a case-control study in a Mediterranean population: an analysis separating histogenetic types. J Natl Cancer Inst 1984; 73:75.
41. Holman CDJ, Armstrong BK. Cutaneous malignant melanoma and indicators of total accumulated exposure to the sun: an analysis separating histogenetic types. J Natl Cancer Inst 1984; 73:75.
42. Wille L, Gefeller O, Kolmel KF. Sunscreens in melanoma protection—pros and cons. In: Altmeyer P, Hoffman K, Stucker M, eds. Skin Cancer and UV Radiation. Berlin: Springer-Verlag, 1997:343-356.
43. Rivers JK. Increased incidence of melanoma: real or epiphenomenon. J Am Acad Dermatol 1999; 41:93-95.
44. Dennis LK. Analysis of the melanoma epidemic, both apparent and real: data from the 1973 through 1994 Surveillance, Epidemiology, and End Results Program Registry. Arch Dermatol 1999; 135:275-280.
45. Surveillance, Epidemiology and End Results (SEER) Program Public Use CD-ROM (1973-1994). Bethesda, Md: National Cancer Institute, Division of Cancer Prevention and Control, Surveillance Program, Cancer Statistics Branch, May 1997. Based on August 1996 submission.
46. Armstrong BK, Kricker A. Cutaneous melanoma. Cancer Surveys: Trends Cancer Incidence 1994; 19:219-239.
47. Dennis LK, White E, Lee JAH. Recent cohort trends in malignant melanoma by anatomic site in the United States. Cancer Causes Control 1993; 4:93-100.
48. Giles G, Thursfield V. Trends in skin cancer in Australia. Cancer Forum 1996; 20:188-191.
49. Greenlee RT, Hill-Harmon MB, Murray T, Thun M. Cancer statistics, 2001. CA Cancer J Clin 2001; 51:15-36.
50. Evans RD, Kopf AW, Lew RA. Risk factors for the development of malignant melanoma, part I: review of case-control studies. J Dermatol Surg Oncol 1988; 14:393-406.
51. Rubenstein R, Hufford D, Downham T II, et al. The health impact of solar radiation and prevention strategies: report of the Environment Council, American Academy of Dermatology, part I: A. Stratospheric ozone depletion: major or minor health risk? J Am Acad Dermatol 1999; 41:82-84.
52. Coldiron BM. Thinning of the ozone layer: facts and consequences. J Am Acad Dermatol 1992; 27:653-662.
53. Herman JR, Bhatia PK, Ziemke J, et al. UV-B increases (1979-1992) from decreases in total ozone. Geophysical Res Lett 1996; 23:2117-2120.
54. Madronich S, de Gruijl FR. Stratospheric ozone depletion between 1979 and 1992: implications for biologically active ultraviolet-B radiation and non-melanoma skin cancer incidence. Photochem Photobiol 1994; 59:541-546.
55. Scotto J, Fears TR, Fraumeni JF Jr. Incidence of nonmelanoma skin cancer in the United States. National Cancer Institute, National Institutes of Health, Public Health Service, US Department of Health and Human Services, Bethesda, Md. NIH Publication No. 83-2433. April 1983.
56. Taylor CR, Stern RS, Leyden JJ. Photoaging, photodamage and photoprotection. J Am Acad Dermatol 1990; 22:1-15.
57. Zitser BS, Shah AN, Adams ML. A survey of sunbathing practices on three Connecticut state beaches. Conn Med 1996; 60: 591-594.
58. Koh HK, Bak SM, Geller AC. Sunbathing habits and sunscreen use among white adults. Am J Public Health 1997; 87:1214-1217.
59. Shovellev JA, Lovato CY, Peters L. Canadian National Survey on sun exposure and protective behaviors: adults at leisure. Cancer Prev Control 1998; 2:111-116.
60. Zinman R, Schwartz S, Gordon K. Predictors of sunscreen use in childhood. Arch Pediatr Adolesc Med 1995; 149:804-807.

61. Vail-Smith K, Felts WM. Sunbathing: college students' knowledge, attitudes, and perceptions of risks. J Am Coll Health 1993; 42:21-26.
62. Leinweber C, Campbell HS. High risk sports—spring skiing and sunburns. Presented at the Third Symposium on the Epidemiology of Melanoma and Non-melanocytic Skin Cancer; May 27-28, 1996; Vancouver.
63. Bourke JF, Graham-Brown RAC. Protection of children against sunburn: a survey of parental practice in Leicester. Br J Dermatol 1995; 133:264-266.
64. Martin R. Relationship between risk factors, knowledge and preventing behavior relevant to skin cancer in general practice patients in south Australia. Br J Gen Pract 1995; 45:365-367.
65. Gilchrest BA. A review of skin ageing and its medical therapy. Br J Dermatol 1996; 135:867-875.
66. Shaath NA. The chemistry of sunscreens. In: Lowe NJ, Shaath NA, Pathak MA, eds. Sunscreens: Development, Evaluation and Regulatory Aspects, 2nd ed. New York: Dekker, 1997:313-351.
67. Wulf H-C, Stender I-M, Lock-Andersen J. Sunscreens used at the beach do not protect against erythema: a new definition of SPF is proposed. Photodermatol Photoimmunol Photomed 1997; 13:129-132.
68. Stenberg C, Larko O. Sunscreen application and its importance for the sun protection factor. Arch Dermatol 1985; 121:1400-1402.
69. Bech-Thomsen N, Wulf H. Sunbathers' application of sunscreens probably inadequate to obtain the sunprotective factor assigned to the preparation. Photodermatol Photoimmunol Photomed 1992; 9:242-244.
70. Pailthorpe M. Apparel textiles and sun protection: a marketing opportunity or a quality control nightmare? Mutation Res 1998; 422:175-183.
71. Stokes R, Diffey B. How well are sunscreen users protected? Photodermatol Photoimmunol Photomed 1997; 13:186-188.
72. Notice of proposed rule-making on sunscreen drug products for over-the-counter human use: tentative final monograph. Federal Register. May 12, 1993; 58:28241.
73. Australian Cancer Society. Policy Statement: Babies and Sunscreen. Sydney, Australia: Australian Cancer Society, 1998.
74. American Academy of Pediatrics, Committee on Environmental Health. Policy statement: ultraviolet light: a hazard to children. Pediatrics 1999; 104:328-333.
75. Walker SI, Young AR. Sunscreens offer the same UVB protection factors for inflammation and immunosuppression in the mouse. J Invest Dermatol 1997; 108:133-138.
76. Garssen J, Goettsch W, deGruijl F. Risk assessment of UVB effects on resistance to infectious diseases. Photochem Photobiol 1996; 64:269-294.
77. Ho KKL, Halliday GM, Barnetson R. Sunscreens protect epidermal Langerhans cells and thy-1 + cells but not local contact sensitization from the effects of ultraviolet light. J Invest Dermatol 1992; 98:720-724.
78. Reeve VE, Boehm-Wilcox C, Bosnic M, et al. Differential photoimmunoprotection by sunscreen ingredients is unrelated to epidermal cis urocanic acid formation in hairless mice. J Invest Dermatol 1994; 103:801-806.
79. Whitmore SE, Morison WL. Prevention of UVB-induced immunosuppression in humans by a high sunprotective factor sunscreen. Arch Dermatol 1995; 131:1128-1133.
80. Wolf P, Donawho CK, Kripke ML. Analysis of the protective effect of different sunscreens on ultraviolet radiation-induced heat and systemic suppression of contact hypersensitivity and inflammatory responses in mice. J Invest Dermatol 1993; 254-259.
81. Lavker RM. Cutaneous aging: chronologic versus photoaging. In: Gilchrest BA, ed. Photodamage. Cambridge, Mass: Blackwell Science, 1995:123-135.
82. Kricker A, Armstrong BK, English DR. Does intermittent sun exposure cause basal cell carcinoma? A case control study in Western Australia. Int J Cancer 1995; 60:489-494.
83. Boyd AS, Naylor M, Cameron GS, et al. The effects of chronic sunscreen on the histologic changes of dermatoheliosis. J Am Acad Dermatol 1995; 33:941-946.
84. Foley P, Nixon R, Marks R. The frequency of reactions to sunscreens: results of a longitudinal population-based study on the regular use of sunscreens in Australia. Br J Dermatol 1993; 128: 512-518.
85. Marks R, Foley PA, Jolley D. The effect of regular sunscreen use on vitamin D levels in an Australian population. Arch Dermatol 1995; 131:415-421.
86. Sollitto RB, Kraemer KH, DiGiovanna JJ. Normal vitamin D levels can be maintained despite rigorous photoprotection: six years' experience with xeroderma pigmentosum. J Am Acad Dermatol 1997; 37:942-947.
87. Matsuoka LY, Wortsman J, Hanifin N. Chronic sunscreen use decreases circulating concentrations of 25-hydroxyvitamin D. Arch Dermatol 1988; 124:1802-1804.
88. Martincigh BS, Allen JM, Allen SK. Sunscreens: the molecules and their photochemistry. In: Gasparro FP, ed. Sunscreen Photobiology. Berlin: Springer-Verlag, 1997:11-45.
89. Knowland J, McHugh PJ, Dunford R. The photochemical potential of some sunscreens to damage DNA. In: Gasparro FP, ed. Sunscreen Photobiology. Berlin: Springer-Verlag, 1997:47-61.
90. Davis S, Capjack L, Kerr N, Fedosejevs R. Clothing as protection from ultraviolet radiation: which fabric is most effective. Int J Dermatol 1997; 36:374-379.
91. Ravishankar J, Diffey B. Laboratory testing of UV transmission through fabrics may underestimate protection. Photodermatol Photoimmunol Photomed 1997; 13:202-203.
92. Pailthorpe M. Apparel textiles and sun protection: a marketing opportunity or a quality control nightmare? Mutation Res 1998; 422:175-183.
93. Gies PH, Roy CR, Toomey S. Protection against solar ultraviolet radiation. Mutation Res 1998; 422:15-22.
94. Marks R, Fraser P. Ozone depletion and human health: fact or fiction? In: Burgdorf WHC, Katz SI, eds. Dermatology: Progress and Perspectives. New York: Parthenon Publishing, 1993:111-114.
95. Jevtic AP. The sun protective effect of clothing, including beachwear. Australas J Dermatol 1990; 31:5-7.
96. Diffey BL, Cheeseman J. Sun protection with hats. Br J Dermatol 1992; 127:10-12.
97. Holly EA, Aston DA, Char DH, et al. Uveal melanoma in relation to ultraviolet light exposure and host factors. Cancer Res 1990; 50:5773-5777.
98. Miller AJ, Gordon S, Gross P, et al. Prevention: public messages. J Am Acad Dermatol 1999; 41:96-99.
99. Threlfall TJ. Sunglasses and clothing—an unhealthy correlation? Aust J Public Health 1992; 16:192-196.
100. Adam SA, Sheaves JK, Wright NH, et al. A case-control study of the possible association between oral contraceptives and malignant melanoma. Br J Cancer 1981; 44:45-50.
101. Autier P, Joarlette M, Lejeune F, et al. Cutaneous malignant melanoma and exposure to sunlamps and sunbeds: a descriptive study in Belgium. Melanoma Res 1991; 1:69-74.
102. Swerdlow AJ, English JSC, MacKie RM, et al. Fluorescent lights, ultraviolet lamps, and risk of cutaneous melanoma. Br Med J 1988; 297:647-650.
103. Walter SD, Marrett LD, From L, et al. The association of cutaneous malignant melanoma with the use of sunbeds and sunlamps. Am J Epidemiol 1990; 131:232-243.
104. Autier P, Dore J-F, Lejeune F, et al. Cutaneous malignant melanoma and exposure to sunlamps or sunbeds: an EORTC multicenter case-control study in Belgium, France, and Germany. EORTC Melanoma Cooperative Group. Int J Cancer 1994; 58: 809-813.
105. Westerdahl J, Olsson H, Masback A, et al. Use of sunbeds or sunlamps and malignant melanoma in southern Sweden. Am J Epidemiol 1994; 140:691-699.

106. Swerdlow AJ, Weinstock MA. Do tanning lamps cause melanoma? An epidemiologic assessment. J Am Acad Dermatol 1998; 38:89-98.
107. Gange RW, Blackett AD, Matzinger EA, et al. Comparative protection efficacy of UVA- and UVB-induced tans against erythema and formation of endonuclease-sensitive sites in DNA by UVB in human skin. J Invest Dermatol 1985; 85:362-364.
108. Kaidbey KH, Kligman AM. Sunburn protection by longwave ultraviolet radiation-induced pigmentation. Arch Dermatol 1978; 114:46-48.
109. Diffey BL, Farr PM. Tanning with UVB or UVA: an appraisal of risks. J Photochem Photobiol 1991; 8:219-223.
110. Goldsmith L, Koh HK, Bewerse B, et al. Proceedings from the national conference to develop a national skin cancer agenda: American Academy of Dermatology and Centers of Disease Control and Prevention, April 8-10, 1995. J Am Acad Dermatol 1996; 34:822-823.
111. AAD joins KaBOOM! to develop a national model for sun-safe playgrounds. Dermatology World. May 1999.
112. Long CS, Miller AJ, Lee HT, et al. Ultraviolet Index forecast issued by the National Weather Service. Bull Am Metereol Soc 1996; 64:792-799.

CHAPTER 5

Beauty and Society

DAVID B. SARWER
TED A. GROSSBART
ELIZABETH R. DIDIE

Beauty is an abstract construct. We all have our own ideas about what is and is not beautiful—a particular song or painting, a man or woman. Accurately describing what exactly "it" is that makes the song, painting, or person beautiful, however, is a daunting task. Dictionaries provide objective definitions, but these descriptions often fail to capture the subjective nature of beauty. Adding to the ambiguity, standards of beauty often seem arbitrary and fluctuating—high hemlines one season, low hemlines the next; Marilyn Monroe one decade, Twiggy the next. Furthermore, we live in a world that holds very disparate views about the nature and importance of physical beauty. On the one hand, we have sayings like, "Beauty is only skin deep," which suggest not only that beauty is subjective but that it extends beyond that which is seen by the human eye. On the other hand, we have sayings such as, "Beauty is a greater recommendation than any letter of introduction," which suggest that physical appearance plays an important role in how we are perceived by others. Whether we believe more in the first group of sayings or the second, the end result is that neither helps us understand the nature of beauty.

In this chapter we will attempt to make the case that beauty and physical attractiveness is a serious matter—that beauty is as fundamental to the practice of cosmetic surgery as knowledge is to science, profit to business, or votes to politics. We begin with a discussion of the role of beauty in evolutionary theory. Next, we turn to theories of the physiology of beauty, which focus on physical characteristics such as pathogen resistance, averageness, physical symmetry, body ratios, and youthfulness. We then describe changes in the societal standards of beauty through a discussion of the relatively recent history of mass media images of beauty. We then use the psychological construct of body image to begin to understand the nature of beauty on an individual level. The chapter concludes with a discussion of the things that we do to make ourselves more beautiful.

BEAUTY AND EVOLUTIONARY THEORY

It is often said that "beauty is in the eye of the beholder." Consistent with that belief, beauty has been described as an individual's subjective assessment of attractiveness that is influenced by current cultural standards. However, Charles Darwin and his intellectual descendants from the field of evolutionary biology offer a different theory of the nature of beauty. In his seminal *The Descent of Man and Selection in Relation to Sex,* Darwin puzzled over the physical characteristics that seemed to act as open lures to predators and therefore interfere with survival maintenance activities. For example, how could (and why did) the brilliant plumage of peacocks evolve? Darwin's answer was sexual selection—that certain characteristics evolved because of reproductive advantage rather than survival advantage.[1]

Are human's concepts of beauty (and perhaps their interest in improving their appearance through means such as cosmetic surgery) also tied to some higher purpose like reproduction? If we are on an evolutionary mission to increase the chances of our genetic material moving to the next generation, what we consider desirable in the opposite sex, or how we sculpt our own appearance, is not simply a matter of taste or arbitrary preference. While the evolutionary mission of reproduction may be universal, research suggests substantial gender differences in humans. For men, fertility and good health are high on the list of determinants of what is considered attractive in a woman. For the International Mate Selection Project, 50 scientists studied 10,047 people in 37 cultures located on six continents and five islands. Without exception, physical cues to youth and health were seen as attractive. "In no known culture do people perceive wrinkled skin, . . . thin lips,

. . . poor muscle tone, and irregular facial features to be attractive."[2] This seems so obvious that we might never ask why.

The evolutionary argument posits that physical signs of youth and health—full lips, smooth, clear skin, clear eyes, lustrous hair, good muscle tone, animated facial expression, high energy level[1]—are at the top of every culture's beauty list because they are the most reliable physical markers of fertility. These characteristics are considered beautiful because, and only because, of their evolutionary advantage. While many other characteristics may make for a good mate, it is hard to imagine obvious physical markers for fidelity, parenting ability, temperament, or intelligence. These qualities certainly make a potential mate more attractive, but they are not components of beauty.

A woman's campaign to select the man to help propel her genetic material into the future requires a very different strategy. What male characteristics are most evolutionarily useful and will therefore define attractiveness? The ability to obtain and defend resources and the willingness to commit them to a particular female and her offspring define attractiveness. Applied to the physical realm, this would seem to require males to be well-muscled and athletic. Yet raw muscle power has been partially replaced by the financial and political equivalent in humans. "Across 36 of 37 cultures from Australia to Zambia women place great(est) value on financial prospects."[2] Henry Kissinger's suggestion that "power is the ultimate aphrodisiac" reflects the same evolutionary verity. If the man's resources are not available to the woman and children, they are irrelevant. Thus, the observation that men are more swayed by beauty, and women by a mix of physical attractiveness and the man's abilities as a provider, may be less a reflection of a more evolved cognitive perspective in women and more the result of fundamental biological differences.

More recent research also supports the idea that perceptions of beauty may be guided by universally shared biological wirings. From this approach, standards of beauty result from fixed neuroanatomical arrangements that have biological relevance.[3] For example, facial features such as symmetry, averageness, and youthfulness not only may indicate attractiveness but more importantly may signal health and reproductive capabilities of potential sexual partners. Similarly, nonfacial features, such as waist-to-hip ratio, may function as indicators of health and reproductive success.[4] Despite some unique cultural variability in aesthetic judgments, evidence has demonstrated that similar patterns emerge across diverse cultures.[2]

A set of compelling studies confirm that our perceptions of attractiveness predate cultural influences.[3] Studies of infants have suggested that the ability to discriminate attractive from unattractive faces may be an innate ability, or at least one acquired at an earlier age than previously believed.[5] Infants 3 to 6 months old appear to be more attentive to "attractive" versus "unattractive" female faces[5]; such preferences occur across sex and race.[6] Similarly, infants express a more positive tone, are less withdrawn, and play more with attractive strangers than with unattractive ones.[7] Infants also play for a longer period of time with attractive dolls than they do with unattractive dolls.[7] These findings challenge the belief that judgments of facial attractiveness are learned through exposure to cultural standards and stereotypes. Thus, beauty may be in not only the eye of a single beholder but rather of many beholders with similar genetic wiring. Or, as suggested by Buss, "Beauty may be in the eyes of the beholder, but those eyes and the minds behind the eyes have been shaped by millions of years of human evolution."[1]

What are the implications of the evolutionary theory of beauty for cosmetic surgery? We would expect that patients would report the greatest unanimity around cosmetic surgical goals that have an evolutionary purpose. Thus, female surgical goals would nearly all seek to simulate youth and health. We would expect more varied agendas around physical features with no implications for fertility. In contrast, we would expect male cosmetic surgery agendas to emphasize economic motives—aiding men in appearing strong and powerful. While these hypotheses may characterize many cosmetic surgery patients, they clearly do not capture the surgical motivations of every patient. Nevertheless, surgeons who recognize the link between surgical goals and these fundamental biological imperatives may better understand their patients' motivations for surgery.

PHYSICAL CHARACTERISTICS OF BEAUTY

Evolutionary theory suggests that an organism's ability to successfully identify a potential mate who will help propel his or her genetic material into the future is a biological imperative. Furthermore, the theory suggests that selection of an ideal, "beautiful" mate is influenced by physiological, rather than cognitive, factors. Contemporary research in this area has attempted to identify the physical features that make an individual attractive. This research has identified several factors: pathogen resistance, facial and body symmetry, averageness, body-size ratios, and youthfulness.

Pathogen Resistance

The pathogen resistance theory of beauty suggests that physical beauty is a "marker" or "signal" that a potential mate is pathogen free.[8] This model of sexual selection indicates that only healthy, pathogen-resistant animals can develop and maintain their secondary sex characteristics. Furthermore, the heritability of parasite resistance increases the chance that mates can provide genetic resistance to their offspring.[8] Therefore, attractiveness may be a visible sign that a prospective partner is pathogen free.

This theory may influence human assessment of potential mates. For example, men and women of cultures with high pathogen and disease prevalence (such as Nigeria, Zambia, and India) rated physical attractiveness as more important in the selection of their long-term mates than men and women from cultures in which the pathogen prevalence was low (such as West Germany, Sweden, and Norway).[9] While certainly open to other interpretations, these findings are not surprising, given that selecting a healthy partner may be more challenging in countries where pathogens are more abundant. However, there is no empirical evidence demonstrating that physically attractive humans have greater parasite resistance than unattractive humans.

Facial and Body Symmetry

Bilateral symmetry has been proposed as one phenotypic indicator of a pathogen-free organism.[10] Animal studies demonstrate that highly symmetrical creatures are at an advantage in competition for sexual partners as compared with their lopsided competitors.[11] For example, female peahens prefer males with long tails containing large numbers of bilaterally symmetrical eye spots.[12] Female barn swallows select male sexual partners with symmetrical tails over those with asymmetrical tails.[11] Female zebra finches also prefer symmetrically leg-banded males.[13] The attraction for symmetrical features has also been found in scorpion flies.[14] It appears that bilateral symmetry may be an advertisement for quality potential mates who may offer a greater probability for reproductive success.

Humans are also thought to respond to visual cues of symmetry to identify potentially desirable mates. Both male and female humans with more bilaterally symmetrical facial features are judged to be more attractive, regardless of the gender of the judges.[10,15,16] Facial symmetry for men and women is positively correlated with judgments of facial attractiveness by cross-sex raters.[16] In one study, for example, body symmetry and facial attractiveness of hundreds of college-aged men and women was examined using right-left disparities of seven body measurements. A positive relationship was found for symmetry and facial attractiveness for men.[15] Furthermore, ratings of attractiveness of faces are increased when bilateral symmetry is enhanced through digital technology that blend images of the normal face and its mirror image.[17] This preference for symmetry was found for both sexes, although the preference for symmetrical faces was stronger for men than for women, as would be expected from the beauty-fertility theory proposed by the evolutionary biologists. In addition, men with the most symmetrical features reported both more sexual experiences and being sexually active at an earlier age than men with more asymmetric features.[18] Thus, it may be that symmetrical facial and body features not only are aesthetically pleasing but also convey a message of reproductive health.

According to evolutionary theorists, facial symmetry is an attractive quality because it signals health and fitness. Under ideal developmental conditions, paired body features (i.e., eyes, ears, elbows) develop in synchronicity, leading to more symmetrical, and therefore more attractive, persons. External factors, such as pollutants, pathogens, and physical trauma, are thought to adversely affect symmetrical development. For many of the same reasons, bilateral symmetry of secondary sexual traits is a difficult developmental accomplishment. As a result, evolutionary theorists believe that only the hardiest and healthiest of the population possess the ability to develop facial and body symmetry in spite of harsh environmental conditions.[10]

Averageness of Appearance

Somewhat surprisingly to many individuals, averageness can equal attractiveness. Averageness is traditionally associated with the ordinary or unexceptional, and certainly does not connote beauty. Studies of averageness in facial appearance have used a mathematical mean of a composite of facial dimensions to generate an "average" appearance.[19,20] To do this, a face is digitally computerized and rated on a scale of 1 to 10, indicating increasing levels of physical attractiveness. The rater then assesses a series of faces that are subsequently "bred" with the preceding face. For both males and females, composite faces of the opposite sex are judged more attractive than the individual faces that made up the composite.[19] Moreover, the more faces that are used to make up the composite, the more attractive the final picture is rated.[20]

The notion that averageness is associated with attractiveness is consistent with evolutionary theory. Arguably, individuals who fall within the mean of the population distribution should be less likely to carry potentially harmful genes or mutations.[20] The parasite theory of sexual selection contends that heterozygosity is greatest among individuals who have the "average expression of continuously distributed, heritable traits."[21] Given this theoretical relationship between heterozygosity and pathogen resistance, averageness may indicate an organism's parasite-resistant genetic composition.[10]

However, while average faces are considered attractive, the most beautiful of the digital faces are certainly not average.[22,23] In fact, these beautiful faces are not common among the general population; rather they are atypical in terms of both the specific facial features and overall facial structure. Studies that have used digital composites of faces have found that the most highly rated composite female faces produced an image that was rated considerably more attractive than the typical face that went into creating the final composite.[22] Overall, the ideal composite female face had facial features that were rather petite. The ideal face had a mouth that was smaller than average but had considerably fuller lips. This face also had a preadolescent's tiny jawline, delicate lower face, and pronounced eyes and cheekbones.[22] In addition, the distance from the eyes to the nose and from the eyes to the mouth, as well as from the mouth to the chin, were smaller than these distances in the individual faces that were used to develop the composite.[22] These findings are consistent with the evolutionary theory that suggests that beauty is characterized by youthfulness, as discussed later.

Body-Size Ratios

Body ratios, specifically the waist-hip ratio (WHR), also are thought to play a role in determining opposite-sex attractiveness for both men and women.[4] The WHR reflects the distribution of fat between the upper and lower body and the relative amount of abdominal fat. Before puberty both males and females have comparable WHRs.[4] During puberty, increased levels of estrogen in females aid in the development of breasts and hips by adding fat deposits to these areas of the body. In males, testosterone stimulates fat deposits in the abdominal region and inhibits fat deposits in the area of the hips and thighs.[4] Therefore, it may be that specific body ratios signal that a prospective mate is sexually mature and has the biological capability to be reproductively active.

Typically, women rated as attractive are normal weight and have a low WHR.[4] Healthy, fertile women typically have a WHR of .60 to .80, meaning waists are 60% to 80% the size of the hips.[24] Female figures with a WHR of greater than .80, independent of overall body weight, were judged less attractive and less healthy than those figures with a WHR of .80 or smaller.[4] The perceptions of attractiveness of men are also influenced by WHR as well as relative weight. Specifically, healthy men have WHRs in the range of .85 to .95.[25] In spite of WHR, underweight and overweight male figures were not judged to be highly attractive or healthy; only normal weight male figures with typical WHRs were perceived as healthy and attractive.[26]

WHR is thought to convey information about both current reproductive and health status of women.[26] Typically, menopausal women have a WHR that is comparable to the WHR of men.[27] Besides being an indicator of reproductive potential, a relatively low WHR also signals health status. The risk factor profile for many obesity-related diseases, such as type 2 diabetes, hypertension, and coronary heart disease, varies with the distribution of fat.[28] A WHR greater than .80 for women and 1.0 for men is considered an independent risk factor for many weight-related illnesses.

Youthfulness

Youthfulness marks an extended period of reproductive potential.[29] Given the theoretical model of sexual selection proposed by the evolutionary biologists, it is not surprising that ratings of facial attractiveness and youthfulness are highly correlated.[30] Ratings of physical attractiveness of men and women declined with age, but the effects were more pronounced for women's faces.[31] Women were rated as less feminine as they aged, whereas ratings of masculinity were unaffected.[32] These findings suggest that standards for attractiveness for men are less stringent and less connected to youth than they are for women, a conclusion again consistent with evolutionary theories of reproduction.

Looking young may be more important than actually being young. Male raters from five populations judged faces that appear to be younger than the actual age of the face to be more attractive than faces that appeared age-appropriate or older than the actual age.[33] Altering facial features in the direction of youth results in higher ratings of attractiveness.[34] Such preferences for youthfulness exist in the real world, where more female models, as compared with female college students, have younger-looking faces.[34] While this quality has been demonstrated to be an asset for ratings of female attractiveness, the same influences have not been found for men. It may be more adaptive for males to prefer youthful female features because of a strong association with fertility.[35]

It appears that specific physical features are deemed attractive because they serve an evolutionary purpose. Throughout the eons, reliance on phenotypic expressions for mate selection has been necessary to result in successful reproduction and survival of the species. While overall facial attractiveness may be interpreted as a sign that an organism is healthy, reliance on this feature alone is inadequate to ensure selection of high-quality mates. Therefore, other facial and bodily features may influence sexual selection. The presence of symmetrical features may indicate that an organism has overcome or avoided developmental stressors and may denote a durable and hardy creature. Averageness may act as an indicator that the organism is safeguarded against potential pathogens. Proportionate body ratios may be the most obvious advertisement that the organism has reproductive potential. Finally, a youthful face has long been associated with fertility.

Taken together, these physical attributes—facial and body symmetry, averageness, body ratio, and youthfulness—not only have aesthetic appeal but very well may guide decisions in successful sexual selection.

SOCIOCULTURAL IDEALS OF BEAUTY

Evolutionary theories of beauty are most compelling when used to explain preferences that are stable across history and culture. Nevertheless, these theories provide only part of the answer to the question of who or what is considered beautiful. Sociocultural approaches to beauty are intuitively pleasing and are helpful in understanding aspects of beauty that change over time. These changes in sociocultural images of beauty are best reflected in a variety of popular beauty icons—from pinup girls, magazine models, and Hollywood stars to Miss America and the *Playboy* centerfold.

Pinup Girls, Magazine Models, and Hollywood Stars

Culture imparts a great deal of variability to ratings of attractiveness.[2] For example, short-lived subcultural variants that are maladaptive in an evolutionary sense, such as the "heroin chic" look of the mid-1990s, can become very popular. Western culture has touted a range of body types as "the ideal" depending on the decade. This is perhaps no better exemplified than through the changes of the ideal Western female figure of the last century.

In the 19th century, two idealized figures of female beauty in the United States were the "steel engraving lady," idolized for her fragile and delicate features, and the "voluptuous woman," whose full, rounded figure epitomized female sexuality. During the late 1890s a new model emerged, the "Gibson Girl," who, in addition to a slender, athletic frame had larger breasts and hips.[36] Following the Victorian era, the 1920s promoted an image that was curveless and almost boyish in shape.[36] While models of the following decade became more curvaceous, these beauties conspicuously lacked extraneous fat. The "Petty Girl," as the icon of the 1930s was known, had a slim lower body and a flat abdomen.[36] This theme continued through the 1940s as depicted by one of the most famed pinups, Betty Grable.

Curves accentuating a woman's breasts and hips made a dramatic return during the 1950s, perhaps most visibly when Marilyn Monroe posed for the first *Playboy* magazine centerfold. The voluptuous hour-glass figure of Monroe, as well as those of Jane Russell and Jayne Mansfield, were glorified as the ideal shape during this decade.[37] Soon after, the waist size of the ideal woman declined sharply, and by the 1960s the ideal torso required an unnatural curvature, with fat distributed away from the waist to the hips and breasts.[36] Similar to the beauty icons of the late 19th century, Western culture during the 1950s also admired the elegant sophisticated lines of Audrey Hepburn and Grace Kelly.

By the late 1960s, thinner fashion icons such as Twiggy replaced the curvaceous figures of the previous decade. This slender trend has endured and has been accentuated by the increasing height and decreasing weights of fashion models and beauty icons since that time.[37] The stringent guidelines for weight and shape relaxed somewhat during the 1970s. Beauty icons such as Farrah Fawcett and Cheryl Tiegs were more curvaceous than models from the previous decade but still remained slender. By the 1980s, another physical characteristic helped define beauty. Media stars such as Christy Brinkley and Bo Derek had not only the desired curves but also well-developed musculature. Moreover, during the 1990s "supermodels" such as Cindy Crawford, Elle McPherson, and Tyra Banks continued to advertise lean and muscular figures that were feminine and curvy as well.

Comparable trends have been evident in models depicted in popular women's magazines. During the period of 1967 to 1987, there was an increase in height and waist measurements of female fashion models, but no increase in hip measurements.[38] The bust-to-waist ratio of models in *Ladies' Home Journal* and *Vogue* has fluctuated greatly over the century, with the combined average of the bust-to-waist ratios of the two magazines remaining at a low through the early 1980s.[39] While this issue has been studied extensively in magazines marketed toward adult women, research on fashion models depicted in magazines geared toward younger female audiences, who may be most susceptible to the influence of such images, has been sparse. One of the few studies that examined teen magazines uncovered trends similar to those found in adult magazines. Guillen and Barr[40] reported that the overall mean hip-to-waist ratio of models in young women's magazines had significantly declined over time, depicting a less curvaceous shape.

Thin ideals are also found in other mass media sources. In a study investigating perceptions of the appearance of popular television characters, 69% of female characters were rated as thin, while only 18% of male characters were rated as thin. In contrast, more male (26%) than female (5%) characters were rated as overweight.[39] Similar thinning trends have been observed in an analysis of popular female movie stars from 1933 through 1978.[39] In the last 5 years, several prominent female television and movie stars (i.e., Jennifer Aniston, Calista Flockhart, and Lara Flynn Boyle) have become dramatically thinner. Many women and men have been openly critical of this current trend in Hollywood, both out of concern for the message this sends to young women and also for the health of the actresses themselves. Nevertheless, there is little to suggest that this trend will change anytime soon.

Miss America and the *Playboy* Centerfold

The Western ideal of physical beauty has changed repeatedly over the past 100 years. However, it has not always been clear that impressions of change have accurately reflected actual change in these standards. To investigate this issue, several researchers have examined changes in the physical features of two of America's most enduring images of physical beauty—Miss America and the *Playboy* centerfold.

In the 1920s, the mean bust-to-hip measurements of Miss America winners were 32-25-35.[36] By the 1930s, waist and hip measurements remained constant but the average bustline grew by 2 inches. This trend continued through the mid-1960s.[36] Over a 20-year period (1959 to 1978), the weights of Miss America contestants gradually declined, while height climbed steadily.[41] Bust and hips were still symmetrical but the height of contestants rose by an average of 1 inch, while weight fell by an average of 5 pounds per decade.[36] Miss America finalists in the 1960s, for example, averaged 66 inches in height and 120 pounds. In contrast, finalists in 1983 and 1984 also weighed 120 pounds but were 2 inches taller on average.[36] Body weight for Miss Americas was 13% to 19% below their expected weight, with 60% of contestants at weights 15% or more below the expected weight for their age and height, a characteristic found in women with anorexia nervosa.[42] In contrast to normal height and weight relationships, which are highly correlated, while Miss America has gotten taller, she has lost weight.

Similar trends have been found for another icon of Western beauty, *Playboy* centerfolds. Over a 20-year period (1959 to 1978), the weight of *Playboy* centerfolds decreased while height rose steadily.[41] A more recent update of this study found that the weight of *Playboy* centerfolds continued to fall during the period 1978 to 1988 and has stabilized at a very low level.[42] For example, during the time period 1979 to 1983 the mean weight of *Playboy* centerfolds was 111.5 pounds, a weight significantly less than the 115.7 pound mean reported by Garner et al. for the years 1959 to 1978.[41] Similar to Miss America contestants, over the 10-year period (1979 to 1988), 69% of the *Playboy* centerfolds weighed 15% or more below the expected weight for their age and height.[42] Troublingly, the current height-weight ratios for both Miss America and the *Playboy* centerfold have reached the point where the majority of these women now reflect an underweight, and potentially unhealthy, body type.

Cross-Cultural Studies of Beauty

Although many argue that Western society establishes the current ideals of beauty, it is often assumed that there are distinct cultural variabilities in aesthetic judgments. Most of the cross-cultural literature on beauty has focused on preferences in facial attractiveness. Across 37 cultures, both males and females prioritized physical attractiveness over personality characteristics like dependability, emotional stability, and maturity in their choice of mates.[2] Furthermore, standards of physical attractiveness are not arbitrarily isolated to certain cultures.[33] Ratings of facial attractiveness of Greek men by women in China, England, and India were consistent across the cultural groups.[43] In a similar study the attractiveness of female faces of international contestants from the Miss Universe pageant were rated by Caucasian males. Those faces that were rated as highly attractive also correlated with young-looking features, such as wide eyes, small chin, and small nose.[33] In addition, features such as prominent cheekbones and narrower cheeks were also associated with high ratings of attractiveness.[33] These findings have been replicated across female faces of Asian, Hispanic, and African American decent,[44] further suggesting the cross-cultural commonalities of certain aspects of beauty.

In looking at the variety of images of Western beauty from the last century, it appears that ideals of beauty have principally "evolved" from the round voluptuous figures of female models to the strikingly linear figures of fashion models and actresses today. Unfortunately, it also appears that many of these images have evolved to the point of projecting a potentially physically unhealthy ideal to society. Given the theoretical relationship between mass media images of beauty and eating disorders and body image problems, the potential influence of these ideals on young women in particular is of great concern to many mental health professionals.

Many people argue that the mass media (magazines, movies, television, and Internet) are influential promoters of beauty ideals. Others contend that the media are simply reflecting a trend of public preferences. Even if this thin ideal did not originate in the media, many believe that the media exploit this ideal and promote the message that thinness is equated with success and popularity. One feminist perspective offered by Naomi Wolf[45] suggests that the multibillion-dollar diet, cosmetics, and cosmetic surgery industries seek to keep women in frantic pursuit of this "beauty myth." As such, the mass media function as a counterfeminist movement that seeks to maintain and extend economic, political, and sexual control over women. Regardless of how one understands the relationship between the mass media and these images, the images themselves are inescapable. While some would argue that these images inspire us to visualize our appearance in the idealized form, others would suggest that they, as one patient put it, "leave me feeling that I look like chopped liver." Given that the vast majority of women will never attain the idyllic standards reflected by media, it is not surprising that women who are dissatisfied with their appearance are motivated to use a variety of methods, including cosmetic surgery, to improve what they perceive as bodily imperfections.

WHAT DO WE THINK ABOUT BEAUTIFUL PEOPLE?

Thirty to 40 years ago, mental health professionals did not give much thought to beauty. If beauty was considered, it was seen as a trivial pursuit of vanity or a misplaced effort at enhancing self-esteem. Women who were interested in changing their appearance through cosmetic surgery during this time were typically seen in a negative light—their motivations for changing their appearance viewed as a misplaced attempt to solve an internal emotional conflict. Since that time, a body of research from the field of social psychology has greatly increased our understanding of the role of physical beauty in daily life. This research has suggested that, whether we like to admit it or not, our appearance really does seem to matter.

One of the first experiments in this area was designed to test the belief first offered by the Greek philosopher Sappho[46] that "what is beautiful is good." To test this idea, men and women were asked to look at pictures of good-looking, average-looking, or unattractive individuals (the pictures were categorized by another group of raters) and rate them on a variety of personality characteristics. As compared with the average and unattractive pictures, good-looking individuals were rated as more kind, interesting, sociable, and outgoing. In addition, they were predicted to have happier marriages, better jobs, and more fulfilling lives.[47] Over the next 25 years, numerous studies found similar results, strengthening the belief that more beautiful individuals are viewed more positively than those who are less attractive.

Not only are beautiful individuals judged more positively than their less attractive peers, but attractive individuals appear to receive preferential treatment from others. Throughout the lifespan, beautiful men and women appear to be treated more favorably. For example, elementary school teachers typically assumed that cute boys and girls were more intelligent and were more likely to achieve academic success than less attractive children.[48,49] Such biases also occur when schooling has been completed. As compared with less attractive persons, attractive individuals are more likely to be hired for jobs and receive higher starting salaries.[50]

Appearance and the Medical, Mental Health, and Legal Systems

Medical and mental health professionals (who we would like to think are immune to such beauty biases) appear to treat attractive and unattractive patients differently. Numerous studies have documented the negative, indifferent, or demeaning behavior that unattractive individuals, such as those who are facially disfigured or who are obese, have received from their physicians. Mental health professionals also fall victim to the same stereotypes about the beautiful and the homely as everyone else. In general, psychotherapists tend to attribute greater psychopathology to their unattractive patients. For years, psychotherapists have acknowledged that they prefer working with YAVIS (young, attractive, verbal, interesting, and successful) clients rather than old, unattractive, and unsuccessful clients.[51] Not surprisingly, several studies have suggested that psychotherapy patients also prefer to work with more attractive therapists.[52,53]

Physical appearance also influences our interactions with the legal system. Reviewing the literature on the relationship between physical appearance and criminal behavior, Hatfield and Sprecher[54] concluded that more attractive individuals are less likely to be caught committing a crime and are less likely to be severely punished by judges and jurors. There is one exception to the benefits of beauty in legal proceedings—if one's physical beauty is used to prey on others. Attractive female defendants, for example, will receive longer prison sentences than less attractive defendants in cases of embezzlement.[55] The benefits of physical beauty apply to victims as well, as attractive victims appear to be more successful in winning their legal cases.[54]

Appearance and Helping Behaviors

Physical beauty also determines who we help and who we ask for help. Across several studies, men have been shown to be more likely to help an attractive woman than an unattractive woman with tasks ranging from mailing letters to providing directions.[56,57] While good-looking individuals appear to be more likely to receive help, they are less likely to be asked for help. Whether it is out of fear of rejection or concern about looking helpless in front of a beautiful person, we are more likely to ask less attractive friends and strangers for help in times of need.[54]

Appearance in Romantic Relationships

Physical appearance obviously plays a central role in the selection of our romantic partners. It is frequently the first bit of information we gather about a potential romantic partner. If the "spark" of physical attraction does not exist, the romantic relationship will most likely not flourish. In a perfect world, almost all men and women would prefer to be with the most physically attractive partner available, even at the expense of exceptional intelligence or a sense of humor. When the possibility of rejection is added to the romantic equation, however, desire for the most attractive partner is balanced by the fear of rejection. The end result is that people will typically end up selecting people who are similar to themselves in attractiveness. For example, if a woman views herself as a "7," she may desire to be with a "10," but the fear of possible rejection by a more attractive partner will lead her to become interested in another "7." In these more realistic settings, the other personality characteristics that attract people to one another, such as intelligence, sense of humor, compassion, and loyalty, play a more central role in romantic relationships. Nevertheless, similarity in physical attractiveness remains important, as couples who are matched on physical attractiveness, as well as on other desirable personality characteristics, are more content in their romantic relationships.[54]

Over the last several decades a significant body of research has demonstrated the benefits of physical beauty. Not only are physically attractive individuals judged more positively by other individuals, but they have been shown to receive preferential treatment in numerous interpersonal encounters across the lifespan. Even in situations where we would like to think our appearance does not matter—when we trust that others will help us—beauty strongly influences how we are treated. Physical attractiveness plays a vital role in our interpersonal interactions, yet it is almost completely unrelated to how we truly feel about our appearance. In fact, no discussion of beauty is complete without an exploration of the inner view of beauty—one's body image.

BODY IMAGE

At the beginning of the new century, body image is clearly one of the hottest topics in the field of psychology. In the 1990s, numerous professional textbooks and hundreds of journal articles were devoted to the study of body image. Unfortunately, as with any rapidly developing area, there is often disagreement as to what exactly "body image" is. In his landmark text, *Exacting Beauty,* Thompson and colleagues[58] suggested that no less than 14 terms can be used to describe body image. In some respects, body image is similar to its closely related construct of self-esteem. That is, we all have an idea of what self-esteem is, but if we were asked to put that idea into words, we would struggle to come up with a concise definition that accurately represents the complexity of the construct. Thompson and colleagues suggest that "body image" has come to be accepted as the internal representation of your own outer appearance.[58] Regardless of the exact definition used, body image plays a significant role in how people feel about both their appearance and themselves.

Dimensions of Body Image

While there is little agreement on the exact definition of body image, there is little disagreement that body image is a multidimensional construct. Relevant psychological influences of body image typically include perceptual, developmental, and sociocultural dimensions.[59,60] Perceptual influences account for an individual's ability to accurately determine the physical features of a given body part. This accounts for our ability to perceive ourselves in time and space, as well as our ability to accurately (or inaccurately) make judgments about the size and shape of our bodies and its features. Developmental influences consider the contribution of childhood and adolescent experiences to the adult body image. The strongest of these influences may be the experience of appearance-related teasing. Recent empirical studies, as well as anecdotal clinical reports, highlight the often devastating effects that childhood and adolescent teasing can have on the adult body image. Each of us, in our psychotherapeutic work, has been struck by patients who, even as highly successful adults, can recall the pain of being teased about their appearance decades earlier as if it had just occurred. These patients often ask cosmetic surgeons to correct the feature that elicited the schoolyard teasing, often years after the last episode of teasing. Finally, sociocultural influences (as discussed in detail earlier) account for the interaction of the mass media and cultural ideals of appearance (which frequently portray unrealistic and exaggerated images of beauty that have been digitally enhanced and airbrushed to perfection) with the tendency of individuals to compare themselves to others. These three factors are thought to play a significant role in the adult body image.

Body Image Valence and Value

Sarwer and colleagues have suggested that attitudes toward the body have at least two dimensions.[60] The first consists of a valence, defined as the degree of importance of body image to one's self-esteem. Persons with a high body image valence, in contrast to those with a low valence, are thought to derive much of their self-esteem from their body image. In addition, body image has a value (i.e., positive or negative), which can also be understood as the degree of satisfaction or dissatisfaction with the body image. Large-scale surveys have indicated that, in general, Americans are dissatisfied with their appearance.[61] Comparisons of survey results conducted in 1972, 1985, and 1996 have suggested that dissatisfaction with overall appearance among women increased from 23% to 56%, and among men increased from 15% to 43%, in just 25 years. One of the greatest concerns for both genders was dissatisfaction with weight. For example, the percentage of women dissatisfied with their weight increased from 48% to

66%, an increase that closely parallels the change in the prevalence of obesity and overweight in the United States. This dissatisfaction is no trivial matter. Weight was so associated with personal happiness that 24% of women and 17% of men said they would give up more than 3 years of their lives to be thinner.[61]

It is difficult, however, to determine the point at which an individual's body image dissatisfaction becomes extreme and problematic. It has been hypothesized that body image dissatisfaction falls on a continuum.[59,60] Such dissatisfaction may range from a dislike of a specific appearance feature to psychopathological dissatisfaction, in which thoughts about appearance distress and preoccupy the individual, and behavior is negatively influenced by these concerns.[59,60] While extreme dissatisfaction may be a symptom of clinically significant psychopathology, mild dissatisfaction may motivate a whole range of behaviors to improve body image.

ADDRESSING BODY IMAGE DISSATISFACTION

As previously discussed, it appears that many women (and some men) desire to achieve increasingly unrealistic body shapes portrayed by the mass media. Not only are these body ideals unattainable for most people, the comparisons between the self and the ideal are thought to contribute to the dramatic increase in discontent about their own appearances.[58-61] This dissatisfaction is thought to motivate many behaviors: dieting and exercise, cosmetics use, and cosmetic surgery.

Dieting and Exercise

Perhaps the most common response to body image dissatisfaction is dieting and exercise. It is estimated that the weight-loss industry contributed $32.6 billion to the nation's economy in 1994.[62] The sale of self-help books, videos, and audiocassettes focusing on dieting topped $380 million in 1994, while commercial weight loss programs, such as Jenny Craig and Weight Watchers, reported earnings of $1.7 billion.[62] Americans also spend billions of dollars annually on health club memberships; fitness club revenue grew from $6.7 billion in 1991 to $8.4 billion in 1994.[62]

Reports of dieting among women are extremely common—such a large percentage of females diet that it can almost be considered "normative eating" in Western cultures. In a sample of 60,860 adults, 38% of women and 24% of men were attempting to lose weight.[63] As many as 81% of high school girls desire to lose weight, and 63% have dieted in the past year.[64] Rosen and Gross[65] found in a sample of 3000 adolescents that 63% of the girls were trying to lose weight. Even some preadolescents are attempting to lose weight. According to the National Heart, Lung, and Blood Institute Growth and Health Study, among 9- and 10-year-olds, 40% of the girls were dieting to lose weight.[66]

Given the increasing prevalence of obesity in the United States, and the well-established relationship between obesity and health conditions such as type 2 diabetes, hypertension, and coronary heart disease, which increase the risk of mortality, one could easily assume that more people are dieting to improve their health status. In reality, the primary motivation for dieting, even among the severely obese, is almost exclusively appearance related. Not surprisingly, women are more likely than men to indicate that their primary concern for trying to lose weight is improving their appearance.[67] Those who engage in frequent physical activity also report that looking good is their primary motivation for exercising.[68] Therefore, even given the benefits of diet and exercise on improving health, improving one's body image appears to be the primary motivation for improving one's diet and being more active.

Cosmetics Use

From the pages of magazines to music videos and television commercials, women are exposed to thousands of messages and images instructing them how to be beautiful. Cosmetics have become a profitable means through which women can attain beauty in Western society. Given the early history of the cosmetics industry, manufacturers have done a phenomenal job at fostering the marketability of their products. Prior to the 1920s, women who "painted their faces" elicited an image of women's sexuality that Victorian society was not ready to acknowledge.[69] Such ideas about cosmetics clearly have not endured, as American consumers spent almost $16 billion on cosmetics, toiletries, and perfumes in 1994.[70]

In her book on the history of the cosmetics industry, Piess suggests that women use makeup to "announce their adult status, sexual allure, youthful spirit, political belief and self-definition."[69] Cosmetics offers women an accessible and affordable means to improve their appearance. It not only provides them with an opportunity to improve their outward appearance; it also can improve their body image and self-esteem. While strains of the feminist movement are often critical of the cosmetic industry and the messages it promotes, women from all walks of life use cosmetics as an acceptable way to enhance desirable facial features and to create the appearance of youth or sexuality.

Cosmetic Surgery

Increasing numbers of women and men use cosmetic surgery to address body image dissatisfaction. In their theory of the relationship between body image and cosmetic surgery, Sarwer and colleagues speculate that it is the interaction between body image valence (the relationship of the body image to self-esteem) and body image value (the degree of body image dissatisfaction) that influences the decision to seek cosmetic surgery.[59,60] One consistent finding of the preoperative studies of cosmetic surgery patients is that persons who seek cosmetic surgery have reported increased dissatisfaction with body image.[71,72] Persons with a high body image valence, for whom body image is an important part of self-esteem, and who have a heightened degree of dissatisfaction with a specific feature, are thought to comprise the majority of cosmetic surgery patients.[60] In contrast, persons with a low body image valence and little body image dissatisfaction are unlikely to seek cosmetic surgery.

The Disfigured

We have spent the majority of this chapter discussing beauty—how we determine what is beautiful, what we think about and how we treat beautiful people, how we think about our own beauty, and what we do to make ourselves more beautiful. Nevertheless, our chapter would be incomplete without a discussion of those who are not beautiful. Whether as a result of a genetic deformity or traumatic insult, there are many members of our society with disfigured appearances who think about beauty in a way that those of us who are not disfigured can probably never understand. While many persons who seek aesthetic surgery hope to improve their "normal" appearance to make it "stand out from the crowd," those who are disfigured often desire nothing more than to have an appearance that allows them to blend into the crowd without being the victims of unwanted stares, looks of disgust, or relentless ridicule.

Compared with the vast literature on beauty available to us for this chapter, relatively little is known about those who are not beautiful. In some respects, this is not particularly surprising, as both the lay public and mass media appear to be much more interested in talking about beauty. Nevertheless, children and adolescents with disfigured appearances are at risk for psychological problems. We also know that disfigured adults may struggle with low self-esteem and poor quality of life, and may experience discrimination in both employment and social settings. Unfortunately, we do not currently know how we can best help those who look different cope with their disfigurement. Between what we do and do not know about disfigurement, one thing is certain. In a society that puts such a premium on physical beauty, while many people have probably dreamed of being more beautiful, probably no one dreams of being disfigured.

CONCLUSION

The role of physical beauty in evolutionary theory suggests that beauty is more than skin deep. Beauty is marked not just by obvious physical features such as hair color and skin tone; rather, it is also marked by more subtle features such as facial and body symmetry, averageness, and body-size ratios, all of which serve as signals for reproductive potential. The intuitively pleasing sociocultural approaches to beauty also reveal some interesting things. We traced the changing trends in ideals of beauty represented in mass media figures and found that many of the current images of beauty are not only unrealistic and unattainable but also potentially unhealthy. The social psychological research on physical attractiveness suggests that not only do we think more positively about beautiful people, we also treat them more favorably in interpersonal situations across the lifespan. The construct of body image can be used to understand physical appearance concerns and our relentless pursuit of an improved body image through diet, exercise, cosmetics use, and cosmetic surgery. Finally, our discussion of beauty and society revealed that, in a world that places such a premium on beauty, we know very little about living with a disfigured appearance. While we continue to learn more about the nature of beauty, it is important for us to continue to learn about the difficulties and challenges of being disfigured.

REFERENCES

1. Buss DM. The Evolution of Desire: Strategies of Human Mating. New York: Basic Books, 1994.
2. Buss DM, Abbot M, Angleitner A, et al. International preferences in selecting mates: a study of 37 cultures. J Cross-Cultural Psychol 1990; 21:5-47.
3. Chen AC, German C, Zaidel DW. Brain asymmetry and facial attractiveness: facial beauty is not simply in the eye of the beholder. Neuropsychologica 1997; 35:471-476.
4. Singh D. Adaptive significance of female physical attractiveness: role of waist-to-hip ratio. J Pers Soc Psychol 1993; 65:456-466.
5. Langlois JH, Roggman LA, Casey RJ, et al. Infant preferences for attractive faces: rudiments of a stereotype? Dev Psychol 1987; 23: 363-369.
6. Langlois JH, Ritter JM, Roggman LA, Vaughn LS. Facial diversity and infant preferences for attractive faces. Dev Psychol 1991; 27: 79-84.
7. Langlois JH, Roggman LA, Reiser-Danner LA. Infants' differential social responses to attractive and unattractive faces. Dev Psychol 1990; 26:153-159.
8. Hamilton WD, Zuk M. Heritable true fitness and bright birds: a role for parasites? Science 1982; 218:384-387.
9. Gangestad SW, Buss DM. Pathogen prevalence and human mate preferences. Ethology Sociobiol 1993; 14:89-96.
10. Thornhill R, Gangestad SW. Human facial beauty: averageness, symmetry, and parasite resistance. Hum Nature 1993; 4:237-269.
11. Moller AP. Female swallow preferences for symmetrical male sexual ornaments. Nature 1992; 357:238-240.
12. Petrie M, Halliday TR, Sanders C. Peahens prefer peacocks with elaborate trains. Animal Behav 1991; 41:323-331.

13. Swaddle JP, Cuthill IC. Preference for symmetric males by female zebra finches. Nature 1994; 367:165-166.
14. Thornhill R. Fluctuating asymmetry and the mating system of the Japanese scorpionfly, Panorpa japonica. Animal Behav 1992; 44:867-879.
15. Gangestad S, Thornhill R, Yeo R. Facial attractiveness, developmental stability and fluctuating asymmetry. Ethology and Sociobiol 1994; 15:73-85.
16. Grammar K, Thornhill R. Human facial attractiveness and sexual selection: the role of symmetry and averageness. J Comp Psychol 1994; 108:233-242.
17. Rhodes G, Proffitt F, Grady JM, Sumich A. Facial symmetry and the perception of beauty. Psychonomic Bull and Rev 1998; 5:659-669.
18. Thornhill R, Gangestad SW. Human fluctuating asymmetry and sexual behavior. Psychol Sci 1994; 5:297-302.
19. Langlois JH, Roggman LA. Attractive faces are only average. Psychol Sci 1990; 1:115-121.
20. Langlois JH, Roggman LA, Mussleman L. What is average and what is not average about attractive faces? Psychol Sci 1994; 5: 214-220.
21. Mitton JB, Grant MC. Associations among protein heterozygosity, growth rate and developmental homeostasis. Anim Rev Ecology and Systematics 1984; 15:479-499.
22. Johnston VS, Franklin M. Is beauty in the eye of the beholder? Ethology and Sociobiol 1993; 14:183-199.
23. Alley TR, Cunningham MR. Averaged faces are attractive, but very attractive faces are not average. Psychol Sci 1991; 2:123-125.
24. Lanska DJ, Lanska MJ, Hartz AJ, Rimm AA. Factors influencing anatomical location of fat tissue in 52,953 women. Int J Obes 1985; 9:29-38.
25. Jones PR, Hunt MJ, Brown TP, Norgan NG. Waist-hip circumference ratio and its relation to age and overweight in British men. Hum Nutr Clin Nutr 1986; 40:239-247.
26. Singh D. Female judgement of male attractiveness and desirability for relationships: role of waist-to-hip ratio and financial status. J Pers Soc Psychol 1995; 69:1089-1101.
27. Kirschner MA, Samojilik E. Sex hormone metabolism in upper and lower body obesity. Int J Obes 1991; 15:101-108.
28. Leibel DJ, Edens NK, Fried SK. Physiologic basis for the control of body fat distribution in humans. Annu Rev Nutr 1989; 9:417-443.
29. Symons D. The Evolution of Human Sexuality. New York: Oxford University Press, 1979.
30. Zebrowitz LA, Olson K, Hoffman K. Stability of babyfaceness and attractiveness across the lifespan. J Pers Soc Psychol 1993; 65: 453-466.
31. McLellan B, McKelvie SJ. Effects of age and gender on perceived facial attractiveness. Can J Behav Sci 1993; 25:135-142.
32. Deutsch FM, Zalenski CM, Clark ME. Is there a double standard of aging? J Appl Soc Psychol 1986; 16:771-785.
33. Cunningham MR. Measuring the physical in physical attractiveness: quasi-experiments on the sociobiology of female facial beauty. J Pers Soc Psychol 1986; 50:925-935.
34. Jones D. Physical Attractiveness and the Theory of Sexual Selection. Ann Arbor: Museum of Anthropology, University of Michigan, 1996.
35. Jones D. An evolutionary perspective on physical attractiveness. Evol Anthropol 1996; 5:97-109.
36. Mazur A. U.S. trends in feminine beauty and overadaption. J Sex Res 1986; 22(3):281-303.
37. Fallon A. Culture in the mirror: sociocultural determinants of body image. In: Cash TF, Pruzinsky T, eds. Body Images: Development, Deviance and Change. New York: Guilford Press, 1990: 80-109.
38. Morris A, Cooper T, Cooper PJ. The changing shape of female fashion models. Int J Eat Disord 1989; 8:593-596.
39. Silverstein B, Perdue L, Peterson B, Kelly E. The role of the mass media in promoting a thin standard of bodily attractiveness for women. Sex Roles 1986; 14:519-532.
40. Guillen EO, Barr SI. Nutrition, dieting, and fitness messages in a magazine for adolescent women, 1970-1990. J Adolesc Health 1994; 15:464-472.
41. Garner DM, Garfinkel PE, Schwartz D. Cultural expectations of thinness in women. Psychol Rep 1980; 47:483-491.
42. Wiseman CV, Gray J, Mosimann JE, Aherns AH. Cultural expectations of thinness in women: an update. Int J Eat Disord 1992; 11: 85-89.
43. Thakerar JN, Iwawaki S. Cross-cultural comparisons in interpersonal attraction of females toward males. J Soc Psychol 1979; 108: 121-122.
44. Cunningham MR, Roberts AR, Barbee AP, et al. "Their ideals of beauty are, on the whole, the same as ours": consistency and variability in the cross-cultural perception of female physical attractiveness. J Pers Soc Psychol 1995; 68:261-279.
45. Wolf N. The Beauty Myth. New York: Morrow, 1991.
46. Sappho. Fragments 101. In: Poems and Fragments. Translation with an introduction by G. Davenport. Ann Arbor: University of Michigan Press, 1965.
47. Dion K, Berscheid E, Hatfield E. What is beautiful is good. J Pers Soc Psychol 1972; 24:285-290.
48. Adams GR. Racial membership and physical attractiveness effects on preschool teachers' expectations. Child Study J 1978; 8: 29-41.
49. Clifford MM, Hatfield E. Research note: the effects of physical attractiveness on teacher expectations. Sociol Educ 1973; 46:248-258.
50. Dipboye RL, Fromkin HL, Wiback K. Relative importance of applicant sex, attractiveness, and scholastic standing in evaluation of job applicant resumes. J Appl Psychol 1975; 60:39-43.
51. Schofield W. Psychotherapy: The Purchase of Friendship. Englewood Cliffs, NJ: Prentice Hall, 1964.
52. Cash TF, Begley PJ, McCown DA, Weise BC. When counselors are heard but not seen: initial impact of physical attractiveness. J Counseling Psychol 1975; 22:273-279.
53. Cash TF, Kehr J. Influence of nonprofessional counselors' physical attractiveness and sex on perceptions of counselor behavior. J Counseling Psychol 1977; 25:336-342.
54. Hatfield E, Sprecher S. Mirror, Mirror . . . The Importance of Looks in Everyday Life. Albany: SUNY Press, 1986.
55. Sigall H, Ostrove N. Beautiful but dangerous: effects of offender attractiveness and nature of the crime on juridic judgment. J Pers Soc Psychol 1975; 31:410-414.
56. Benson PL, Karabenick SA, Lerner RM. Pretty pleases: the effects of physical attractiveness, race, and sex on receiving help. J Exp Soc Psychol 1976; 12:409-415.
57. Wilson DW. Helping behavior and physical attractiveness. J Soc Psychol 1978; 104:313-314.
58. Thompson JK, Heinberg LJ, Altabe M, Tantloff-Dunn S. Exacting Beauty: Theory, Assessment and Treatment of Body Image Disturbance. Washington, DC: American Psychological Association, 1999:19-47.
59. Sarwer DB, Pertschuk MJ, Wadden TA, Whitaker LA. Psychological investigations of cosmetic surgery patients: a look back and a look ahead. Plast Reconstr Surg 1998; 101:1136-1142.
60 Sarwer DB, Wadden TA, Pertschuk MJ, Whitaker LA. The psychology of cosmetic surgery: a review and reconceptualization. Clin Psychol Rev 1998; 18:1-22.
61. Garner DM. The 1997 body image survey results. Psychol Today 1997; 31:30-87.
62. Johnson CA. Bound by culture. In: Self-esteem Comes in All Sizes. New York: Doubleday, 1995:37-53.
63. Serdula MK, Collins E, Williamson DF, et al. Weight control practices of U.S. adolescents and adults. Ann Int Med 1993; 119:667-671.

64. Whitaker AH. An epidemiological study of anorectic and bulimic symptoms in adolescent girls: implications for pediatricians. Pediatr Ann 1992; 21:752-759.
65. Rosen JC, Gross J. Prevalence of weight reducing and weight gaining in adolescent girls and boys. Health Psychol 1987; 26:131-147.
66. Schreiber GB, Robins M, Striegel-Moore R, et al. Weight modification efforts reported by black and white preadolescent girls: national heart, lung, and blood institute growth health study. Pediatrics 1996; 98:63-70.
67. Levy AS, Heaton AW. Weight control practices of US adults trying to lose weight. Ann Intern Med 1993; 119:661-666.
68. Cash TF, Novy PL, Grant JR. Why do women exercise? Factor analysis and further validation of the reasons for exercise inventory. Percept Mot Skills 1994; 78:539-544.
69. Peiss K. Hope in a Jar: The Making of America's Beauty Culture. New York: Metropolitan Books, 1998.
70. Department of Commerce, Bureau of Economic Statistics, sections: toilet articles and preparation, clothing and shoes. In: Survey of Current Business, April 1995.
71. Pertschuk MJ, Sarwer DB, Wadden TA, Whitaker LA. Body image dissatisfaction in male cosmetic surgery patients. Aesthetic Plast Surg 1998; 22:20-24.
72. Sarwer DB, Wadden TA, Pertschuk MJ, Whitaker LA. Body image dissatisfaction and body dysmorphic disorder in 100 cosmetic surgery patients. Plast Reconstr Surg 1998; 101:1644-1649.

CHAPTER 6

Psychosocial Issues and Their Relevance to the Cosmetic Surgery Patient

TED A. GROSSBART
DAVID B. SARWER

Psychosocial issues permeate the field of cosmetic surgery:

- The preoperative psychological profile of cosmetic surgery patients is likely to differ from that of people who don't come for surgery. Despite several decades of research, this difference is not well understood.
- Cosmetic surgery patients often look for more than changes in their physical appearance. If these procedures do not lead to improvements in body satisfaction, self-esteem, or quality of life, then what is their purpose?
- Patient-surgeon rapport is not simply a nice plus if it happens. Patient satisfaction, reduced legal liability, and improved surgical outcome can all be direct reflections of the surgeon's mastery of relationship-building techniques.
- Identifying and screening out patients who should not have cosmetic surgery can prevent both patient and surgeon frustration and more extreme adverse outcomes.
- A wide range of studies document the use of psychological techniques to improve surgical outcome.

Increasing numbers of physicians from a variety of specialties, and nonphysicians as well, now perform cosmetic surgery. For example, the American Society of Plastic and Reconstructive Surgeons reported that its membership performed over 1 million cosmetic procedures in 1998. These numbers represent an increase of 50% since 1996 and 153% since 1992.[1]

This increasing demand for cosmetic surgery has been accompanied by greater coverage of procedures in the mass media. Stories on cosmetic surgery regularly appear on daytime talk shows and evening news magazine programs. Newspaper and magazine articles on cosmetic surgery typically highlight recent innovations in cosmetic procedures while tapping the readers' or viewers' dissatisfaction with their physical appearance. Color advertisements featuring beautiful models often promise improvement in physical appearance, self-esteem, and quality of life. As the demand for cosmetic surgery continues to grow, it becomes increasingly important to understand the psychological factors that motivate people to seek surgery and to determine if cosmetic surgery leads to psychological benefit.

WHO COMES FOR COSMETIC SURGERY?

The accelerating growth in both the number of procedures performed and the number of physicians performing them reflects the American public's rapidly growing acceptance of cosmetic surgery as a means of self-improvement.[2] Stereotypes endure. Cosmetic surgery patients are cast as jet-setters with more money than taste or judgment, relentlessly trying to polish their exteriors because there isn't much going on in their interiors. Other common clichés are "neurotic narcissists searching for the Fountain of Youth" or "relentless improvers" frantically obsessed with minor flaws, perfectionistically motivated to wear the latest fashions and hair styles, running to the gym, the tanning parlor, and the cosmetic surgeon. Do these stereotypes of narcissistic or perfectionistic patients accurately represent the majority of cosmetic surgery patients?

A collaboration of psychiatrists and plastic surgeons at Johns Hopkins in the 1950s and 1960s produced the first significant body of research on the psychological functioning of cosmetic surgery patients. For the most part, these studies relied on clinical interviews of patients conducted by psychoanalytically trained psychiatrists. Regardless of the type of surgical procedure,

Portions of this chapter appeared in Grossbart TA, Sarwer DB. Cosmetic surgery: surgical tools—psychosocial goals. Semin Cutan Med Surg 1999; 18(2):101-111.

the majority of patients were seen as having significant psychopathology.[3-5] The most common diagnoses were personality disorders, with smaller percentages (10% to 20%) of patients being characterized as neurotic or psychotic.[3,6,7]

In one example, a study of 72 patients seeking face lifts or blepharoplasty to remove signs of aging showed intriguing consistencies according to age. The 29- to 39-year-old group had more childhood disturbance, more difficulty assuming parental roles, and more strained relationships with their own parents. The 40- to 50-year-olds were intensely committed to their work lives and sought occupational advantages from a more youthful appearance. Their personal relationships were given less priority. In the over-50 group, 90% had lost close relatives within 5 years, and many showed symptoms of unresolved grief reactions. Their desire to mask the warded-off sadness went beyond trying to act perky and upbeat. Some were explicit about the hope that the surgery would remove the physical signs of the sadness.[7]

During the 1970s, other interview research also found high rates of psychopathology. Prospective patients in several studies were described as experiencing increased symptoms of depression and anxiety, as well as low self-esteem.[8-10] Although these interview studies have been consistent in their outcomes, they typically have suffered from significant methodological problems. The majority have lacked both uniform diagnostic criteria and control or comparison groups. Therefore it is impossible to determine if the reported level of psychological disturbance is greater than that found in the general population or in other medical patients.[11,12] While these studies do not give us an overall picture of the cosmetic surgery population, their findings may help us understand some cosmetic surgery patients' individual issues.

In contrast with the interview investigations, most studies that have used standardized paper and pencil psychometric tests have found dramatically less psychopathology. Female rhinoplasty, rhytidectomy, and breast augmentation patients reported few symptoms of psychopathology.[13-18] Although these psychometric investigations present a more favorable view of cosmetic surgery patients, they also have significant methodological problems. Some studies used only postoperative assessments and others failed to use control groups or made comparisons only to normative groups, limiting the conclusions that can be drawn from them.[11,12]

This contradictory research makes it difficult to draw firm conclusions about the psychological status of cosmetic surgery patients.[11,12] Initial interview-based studies suggested that cosmetic surgery patients are highly psychopathological. In contrast, studies that have used valid and reliable (but, some might argue, more superficial) psychometric measures have found little psychopathology. Both sets of studies, however, have suffered from a myriad of methodological problems. The shifting characteristics of the cosmetic surgery population over time could result in more of the earlier studies having found significant psychopathology.

Studies suggesting that the majority of cosmetic surgery patients have little psychopathology are more consistent with the experiences of the present-day cosmetic surgeon. But to accept that people who undergo cosmetic surgery are no different from those who do not seek surgery does not make intuitive sense.[11] Although the popularity of cosmetic surgery is increasing rapidly, only a small percentage of people currently seek surgery. This suggests that there must be personality characteristics that differentiate those who seek cosmetic surgery from those who do not. The most distinguishing characteristics of people who seek surgery are likely to be aspects of their thoughts and feelings about their physical appearance. Obviously, men and women seek cosmetic surgery because they are not satisfied with an aspect of their appearance. Deeper understanding of this dissatisfaction may help in defining these individuals.[11,12] Another possible differentiator is being "action oriented." Assuming equal dissatisfaction, one person frets, another calls the cosmetic surgeon.

BODY DISSATISFACTION AND COSMETIC SURGERY

Fifty-six percent of American women and 43% of American men report dissatisfaction with their overall appearance.[19] This epidemic of dissatisfaction probably motivates many behaviors—weight loss, exercise, cosmetic use, and cosmetic surgery. Do prospective cosmetic surgery patients' body concerns differ from the general population? The research results fall into two groups. The most consistent finding is that women who seek cosmetic surgery report increased dissatisfaction with their bodies[8,13,16,17] and report improvements in body evaluation postoperatively.[10,13,16,20]

In contrast, other studies examined this dissatisfaction in more detail, finding that prospective patients (across a range of procedures) did not report a greater investment nor increased dissatisfaction with their overall body. Yet they did report heightened dissatisfaction with the specific body feature for which they were pursuing surgery.[11,12,21,22]

Studies of breast augmentation patients using physically similar women as controls suggest that not only do these women have greater dissatisfaction with their breasts, they also have greater investment and overall dissatisfaction with their bodies, as well as a history of more appearance-related teasing.[21,23] The breast augmentation patients also report increased symptoms of both anxiety and depression. We don't know if these symptoms are a cause or a result of their dissatisfaction with their breasts. The pursuit of cosmetic surgery to address body dissatisfaction may be an adaptive coping strategy in a culture that emphasizes the importance of physical appearance. However, these findings suggest that we should be asking if, for some patients, body dissatisfaction may be related to general psychopathology more appropriately addressed by psychotherapy than cosmetic surgery. This research also underscores the importance of listening carefully to prospective patients' need and hopes, which often go well beyond the requested physical changes.

WHAT DO COSMETIC SURGERY PATIENTS WANT?

Cosmetic surgery may produce other results, patients may have other agendas, but let's begin with the top priority: increasing physical beauty or attractiveness.*

Chapter 5 examines the wide range of forces that sculpt our views of beauty—as an experience, a commodity, and as an evolutionary imperative. Media images, social forces, peer reactions, and spousal or family pressures often influence patients' estimates of their attractiveness. The aggregate of these influences becomes the patients' view of themselves. The motivation for surgery can be largely *external.* Ethnic prejudice or fear of age discrimination alone may motivate surgery that would otherwise be of no interest. In extreme instances the patients may have been coerced into surgery, asking the surgeon to turn them into a spouse's, a parent's, or a boss's vision of what they should look like. Patients are also typically very receptive to the surgeon's professional evaluation of their presurgical appearance. At an extreme, the surgeon may feel pressure to prescribe procedures to a patient who is unable to present his or her own preferences. More typically the patient's motivation is *internal,* and we will focus on these cases. Ideally, the patient has flexibly chosen which external influences to heed and integrate with his or her own desires, culminating in the decision to seek surgery. While a spouse's, friend's, or parent's feedback may be quite influential, the patient's own evaluation of postsurgical appearance is rightfully the ultimate yardstick or outcome measure.

What is the scientific status of patients' judgments of their own attractiveness? What of their reliability, their validity? On the surface, what could be more straightforward? The patient says, "I look better than I have in years," or "I have the thighs (or nose, or breasts) that I've always wanted." If the feeling endures, this self-report measure seems both reliable and sensible. Who would presume to argue with it?

How much overlap would you expect between peoples' own views of their appearance and ratings of a more objective "jury of their peers"—80%? 60%? In fact, multiple studies suggest that normal human beings have so little awareness of their own attractiveness that we must regard the inner and the outer realities as two almost completely disconnected entities.

Feingold's meta-analysis of 93 studies of self-ratings of attractiveness vs. objective measures found correlations of .24 for men and .25 for women.[25] This means that just over 6% of our view of our appearance is predictable from our actual appearance, and that 94% is accounted for by other factors! (This 6%+ figure comes from squaring the correlation coefficient to calculate the percentage of variance accounted for.)[26] We know that some patients, especially those with body dysmorphic disorder (discussed later) present with striking and poignant discrepancies between their experience of their own attractiveness and how the rest of us see them, but these 93 studies were all of normal people, mostly college students. (One could question labeling a cross-section of American college students as normal adults.)

These figures dramatically underscore how radically different cosmetic surgery is from most other medical specialties. We could hardly imagine a drug study, new procedure, or intervention being measured by a yardstick that was 6% accurate. Do we need more objective measures of cosmetic surgery outcomes? Most likely, the pursuit of objective aesthetic standards would lead us down an absurd path. Imagine a surgeon's postoperative discussion with a patient if such measures were used:

> Mrs. Jones, I'm terribly sorry that you are unhappy with the results of your surgery, and I fully understand that you are convinced you look less attractive than before I operated. I am very concerned about this outcome. I have called in both a panel of beauty experts and a group of your peers to help us in this difficult situation. They both agree that my surgery made you look *more* attractive. This is objective, statistically valid data, gathered according to every accepted scientific procedure. Clearly you are mistaken.

While this might be an effective defense if Mrs. Jones sought legal redress, and might effectively intimidate her into going away, her inner reality has not been addressed. Assuming no issues of mental competence, we cannot dismiss her view. Beauty is in the eye of the beholder—but when the beholder is also the beheld, we cannot escape a conclusion with wide implications. Patients come to the cosmetic surgeon seeking an objective enhancement of attractiveness; but they measure the success of the surgery by the inner experience of feeling more physically attractive, and this experience has a minimal relationship to the objective reality.

*We will use beauty and attractiveness interchangeably, but clearly one can be beautiful but unattractive, or not particularly beautiful but very attractive. This discussion will be limited to the types of beauty and physical attractiveness that are "skin deep."[24]

What keeps the extreme disparity between perceived and actual attractiveness from being more troublesome in daily clinical practice? The studies deal with global assessments at one point in time. Surgery patients are presumably more focused on a specific body part and its presurgical vs. postsurgical appearance. When they seek outside feedback from the surgeon, spouse, or friends (all of whom are likely to be favorably predisposed), the focus is similarly on the specific part and the change because of the surgery.

If the inner experience of being more or less beautiful is not a natural consequence of external physical reality, what does it reflect? In the meta-analysis, three dimensions were consistently linked to self-judged attractiveness: self-esteem, emotional stability, and dominance. Note that these three dimensions were not linked to outside judgments of physical attractiveness. Social skill levels and freedom from social self-consciousness were related to the outside measure but not to self-ratings. Both measures correlated with freedom from loneliness, opposite-sex popularity, and sexual experience.[25]

WHY DO PATIENTS WANT THE CHANGES THEY ARE SEEKING?

The desire for thinner thighs or smoother skin may seem so self-evident that asking "why?" could easily seem superfluous. In a previous paper[27] we conceptualized cosmetic surgery as "the use of surgical procedures, in the absence of disease or physical trauma, to alter the physical appearance of the body in pursuit of psychosocial benefit." We hypothesized that improvement in physical appearance is only part of the motivation for cosmetic surgery. These changes, though central, are a means to other psychological goals. Patient satisfaction is, ultimately, a direct reflection of the degree to which the surgery has met the patient's expectations of the costs (physical, emotional, and financial) and benefits (physical and psychosocial) of the procedure. Determination of a "successful" surgical result can be influenced by a variety of factors that may never become apparent to the surgeon.

Physicians and staff routinely help patients shape their expectations of the physical impact of surgery. Helping patients articulate and refine psychosocial goals is a less familiar process. Individual objectives vary but frequently share an origin in recurrent painful feelings, thoughts, or experiences. Helping patients establish realistic psychosocial expectations is as essential to patient satisfaction as having realistic physical expectations. Patients may present with a variety of agendas:

1. *Psychological Agendas:* Is the patient seeking surgery as a means to improve emotional state, to diminish feelings of appearance-focused depression, shame, social anxiety, or unlovability? Other patients are motivated by ideas like, "People are put off by my nose," or "I am really so much younger than I look."
2. *Interpersonal Agendas:* Is the patient hoping surgery will improve some aspect of a close relationship? Patients often hope that surgery will rekindle a present relationship or save a marriage, or that improving their appearance will facilitate future relationships.
3. *Social Agendas:* Goals that focus on the larger society may center on employability or perceived suitability for promotion. The desire to be perceived as an individual rather than a member of a specific stereotyped age, ethnic, or other group is best spelled out explicitly whenever possible.

The experience of teamwork and collaboration between patient and surgeon is difficult if the surgeon is not attuned to the patient's deeper motivation for undertaking the procedure.[27]

DOES COSMETIC SURGERY PRODUCE PSYCHOLOGICAL BENEFITS?

The psychosocial impact of cosmetic surgery may be the most central question in the field. If these procedures do not lead to improvements in body image, self-esteem, and quality of life, then what is their purpose? The majority of clinical interview investigations, surveys, and anecdotal reports strongly indicate high levels of patient satisfaction and generally favorable psychological outcomes, including improvements in depression and anxiety.[9,28]

Studies using standardized tests, however, have found very mixed results. Four found favorable changes postoperatively,[15,16,29,30] three reported no change,[18,31,32] and two described a modest increase in depressive symptoms.[14,33]

Preliminary studies suggest that many patients experience postoperative improvements in body image.[22,34] While these results are encouraging, considering the postoperative literature as a whole, it is premature to confidently conclude that cosmetic surgery leads to psychological benefit in the majority of patients.[12,23,27,35]

PSYCHOLOGICAL CONTRAINDICATIONS: ARE THERE CLEAR DANGER SIGNS?

Given the increasing numbers of individuals who now pursue cosmetic surgery, it is likely that all of the major psychiatric diagnoses occur in this population. However, certain disorders, particularly those with a body image component, may be more prevalent in cosmetic surgery patients and may contraindicate surgery. These disorders include body dysmorphic disorder, thought disorders, and eating disorders.

Body Dysmorphic Disorder

Extreme body image dissatisfaction is a central component of body dysmorphic disorder (BDD). BDD is defined as a preoccupation with an imagined or slight defect in appearance that leads to significant impairment in functioning.[36] Any area of the body may be the focus of concern; the skin, hair, and nose are the most common targets.[37,38] BDD has several characteristics that distinguish it from more normal body dissatisfaction. Persons with BDD are often so preoccupied with some aspect of their appearance that they will examine, check, or alter their appearance repeatedly. These activities can totally consume waking life, preventing holding a job or maintaining romantic and social relationships. Often all pain in the person's past and present life is attributed to the physical defect.

Cosmetic surgery or other medical treatments may feel like the only salvation. Phillips and Diaz[38] reported that in a sample of 93 women with BDD, 73% sought and 66% received nonpsychiatric treatments including plastic surgery and dermatologic care. A study of women who sought cosmetic surgery found that 7% met diagnostic criteria for BDD,[39] a prevalence greater than the 2% prevalence thought to exist in the general population. BDD, however, may be particularly difficult to diagnose in cosmetic surgery patients.[35,39] Given the newness of BDD to American psychiatry (it was first introduced in *DSM-III-R* in 1987), many cosmetic surgeons are unfamiliar with the diagnosis. In addition, an objective of cosmetic surgery—to improve the appearance of a person with a "normal" appearance—may make diagnosis difficult. Cosmetic surgery patients frequently seek to improve slight defects in their appearance that are frequently judged as observable and correctable by the surgeon. As a result, judgment of a defect as "slight" becomes highly subjective. We have suggested that the degree of emotional distress and behavioral impairment, rather than the size or nature of the physical defect, may be more accurate indicators of BDD in plastic surgery patients.[23,39]

Preliminary clinical reports have found that the vast majority of patients with BDD do not benefit from cosmetic surgery if the underlying emotional issues are not addressed.[37,38] Following surgery, they often remain focused on the same feature or become focused on a different feature. There is also some concern that these individuals may become violent toward themselves or the surgeon. These reports suggest that BDD may contraindicate cosmetic surgery.[23,27,35]

Psychotic Disorders

Cosmetic surgery patients with schizophrenia and other psychotic disorders have been of particular interest to cosmetic surgeons. Like patients with BDD, cosmetic surgeons frequently fear that individuals with psychotic disorders are likely to threaten or become violent following unsuccessful cosmetic surgery. The presence of an active psychotic disorder is commonly thought to contraindicate cosmetic surgery.[23,35,39]

Edgerton and colleagues have made a case against screening out patients with significant psychopathology, as long as appropriate mental health care precedes or is integrated with the surgery.[40] They report successful outcomes using a combined approach for the treatment of patients who are the most psychologically disturbed, with diagnoses including severe neurosis, character pathology, and psychosis. (Some of these patients appear to be similar to those today diagnosed with BDD.) Initial indicators of disturbance included "extreme intensity of desire for surgery, major disruption in psychological or social functioning, exaggerated response to deformity, request for 'unusual' type of surgery, or major difficulties in communicating with the surgeon." Significantly, 60.9% had a history of previous surgery elsewhere that had left them unsatisfied. Typically, patients received an initial evaluation and a brief course of psychotherapy focusing on feelings of deformity. More extended evaluations, medication, and psychotherapy were available as necessary. Of the 87 who received an average of 3.7 varying surgical procedures each, 82.8% reported clear psychological benefit, including reduced self-consciousness, anxiety, depression, and social isolation. There were no lawsuits, suicides, or psychotic decompensations within this sample of patients. This clinical report lacks many of the attributes of a research study, including standardized diagnoses and procedures, control groups, and more objective and blind outcome measures. We have no indication of the relative impact of the psychological interventions without surgery. Yet this impressive "real world" experience suggests that many patients who might be poor candidates for surgery alone can receive lasting psychological benefits from combined surgical-psychological intervention.

Eating Disorders

Given the extreme body image concerns of people with anorexia and bulimia, these disorders may be disproportionately represented among cosmetic surgery patients. There are case reports of women with both disorders who have experienced an exacerbation of symptoms following both face and body procedures.[41,42] Eating disorders may be a particular concern for women interested in liposuction and breast augmentation surgery. Willard and colleagues[43] described two cases of women with bulimia who underwent liposuction in an attempt to lose weight, only to experience an exacerbation of their bulimic symptoms postoperatively. Breast augmentation patients are frequently of below average weight, leading to speculation that they are at risk for eating disorders.[21,33] Both anorexia and bulimia may be potential contraindications to cosmetic surgery.

PSYCHOSOCIAL DETERMINANTS OF SURGICAL OUTCOME

A substantial literature documents the impact of psychological variables and interventions on surgical outcome across a wide range of procedures. Observational studies of pain level and wound healing time suggest that highly anxious patients experience increased pain, require more anesthesia, have longer hospital stays, and comply more poorly with postoperative instructions. Two hundred studies of interventions addressing surgical patients' psychological needs document more rapid physical recovery, decreased anxiety, reduced hospital stays, fewer postoperative complications, increased compliance, and reduced pain and need for pain medication.[44] Multiple meta-analyses found that a wide range of interventions were effective, including education, coping skills training, relaxation, and hypnotic, behavioral, cognitive, and emotionally focused techniques. Many different formats were effective, including individual and group administration, audiotapes, videotapes, and printed materials. With very modest interventions, 79% to 84% of studies showed significantly reduced pain, psychological distress, and improvements in relevant indexes of recovery. Typical rates of improvement ranged from 20% to 28%.[45-47]

Is it fair to generalize from studies of major surgery to more typical outpatient cosmetic procedures? Studies of the effect of emotional state on healing of more minor wounds suggest that it is. Family members who care for a relative with Alzheimer's disease demonstrate poorer immune function than well-matched controls. These caretakers took an average of 9 days or 24% longer to completely heal a small standardized wound.[48] Wikesjo and colleagues found wound healing in dental students during summer vacation, a time of minimal emotional stress, was 40% faster than 3 days before a major exam.[49]

SPECIAL CONCERNS FOR AGING PATIENTS

With many cosmetic procedures targeting the effects of aging throughout the life span, we must look especially carefully at the effects of psychosocial variables on surgical recovery later in the life span. The increasing risk of surgery with age is probably due in part to declining immune function increasing the risk of infectious complications, which in turn increase surgical mortality.[44] At least one study addressed the interplay between increased surgical risk from both aging and anxiety. Not surprisingly, in a sample of elective hernia repair patients, the patients who were both older and highly anxious had less favorable outcomes.[50] It is not clear if physiologic aging produces unique vulnerability to anxiety, or anxiety uniquely contributes to heightened risks from aging, or if this group simply had the additive impact of the two risk factors.

DOES THE PATIENT-SURGEON RELATIONSHIP INFLUENCE SURGICAL SUCCESS?

What is the medical and psychological impact of the rapport between patient and cosmetic surgeon? We have little data on this important question, but at least one study found a significant link between the surgeon's emotional reaction to the patient and the postoperative course in 50 female face lift patients.[51]

A survey of 115 experienced cosmetic surgeons found that nearly half had been sued for malpractice. Of this group, 51.6% attributed the suit to lack of rapport (vs. 17% for the next highest cause: unrealistic expectations), and only 14.5% attributed the suit to poor surgical results.[52] We can easily imagine these results being skewed by the fact that a surgeon filling out a survey would be much more likely to confess poor relationship skills than botched surgical results. Poor surgeon-patient relationships may well independently reduce surgical success and set the stage for litigation. The surgeon who does not successfully build rapport with patients heightens both medical and legal risks.

BETTER THAN WELL: MORAL AND ETHICAL ISSUES IN COSMETIC SURGERY

World War I trench warfare produced unprecedented numbers of soldiers with massive facial trauma. The "first generation" of plastic surgeons who came to their aid were able to develop their craft in a morally unambiguous, even heroic, context.[53] Seeds of many of the controversies that were to face surgeons for decades to come originated when they brought their skills back to civilian life. In 1916, surgeon John Staige Davis declared, "True plastic surgery, without question . . . is absolutely distinct and separate from what is known as cosmetic or decorative surgery."[54] As late as 1958, Pope Pius XII cautioned that although cosmetic surgery had many legitimate uses, using surgery to increase the "powers of seduction, thus leading others more easily into sin . . . or to satisfy vanity or the caprice of fashion" was morally unlawful.[55]

Performing medical procedures in the absence of undisputed pathology and measuring outcomes by aesthetics or patient satisfaction raises complex ethical issues. Ringel[56] provocatively revisits some of these ethical quandaries that have made regular appearances in the history of cosmetic surgery (she limits her case to aging skin, but most of her arguments are directly exportable to any alteration of physical features that do not fit the prevailing societal notion of beauty). Assuming that the essence of medicine is to promote health and healing, Ringel examines three attempts to bring the treatment of aging skin into this framework.

1. Define skin aging as illness: "Treatment of the aging face" is then on a par with treatment of any other disorder. The historical parallel with cosmetic surgeons of the early 1930s creating pseudomedical entities like "hook nose" is clear. Once a condition is designated pathological, all moral ambiguities vanish. But Ringel suggests that, "in defining aging as an illness, we implicitly define life as an illness." She suggests that surgeons have a responsibility to fight ageism, the stigma of old age, and the incessant media image that the elderly must be "sick, jaded, and spent."
2. Define the treated disease as low self-esteem that is triggered by the physical feature: This view permits the surgeon to proceed with moral clarity, performing a sort of surgical psychotherapy. (Surgical treatment of a so-called inferiority complex is the historical analog here).[53] But Ringel counters, "The self who benefits from cosmetic surgery is necessarily an impostor. Cosmetic surgeons are in the business not of enhancing who we are, but of replacing who we are with who we or they think we should be. The prescription for low self-esteem is to change the packaging rather than the package, to get a new look rather than a new awareness." She concludes, "Cosmetic surgery cannot have it both ways. If a request for cosmetic surgery implies a significant psychiatric illness, the illness should be evaluated and treated."
3. Redefine the goal of medicine as patient satisfaction or happiness rather than promotion of health and healing: Ringel suggests that this model is dubious and inevitably reduces cosmetic surgeons to "technical entrepreneurs," little different from cosmetologists. If a patient wants decorative scars on the face, removal of a healthy organ, or, even as technology permits, one might add, a second head or a bionic arm, that would be a matter between patient and surgeon alone. She makes the case that what separates the professional from the businessperson is the "willingness to use clinical judgment on behalf of the welfare of patients."

She concludes, "Perhaps physicians cannot change society's preoccupation with physical appearance, but they need not promote it."

Replies to this provocative challenge were also direct and spirited, including the observation that our beauty standards have a likely evolutionary basis (see Chapter 5) rather than being more arbitrary societal or personal whims. The article triggered vigorous defenses of the legitimacy of wanting to look one's best during an increasing life span, either for personal reasons or to avoid the impact of social discrimination, ageism, or ethnic bias. Several respondents made the case that photoaged skin is damaged and at risk. "Degenerative joint disease, dementia, and osteoporosis are all natural consequences of aging in the predisposed population. Would Ringel have us simply accept this type of degeneration and not offer treatment for these disorders?"[57] Body piercing and tattooing underscore individuals' right to decide the fate of their own bodies as a fundamental democratic value.

Glogau counters (and data quoted in his paper support), "it is self-esteem that leads many of our patients to seek help for their photodamage." He suggests patients' motivation, "is not that they want to look young but that they do not look the way that they feel." He also notes that medical decision making is now "patient centered rather than physician centered, . . . so it is for the physician to provide information, the patient to wrestle with the practical and moral dilemmas." He concludes, "there is nothing wrong with the pursuit of happiness as a goal of professional medicine. Should misery be the goal instead?"[58]

This debate has parallels in other fields of medicine. Cosmetic surgery is not unique in grappling with the application of medical procedures in the absence of pathology. Psychiatry struggles with the use of psychotropic drugs to make people "better than well." Prozac for people who don't meet the criteria for clinical depression or Ritalin to enhance performance in patients who really could not be diagnosed with attention deficit disorder raises many of the same ethical issues.

Genetics has its own version of this discussion, as the morality of Nobel prize winner sperm banks stimulates debate. In the fall of 1999 an on-line auction of eggs from medically screened California models began. The bidding began at $15,000, up to a maximum of $150,000. A spokesman for the American Society of Reproductive Medicine states, "It's unethical and distasteful," but is anyone listening?[59]

ADOLESCENT COSMETIC SURGERY

Adolescent cosmetic surgery is a frequent, and often controversial, mass media topic. Over the course of several weeks, one of us (DBS) saw stories on teens and cosmetic surgery on two major television magazines. It was a central feature of an article on cosmetic surgery in *Newsweek* during the summer of 1999. Each of these stories debated the appropriateness of cosmetic surgery on adolescents whose bodies have not reached physical maturity. An equally important issue is the potential effects of surgery on the developing body image. Adolescents' thoughts and feelings about their ap-

PART II

ANESTHESIA

CHAPTER 7

Regional Anesthesia for Aesthetic Surgery

JOHN BRAMHALL

SECTION ONE

History and Scientific Review

BACKGROUND AND HISTORY

What we now refer to as aesthetic or cosmetic surgery was not commonly practiced until the advent of effective, reliable, and safe anesthetic techniques. The extensive use of tattooing, scarring, piercing, and other emblematic surgical interventions across a wide variety of cultures, generally without any attempt at pain control, is perhaps testimony to the strong and pervasive social motivation underlying attempts at manipulation of body image. Nevertheless, except under the most compelling motivating circumstances, people are generally reluctant to submit to excruciatingly painful life-enhancing (in contrast to life-sustaining) surgical procedures without some form of functional, safe analgesia.

As recently as the early 1940s mortality attributable to the effects of general anesthesia could be as high as 1:1000—even in the United States, and few rational physicians would expose patients to such risk unless the perceived gains were large enough to balance the equation. As a consequence of this insecurity surrounding general anesthesia, throughout the first half of the twentieth century there was considerable emphasis placed on, and expertise developed in, alternative strategies for painless elective surgery, in particular techniques for selectively anesthetizing specific, isolated anatomic regions. The term *regional anesthesia* was formally introduced by Harvey Cushing in 1901 when describing pain relief by the use of nerve block. The risk of mortality and major morbidity associated with these approaches was considered to be vastly lower than that associated with general anesthesia, and there was a great deal of enthusiasm among surgeons for the development of specific sensory nerve blocks of every conceivable anatomic structure.

Modern techniques of local anesthesia derive from the use of cocaine for nerve blocks. Cocaine, introduced into medical practice in 1884 when Carl Koller of Vienna used it for topical analgesia of the eye, was subsequently used for infiltration analgesia of the upper extremity by Halsted and Hall in New York in the 1880s. In early practice the skin was anesthetized with cocaine, the trunks of the brachial plexus were dissected out, and then each was individually anesthetized. By 1899, Barker had introduced infiltration analgesia using needle injection. (The hypodermic needle was described by Rynd in 1845 and popularized by Alexander Wood of Edinburgh, who also devised an effective syringe in 1855.)

Substitutes for cocaine were sought actively because of the addictive potential and toxicity of cocaine. (Halsted became addicted, presumably as a result of acting as his own guinea pig during his evaluations of the new drug.) Several synthetic agents were developed around the end of the nineteenth century, including procaine, which was synthesized by Einhorn in 1904. Tetracaine was synthesized in 1931 and lidocaine in 1943, although it was not put to clinical use until 1948. Regional anesthesia performed by surgeons at that time obviated the need for an individual dedicated to administering inhalational anesthesia and eliminated the consequences of toxic effects of agents such as ether, ethyl chloride, cyclopropane, and chloroform. Robert Macintosh, in the forward to Winnie's text on plexus anesthesia[1] notes that much of the subsequent development of regional anesthetic technique was carried out on the mainland of Europe where the "art and science of general anesthesia had been strangely disregarded."

Moving from a historical perspective to current medical practice, as the clinical risks and subjective unpleasantness of general anesthesia have declined over the latter half of the twentieth century, general anesthesia increasingly has become the most widely used technique for hospital-based surgery. Techniques have been developed making general anesthesia safe for all but the most debilitated patients (with mortality attributable to anesthesia alone now approaching 1:250,000). This safety, coupled with a very high degree of patient acceptance (with the widespread incorporation of agents that have dramatically reduced such anesthetic

Table 7-1 Properties of Specific Local Anesthetics

Anesthetic	Properties
Esters	
Tetracaine Benzocaine	Useful for topical analgesia, long-acting, possibility of methemoglobin formation (cyanosis)
Procaine	Low potency, low toxicity, short duration, often favored for oral anesthesia
2-Chloroprocaine	Used in Europe for Bier block, not used much in the United States for this purpose
Cocaine	Naturally occurring, vasoconstriction effect, potential for abuse and addiction
Amides	
Bupivacaine	Sensory block>motor block, cardiotoxicity potential, delayed onset, long duration
Mepivacaine Ropivacaine	Similar to bupivacaine, less cardiotoxic, widely used for arm blocks
Etidocaine	Motor block>sensory block, very rapid onset, long duration
Prilocaine	Similar to lidocaine, may have slightly less CNS toxicity
Lidocaine	Most versatile local anesthetic
Eutectic mixture of local anesthetic (EMLA) (lidocaine/prilocaine)	Useful topical anesthetic

comorbidities as nausea and dysphoria), has made it common for many reputable and well-managed North American anesthetic practices to use regional techniques hardly at all. With general anesthesia so safe and pleasant, why bother with anything else? In fact, it is abundantly clear that for certain categories of surgical practice, including a variety of aesthetic procedures, the use of regional anesthesia offers profound advantages both to the practitioner and to the patient. This observation does not, however, seem to hamper debates in the anesthesiology literature regarding the relative merits of regional vs. general anesthetic techniques for any given surgical intervention. Although there frequently is less than compelling scientific or clinical evidence favoring one over the other, the lines of discussion are often quite sharply drawn.

Clearly, the modern practice of aesthetic surgery encompasses a very wide range of procedures, from major plastic or reconstructive techniques involving rotational or free tissue flaps and major reorganization of tissues to relatively noninvasive cosmetic procedures such as skin tag removal. For the most part, the more invasive techniques are likely to be performed in hospital settings with anesthesia provided by the in-house anesthesia service. For large reconstructive cases, there are significant advantages in general anesthesia with invasive monitoring, although there may well be benefit from the application of specific regional blocks for the purposes of increasing blood supply to specific tissue sites.[2,3] We are concerned, in this review, with the more limited procedures that make up the majority of cases performed in free-standing procedure suites and lend themselves to local or regional anesthesia administered by the operating surgeon.

The basic requirements for elective surgical procedures are that the patients be safe, comfortable, and stable; it also helps if they are immobile and not too talkative. The technique of anesthesia selected must be one that facilitates surgery and that is acceptable to the patient. As we have stated, regional anesthesia has profound advantages in many situations and is often an ideal approach to painless surgery in free-standing ambulatory surgery facilities; many blocks can be placed by the surgical practitioner without recourse to specialized anesthesia services. However, knowing when to seek expert guidance is the hallmark of professional judgment, and there will be some procedures, some patients, some settings where regional anesthesia practiced solo or with minimal professional backup is ill advised.

BASIC SCIENCE

When applied to peripheral nerves, local anesthetics reversibly inhibit signal transmission by blocking sodium influx via membrane sodium channels.[4] The agents used are marketed as water-soluble hydrochloride salts. In an aqueous solution, the local anesthetic's fixed dissociation constant (pK_a) determines the equilibrium between the charged local anesthetic cation and the uncharged base. It is the uncharged base that freely diffuses through the lipid bilayer of neurons. After crossing a neuron's lipid bilayer, the local anesthetic molecule again dissociates into its basic and cationic forms with the charged cation entering the protein-based sodium channel. It is

Table 7-2 Speed of Onset

Onset	Agent
Fast	Chloroprocaine Lidocaine Prilocaine Mepivacaine Etidocaine
Moderate	Ropivacaine Bupivacaine
Slow	Procaine Tetracaine

the presence of the local anesthetic molecule within the ion channel that renders the channel impermeable to sodium, thus preventing the propagation of action potentials and impulse conduction.[5] With time, the local anesthetic diffuses out of the channel, rendering the neurons once again susceptible to depolarization.

All local anesthetics in clinical use consist of a benzene ring connected to a hydrocarbon chain; the linkage can be an ester or amide. This distinction between ester and amide may seem arcane, but it is of clinical value because allergic reactions can occur, quite frequently, with esters, whereas allergic reactions to amides are rare. Esters such as benzocaine and procaine break down to structures similar to PABA (*p*-aminobenzoic acid), a common component of cosmetics and sunscreens, and should be avoided in patients with known sensitivity to such compounds. Clinical properties of local anesthetics are structure-dependent (Table 7-1).

The lipid solubility of clinically useful local anesthetics is usually quite high, but is pH-dependent, with high pH favoring increased lipid solubility, anesthetic potency, and speed of onset (Table 7-2). Ester-linked anesthetics are tetracaine, procaine, 2-chloroprocaine, and cocaine. Amide-linked anesthetics include bupivacaine, mepivacaine, prilocaine, etidocaine, ropivacaine, and lidocaine. Substitutions on the benzene ring or tertiary amine portion of the local anesthetic molecule alter its pK_a, lipid solubility, and protein binding, determining respectively the speed of onset, potency, and duration of action.

CLINICAL STUDIES

General Techniques of Regional Anesthesia

Topical Application. There is only one local anesthetic that will readily penetrate intact skin; this is the combination of 5% lidocaine and 5% prilocaine known as EMLA, an acronym for eutectic mixture of local anesthetics.[6] It is a white, oily cream that is smeared over the target area and then covered with an occlusive dressing (such as Tegaderm); after 20 to 40 minutes, profound anesthesia of the superficial skin layers (to a depth of 5 to 6 mm) can be anticipated. Although the technique is useful for procedures such as tattoo removal or laser ablation of portwine stains, the area of skin treated should probably be modest. There are reports of facial procedures such as dermabrasion being performed after "facial anesthesia" effected by application of a form-fitting plastic mask slathered in EMLA, an approach that would seem to be time consuming, expensive, and subject to the consequences of prilocaine toxicity (see subsequent discussion).

For mucous membranes, topical anesthesia can be obtained using proprietary aerosol formulations of benzocaine or paste/gel formulations of lidocaine-epinephrine-tetracaine or bupivacaine-epinephrine.[7-11] These products are useful, in particular, for providing topical analgesia as a precursor to the placement of regional nerve blocks at sensitive mucous membrane sites such as the oral mucosa, and also for incision and suture lines involving mucosal tissues.

Local Infiltration. Anesthetic solutions such as bupivacaine or lidocaine are injected into the soft tissues surrounding a wound or surgical site; the technique is effective, for example, for the excision of small superficial cysts or lipomas, or for painless suturing of lacerations. It is not particularly useful for large wounds because of safety limitations on the amount of anesthetic agent that can be used. Table 7-3 lists approximate maximum doses for local anesthetics administered by this route to a normal adult.

Intravenous Anesthesia. The anesthetic solution is injected into a major vein draining an extremity. This technique is commonly used for short surgical procedures on the arm: the limb is first squeezed free of blood (elastic bandage), then isolated (tourniquet), and the anesthetic (almost always lidocaine 0.5%; *never* bupivacaine[12]) is injected into a distal vein. This is an excellent technique for surgeries such as contracture release or joint mobilization.

Peripheral Nerve Block. A major nerve supplying a limb or specific area of the body is identified (anatomy, paresthesias, nerve stimulator) and a solution of local anesthetic is injected very close to, but not inside, the nerve, yielding a sensory (and often motor) block dense enough for painless surgery. The block may last up to 24 hours depending on the amount and type of anesthetic agent used, or may be prolonged indefinitely by use of a continuous infusion of agent directed through a fine plastic catheter.

Neuraxial Block. *Neuraxial block* is a term used to describe epidural and spinal analgesia in which small

Table 7-3 Potency of Local Anesthetics

Duration	Ester	Amide	Potency	Maximum Recommended Dose
Short	Procaine		1	1000 mg
	Chloroprocaine		1	
Moderate		Lidocaine	2	500 mg
		Prilocaine	2	
		Mepivacaine	2	
Long	Tetracaine	Etidocaine	6	250 mg
		Ropivacaine	6	
		Bupivacaine	8	

amounts of local anesthetic are injected or infused into the epidural space (yielding a segmental blockade of the nerves supplying a large territory) or into the subarachnoid space (yielding a spinal blockade of the lower half of the body). Note: although it is completely acceptable for local, intravenous, and peripheral blocks to be administered by nonanesthesiologists, neuraxial blocks must be placed only by specialists who have undergone intensive training both in the techniques of block placement and also in resuscitation and airway management.

Complications of Regional Anesthesia[13]

Neurotoxicity. Local anesthetics are potentially neurotoxic, and in clinical practice injected doses are frequently much greater than those thought capable of producing neurotoxicity. It is the presence of the perineurium acting as a diffusion barrier that prevents excessively high concentrations of local anesthetic from reaching the intraneural structures.[14] Neurotoxicity, in practice, is likely to occur only with intraneural injection, which is generally accompanied by intense pain. Indeed, pain may be the only initial indication of trouble to come, and many conservative practitioners will avoid performing nerve blocks on patients who are excessively sedated or otherwise uncommunicative and who may not be able to give warning of nerve penetration by the needle or of the intraneural injection. For similar reasons, care should be exercised when supplementing preexisting nerve block.

Allergy. As noted, allergic reactions to amide local anesthetics are rare; careful history elicited from those with a history of an allergic reaction to amides quite often reveals symptoms of tachycardia, chest tightness, and lightheadedness—the consequence of intravascular injection of epinephrine, a common additive to a local anesthetic mixture. True allergies to ester local anesthetics are also not common, but do occur.[15] Ester local anesthetics should certainly be avoided in individuals with allergies to PABA. If signs or symptoms of allergic response occur, then standard medical interventions need to be implemented immediately: get assistance, support the airway, administer fluids, and don't delay giving epinephrine in the event of hypovolemic shock or severe bronchospasm or both.

Systemic Toxicity. Most systemic reactions occur as a result of inadvertent intravascular injection or injection into a highly vascular tissue bed with resultant rapid local anesthetic uptake into the circulating system; the danger sites are the brain and the heart. Incorporation of epinephrine 5 μg/ml into the local anesthetic dose (1:200,000 dilution) both delays systemic absorption and, more significantly, when used as a test dose can warn of intravascular injection by eliciting tachycardia.[16] Central nervous and cardiovascular system toxicity are dose and time dependent. The faster plasma levels of local anesthetic rise, the more likely that an adverse reaction will occur. Prevent high blood levels by always using the lowest dose or weakest concentration compatible with desired effect, and by injecting slowly or in divided doses; minimize redistribution by incorporating epinephrine or phenylephrine in the mix.

Initial symptoms of central nervous system (CNS) toxicity are tinnitus, metallic taste, difficulty focusing, lightheadedness, circumoral numbness, and intellectual confusion. Note that these responses can be detected only in an awake, alert patient; as a consequence, performing regional blocks on comatose subjects takes away one level of safety. If brain tissue levels continue to rise, the patient will experience muscle twitching, tremors, and then generalized tonic-clonic convulsions resulting in loss of consciousness, generalized CNS depression, and respiratory arrest.[17] If seizures occur, the airway should be protected and the patient mask ventilated with oxygen until the seizure abates. If necessary, the seizure can be aborted with diazepam or sodium pentothal and the patient intubated and ventilated.

Cardiovascular toxicity is most frequently associated with the use of bupivacaine; however, all local anesthetics affect the cardiac electrical conducting system and depress the myocardium and peripheral vascular smooth muscle. As in the nerve, they reduce the action potential in the heart by limiting the inward flow of sodium current. Lidocaine is a "fast-in, fast-out" sodium channel blocker that reaches steady-state block in one or two beats. Bupivacaine, conversely is "fast-in, slow-out" and channel inhibition increases with successive beats and with faster heart rates.[18] The reason is that several local anesthetics, bupivacaine included, will penetrate the ion channel only when it is in the "open" conformation.

Local anesthetics prolong conduction time in the heart (lengthened PR and QRS intervals). Increasing plasma levels will suppress the sinoatrial and atrioventricular nodes, causing sinus bradycardia, conduction block, electrical inexcitability, and cardiac arrest. Bupivacaine's "fast-in, slow-out" action makes the heart vulnerable to malignant reentry cardiac arrhythmias. The ratio of the dosage required for irreversible cardiovascular collapse and the dosage that will produce CNS toxicity, CC/CNS ratio, is approximately 7:1 for lidocaine and 4:1 for bupivacaine, indicating that bupivacaine has greater cardiovascular toxicity than lidocaine (the heart is further sensitized to bupivacaine during pregnancy). Commercially available bupivacaine is the racemic mixture of its *r* and *s* enantiomers. The pure *s* isomeric form of bupivacaine is now commercially available (as chirocaine), and it complements ropivacaine, a relatively new homologue of *s*-bupivacaine. Early studies with ropivacaine suggested that it might be significantly less cardiotoxic than bupivacaine; however, adjusting for ropivacaine's lesser potency, equipotent doses seem to confer approximately the same degree of cardiotoxicity as bupivacaine. Similar, preliminary, data have now been obtained with chirocaine, although clinical trials with this drug are in their infancy.

Little is known about the most appropriate antiarrhythmic to use during local anesthetic-induced cardiac arrest. High doses of epinephrine and atropine may be appropriate; bretylium may be of benefit in cases of bupivacaine toxicity.[19] In the cardiac arrest situation, one must pay particular attention to oxygenation and ventilation and be prepared to perform cardiopulmonary resuscitation for an indefinite period of time. In extreme situations, cardiopulmonary bypass may have to be implemented until the effects of the local anesthetic have dissipated. Understand that if organ oxygenation and perfusion can be maintained effectively until local anesthetic levels diminish, the patient *will* recover fully.[20]

One final note on toxicity: both benzocaine and prilocaine (more correctly its *o*-toluidine metabolite) produce methemoglobinemia, which both reduces the oxygen-carrying capacity of hemoglobin and impairs oxygen release, and promotes a noticeable cyanosis when present in high doses.[21] In patients monitored by pulse oximetry probes methemoglobinemia causes the probe to read 85%, regardless of the actual SaO_2 (i.e., a falsely low saturation reading when SaO_2 is actually >85%, and a falsely high reading when it is actually <85%). Treatment of this complication involves administration of methylene blue or ascorbic acid. Prilocaine is no longer available in the United States as the pure drug, but it is present in the topical anesthetic mixture EMLA (see above) and as a prilocaine-phenylephrine formulation for topical use on mucous membranes.[22]

DISCUSSION

There are relatively few types of surgery where regional anesthesia is absolutely indicated (as opposed to merely being an option), but certain surgeries lend themselves in particular to regional techniques, and there can be compelling reasons either for avoiding general anesthesia or, more commonly, for supplementing general anesthesia with some form of regional block. In general terms, the types of advantages to be expected from regional techniques are a reduction in overall stress of surgery, better postoperative pain control, decreased incidence of postoperative nausea and dysphoria, and, in many situations, improved wound healing.

Reduced Surgical Stress. Postoperative complications such as myocardial infarction, pulmonary infection, thromboembolism, and fatigue are probably related to increased demands, hypermetabolism, catabolism, and other physiologic changes included in the global surgical stress response.[23] Stress can sometimes be monitored by looking at changes in heart rate or blood pressure, or, in more sophisticated ways by monitoring cerebral blood flow or the release into the blood of specific markers of stress reactions such as cortisol. Transcranial Doppler (TCD) studies show that cerebral blood flow through major vessels such as the middle cerebral artery increases significantly for several minutes after skin incision in patients under apparently adequate general anesthesia (2% minimum alveolar concentration isoflurane). There is evidence, in children at least, that this effect is abolished or attenuated when there is effective concomitant epidural regional anesthesia. The relevance of these observations to aesthetic surgical procedures performed under regional anesthesia alone are that the same reductions in stress are present even when the patient is fully awake; decreased stress is almost always beneficial.

Reduced Postoperative Pain. Some procedures are particularly painful, for example, many surgical procedures involving bone shaping. Patients who have this type of surgery will need a high level of analgesia postoperatively, and although this can be provided by simple techniques such as morphine injections, these tend to produce nausea, constipation, sleep disturbances, and sometimes mood changes and dysphoria. By incorporating a regional nerve block into the anesthetic regimen all these complications can be reduced or eliminated. Even in procedures performed under general anesthesia, the period of awakening *(emergence)* is typically much smoother, less stressful, and more comfortable when all pain from the surgical site has been eliminated by a regional nerve block, rather than simply masked by systemic opioids.

Reduced Postoperative Infection. Inactive postsurgical patients lying in hospital beds are at significant risk for acquiring pneumonia. In general, opioids such as morphine cause *respiratory depression* and patients tend to ventilate less energetically than they should, exacerbating this risk. This is the reason why many posttrauma patients need routine respiratory therapy or incentive spirometry during convalescence. Reducing the amount of morphine needed generally reduces the incidence of respiratory depression and consequent pulmonary complications, and patients with good pain control provided by peripheral nerve blocks or epidural infusions require dramatically less morphine than they would otherwise.

The specific group of patients who have undergone painful chest or abdominal procedures or who have had irritating drainage tubes placed are at even greater risk of postoperative pneumonia. Painful chest wounds make it very difficult to cough or breath deeply, and patients will often sit up in bed panting shallowly because it hurts to take proper breaths. This is a setup for atelectasis, pulmonary infection, and reduced oxygen supply; in many cases the appropriate use of regional techniques such as intercostal blocks can make a significant positive difference and can even make the difference between a successful recovery or death in elderly or frail patients.

Improved Healing. The body has a natural defense against blood loss after surgical incision and that is *vasospasm,* intense vasoconstriction causing arteries to clamp down in response to the stress of injury to reduce the amount of blood loss. Although this is beneficial acutely at the time of injury, it is generally unhelpful in the immediate postoperative period, and vasospasm or vasoconstriction is a feared complication of aesthetic surgical procedures involving rotational or translational flaps, starving the surgical wound of the blood needed for healing. One of the effects of regional nerve blocks using local anesthetics is *sympathectomy,* the elimination of vasoconstriction provoked by sympathetic responses to stress. For this reason, many surgeons request that regional blocks be used in patients undergoing reimplantation or reconstructive procedures in order to improve wound healing and to increase the chances of a successful graft.[2,3]

SECTION TWO

Atlas of Surgical Procedures

PREOPERATIVE CLINICAL CONSIDERATIONS

Patient Selection and Evaluation

Not every aesthetic surgical procedure is appropriate for execution under regional anesthesia; long cases and uncomfortable positioning can tax even the most motivated of patients. Not every patient is an appropriate candidate for regional anesthesia, and difficulties are going to be encountered during surgery if awake patients are unable to stay calm, quiet, and still during the procedure. Difficult patients are those with anxiety disorders or developmental delay, some children, and intoxicated or belligerent patients. Avoid the temptation to oversedate in an attempt to gain cooperation. Even modest sedation in some patients can result in *disinhibition,* converting a reasonable and rational person into a talkative, agitated, seductive, or dysphoric one.[24-26] There are very real dangers in sedating to the point of unconsciousness unless a vigilant, trained patient monitor (physician or nurse), whose sole attention is to the patient's vital signs, is present throughout the planned procedure and specific resuscitation equipment (together with people who know how to use it properly) are available at a moment's notice. Thus, the prudent surgeon contemplating procedures under regional anesthesia will ensure the patient understands what is to be undertaken (its risks and requirements), is competent to cooperate, has no stated allergies to agents likely to be used, and can assume the operative position required without undue discomfort or hazard. (Some patients find it difficult to lie flat because of congestive heart failure, chronic obstructive pulmonary disease, arthritis, or obesity; others are claustrophobic under drapes or masks.) It is prudent to require patients to refrain from eating solid food for 6 hours and from drinking clear liquids for 2 hours prior to surgery if the use of sedatives is anticipated.

As with all anticipated elective surgery, the patient's medical condition should be optimized; it is unwise to perform even modestly invasive procedures on raging hypertensives, out-of-control diabetics, or patients in florid heart failure. In general, the patient who is an appropriate candidate for the surgery is probably also an appropriate candidate for consideration of regional anesthesia. Remember, however, that blocks can go wrong, sensitivities to drugs can suddenly be revealed, bronchospasm can suddenly appear, and panic can suddenly emerge; have the appropriate backup plans well rehearsed and ready to execute. Be alert to preoperative medication intake (aspirin, metformin, coumadin, etc.) and also to the existence of preexisting cognitive, motor, or sensory deficits; chart them prior to initiation of procedures and discuss any concerns frankly with the patient. If the left side of the face is still numb 2 days after surgery, it's comforting to have recorded the fact that it was numb prior to surgery too before exploring the possibility of persistent nerve deficits attributable to surgery or anesthesia.

PROCEDURAL TECHNIQUES

With respect to the placement of regional anesthetic blocks, there are a number of points to be borne in mind. It is dangerous to exceed safe doses of local anesthetics; they are all toxic to some degree, and some (e.g., bupivacaine) present a very real risk of death if they are inadvertently injected intravascularly. Some injection sites are inherently more dangerous than others (e.g., trigeminal ganglion), some sites are technically more difficult to reach (e.g., sciatic nerve). Correct selection of agent, meticulous attention to needle position, careful test dosing, constant vigilance to patient vital signs, appropriate patient sedation, sensible patient selection and preparation, and a practiced confidence in technique will all tend to improve the success of regional anesthetic approaches provided by the surgical practitioner. Knowing when to invite the assistance of an anesthesiologist (for neuraxial block, general anesthesia or unconscious sedation, or advice on block placement) is another hallmark of a successful surgical practice. The regional blocks described in this chapter are selected for their simplicity; the list is not exhaustive, but concentrates on those blocks most likely to be practically useful to freestanding practices of aesthetic and cosmetic surgery.

As a final caveat, skillful and comfortable execution of regional anesthesia demands training and dedicated practice. There is a world of difference between painfully flooding a tissue site with local anesthetic and crisply anesthetizing a specific nerve to render a wide area devoid of sensation. Patients recognize and appreciate the difference. Before attempting complex blocks it is prudent to search out experienced practitioners who can guide and advise; it may also be beneficial to undertake formal training in specific blocks at a regional meeting. For more detailed descriptions of the techniques discussed here I recommend the four referenced procedural guides[27-30] and two collateral texts dealing with specifics of plastic and aesthetic surgery.[31,32]

Head and Neck

Many surgical procedures on superficial tissues in this region can be performed readily under effective regional block. Sensory innervation to the posterior neck and scalp is from the dorsal rami of the cervical nerves; and that to the anterior and lateral cutaneous neck tissues is from their ventral rami. Sensory innervation of the face is via the trigeminal nerve, whose three major divisions leave the cranial vault through three major foramina: superior orbital fissure (ophthalmic nerve), foramen rotundum (maxillary nerve), and foramen ovale (mandibular nerve). The terminal branches of these three nerves become cutaneous by passing through the supraorbital, infraorbital, and mental foramina to form the supraorbital, infraorbital, and mental nerves respectively.

Scalp

Occipital Nerve Block. Effective scalp anesthesia can be attained by occipital nerve block. The greater occipital nerve becomes subcutaneous on the superior nuchal line at a point approximately one third of the way between the occipital protuberance and the mastoid process. If the occipital artery can be palpated at the superior nuchal line, it provides a useful landmark—the nerve is generally just medial to it. The patient should be sitting, neck modestly flexed. Palpate the occipital process, then move laterally along the superior nuchal line, ipsilateral to surgical site, until the pulsation of the occipital artery is felt. Using a short, sharp bevel 25- to 30-gauge needle, form a subcutaneous wheal of anesthetic around the artery using 5 ml 1% lidocaine or 0.25% bupivacaine. If the arterial pulsation cannot be appreciated—and this will often be the case—then infiltrate along the superior nuchal line midway between occipital protuberance and mastoid (Fig. 7-1). The block should take less than 5 minutes to set up, will last 4 to 6 hours if bupivacaine with epinephrine supplement is used, and is not particularly

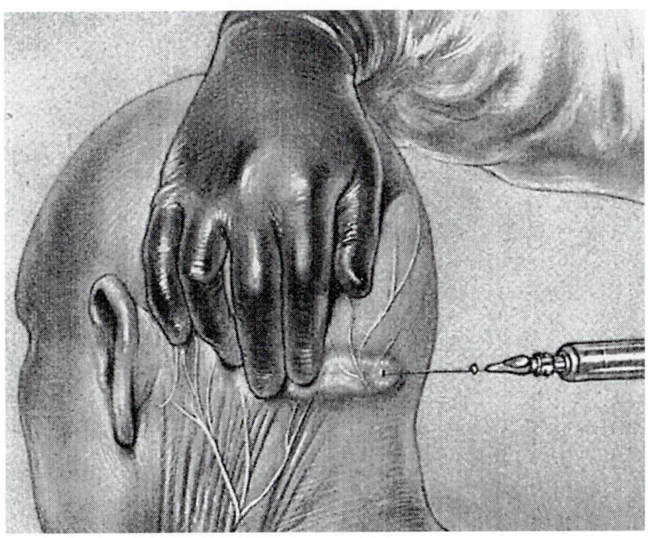

FIG. 7-1 Occipital Nerve Block
Infiltration along the superior nuchal line midway between occipital protuberance and mastoid. (Modified from Pitkin GP. Conduction Anesthesia. Philadelphia: Lippincott, 1946:315.)

hazardous provided direct intravascular injection is avoided and the needle is never advanced under the occipital ridge and into the foramen magnum.

Face

The sensory supply to the face and anterior regions of the scalp is provided by the trigeminal nerve; consequently, trigeminal blockade will provide cutaneous anesthesia over this entire region. However, a much safer, and better-tolerated, approach is to anesthetize specific facial regions by blockade of the ophthalmic, maxillary, or mandibular branches or by blockade of the distal trigeminal nerve fibers. The planned surgical procedure will normally dictate which approach is appropriate. It is important to appreciate that some elements of the trigeminal nerve (third division) are motor fibers; if these are inhibited, there may well be facial drooping or asymmetry that may complicate assessment of aesthetic procedures.

Trigeminal Ganglion Block. Trigeminal ganglion block anesthetizes the entire face when performed bilaterally but is not without risk and can be uncomfortable for the unsedated patient; minor needle position error can result in subarachnoid injection of anesthetic. Because of the serious consequences of misdirected injection, many practitioners would insist that this block should be carried out only under radiographic guidance. The surgeon should be thoroughly familiar with the local anatomy and should not attempt to place the block particularly quickly—a slow, steady, gentle, careful approach is needed. Be ready to support or resuscitate if necessary.

The subject should be supine, comfortable and relaxed, lightly sedated. The ganglion lies lateral to the carotid artery, superior to the foramen ovale; it is reached from a skin insertion site anterior and inferior to this point at the anterior margin of the masseter muscle, level with the corner of the mouth. Use a standard 23- to 25-gauge Quincke-type spinal needle (sharp bevel, not pencil-point) inserted just medial to the masseter muscle and in a vertical plane passing through the lateral margin of the pupil (Fig. 7-2); the needle tip should contact the sphenoid bone just anterior to the foramen ovale at a depth of 4 to 6 cm. The tip should now be withdrawn slightly and redirected caudally until it steps off the superior margin of the foramen and penetrates the cranial vault. Now the tip should be advanced gently, perhaps a further 1 cm, until paresthesias in the trigeminal distribution are announced. Look for paresthesias in regions V1 and V2 to ensure that the needle is adjacent to the ganglion and not simply the mandibular nerve root. The posterior part of the trigeminal ganglion is adherent to a reflection of dura mater (Meckel's cave), so subarachnoid injection is a very real possibility. Aspirate carefully to ensure that no cerebrospinal fluid (CSF) draws back, then slowly inject 2 ml 1% lidocaine or 0.125% mepivacaine; the block should set up in 5 minutes. Clearly, unilateral block will provide only unilateral anesthesia, so for many plastic procedures the technique will have to be applied bilaterally.

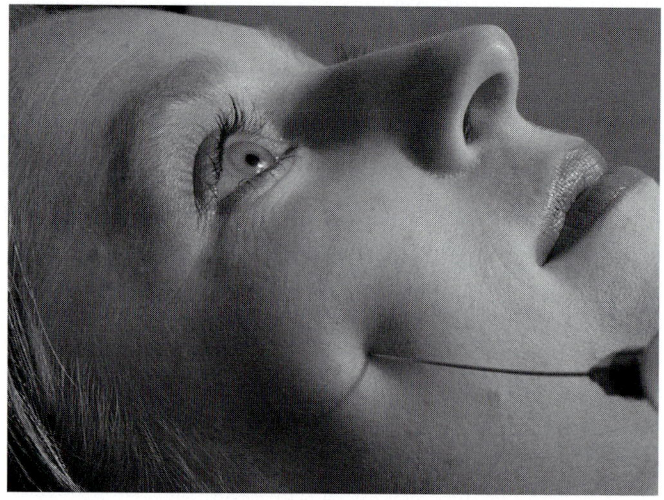

FIG. 7-2 Trigeminal Nerve Block
The needle is inserted just medial to the masseter muscle and in the vertical plane passing through the lateral margin of the pupil. Use extreme caution when attempting this block; radiographic guidance is strongly suggested.

Ophthalmic Block. Ophthalmic block has relatively few indications in aesthetic surgery and there are dangers inherent in its placement (corneal ulceration from persistent anesthesia). Most ophthalmic procedures involving the globe of the eye are performed using retrobulbar or peribulbar blocks if regional techniques are selected. Blockade of the more distal branches of the ophthalmic nerve, supplying the lateral margins of the nose, the upper eyelids, and the forehead, is much more useful in plastic surgery, as described below under *distal trigeminal block.*

Maxillary Block. Maxillary block is appropriate for establishing anesthesia over the cheeks, the inferior margins of the orbit, and the lateral aspects of the nose. The patient lies supine, the zygomatic arch is palpated, and its midpoint is marked with a skin pen. The mandibular notch is appreciated by gentle but firm palpation of the upper margin of the mandible as the patient is invited to mimic chewing; try to identify the deepest part of the notch, mark it with a pen, then prepare the area and raise a skin wheal at the marked site. Using a 23-gauge Quincke-type spinal needle (sharp bevel), penetrate the skin at the marked point, then an-

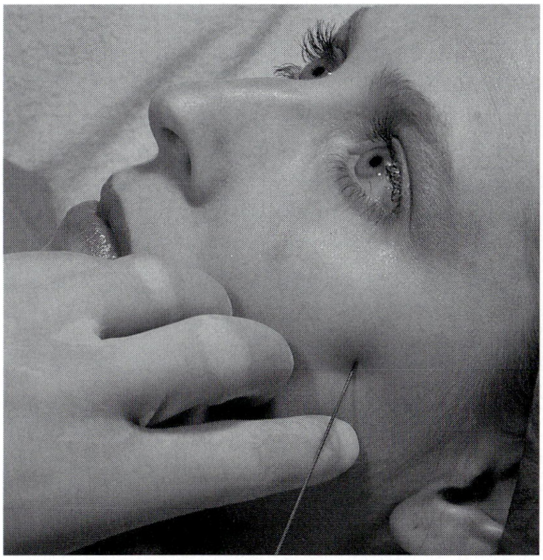

FIG. 7-3 Maxillary Nerve Block
Palpate the mandibular notch and penetrate the skin over that point, angling the needle toward the ipsilateral eye. The pterygoid plate will be encountered at a depth of approximately 5 cm; the needle is then "walked off" this plate in an anterior direction until the pterygopalatine fossa is encountered.

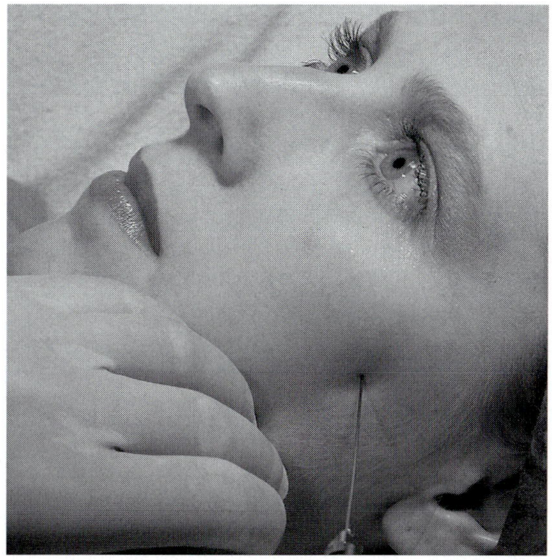

FIG. 7-4 Mandibular Nerve Block
Positioning is similar to that for the maxillary block except that the needle is maintained perpendicular to the skin plane as it is advanced toward the pterygoid plate.

gle the needle toward the center of the eye (i.e., superior and anterior) (Fig. 7-3). The pterygoid plate should be encountered at a depth of approximately 5 cm; now gently "walk off" the plate in an anterior direction until the needle advances approximately 1 cm into the pterygopalatine fossa. Aspirate, inquire about paresthesias (to the teeth or nose), then inject 5 ml 2% lidocaine or 0.5% bupivacaine. Because of the close proximity of the injection site to the orbit it is quite possible for ocular movements to be impaired and also for periorbital hematomas to develop; I would recommend not actively probing for paresthesias with this block, but relying on anatomic landmarks alone; a modest degree of sedation will enhance patient comfort and tolerance.

Mandibular Block. Mandibular block is appropriate for procedures along the line of the lower jaw, lip, and chin considered too extensive for simple infiltration anesthesia. Positioning and initial skin penetration is the same as for the maxillary block, except that the needle should be kept perpendicular to the skin in all planes as it is advanced medially to engage the pterygoid plate (Fig. 7-4); the needle is then gently walked off the bony plate in a posterior direction to encounter the mandibular nerve a little less than 1 cm deep to the plate. After careful aspiration, and gentle probing for paresthesias to the jaw or lower teeth, 5 ml 2% lidocaine or 0.5% bupivacaine should induce anesthesia (as well as weakness of the masseter muscle because of the motor component of the mandibular nerve).

Distal Trigeminal Block. Distal trigeminal block is useful for minor, superficial surgical procedures too extensive for infiltration anesthesia; the general approach is appropriate for almost any patient who is a good candidate for regional technique, and the distal blocks are relatively easy to perform because of the readily identifiable nature of the principal landmarks—the supraorbital, infraorbital, and mental foramina. In general, for distal trigeminal block the subject is supine with head supported on a small towel roll. The appropriate foramina are palpated and 2 ml anesthetic solution is injected immediately adjacent, avoiding injection actually into the foramen itself, which can increase the risk of intraneuronal injection. The three foramina are aligned vertically in the paramedian sagittal plane passing through the center of the pupil; specific landmarks are described below.

Forehead

Supraorbital Block. The frontal nerve bifurcates to form the supraorbital nerve, which emerges from the supraorbital notch (palpated easily on the superior rim of the orbit approximately 2 to 3 cm from the midline) and the supratrochlear nerve, which exits more medially. To anesthetize the proximal branches of these two nerves, first palpate the superior rim of the orbit, identify the supraorbital notch, and insert a 25- or 30-gauge needle immediately above and lateral to this notch (Fig. 7-5). In a sequence of gentle injections, infiltrate subcuta-

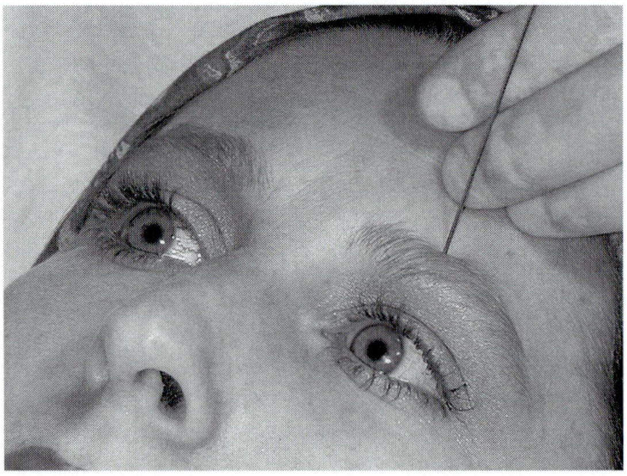

FIG. 7-5 Supraorbital Nerve Block
The supraorbital notch is readily palpated on the superior rim of the orbit; needle insertion is immediately above and lateral to this notch.

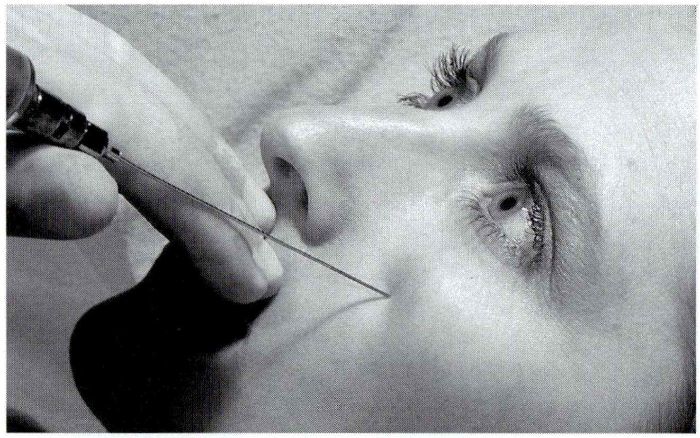

FIG. 7-6 Infraorbital Nerve Block
The percutaneous approach involves gentle probing for the infraorbital foramen—generally lying 1 cm caudal to the inferior margin of the orbit in the same sagittal plane as the pupil of the eye.

neously and down to the periosteum, advancing the needle superiorly and medially until the midline is reached. Repeat the process on the contralateral side if it is necessary to attain bilateral anesthesia. With 0.25% bupivacaine or 1% lidocaine solution, 2 to 5 ml should be sufficient injectate to cover the entire forehead region.

Cheek

Infraorbital-Zygomatic Block (Percutaneous). The infraorbital nerve becomes superficial at the infraorbital foramen, which is palpable directly in some patients or may be located by careful exploration with a fine (25-gauge) needle approximately 1 cm below the inferior margin of the orbit, in the same vertical plane as the pupil of the eye (Fig. 7-6). Note that the bony canal runs cephalad from the foramen, so a rostral orientation of the probing needle may facilitate identification; however, when the injection is made, the needle should be directed caudally, toward the mentum to minimize the risk of intraneuronal injection of local anesthetic. The zygomaticofacial nerve becomes subcutaneous at a point 1 to 2 cm below the lateral margin of the infraorbital rim; injecting local anesthetic solution over the periosteum, directing the needle laterally toward the zygomatic bone will augment anesthesia of the upper cheek. Again, a total of 2 to 5 ml 0.25% bupivacaine or 1% lidocaine should be sufficient to provide full coverage of the cheek.

Infraorbital Block (Oral). For intraoral blockade of the infraorbital nerve, the upper lip is retracted firmly, and topical anesthetic is applied to the mucosa directly above the second bicuspid. The needle (25- or 27-gauge) should be inserted into the mucosa at this point and advanced in line with the long axis of the tooth, generally directed toward the pupil of the ipsilateral eye (Fig. 7-7). The infraorbital foramen will usually be reached when the needle tip is lying about one fingerbreadth below the inferior orbital margin (a point readily marked using the fingers of the hand retracting the upper lip). Generally, 2 to 3 ml 0.5% bupivacaine with 1:200,000 epinephrine will give a profound sensory block of the upper cheek within 5 minutes of injection.

Chin (Soft Tissues)

Mental Block (Percutaneous). The mental foramen lies on the vertical line passing through the mandible, the pupil, and the second premolar, approximately at the midpoint of the vertical depth of the mandible. A palpating finger is pressed on the inferior rim of the mandible to stabilize soft tissues and identify the injection site (Fig. 7-8). The foramen is located by gentle probing, this time keeping the needle perpendicular to the skin, and 1 to 2 ml solution is injected over the periosteum after gentle aspiration, avoiding direct injection into the foramen to minimize the risks of nerve trauma.

Mental Block (Oral). All four branches of the mental nerve can be blocked by an intraoral approach, using the mandibular first and second bicuspid teeth as a landmark (Fig. 7-9). With the patient's mouth gently opened, the bicuspid teeth are exposed by firm retraction of the lower lip. The mental foramen lies just inferior and lateral to the gingival margin of the bicuspid teeth. After local application of topical anesthetic and insertion of the needle through the mucosa at this site, the mental foramen may sometimes be palpated directly with the needle tip. Regardless, injection of 2 to 4 ml anesthetic over

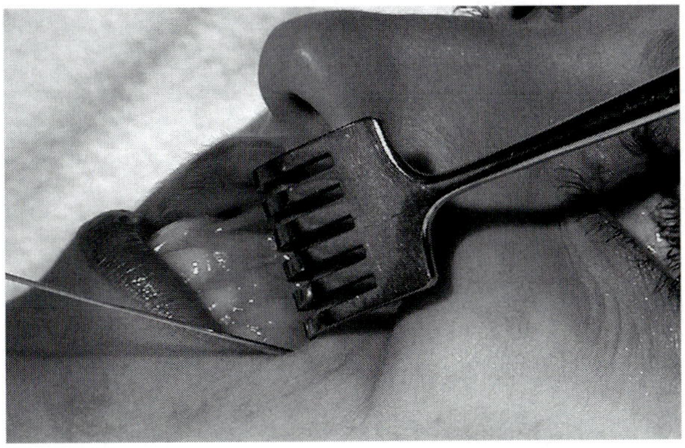

FIG. 7-7 Infraorbital Nerve Block
The upper lip is firmly retracted (either by rake, as here, or by gloved finger), and the needle is inserted into the mucosa directly above the second bicuspid, advancing in line with the long axis of the tooth (generally in the direction of the pupil of the ipsilateral eye).

FIG. 7-8 Mental Nerve Block
The foramen lies on the line connecting mandible, pupil, and second premolar; this line also passes through the infraorbital and supraorbital foramina as indicated here. Percutaneous probing at the midpoint of the vertical depth of the mandible usually locates the mental foramen at an intersection of this imaginary line.

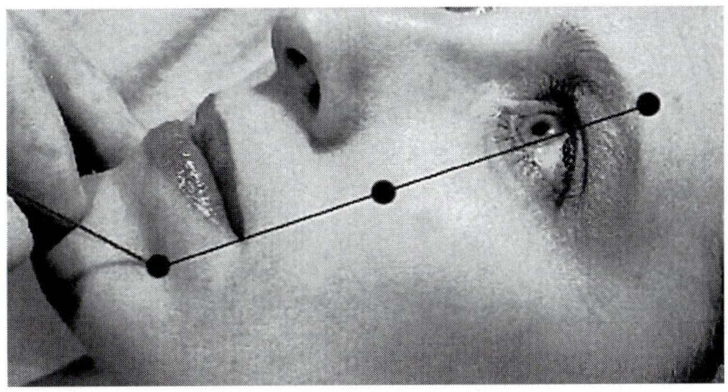

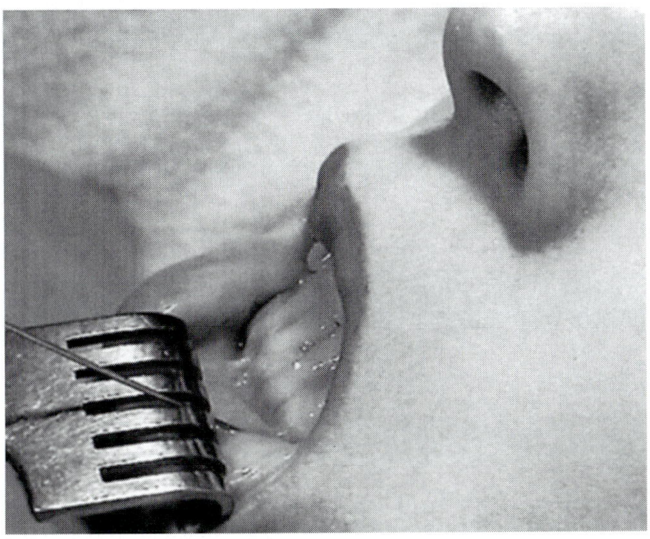

FIG. 7-9 Mental Nerve Block
For the intraoral approach, the bicuspid teeth are exposed by gentle retraction of the lower lip; the foramen lies just inferior and lateral to the gingival margin of the bicuspids.

the periosteal plane at this site will provide solid anesthesia of the mental symphysis–related soft tissues.

Chin (Bone)

Combined Mental–Inferior Alveolar Block (Oral). For more extensive procedures on the chin, such as mental advancement and genioplasty, the sensory innervation of the skeletal structures must also be blocked. The inferior alveolar nerve supplies the body and ramus of the mandible and the posterior mandibular teeth; the mental nerve supplies the soft tissues of the lower lip and chin (above) and the anterior mandibular teeth. The principal landmark for inferior alveolar nerve block is the anterior border of the mandibular ramus. The patient's mouth is opened as widely as possible; the anterior border of the mandibular ramus is palpated firmly and the sulcus formed between the ramus and the temporalis muscle is appreciated. After topical anesthetic has been applied to the mucosa, a medium-length 25-gauge needle is inserted as high in the sulcus as possible, angled at about 45 degrees medial to the plane of the ramus (Fig. 7-10). After aspiration, and with very gentle local reorientations of the needle tip, 2 ml 0.5% bupivacaine (containing 1:200,000 epinephrine) is injected.

Eyelids

Sensory Block. Sensory blockade of the eyelids can be attained by anesthesia of the supraorbital and supratrochlear nerves as they emerge from the orbit. For supraorbital block, palpate the supraorbital foramen at the midpoint of the upper margin of the orbit and raise a skin wheal using 2 to 3 ml of local anesthetic (1% lidocaine or 0.25% bupivacaine) at that point, under the eyebrow and with the needle oriented upward; avoid injecting directly into the foramen (see Fig. 7-5). The supratrochlear nerve can be blocked in a similar fashion, although the site of emergence is not so readily palpated. Using a short, sharp bevel 25-gauge needle, raise a small skin wheal at the medial upper segment of the orbit just lateral to the root of the nose (Fig. 7-11). Contact bone with the needle oriented superior and medial and deposit 2 to 3 ml local anesthetic over the periosteum. An alternative (or supplemental) approach often used for blepharoplasty is the subcutaneous infiltration of the upper or lower lids. This is best accomplished with a short 27-gauge needle, using multiple small injections into the plane between skin and muscle. The addition of hyaluronidase will encourage tissue spread of the injectate and reduce anatomic distortion, and the use of 0.5% bupivacaine solution will reduce the volume of injectate needed to a minimum, but may well necessitate generous patient sedation if the pain of injection is not to intrude too forcefully.

Motor Block. Lateral blockade of the facial nerve generates motor blockade of the eyelids, useful during procedures on the awake patient.[33] The easiest way to effect this is by subcutaneous injection of anesthetic along the

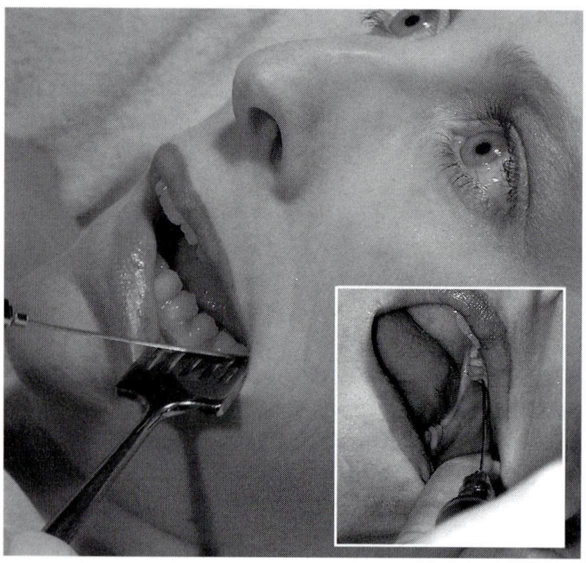

FIG. 7-10 Inferior Alveolar Nerve Block
The patient's mouth is opened widely to allow access to the sulcus formed between the mandibular ramus and the temporalis muscle. Inject as high in the sulcus as possible with the needle angled at about 45 degrees medial to the plane of the ramus.

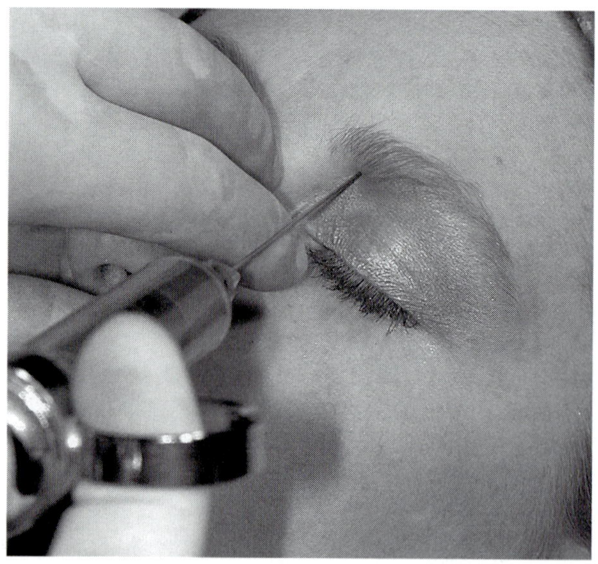

FIG. 7-11 Supratrochlear Nerve Block
A periosteal infiltration at the medial upper segment of the orbit just lateral to the root of the nose.

inferior and lateral margin of the eye approximately 4 cm lateral to the lateral canthus: using a medium-length, sharp 25-gauge needle a skin wheal is raised 2 to 3 cm lateral to the orbital rim. The needle is then directed, via the wheal, in both superior and inferior directions to generate a subcutaneous "wall" or field of anesthetic; patients find this procedure painful unless it is performed very gently and slowly. If the injections are made even more laterally there is increasing chance that a more proximal block of the facial nerve may occur, with resultant distortion of facial features. Appropriate anesthetics for this block are 1% lidocaine or mepivacaine or 0.25% bupivacaine, using a total volume of 4 to 6 ml.

Ears

Sensory Block. Although it is possible to anesthetize the inner ear structures with regional block, most aesthetic procedures on the ear region are likely to involve only the soft tissues of the auricle and immediately surrounding cutaneous surfaces of the external ear. The great auricular, the auriculotemporal, the lesser occipital, and the auricular branch of the vagus innervate the external ear. A variety of complicated field blocks have been described in the past[34,35] but effective block can, in fact, be attained by four oriented injections from a single skin puncture site. The patient should be supine, lightly sedated, head tilted slightly away from the surgeon. Using a 4 cm 25- to 27-gauge needle raise a cutaneous wheal over the tip of the mastoid bone and then inject subcutaneously 2 to 3 cm anterior and 2 to 3 cm posterior from this point to form a line of anesthetic over the surface of the mastoid bone (blocking the posterior auricular and lesser occipital nerve fibers). Withdraw the needle almost to the skin and reorient to make two further injections: first to form a line of anesthetic along the anterior margin of the mastoid, advancing the needle posterior to the auditory canal until bone is encountered; second, withdraw the needle to skin, reorient toward the posterior margin of the temporomandibular joint, advance the needle anterior to the auditory canal, until the tip gently engages the tympanic part of the temporal bone, and inject 2 to 3 ml anesthetic into the posterior mandibular fossa to block the auricular fibers of the auriculotemporal nerve. Effective sensory blockade of the soft tissues of the ear is obtained using a total of 8 to 10 ml anesthetic equally distributed between the four injection tracks. All injections are relatively superficial and, provided inner ear structures are not engaged, the block is relatively free of complications. As with other blocks involving tracking of needles through the subcutaneous tissues, the block will be better appreciated and tolerated by the patient if the injections are made slowly, using a sharp, thin needle, with incremental injection of small amounts of anesthetic as the tip of the needle is advanced through the tissues.

Nose

Sensory Block. Although the infraorbital and infratrochlear branches of the maxillary nerve supply sensory innervation to the cutaneous tissues of the nose, sensory innervation of the deeper structures of the nose is principally by maxillary nerve fibers projected to the sphenopalatine ganglion. Infraorbital nerve block has been described (above) and can be extended medially (with a subcutaneous ridge of anesthetic) to block the infratrochlear fibers supplying the lateral aspects of the bridge of the nose. In older texts[35] there are descriptions of lateral and medial orbital injection routes to the anterior ethmoidal and infratrochlear nerves and to the infraorbital nerve. These are effective blocks for rhinoplasty and nasal reconstruction but, in my opinion, they pose an unnecessary risk to the globe and orbital structures. Sphenopalatine ganglion block is much more safely, and pleasantly, achieved by transmucosal diffusion of anesthetic agent; this is safe and well tolerated by the patient, but requires appreciable soak time to be fully effective. Cotton-tipped applicators ("Q-tips") are soaked in anesthetic solution (4% cocaine solution or proprietary tetracaine-phenylephrine solution), then two or three are gently inserted into each nare and pushed along the superior margin of the middle turbinate until the applicator tips are in contact with the mucosa overlying the ganglion. The swabs are left in place for 5 minutes, then replaced with fresh anesthetic-soaked applicators; this process is repeated three to four times to allow sufficient opportunity for the anesthetic to diffuse through 3 to 5 mm of connective tissue and mucous membrane and reach the ganglion. Note that the direction of insertion of applicator is cephalad in a slightly posterior orientation; it is not the same direction as would be used for topical anesthesia of the nasopharynx or for passage of a nasogastric tube. My choice of anesthetic agent would be 4% lidocaine, but 1% tetracaine can be used to provide a longer-lasting block. On rare occasions, patients with successful sphenopalatine ganglion block will experience orthostatic hypotension; use appropriate monitors, be vigilant for signs, and be ready to provide assistance with standing and ambulation after block placement. After sphenopalatine block, supplemental anesthesia of nasal structures (septal mucosa, lateral wall, nasal tip) can be comfortably established with limited local infiltration of local anesthetic using a 27-gauge needle.

Lips

Infraorbital–Mental Nerve Block. Anesthesia of the lips can be effected by distal trigeminal block at the infraorbital (upper lip) and mental (lower lip) foramina. For aesthetic surgical procedures on the lips, it is helpful to avoid asymmetric muscle paralysis and also to avoid confusing engorgement of tissues by injections directly into the labial tissue. The approach to anesthesia described here will minimize these complications. The foramina are not easily palpated by touch alone; the better technique is to identify the approximate location of the foramina by anatomic landmarks (above), then raise a small skin wheal at the site and gently probe the bony surfaces of the maxilla or mandible or both until the needle tip engages a foramen. As noted previously, avoid injecting anesthetic directly into the foramen; pull the needle tip back a little (1 to 2 mm) before injecting 3 to 5 ml anesthetic solution.

Jaw

Mandibular Nerve Block. For contouring and alloplastic procedures on the angle of the jaw and chin, solid anesthesia of the mandible and associated soft tissue structures can be effected by mandibular nerve block, described above.

Neck

Superficial Cervical Plexus Block. Blockade of the superficial fibers of the cervical plexus yields anesthesia of the superficial structures of the neck sufficient for many aesthetic surgical procedures. The fibers emerge superficially along the posterior margin of the sternocleidomastoid muscle and then redistribute anterior and posterior to supply the skin of the neck. The deep cervical branches are predominantly motor fibers and need only be blocked if major muscular, bony, and articular structures are to be invaded.

For superficial cervical blockade, place the patient in the "sniffing position" (head extended, neck slightly flexed) with the head turned well away from the surgeon. Identify the posterior margin of the sternocleidomastoid muscle; locate the point at which the external jugular vein crosses this margin (Fig. 7-12); insert a 25-gauge bevel tip spinal needle through a skin wheal made at this point and redirect the needle caudad and then cephalad with slow, continuous injection of agent (1% lidocaine or 0.25% bupivacaine) to form a line of anesthetic along the posterior border of the sternocleidomastoid muscle; 10 ml anesthetic solution should be adequate. Because of the superficial nature of the block, complications should be rare, the most common being hematoma formation if the external jugular is punctured. (Phrenic nerve block is a feature only of deep cervical plexus blockade, so even patients who are diaphragm dependent for ventilation are candidates for superficial block.)

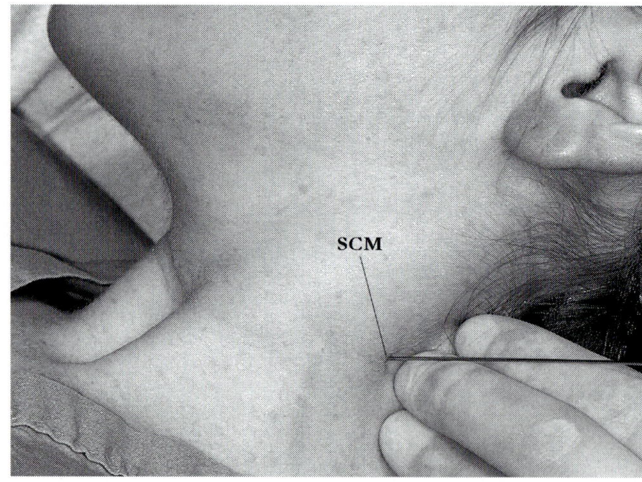

FIG. 7-12 Superficial Cervical Nerve Block
Identify the posterior margin of the clavicular head of the sternocleidomastoid (SCM) muscle approximately at the point where the external jugular vein crosses it; then insert the needle superficially and make a caudal pass and a rostral pass along the muscle margin to form a line of anesthetic along this posterior border of the SCM.

Breast

Although minor breast surgery can be carried out under infiltration anesthesia, more extensive procedures such as augmentation or reduction surgery demand more extensive anesthesia. Although neuraxial blockade can be effective (cervical epidural yielding a segmental thoracic block), this is an approach that should be performed only by anesthesiologists with considerable experience of neuraxial blockade; it is not an approach for the office-based surgeon. An alternative, particularly for surgery that does not encroach on the axillary fossa or involve extensive chest wall dissections, is the so-called *breast block,* which is, in reality, a series of intercostal nerve blocks performed at thoracic dermatomal levels 2 to 7. Success with this approach is more likely with a calm, motivated patient who is not obese; there are two principal approaches that can be employed, and each will be described.

Intercostal Nerve Block (Lateral Approach). Place the patient supine with hands clasped behind the head, to reveal the axillary fossa; prep the flank from the axilla to the costal margin, then mark the mid-axillary line. Palpate ribs 2 to 7 and mark the points where each rib's lower margin intersects the midaxillary line. Using a short, sharp bevel 25-gauge needle and 5 ml syringe filled with 2% lidocaine, make a small skin wheal at each of the points identified (above); do this gently and stay superficial. Now, taking a 10 ml control syringe equipped with 3 cm short bevel 22-gauge needle, identify the midpoint of the second rib in the axillary line by retracting the skin cephalad to position the skin wheal over the body of the rib. Stabilize the operative hand well, then gently insert the needle through the skin, keeping perpendicular to the skin surface in all planes,

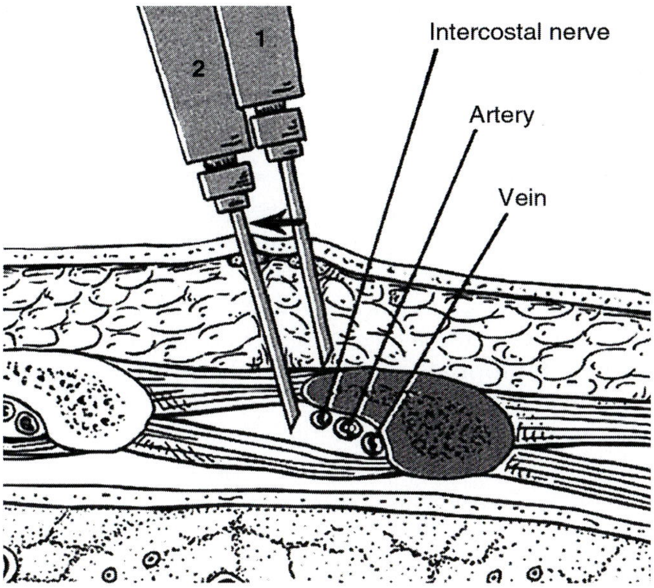

FIG. 7-13 Intercostal Nerve Block
Showing the process of identifying the inferior margin of the rib and "walking off" into the space adjacent to the subcostal groove. (From Morgan GE Jr, Mikhail MS, eds. Clinical Anesthesiology. 3rd ed. Stamford, Conn: Appleton & Lange, 1996.)

and touch the bone. Release skin traction and gently, very gently, walk the needle tip caudad until it just drops over the inferior margin of the rib (Fig. 7-13). Advance the needle tip a further 2 to 3 mm, aspirate to ensure that the tip is not intravenous or subpleural, then inject 2 to 3 ml 0.25% bupivacaine or 1% mepivacaine to suffuse the subcostal groove. Repeat this procedure for each dermatome to be blocked (typically T2-7).

Intercostal Nerve Block (Paravertebral Approach). Place the patient prone on a relatively narrow padded surface (gurney, operating table) with arms loosely hanging at each side so as to rotate the scapulas laterally. Prepare the back over the thoracic midline, then draw two paramedian lines to pass through the posterior angles of the ribs and medial to the medial margins of the scapulas. Palpate and mark the inferior edge of each rib, then follow the general procedures noted above. First raise skin wheals at the intersections of the marking lines, displace the wheals slightly cephalad, insert the regional block needle (22-gauge, 3 cm, short bevel) at the wheal point, then gently walk off the inferior margin of each rib as skin traction is released. Advance the needle a further 3 to 4 mm, aspirate for blood or air, and inject agent adjacent to the subcostal groove (2 to 3 ml 0.25% bupivacaine or 1% mepivacaine).

There are several comments to make about these two approaches to breast anesthesia. Although not technically difficult to perform, both blocks have certain inherent hazards; pneumothorax is a possibility if needle placement is too deep; systemic absorption of local anesthetic is relatively rapid from the subcostal route of injection and blood levels of bupivacaine can be significantly elevated some time (minutes) after placement of an extensive blockade. The approach is difficult in obese patients and is generally uncomfortable even for normal women with normal anatomy; for this reason it is common to provide relatively generous intravenous sedation. Midazolam-fentanyl combinations or propofol are likely to work well for most patients undergoing aesthetic surgery; there is less likely to be a role for droperidol or ketamine in this setting. However, the practitioner must be alert to the consequences of oversedation, particularly in the prone patient, and the usual array of anesthetic monitors must be applied and observed throughout. After placement of intercostal blocks there may be a subjective feeling of dyspnea because of elimination of sensory feedback from the intercostal structures; this is best treated with reassurance and explanation.

The anatomic distribution of the intercostal nerves suggests that the posterior, paravertebral technique is likely to block all branches of each nerve, whereas the midaxillary, lateral technique may spare the anterior and posterior lateral cutaneous branches. Clinically this does not seem to be the case, presumably because there is significant spread of local anesthetic along the inferior margin of the rib in the subcostal groove. Even for surgical procedures limited to cutaneous tissues of the breast it may be necessary to supplement the basic breast block with either a superficial cervical plexus block (as described earlier) or, alternatively, a simple subcutaneous infiltration of local anesthetic along the infraclavicular margin and over the manubrium; this is because fibers from the cervical plexus provide sensory innervation to the upper chest wall and fibers from the contralateral intercostal nerves cross the midline. Again, to emphasize, the breast block is not appropriate for extensive surgery involving axillary structures or deep elements of the chest wall.

Abdomen

Intercostal Nerve Block. Body-contouring procedures such as abdominoplasty or belt lipectomy can be performed under regional anesthesia using a combination of local infiltration at wound margins and regional blockade provided by intercostal blocks. Although it is possible to carry out superficial surgery of the abdominal wall with this combination of anesthetic blockade, some form of systemic supplementation is frequently necessary. Again, this may take the form of bolus administration of modest amounts of midazolam and fentanyl, or may be provided with propofol or methohexital infusion. The approach to abdominal wall block is as described above, except that the dermatomes to be blocked will generally be T6-12. If abdominal wall relaxation is required, then the intercostal injections should be made using 0.5% bupivacaine or 1.5% to 2% mepivacaine; if purely sensory anesthesia is required, 0.25% bupivacaine or 1% mepivacaine will suffice. The same caveats previously noted for breast block apply to the abdominal block; in particular, it may be quite difficult to effect with obese patients (who may, paradoxically, represent a fairly significant proportion of candidates for abdominal contouring).

Thigh

Sensory Block. Sensory innervation of the lateral thigh is by the iliohypogastric and lateral femoral cutaneous nerves. In practice, these can both be readily blocked with a single injection of local anesthetic. With patient supine, identify the anterior superior iliac spine; raise a small skin wheal approximately 2.5 cm medial and caudal to this spine using a sharp, short 30-gauge needle. Using a 3 to 4 cm 23-gauge needle penetrate the skin perpendicularly at the wheal and infiltrate the oblique muscles in a fanlike manner (medial to lateral) using 5 to 10 ml 0.25% bupivacaine. Advance the needle a little deeper to identify fascia lata (by feeling the "pop" as the fascia is penetrated) and inject a further 5 ml anesthetic just deep to the fascial plane, again in a fanwise pattern. Despite the relatively blind approach, the block is generally free of complications and provides excellent sensory anesthesia over the lateral thigh.

Leg

Clearly, sensory anesthesia to the lower extremities (and to the buttocks or inguinal and perineal structures) can be provided very easily and effectively with neuraxial block; equally clearly, these blocks are not to be undertaken other than by anesthesiologists trained in neuraxial anesthetic techniques. Although they are in most cases relatively straightforward to place, spinals and epidurals are never to be attempted by unqualified practitioners. There are, however, safe alternatives appropriate for many aesthetic procedures on the lower extremities. Sensory anesthesia to the anterior thigh and knee region can be provided by femoral nerve block, to the posterior thigh by sciatic nerve block, and to the leg below the knee by a combination of saphenous and popliteal nerve block (for procedures such as vein stripping, etc.). Femoral and saphenous blocks can be placed by anatomic guidance alone; sciatic and femoral blocks generally need to be guided either by elicited paresthesias or by use of a nerve stimulator (Fig. 7-14). A straightforward technique for each block is described next.

Anterior Leg

Femoral Nerve Block. With patient supine, prep the inguinal area, palpate the femoral artery, and raise a skin wheal 1 cm lateral and 1 cm inferior to the point of pulsation using a short, sharp bevel 25-gauge needle. Advance the needle to a depth of 1 cm, maintaining a

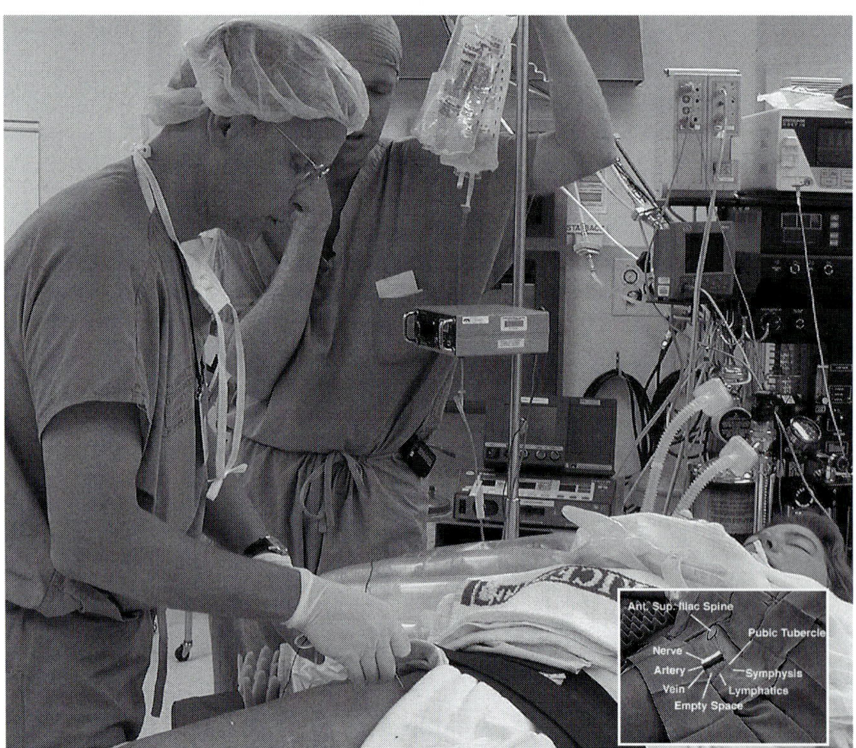

FIG. 7-14 Femoral Nerve Block
General positioning used for location of the femoral nerve using a nerve stimulator, with the local anatomy indicated in the inset. This technique is well tolerated by unsedated, but cooperative, patients provided the nerve stimulator is manipulated with finesse.

slightly cephalad angulation, aspirate for blood, then inject 8 to 10 ml 1% lidocaine or mepivacaine while slowly withdrawing the needle to a depth of 0.5 cm. This is a "blind" technique; results can be improved (or made more certain) by eliciting paresthesias to the anterior thigh or knee. After this block, knee extension will be weakened and ambulation will be difficult until the block has dissipated; use of lidocaine rather than bupivacaine or mepivacaine may permit earlier discharge after day surgery.

Medial Lower Leg and Foot

Saphenous Nerve Block. Place the patient supine, prepare the medial aspect of the knee, and raise a skin wheal 2.5 cm inferior to the medial condyle using a 30-gauge needle. Then, through the wheal, insert a sharp bevel 25-gauge spinal needle and advance the needle tip first anterior and then posterior, injecting 4 to 5 ml anesthetic (0.25% bupivacaine) in each direction, to provide a subcutaneous wall of anesthetic. This provides sensory anesthesia over some of the same territory supplied by the femoral nerve (the saphenous is the terminal branch of the femoral nerve) but spares the knee extensor muscles and facilitates ambulation.

Posterior Leg and Foot

Sciatic Nerve Block. Several eponymous approaches have been described for this somewhat complicated but highly effective method for providing surgical anesthesia to the posterior elements of the leg, the heel, and much of the foot. It is one of the more technically demanding blocks to perform because of the distance the needle must travel from the skin surface to the nerve, which ensures that anatomic guidance alone is seldom successful. Searching for paresthesias can be quite uncomfortable for the patient, so the use of a nerve stimulator is highly recommended (in fact, almost mandatory).

The simplest way to perform the block is to position the patient supine with the leg to be blocked elevated on a padded Mayo stand with 90-degree flexion at hip and knee. After prepping the posterior thigh/buttock, palpate the buttock deeply over the region medial to the greater trochanter of the femur; invariably—even in well-nourished patients—one will feel a distinct groove deep to the superficial fat at the medial margin of gluteus maximus. This groove or sulcus is generally at the midpoint of the imaginary line joining the greater trochanter and ischial tuberosity. Using a 10 to 12 cm nerve stimulator needle, with the negative electrode of the stimulator attached to the needle, puncture the skin over the identified groove and advance the needle tip a short distance into the subcutaneous tissue, orienting the needle tip approximately toward the patient's contralateral shoulder (Fig. 7-15). Adjust the nerve stimulator to give a current of 2 mA, then begin advancing the needle in search of the nerve. The depth to be traveled varies extensively from patient to patient, but typically the

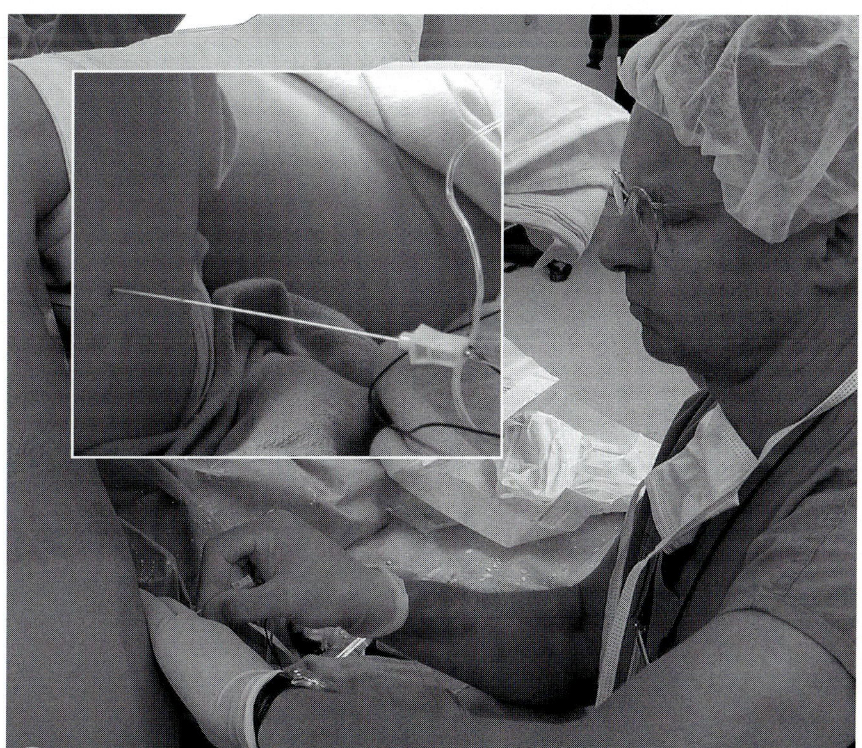

FIG. 7-15 Sciatic Nerve Block
The patient is lying supine with operative leg supported by a padded stand to give 90-degree flexion at hip and knee. The nerve stimulator needle is inserted through the skin lying over the medial margin of gluteal muscle and advanced toward the contralateral shoulder until motor response is encountered. The inset shows that the needle is maintained parallel to the table and may need to be inserted quite some distance in this plane before encountering the sciatic nerve.

nerve will be found at a depth of 8 to 10 cm; plantar flexion and inversion of the foot indicate proximity to the tibial nerve fibers; dorsiflexion and foot eversion are associated with the peroneal fibers. As the needle tip comes closer to the nerve, the muscle movements become stronger and the stimulating current should be reduced; optimal placement of the needle is generally indicated when toe movements (up or down) are just discernible at a current of 0.5 mA. At this point aspirate for blood, then inject 1 ml of local anesthetic; immediate cessation of rhythmic stimulated muscle contractions indicates that the needle tip is in the correct plane. Rapidly inject a further 2 ml anesthetic and watch carefully for relative tachycardia (indicative of intravascular injection of the epinephrine-containing local anesthetic solution[16]); if this test dose is negative, then slowly inject 30 to 35 ml local anesthetic solution (1% lidocaine with 5 μg/ml epinephrine). If this block is performed with bupivacaine, the result will be motor weakness of the affected leg for 12 to 24 hours; lidocaine is a far better choice for day surgery cases.

Problems with this block include failure, necessity for excessive sedation for the patient to tolerate probing with stimulator needle, and intravascular injections (or rapid absorption into the blood) of local anesthetic. These problems all become rare when the practitioner is experienced in the technique. Have an experienced monitor watch the patient carefully while the block is placed and for several minutes after; be very careful not to move the needle once final positioning has been attained (e.g., during injection); pay attention to test doses and the information they yield; stick to lidocaine.

Distal, Posterior Leg and Foot

Popliteal Nerve Block. It is probably optimal to have the patient prone for this block, but lateral positioning may be acceptable in most cases. The terminal branches of the sciatic nerve—the tibial and peroneal nerves—course quite superficially through the popliteal fossa lateral to the popliteal artery. The bifurcation of the sciatic nerve occurs, on average, approximately 7 to 8 cm superior to the popliteal crease, but there is an enormous degree of anatomic variability to this bifurcation. Although the block can be placed "blind," it is probably much more effective to elicit paresthesias and, for this reason, an awake, cooperative, lightly sedated patient is likely to facilitate rather than hinder block placement.

Identify the skin crease behind the knee joint and mark it with a line joining the medial and lateral epicondyles of the femur; identify also the apex of the triangle formed by the lateral margin of the semitendinosus muscle and the medial margin of the biceps femoris muscle. Note these two muscle margins, then bisect the resulting imaginary triangular space with a line running from apex to popliteal crease. At a point 5 to 7 cm superior to the crease and 1 cm lateral to the line just drawn, make a skin wheal. Using a 4 to 6 cm 22-gauge regional needle, pop through the skin wheal, keeping the needle perpendicular to the skin, advance 1 to 2 cm until a paresthesia (to the calf, heel, or ankle) is announced. The needle tip should be lateral to both the popliteal artery and vein at this point; aspirate to confirm no intravascular placement, then inject 25 to 40 ml 1% mepivacaine. If the patient complains of significant pain during injection, stop immediately, since this symptom could herald intraneuronal injection, which is to be avoided. Complications are rare with this block; although ambulation is somewhat hampered by loss of plantar flexion ability, patients are usually mobile enough after unilateral block to ambulate effectively while the block is still in effect.

Foot

Ankle Block. For procedures restricted to the foot, with no tourniquet use, simple ankle block provides excellent anesthesia. Most patients will accept ankle block readily but will appreciate a little sedation for block placement, which can be somewhat painful if the procedure is rushed. Optimal positioning involves having the patient first supine, then prone, but most practitioners become adept at working with seated or supine recumbent patients.

There are five nerves to be blocked if complete foot anesthesia is required: sural, posterior tibial, saphenous, superficial, and deep peroneal. All injections can be made using 4 cm 25-gauge sharp bevel needle with a small skin wheal being made at each site prior to deeper insertion; gentle manipulation with incremental injection of small amounts of anesthetic will minimize the sedation requirements; paresthesias are not sought. Because of frequent need for extended analgesia after foot surgery, 1% mepivacaine is a good choice here; some practitioners mix bupivacaine with lidocaine or prilocaine in order to get a fast-acting, long-acting solution, but this is probably not necessary. Avoid epinephrine if a full circumferential block is planned.

To provide complete ankle block, first prep the entire ankle at the level of the malleoli, then make the following four injections: (1) Just anterior and lateral to the Achilles tendon, insert the needle toward the (lateral) malleolus, touch bone, withdraw 2 to 3 mm, then inject 5 ml while slowly withdrawing the needle to the skin (sural). (2) Repeat on the medial side (posterior tibial). (3) Raise a subcutaneous wheal from medial to lateral malleolus over the dorsum of the foot using 5 to 10 ml anesthetic solution (superficial peroneal and saphenous). (4) Finally, palpate the extensor hallucis longus tendon, identify the dorsalis pedis arterial pulse just lateral to this tendon, and inject 2 to 3 ml anesthetic solution deep to the fascia on both sides of the artery (deep peroneal). This is a safe block, with very few reported complications.

Upper Extremity

As with the sciatic nerve block, many approaches have been described, all with good anatomic rationale. For the majority of aesthetic surgical procedures on the upper extremity (keloid and scar removal, for example), infiltration anesthesia will suffice; for those few occasions when more extensive regional anesthesia is required I would recommend either a periarterial or transarterial axillary nerve block or intravenous (Bier) block as the simplest effective way to attain good results. Interscalene, supraclavicular, and infraclavicular brachial plexus blocks are all widely practiced by anesthesiologists, but they take time to learn and have inherent risks of pneumothorax, intravascular injection, or nerve damage that make them less suited to office-based practices.

Axillary Nerve Block. The upper extremity is innervated by projections from the brachial plexus. At the level of the axilla the plexus has already organized itself into branches and three of these (radial, median, and ulnar) surround the axillary artery where it can most readily be palpated in the groove between the triceps and coracobrachialis muscles just under the lateral margin of the pectoralis muscle. The radial nerve usually lies deep to the artery, the median superior, and the ulnar inferior, and injecting local anesthetic solution adjacent to the axillary artery on all sides has a reasonable chance of eliciting surgical anesthesia of the distal arm and hand. To perform the block, position the patient supine, head turned slightly away, operative arm abducted with elbow flexed and hand tucked behind head. Prep the axilla, palpate the axillary arterial pulse just under the margin of the pectoralis muscle, raise a skin wheal over the pulse, and then use a 23-gauge short bevel regional needle to puncture the skin, directing the needle tip first to the superior side, then the inferior side of the vessel. The objective is to inject approximately 20 ml anesthetic agent just slightly deep to the vessel, delivering approximately 10 ml to the neurovascular sheath at each side of the vessel using a fine, incremental fanning technique and aspirating prior to each incremental injection. If paresthesias are elicited, use the information to determine needle position; if arterial blood is aspirated, again use the information to confirm needle location and inject either deep or superficial to the artery, obviously avoiding intraarterial injection.

Most practitioners of the block use a 10 ml three-ring control syringe; I personally favor the use of narrow-bore extension tubing to connect the regional needle to a 20 ml syringe containing anesthetic solution. I find that this allows good stabilization of the needle while aspirating and injecting, and avoids having to change syringes when >10 ml agent is delivered. The use of a fanning technique is particularly advocated when a "blind" technique is used (although the anatomic rationale for this is endlessly debated in the anesthesia literature).[36]

Intravenous (Bier) Block. The upper extremity to be invaded is identified; a 20-gauge intravenous cannula is inserted into a vein on the dorsum of the hand, taped securely, and fitted with a heparin lock. A double-cuff tourniquet is positioned over the upper humeral region. The arm is elevated and exsanguinated by the very firm application of an Eschmarch bandage wrapped from fingers to axilla. The *proximal* cuff of the tourniquet is inflated to 300 mm Hg, the Eschmarch bandage is removed, the arm is lowered and (typically) 50 mL 0.5% lidocaine solution is slowly injected into the distal intravenous cannula. The cannula is removed and the puncture site dressed. Within 5 minutes the patient should acknowledge essentially complete anesthesia of the upper extremity, which will generally last for 45 to 60 minutes. If, during the course of surgery, the patient begins to complain of tourniquet pain, the following maneuver may prove useful. First, inflate the *distal* cuff to 300 mm Hg, then immediately deflate the *proximal* cuff; this will effectively shift the tourniquet pressure to a region of the arm exposed to intravenous anesthetic, and may well buy enough time for completion of surgery. The total amount of lidocaine used should never exceed 250 mg, and should be prorated for smaller patients; this ensures that accidental deflation of the tourniquet (or early completion of surgery) does not lead to the release of toxic amounts of lidocaine into the general systemic circulation. Do not use any agent other than lidocaine in an attempt to increase the duration of block.

Liposuction

Liposuction is a common approach to removal of unwanted subcutaneous lipid stores; the most frequently treated areas in women are the abdomen, hips, thighs, knees, calves, ankles, and beneath the chin. In men the most commonly treated areas include the waist, the abdomen, breast, and the neck/chin area. In many instances the technique can be performed without invoking general anesthesia, using an approach termed tumescent local anesthesia, involving subcutaneous infiltration of dilute lidocaine solution containing epinephrine—to produce subcutaneous swelling with profound local anesthesia and intense vasoconstriction—followed by aspiration of fat through small cannulae. Although the recommended doses of lidocaine are as high as 55 mg/kg, few safety data are available, and the technique has been the subject of extensive review in the literature.[37] Nevertheless, the general experience with tumescent liposuction is now very extensive and the few catastrophic complications reported seem to have been associated with inadequately monitored heavy sedation or general anesthesia. The possibility of lidocaine toxicity is real, given the very large absolute doses involved, but most of what is administered in the irrigating fluid is not absorbed. Note, however, that systemic toxicity involving high cerebral levels of lidocaine is the most frequent serious adverse outcome associated with its use and that toxic levels can rapidly be established with unintentional intravascular injection. Remember the sequential progression of symptoms of lidocaine toxicity, which usually follow a predictable course: metallic taste — tongue numbness — dizziness — diplopia and visual halos — muscle spasm — unconsciousness — convulsions — coma — respiratory arrest — cardiac depression — anoxic brain damage/death. To emphasize again, an alert and communicative patient may be one of the best monitors of developing toxicity, and for this reason it is probably wise to restrict patients to minimal sedation during liposuction procedures. Although lidocaine is often considered relatively benign, all local anesthetics have similar toxic/therapeutic ratios with respect to CNS inhibition.[38] Lidocaine itself causes dizziness and visual changes at plasma concentrations around 5 μg/ml, convulsions at 10 μg/ml, and respiratory arrest at 20 μg/ml. With tumescent liposuction techniques, it is difficult to predict precise blood levels of lidocaine from the clinical dosage used, so a careful watch must be maintained for the early symptoms of toxicity. The local anesthetics do not themselves cause permanent CNS damage, but cerebral hypoxia during coma and decreased perfusion states is exacerbated by acidosis, hyperkalemia, and hypoxemia generated by seizure activity. Therefore, if toxicity is noted, stop administration of agent at once, provide supportive measures (airway maintenance, oxygen supplementation, etc.) and treat seizures. Generally, thiopental (2 to 4 mg/kg) or diazepam (0.1 mg/kg) will break seizure activity; if muscle spasm interferes with ventilation, then succinylcholine (1 mg/kg) can be used, but this is not a trivial intervention and should not be undertaken unless endotracheal intubation could be performed *immediately* if ventilation remains problematic. Again, to emphasize, appropriate resuscitation equipment should be available at every location where regional anesthetics are administered, and appropriate monitors must be used for every case.[39]

POSTOPERATIVE CLINICAL CONSIDERATIONS

Postoperative considerations relating to the provision of anesthesia for day surgery cases focus on sequelae of regional anesthesia such as persistent motor or sensory blockade, urinary retention, unsteady ambulation, and emerging pain as blocks dissipate; also on sequelae of sedation such as dysphoria, nausea, residual drowsiness, and mental confusion. Nausea is quite common after certain surgical procedures,[40] is occasionally resistant to treatment, but is frequently minimized by prophylactic medication such as metaclopramide with droperidol[41] and by adequate analgesia.[42] Dysphoria, drowsiness, and confusion generally clear with time, but patients should be watched closely for signs of hypoperfusion or stroke, both of which can masquerade as delayed recovery from sedative hypnotics.

Patients undergoing day surgery will generally have, as a matter of course, a follow-up appointment for a clinic visit made as part of their standard discharge protocol. If regional anesthetic techniques have been used (and as a matter of good clinical practice in general), it is prudent also to contact the patient at home within 24 hours of the surgery to ascertain that all is well. Persistent nerve blockade, resulting in subjective symptoms of muscle weakness or sensory deficit, should arouse suspicion of nerve damage. This damage might have originated during execution of a nerve block, or, alternatively, might be a consequence of surgical positioning, or even of surgical trauma. It is difficult to be categorical about when to be concerned, but nerve blocks lasting for greater than 12 hours when mepivacaine or lidocaine have been used, or greater than 24 hours in the case of bupivacaine, may well warrant neurologic evaluation. For medicolegal reasons, as well as for reasons of professional thoroughness, the evaluation should ideally be performed, and charted, by a neurologist.

REFERENCES

1. Winnie AP. Plexus Anesthesia: Perivascular Techniques of Brachial Plexus Block. Philadelphia: WB Saunders, 1983.
2. Blake DW. The general versus regional anaesthesia debate: time to re-examine the goals. Aust N Z J Surg 1995; 65:51-56.
3. O'Toole DP, Cunningham AJ. Regional anesthesia for major vascular surgery. Yale J Biol Med 1993; 66:447-456.
4. Butterworth JF, Strichartz GR. Molecular mechanisms of local anesthesia: a review. Anesthesiology 1990; 72:711-734.
5. Caterall WA. Structure and function of voltage-gated ion channels. Ann Rev Biochem 1995; 64:493-531.
6. Gajraj NM, Pennant JH, Watcha MF. Eutectic mixture of local anesthetics (EMLA) cream. Anesth Analg 1994; 78:574.
7. Keyes PD, Tallon JM, Rizos J. Topical anesthesia. Can Fam Physician 1998; 44:2152-2156.
8. Smith GA, Strausbaugh SD, Harbeck-Weber C, Cohen DM, Shields BJ, Powers JD. Tetracaine-lidocaine-phenylephrine topical anesthesia compared with lidocaine infiltration during repair of mucous membrane lacerations in children. Clin Pediatr 1998; 37:405-412.
9. Kuhn M, Rossi SO, Plummer JL, Raftos J. Topical anaesthesia for minor lacerations: MAC versus TAC. Med J Aust 1996; 164:277-280.
10. Hallen A, Ljunghall K, Wallin J. Topical anaesthesia with local anaesthetic (lidocaine and prilocaine, EMLA) cream for cautery of genital warts. Genitourin Med 1987; 63:316-319.

11. White WB, Iserson KV, Criss E. Topical anesthesia for laceration repair: tetracaine versus TAC (tetracaine, adrenaline, and cocaine). Am J Emerg Med 1986; 4:319-322.
12. Albright GA. Cardiac arrest following regional anesthesia with etidocaine or bupivacaine. Anesthesiology 1979; 51:285-291.
13. Auroy Y, Narchi P, Messiah A, Litt L, Rouvier B, Samii K. Serious complications related to regional anesthesia: results of a prospective survey in France. Anesthesiology 1997; 87:479-486.
14. Lambert LA, Lambert DH, Strichartz GR. Irreversible conduction block in isolated nerve by high concentration of local anesthetics. Anesthesiology 1994; 80:1082-1093.
15. Incaudo G, Schatz M, Patterson R, Rosenberg M, Yamamoto F, Hamburger RN. Administration of local anesthetics to patients with a history of prior adverse reaction. J Allergy Clin Immunol 1978; 61:339-345.
16. Moore DC, Batra MS. The components of an effective test dose prior to epidural block. Anesthesiology 1981; 55:693-696.
17. Moore DC, Mater LE, Bridenbaugh PO. Severe hypoxia and acidosis following local anesthesia-induced convulsions. Anesthesiology 1980; 53:259-265.
18. Clarkson CW, Hondeghem LM. Mechanism for bupivacaine depression of cardiac conduction: fast block of sodium channels during the action potential with slow recovery from block during diastole. Anesthesiology 1985; 62:396-405.
19. Kasten GW, Martin ST. Bupivacaine cardiovascular toxicity: comparison of treatment with bretylium and lidocaine. Anesth Analg 1985; 64:911-915.
20. Kasten GW, Martin ST. Successful cardiovascular resuscitation after massive intravenous bupivacaine overdose in anesthetized dogs. Anesth Analg 1985; 64:491-496.
21. Kuschner WG, Chitkara RK, Canfield J Jr, Poblete-Coleman LM, Cunningham BA, Sarinas PS. Benzocaine-associated methemoglobinemia following bronchoscopy in a healthy research participant. Respir Care 2000; 45:953-956.
22. Smith GA, Strausbaugh SD, Harbeck-Weber C, Cohen DM, Shields BJ, Powers JD. Prilocaine-phenylephrine topical anesthesia for repair of mucous membrane lacerations. Pediatr Emerg Care 1998; 14:324-328.
23. Kehlet H. The surgical stress response: should it be prevented? Can J Surg 1991; 34:565-567.
24. Nguyen HN. [Recovery after anesthesia with Diprivan]. Ann Fr Anesth Reanim 1994; 13:519-523.
25. Fiset L, Milgrom P, Beirne OR, Roy-Byrne P. Disinhibition of behaviors with midazolam: report of a case. J Oral Maxillofac Surg 1992; 50:645-649.
26. Lieberherr S, Scollo-Lavizzari G, Battegay R. [Confusional states following administration of short-acting benzodiazepines (midazolam/triazolam)]. Schweiz Rundsch Med Prax 1991; 80:673-675.
27. Brown DL. Atlas of Regional Anesthesia. Philadelphia: WB Saunders, 1999.
28. Hahn MB, McQuillan PM, Sheplock GJ. Regional Anesthesia. St Louis: Mosby, 1996.
29. Mulroy MF. Regional Anesthesia. Boston: Little, Brown, 1996.
30. Scott DB. Techniques of Regional Anesthesia. East Norwalk, Conn: Appleton & Lange, 1989.
31. Abadir AR, Hymayun SG. Anesthesia for Plastic and Reconstructive Surgery. St Louis: Mosby, 1991.
32. Nique TA, Tu HK. Anesthesia for Facial Plastic Surgery. New York: Thieme, 1993.
33. Atkinson WS. The development of ophthalmic anesthesia. Am J Ophthalmol 1961; 51:1.
34. Braun H. Local Anesthesia. Philadelphia: Lea & Febiger, 1924.
35. Pitkin GP. Conduction Anesthesia. Philadelphia: Lippincott, 1946.
36. Winnie AP, Radonjic R, Akkineni SR, Durrani Z. Factors influencing distribution of local anesthetic injected into the brachial plexus sheath. Anesth Analg 1979; 58:225-234.
37. Rao RB, Ely SF, Hoffman RS. Deaths related to liposuction. N Engl J Med 1999; 340:1471-1475.
38. Liu PL, Feldman HS, Giasi R, Patterson MK, Covino BG. Comparative CNS toxicity of lidocaine, etidocaine, bupivacaine, and tetracaine in awake dogs following rapid intravenous administration. Anesth Analg 1983; 62:375-379.
39. Eichhorn JH. Prevention of intraoperative anesthesia accidents and related severe injury through safety monitoring [see comments]. Anesthesiology 1989; 70:572-577.
40. Pataky AO, Kitz DS, Andrews RS. Nausea and vomiting following ambulatory surgery: are all procedures created equal? Anesth Analg 1988; 67:S163.
41. Doze VA, Schafer A, White PF. Nausea and vomiting after outpatient anesthesia: effectiveness of droperidol alone and in combination with metoclopramide. Anesth Analg 1987; 66:S41.
42. Anderson R, Crogh K. Pain as a major cause of postoperative nausea. Can Anaesth Soc J 1976; 23:366-372.
43. Rowlingson JC. Toxicity of local anesthetic additives. Reg Anesth 1993; 18:453-460.

APPENDIX A

Patient Instructions

CONSENT

Consent for anesthesia is generally included in the rubric of consent for surgery used in most standardized forms. Patient consent needs to be *informed* consent, meaning that patients have been offered a full, although not necessarily exhaustive, description of what it is that will be done to them, the risks they run, and the benefits they stand to gain. When dealing with issues of anesthesia and pain control, avoid the use of jargon and platitudes ("risks discussed, dental to death") but instead talk reassuringly to the patients, telling them in lay terms what measure of discomfort they may reasonably expect during the various stages of the planned procedure and outlining the possible complications that might be expected. I think it is reasonable to ignore discussion of specific complications that occur in less than 1% to 5% of cases in *your* practice unless the patient is particularly inquisitive.

PREOPERATIVE INSTRUCTIONS

Patients should arrive for surgery with an empty stomach and empty bladder; they should abstain from food for 6 hours and water for 2 hours prior to surgery. They should take all their normal medications at the appointed time, but should be given specific instructions about aspirin, coumarin, metformin, and insulin intake. Arrangements need to be made for timely arrival on the day of surgery, and for escort home later in the day.

POSTOPERATIVE INSTRUCTIONS

In addition to the postoperative protocols for the surgical procedure, the patient should be encouraged to report any complications with regional anesthetics. These include persistent sensory or motor block, paresthesias, unexpected pain, difficulties with voiding, persistent nausea, visual or cognitive disturbances, or general malaise. Take careful note of any complaints reported postoperatively, record them accurately, and deal with them promptly and with sensitivity. Having the patient evaluated by a neurologist can often be a wise move in the event of possible neurologic sequelae of surgery or anesthesia.

APPENDIX B

Additives Commonly Mixed with Local Anesthetics

SODIUM BICARBONATE

Because the free base form of most local anesthetics is poorly soluble in water, they are prepared as hydrochloride salts with commercial solutions having a pH in the range of 4 to 6. Addition of bicarbonate can increase the rate of onset of some local anesthetics by shifting the equilibrium to the uncharged base form, which readily penetrates into nerve tissue. Neutralizing the pH of a local anesthetic solution may also decrease the associated pain on injection. Using an 8.4% sodium bicarbonate solution, 1 ml can be added to a lidocaine 30 ml vial or 0.2 ml can be added to a bupivacaine 30 ml vial. Attempts to add further bicarbonate will result in precipitation of the local anesthetic from its solution.

PRESERVATIVES

Antimicrobial preservatives are added to multidose vials of local anesthetics. Preservative-containing local anesthetic solutions must not be used in spinal or epidural anesthesia because of their potentially cytotoxic effects. The most frequently used antimicrobials are methyl- ethyl- and propyl-*para*benzoates. Antioxidants or ion chelating agents such as sodium ethylenediaminetetraacetic acid (EDTA) are added to commercially available local anesthetics to prevent oxidation or to scavenge divalent cations and thus retard their degradation. Preservative-free preparations are available for patients suspected of having allergies to any of these preservatives.

EPINEPHRINE

Low concentrations of epinephrine can be added to local anesthetics in order to retard their systemic absorption. This has the effect of decreasing blood levels, thus minimizing toxic reactions and prolonging the duration of anesthesia they produce. Addition of 5 μg epinephrine to each 1 ml of local anesthetic produces the commonly used 1:200,000 concentration. Caution is exercised with patients known to suffer from coronary vascular disease, and epinephrine-containing solutions should never be injected into areas with no collateral circulation, such as fingers, toes, ears, penis, and nose.[43]

CHAPTER 8

Office-Based Sedation and Monitoring

RODNEY L. TRYTKO

SECTION ONE

History and Scientific Review

BACKGROUND AND HISTORY

In the past few years, the number of office-based procedures has risen dramatically. Some experts predict that within 5 years, 10 million office-based surgical procedures will be performed each year.[1] The factors driving this growth include patient preference, cost containment, physician autonomy, and advances in anesthesia. Today, a growing number of patients can have anesthesia and surgery in offices with minimal postoperative pain, bleeding, and side effects.

Because many of these procedures are also uncomfortable or painful, the need has grown rapidly for office-based conscious sedation and general anesthesia. Anesthesiologists have responded to this new office-based setting by applying expertise gained in ambulatory settings. New anesthetic medications are extremely short acting and have minimal side effects. Fast emergence and early discharge have become the norm. Industry interest in developing smaller and more portable monitoring and resuscitation equipment has created a safer environment for conscious sedation and anesthesia.

Despite all the advances and enthusiasm, serious concerns regarding safety are now being raised. Conscious sedation is no longer considered completely safe. The American Society of Anesthesiology (ASA) Closed Claims Study demonstrates a rapid growth in malpractice claims and injury severity associated with conscious sedation among anesthesiologists.[2] In fact, this study demonstrates a greater proportion of permanent injuries and a lower proportion of temporary injuries than in claims associated with general or regional anesthesia.

For this reason, a number of entities have developed office-based guidelines for conscious sedation and general anesthesia. The ASA has developed guidelines for "Sedation and Analgesia for Non-anesthesiologists"[3] and "Office-Based Anesthesia"[4] (Appendixes B and C). The American College of Surgeons has developed guidelines for office-based surgery, and the recommendations for conscious sedation and general anesthesia are very similar to the ASA's guidelines.[5] The Accreditation Association for Ambulatory Health Care has established new quality standards for office-based anesthesia organizations.[6] Finally, several states have passed legislation (California, Florida, Texas, and New Jersey) to regulate conscious sedation and anesthesia in the office-based setting.

BASIC SCIENCE

A continuum exists for sedation that ranges from conscious sedation to general anesthesia (Fig. 8-1). No discrete interval exists between the various levels of sedation. Too much medication can rapidly convert conscious sedation into general anesthesia and expose the patient to the risks associated with an unsecured airway and a lack of protective reflexes.

Conscious sedation* describes a state that allows patients to tolerate unpleasant procedures while maintaining adequate cardiorespiratory function and the ability to respond purposefully to verbal commands and tactile stimulation. Conscious sedation provides three general types of benefits. First, it allows patients to tolerate (and sometimes forget) unpleasant procedures by relieving anxiety, discomfort, or pain. Second, conscious sedation may expedite the conduct of procedures in uncooperative patients who are not particularly uncomfortable but are required to not move. Finally, conscious sedation permits many uncomfortable procedures to be performed without the need for general anesthesia.

Deep sedation is a medically controlled state of decreased consciousness or unconsciousness from which

*Conscious sedation, monitored anesthesia care (MAC), and "sedation and analgesia" are all equivalent terms.

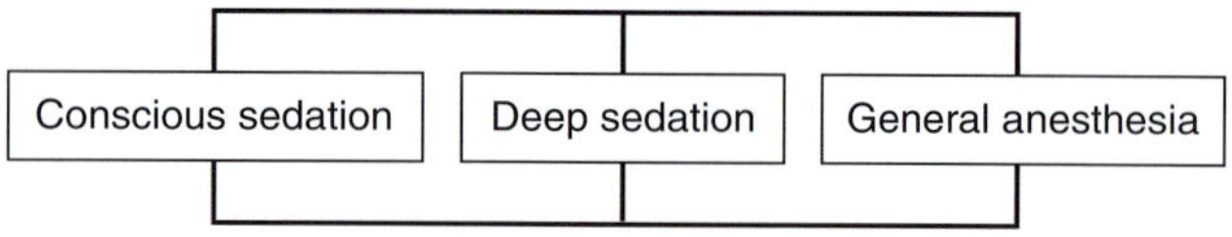

FIG. 8-1
Sedation continuum.

the patient is not easily aroused. It is associated with the possible loss of protective airway reflexes, the possible inability to maintain a patent airway independently, and the inability to respond purposefully to tactile or verbal stimulation. If the only response to stimulation is withdrawal, a condition of deep sedation exists. Deep sedation is never a desirable state in an office-based setting and should be converted either to conscious sedation or general anesthesia.

General anesthesia is a medically controlled state of unconsciousness and amnesia. It is associated with a loss of protective airway reflexes, the inability to maintain a patent airway independently, and the inability to respond to tactile or verbal stimulation. General anesthesia can be administered with potent inhalational anesthetic gases (e.g., Forane, Sevoflurane, and halothane), total intravenous anesthesia (TIVA), or a combination of both. The patient under general anesthesia is completely dependent upon the anesthesiologist to resuscitate him or her from the anesthesia after the surgical procedure. For this reason, general anesthesia should be administered only by an anesthesiologist.

Providing general anesthesia in an office-based setting can be time consuming, risky, and expensive. Many offices lack noninvasive monitoring equipment, emergency resuscitation equipment, recovery facilities, or appropriate perioperative nursing personnel. Many offices also lack adequate suction for anesthetic trace gas scavenging; therefore, the utilization of an anesthesia machine is problematic. TIVA techniques with minimal complications and extremely rapid recoveries have become the standard anesthetic technique in the office-based setting. For those offices with capabilities to support an anesthesia machine, general anesthesia can be administered as in any ambulatory surgery center or hospital.

CLINICAL STUDIES

Conscious Sedation

Conscious sedation techniques for office-based procedures typically combine a short-acting sedative-hypnotic (midazolam or propofol) and a short-acting narcotic (fentanyl). The goal is to provide a comfortable situation for the patient and the operating practitioner while minimizing recovery times and unintended admissions. Specifically, the pain associated with injection of the local anesthetic should be eliminated. Also, patient apprehension and recall should be reduced or eliminated. In order to achieve these goals, a combination of medications is usually necessary.

The simplest technique involves incremental doses of midazolam (Versed) and fentanyl.[7] An alternative is to infuse propofol in order to titrate the level of sedation.[8] The typical total dosages of medication correlate significantly with procedure duration. Recovery typically is rapid (<10 min) with a minimum of delirium and confusion. The most common complication is nausea and emesis, which occur in a minority of patients. Discharge times are longer for patients who developed nausea or emesis, younger patients, and patients receiving preoperative oral sedation.[7]

Propofol infusions require heightened surveillance for the monitoring individual because of propofol's propensity to rapidly produce anesthesia as well as apnea. Slow and careful titration of the propofol by individuals experienced with this technique will result in a very favorable and safe conscious sedation experience for the patient.

General Anesthesia

General anesthesia can be administered with potent inhalational anesthetic gases (e.g., Forane, Sevoflurane, and halothane), total intravenous anesthesia, or a combination of both. Administering potent inhalational anesthetics requires an anesthesia machine and suction capabilities to scavenge trace anesthetic gases. For this reason, most office-based general anesthesia techniques involve TIVA.

Many TIVA techniques with minimal complications and extremely rapid recoveries have been described.[9-18] TIVA offers advantages over inhalational anesthesia in terms of patient satisfaction, lower costs, and improved recovery profile.[9,16,17] Most TIVA techniques utilize a propofol infusion that is supplemented with fentanyl or ketamine (Appendix E). With TIVA, the patients are asleep and hemodynamically stable, the surgical field is steady, the time requirements for the operating practitioner are substantially decreased, and the postoperative complications are minimal. Since the patients are under general anesthesia, an anesthesiologist should be present at all times. While the absence of a local or regional block does not affect the operative procedure when the patients are under general anesthesia, blocks may dramatically reduce postoperative pain. Finally, after short TIVA techniques the patients typically are ready to be safely discharged after a minimal recovery period.[15-17]

Dissociative anesthesia is a TIVA technique that was first popularized almost 20 years ago.[18] While the original dissociative technique involved diazepam and ketamine, newer techniques have replaced diazepam with propofol infusions. The propofol-ketamine technique is

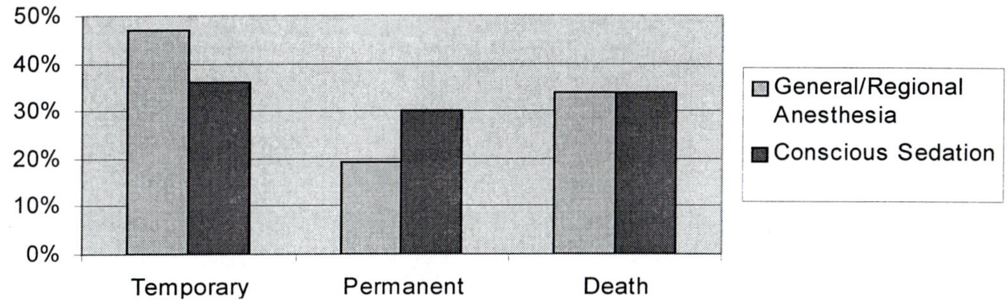

FIG. 8-2
Proportion of claims resulting from various types of injury based on type of anesthetic in the ASA Closed Claims Study.[2]

an opioid-avoidance, room air, and spontaneous ventilation dissociative anesthesia technique that has been extensively studied[17] (Appendix E). While most anesthesiologists rarely utilize ketamine, these studies all seem to demonstrate the efficacy and safety of dissociative anesthesia in those centers experienced with this technique. While some disagreement currently exists as to whether this technique is general anesthesia or conscious sedation, the conduct of all TIVAs, including propofol-ketamine, should be only in the presence of an anesthesiologist.

Postoperative Care

Recovery is a continual process. Patients cannot be considered fully recovered until they have returned to their preoperative physical and mental status. Respiratory depression in the early postoperative period is a significant risk to all patients after sedation.[19] Postoperative monitoring must continue until the patient meets accepted discharge criteria.[20] The best method for determining discharge readiness after an office-based procedure is to utilize the Post Anesthesia Scoring System[21] (Appendix F). In the last few years, the requirement for oral intake and voiding has been questioned; however, this issue remains unresolved. Quality postoperative nursing care is the single most important factor to ensure rapid discharge.[22]

Sedation and Anesthesia Risk

The risk of general anesthesia has dramatically declined because of the advances in airway management, monitoring standards, and improved supervision. Currently the risk of death from anesthesia is less than 1 in 185,000.[23]

Contrarily, the ASA Closed Claims study has demonstrated an increasing number of annual malpractice litigation actions involving serious injuries associated with conscious sedation in the last decade[2] (Fig. 8-2). In addition, these claims demonstrate that the risk associated with permanent injury for conscious sedation exceeds that of general anesthesia.

Recently, a particularly disturbing study described the mortality associated with liposuction.[24] In a large survey of plastic surgeons, 95 liposuction-related fatalities in nearly half a million procedures yielded a normalized fatality rate of 19.1 per 100,000. The most common location of the procedures resulting in death was an office (45%). The most commonly identified cause of death was thromboembolism (23.1%). Although several different techniques for performing liposuction (with varying safety records) are available to the surgeon, a distinct trend in deaths during the first postoperative night following sedation and anesthesia suggests that better postoperative monitoring may prove to be beneficial.

DISCUSSION

Conscious sedation and general anesthesia can be safely administered to healthy adults in an office-based setting. For conscious sedation, the ASA's sedation and analgesia guidelines[3] should be meticulously followed in order to ensure patient safety. General anesthesia with TIVA can be safely administered by an anesthesiologist to healthy office-based adult patients for procedures while enabling a rapid discharge to home. The practice of office-based pediatric sedation is controversial and probably should be avoided.

Unfortunately, private physician offices have been relatively insulated from the quality improvement movement that has swept the rest of the country. The public will likely become more educated on the problems associated with quality in the office-based setting. Eventually, they will demand outcome studies, quality equivalent to the hospital setting, and economic evaluations. Certainly, the risks associated with sedation warrant further study; however, the future will demonstrate that many procedures now performed in an ambulatory surgery center or a hospital can be safely performed in the office-based setting.

SECTION TWO

Atlas of Surgical Procedures

PREOPERATIVE CLINICAL CONSIDERATIONS

Patient Selection

The ASA classifies patients according to preoperative physical status with classes I to V (Table 8-1). Conscious sedation should be limited to adult patients younger than 70 years old with ASA physical status I to III. The ASA Closed Claims study has demonstrated that for conscious sedation, age greater than 70 years and ASA physical status III to V result in a higher risk of litigation.[2] General anesthesia should be limited to ASA physical status I to III. Physical status has been demonstrated to correlate with anesthetic outcome in at least one study.[25]

Preprocedure Preparation

Patients should be informed of the associated risks and agree to the administration of conscious sedation or anesthesia before the procedure begins. All reasonably possible complications should be discussed.

Table 8-1 ASA Physical Status Classification

Category	Description
I	Healthy patient
II	Mild systemic disease; no functional limitation
III	Severe systemic disease; definite functional limitation
IV	Severe systemic disease that is a constant threat to life
V	Moribund patient unlikely to survive 24 hours with or without operation

A preoperative history should include the following:

1. Abnormalities of the major organ systems
2. Previous adverse experience with conscious sedation, and regional and general anesthesia
3. Current medications and drug allergies
4. Time and nature of last oral intake
5. History of tobacco, alcohol, or substance use or abuse

ASA guidelines for preoperative fasting and the use of pharmacologic agents to reduce the risk of pulmonary aspiration were recently developed for all patients undergoing conscious sedation or general anesthesia.[26] These guidelines state that the preoperative fast should be at least 2 hours for clear liquids, 4 hours for breast milk, and 6 hours for all other liquids and solid foods. Medications may be given at their usual times with a sip of water. The routine use of medications to reduce the risk of pulmonary aspiration is not recommended.

Patients should undergo a focused physical examination including auscultation of the heart and lungs, and evaluation of the airway. Airway evaluation is performed in order to identify patients who are likely to be difficult to intubate. Such patients should be sedated with extreme caution, and general anesthesia should be avoided in the office setting (Fig. 8-3). Airway evaluation includes the following three criteria:

1. Relative tongue size. Mallampati utilized three classifications for describing the relative size of the tongue.[27] The Mallampati classification is best obtained with the patient in the sitting position with the head in full extension, tongue out, and with phonation.[28]
2. Mandibular space (space anterior to the larynx) size. This is the space where the tongue must be displaced in order to intubate the patient under direct vision.
3. Atlanto-occipital joint extension. Such extension aligns the laryngeal and oral axes.

Only patients who are Mallampati class I or II, possess a mandibular space greater than 6 cm, and demon-

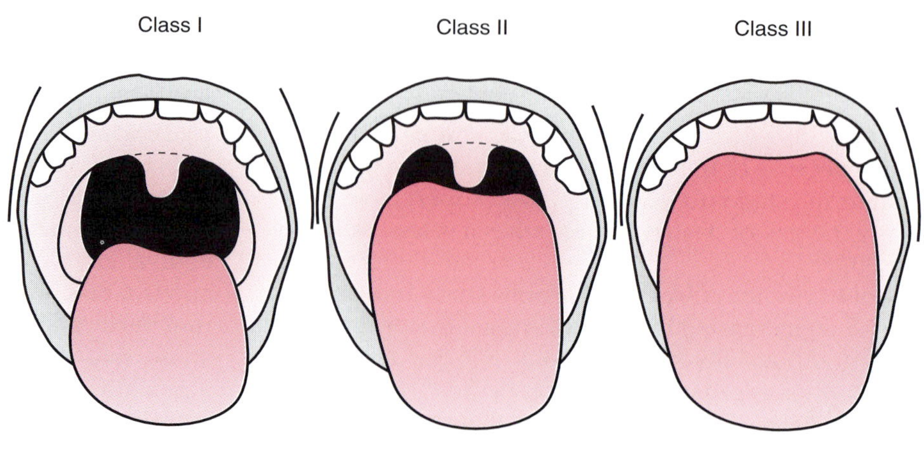

FIG. 8-3
Mallampati classification.[27]

strate an atlanto-occipital extension greater than 35% should be considered candidates for office-based procedures.[29]

Preprocedure testing should be guided by the patient's underlying medical condition and the likelihood that the results will affect the management of conscious sedation and general anesthesia. ASA physical status I patients scheduled for noninvasive surgery do not need laboratory tests before the procedure.[30] Other testing (laboratory, ECG, and chest x-rays) should be considered only for specific indications.

PROCEDURAL TECHNIQUES

Procedure Guidelines and Standards

Basic monitoring standards for anesthesiology were first developed at the Harvard Medical School and then adopted 1 year later by the ASA.[31,32] The ASA has also promulgated a number of guidelines and standards pertinent to office-based conscious sedation and general anesthesia, and these are listed in Appendixes A to C. In addition, suction, emergency equipment of the proper size, narcotic and benzodiazepine antagonists, emergency medications, oxygen, and a positive pressure delivery device should be immediately available.

Conscious Sedation

A designated individual should be present to monitor the patient throughout procedures. This individual should understand the pharmacology of the agents that are administered, understand the role of pharmacologic antagonists for opioids and benzodiazepines, and recognize the associated complications. At least one individual capable of establishing a patent airway and positive pressure ventilation, as well as a means for summoning additional assistance, should be present whenever conscious sedation is administered. It is recommended that an individual with advanced life-support skills be immediately available.

Most techniques involve the following steps:

1. Establish an intravenous line.
2. Administer fentanyl 0.05 to 1 μg/kg IV prn
   and
3. Administer midazolam 0.5 to 1 mg IV prn
   and/or
4. Administer continuous propofol infusion (25 to 50 μg/kg/min), increasing at increments of 5 μg/kg/min prn. Rarely more than 150 μg/kg/min is needed.

All medications (see Appendix D) should be carefully titrated in order to achieve the desired level of conscious sedation. The typical total dosages of medication correlate significantly with procedure duration as well as patient age, sex, and weight.

General Anesthesia

General anesthesia should be conducted only by an anesthesiologist. General anesthesia techniques utilize either a potent inhalational anesthetic gas, TIVA, or some combination of both. TIVA does not require an anesthesia machine or the need for trace anesthetic gas scavenging equipment. Since most offices do not have such equipment, TIVA offers a cost-effective alternative for providing general anesthesia in an office-based setting.

Two TIVA protocols are listed in Appendix E. A picture of an office-based laser facial resurfacing under TIVA is in Figure 8-4. Please note that all of the ASA Basic Monitoring Standards can easily be followed in an

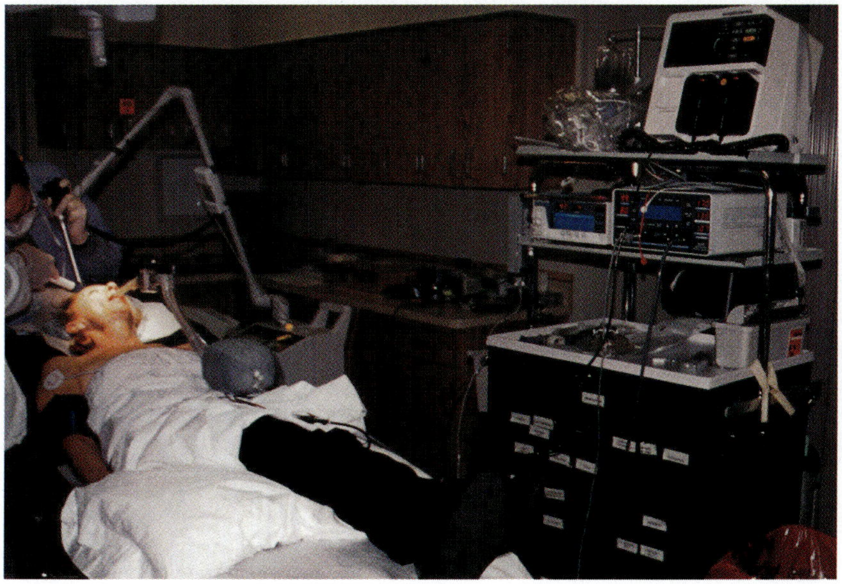

FIG. 8-4
W. Phillipa Werschler, MD, is performing laser facial resurfacing under total intravenous anesthesia (TIVA) at the Spokane Dermatology Clinic, Spokane, Washington.

office-based setting and that an anesthesia machine is not required.

Perioperative Risk Management

The primary complication associated with conscious sedation and general anesthesia in an office-based setting is airway mismanagement. A particularly dangerous combination of apnea and unresponsiveness occurs when sedative-hypnotics and narcotics are utilized simultaneously. Another common problem is airway obstruction at the level of the oral pharynx caused by the relaxation of the normal tone of the genioglossus muscle.

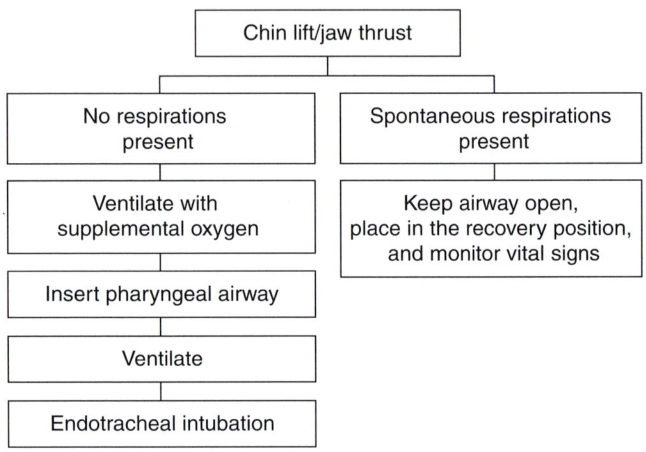

FIG. 8-5
Open airway algorithm.

Upon recognizing hypoventilation or apnea, the open airway algorithm should be followed until the patient returns to a stable state of unassisted respiration and adequate oxygen saturation (Fig. 8-5).

The first response to a suspected hypoventilation or apnea should be an immediate attempt to open the airway. Most of the time, a simple chin lift will either relieve the obstruction or stimulate the patient to begin breathing. If the problem persists, the next steps include pharmacologic reversal agents and positive pressure ventilation. As previously stated, combinations of sedatives and narcotics are much more likely to cause hypoventilation or apnea. While pharmacologic reversal agents are available for narcotics and benzodiazepines, usually only reversing the narcotic is necessary to restore adequate ventilation. Small doses of Narcan (see Appendix D) are usually effective.

If positive pressure mask ventilation is attempted, one person should hold the face while maintaining a mask seal and a chin lift/jaw thrust, while the other person squeezes the bag. In those rare situations in which the open airway algorithm is followed and the patient cannot be intubated, an obturator airway (laryngeal mask airway or Combitube) should be immediately inserted and positive pressure ventilation with 100% oxygen should be administered. Laryngeal mask airways (LMA) are placed blindly and obturate the airway at the level of the larynx (Fig. 8-6). Adult LMAs typically are sizes 3 to 5.

These situations are true emergencies, and airway management experts should be immediately summoned.

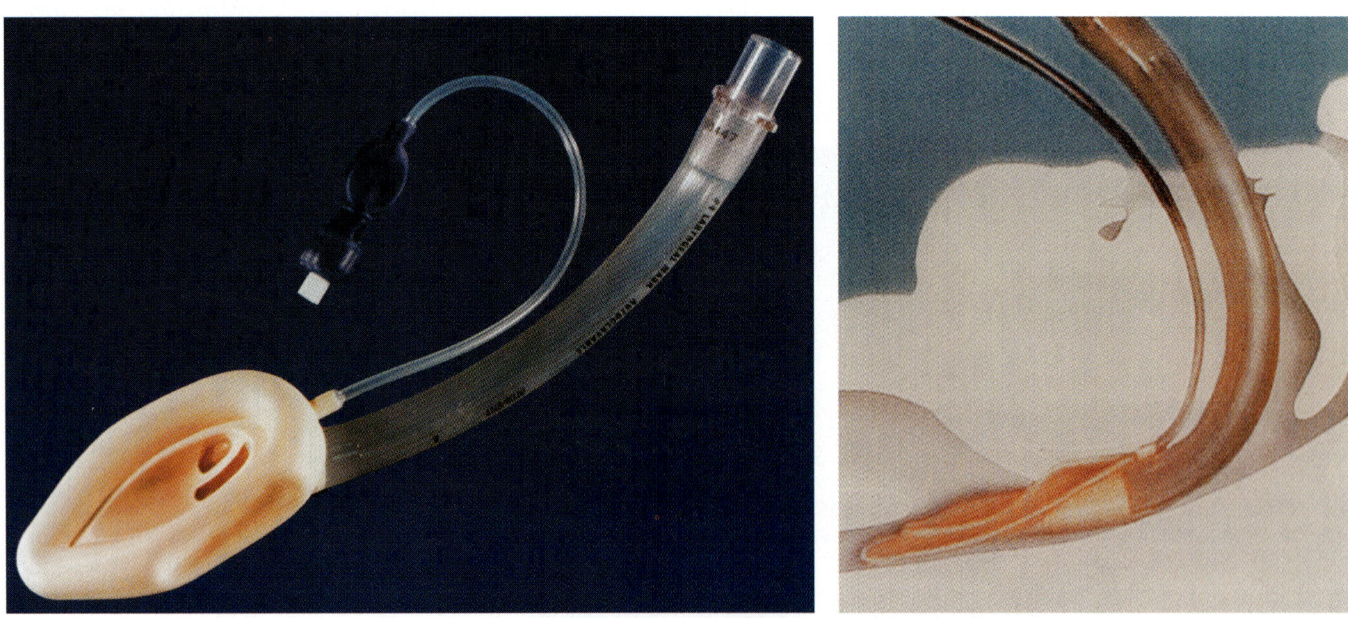

FIG. 8-6
Laryngeal mask airway (LMA). *Left,* An LMA. *Right,* Diagram of an LMA in proper position to obturate the airway at the level of the larynx.

POSTOPERATIVE CLINICAL CONSIDERATIONS

Postoperative care of the patient encompasses three phases of recovery care: early recovery as the patient emerges from sedation, intermediate recovery where the patient achieves criteria for discharge home (see Appendix F), and late recovery or postdischarge recovery when the patient achieves full recovery from both surgery and sedation. Intraoperative monitoring should be continued into the recovery period at regular intervals during the first two of these phases until the patient is discharged.

With the development of newer anesthetic agents and techniques, extremely rapid recovery from anesthesia can be expected. Patients should be assessed immediately upon emergence to determine which phase of recovery should be initiated. Objective discharge criteria (Appendix F) should be documented before phase 3 is initiated and appropriate monitoring is terminated. While it is the physician's responsibility to ensure that patients satisfy criteria for discharge, the nursing staff in discharging patients may utilize a written policy establishing specific criteria.

Common problems in the postoperative period are pain, nausea, and vomiting. The management of these problems is covered in Chapter 9. These problems must be effectively treated before discharge. Those rare patients who do not meet the discharge standards in a reasonable amount of time should be transferred to a hospital under continuous monitoring. Fortunately, hospital admissions after ambulatory surgery are extremely uncommon.[33]

REFERENCES

1. SMG Group. SMG forecast of surgical volume in hospital/ambulatory settings: 1981-2006. Chicago: SMG Marketing Group, Inc., 1999.
2. Domino KB. Trends in anesthesia litigation in the 1990's: monitored anesthesia care claims. ASA Newsletter 1997; 61:15-17.
3. Practice guidelines for sedation and analgesia by non-anesthesiologists: a report by the American Society of Anesthesiologists task force on sedation and analgesia by non-anesthesiologists. Anesthesiology 1996; 84:459-471.
4. Guidelines for Office-based Anesthesia. Approved by the American Society of Anesthesiologists' House of Delegates on October 13, 1999.
5. Guidelines for Optimal Office-based Surgery. 2nd ed. Chicago: American College of Surgeons, 1996.
6. Accreditation Association for Ambulatory Health Care Association creates new standards for anesthesia. Healthcare Benchmarks 1999; 6:78-79.
7. Marcus JR, Tyrone JW, Few JW, et al. Optimization of conscious sedation in plastic surgery. Plast Reconstr Surg 1999; 104:1338-1345.
8. Abeles G, Warmuth IP, Sequeira M, et al. The use of conscious sedation for outpatient dermatologic surgical procedures. Dermatol Surg 2000; 26:121-126.
9. Tang J, Chen L, White PF, et al. Recovery profile, costs, and patient satisfaction with propofol and sevoflurane for fast-track office-based anesthesia. Anesthesiology 1991; 91:253-261.
10. Chan VW, Chung FF. Propofol infusion for induction and maintenance of anesthesia in elderly patients: recovery and hemodynamic profiles. J Clinical Anesth 1996; 8:317-323.
11. Jellish WS, Leonetti JP, Murdoch JR, Fowles S. Propofol-based anesthesia as compared with standard anesthetic techniques for middle ear surgery. Otolaryngol Head Neck Surg 1995; 112:262-267.
12. Dyer RA, Llewellyn RL, James MF. Total I.V. anaesthesia with propofol and the laryngeal mask for orthopaedic surgery. Br J Anaesth 1995; 74:123-128.
13. Candelaria LM, Smith RK. Propofol infusion technique for outpatient general anesthesia. J Oral Maxillofac Surg 1995; 53:124-128.
14. Collins SJ, Robinson AL, Holland HF. A comparison between total intravenous anesthesia using a propofol/alfentanil mixture and an inhalational technique for laparoscopic gynaecological sterilization. Eur J Anaesthesiol 1996; 13:33-37.
15. Blakely K, Klein K, White, P, et al. A total intravenous anesthetic technique for outpatient facial laser resurfacing. Anesth Analg 1998; 87:827-829.
16. Trytko RT, Werschler WP. Total intravenous anesthesia for office-based laser facial resurfacing. Lasers Surg Med 1999; 25:126-130.
17. Friedberg BL. Propofol-ketamine technique: dissociative anesthesia for office surgery. Anesth Plast Surg 1999; 23:70-75.
18. Vinnik CA. An intravenous dissociative technique for outpatient plastic surgery: tranquility in the office surgical facility. Plast Reconstr Surg 1981; 67:799.
19. Tiret L, Hatton F, Desmonts JM, Vourc'h G. The implications of a national study of risk of anesthesia. Health Policy 1988; 9:331-336.
20. Marshall SI, Chung F. Discharge criteria and complications after ambulatory surgery. Anesth Analg 1999; 88:508-517.
21. Chung F. Recovery pattern and home-readiness after ambulatory surgery. Anesth Analg 1995; 80:896-902.
22. Pavlin DJ, Rapp SE, Polissar NL, et al. Factors affecting discharge time in adult outpatients. Anesth Analg 1999; 89:75.
23. Bodenheimer T. The American health care system—the movement for improved quality in health care. N Engl J Med 1999; 340: 488-492.
24. Grazer FM, de Jong RH. Fatal outcomes from liposuction: census survey of cosmetic surgeons. Plast Reconstr Surg 1999; 105:436-446.
25. Schneider AJL. Assessment of risk factors and surgical outcomes. Surg Clin North Am 1983; 63:1113.
26. American Society of Anesthesiologists' task force on preoperative fasting. Practice guidelines for preoperative fasting and the use of pharmacologic agents to reduce the risk of pulmonary aspiration: application to healthy patients undergoing elective procedures. Anesthesiology 1999; 90:896-905.
27. Mallampati SR, Gatt SP, Gugino LD, et al. A clinical sign to predict difficult intubation: a prospective study. Can J Anaesth 1985; 32:429-434.
28. Lewis M. What is the best way to determine oropharyngeal classification and mandibular space length to predict difficult intubation? Anesthesiology 1994; 81:69-75.
29. Tse JC. Predicting difficult endotracheal intubation in surgical patients scheduled for general anesthesia: a prospective blind study. Anesth Analg 1995; 81:254-258.
30. Narr BJ, Warner ME, Schroeder DR, et al. Outcomes of patients with no laboratory assessment before anesthesia and a surgical procedure. Mayo Clin Proc 1997; 72:505.
31. Eichhorn JH, Cooper JB, Cullen DJ, et al. Standards for patient monitoring during anesthesia at Harvard medical school. JAMA 1986; 256:1017-1020.
32. Basic Monitoring Standards. Approved by the American Society of Anesthesiologists' House of Delegates on October 21, 1986 and last amended on October 23, 1996.
33. Twersky RS. Admissions following ambulatory surgery: outcome in seven urban hospitals. Ambulatory Surg 1995; 3:141-146.

APPENDIX A

Basic Monitoring Standards[32]

STANDARD I

Qualified anesthesia personnel shall be present in the room throughout the conduct of all general anesthetics, regional anesthetics, and monitored anesthesia care.

STANDARD II

During all anesthetics, the patient's oxygenation, ventilation, circulation, and temperature shall be continually evaluated.

1. Oxygenation:
   - An oxygen analyzer shall measure the concentration of oxygen in the patient's breathing system with a low oxygen concentration limit alarm in use.
   - A quantitative method of assessing oxygenation, such as pulse oximetry, shall be employed.
2. Ventilation: Adequacy of ventilation shall be continuously monitored. If an endotracheal tube is placed, its correct positioning must be verified by clinical assessment and by identification of carbon dioxide in the expired gases.
3. Circulation:
   - Electrocardiogram shall be continuously displayed.
   - Arterial blood pressure and heart rate shall be determined and evaluated at least every five minutes.

   In addition to the above, circulatory function shall be continually evaluated by at least one of the following: palpation of a pulse, auscultation of heart sounds, monitoring of a tracing of intra-arterial pressure, ultrasound peripheral pulse monitoring, or pulse plethysmography or oximetry.
4. Body Temperature: There shall be a readily available means to continually measure the patient's temperature.

APPENDIX B

Practice Guidelines for Sedation and Analgesia by Non-anesthesiologists[3]

I. PATIENT EVALUATION

Clinicians administering sedation and analgesia should be familiar with relevant aspects of the patient's medical history including: (1) abnormalities of the major organ systems, (2) previous adverse experience with sedation/analgesia, as well as regional and general anesthesia, (3) current medications and drug allergies, (4) time and nature of last oral intake, and (5) history of tobacco, alcohol, or substance use or abuse. Patients presenting for sedation and analgesia should undergo a focused physical examination including auscultation of the heart and lungs and evaluation of the airway. Pre-procedure laboratory testing should be guided by the patient's underlying medical condition and the likelihood that the results will affect the management of sedation and analgesia.

II. PREPROCEDURE PREPARATION

Patients should be informed of and agree to the administration of sedation and analgesia before the procedure begins. Patients undergoing sedation and analgesia for elective procedures should not drink fluids or eat solid foods for a sufficient period of time to allow for gastric emptying before their procedure.

III. MONITORING

Level of Consciousness: The response of patients to commands during procedures performed with sedation and analgesia serves as a guide to their level of consciousness. Spoken responses also provide an indication that the patients are breathing. Patients whose only response is reflex withdrawal from painful stimuli are likely to be deeply sedated, approaching a state of general anesthesia, and should be treated accordingly.

Pulmonary Ventilation: Ventilatory function usually can be effectively monitored by observation of spontaneous respiratory activity or auscultation of breath sounds. Impedance plethysmography may fail to detect airway obstruction.

Oxygenation: Hypoxemia during sedation and analgesia is more likely to be detected by oximetry than by clinical assessment alone.

Hemodynamics: Early detection of changes in patients' heart rate and blood pressure may enable practitioners to detect problems and intervene in a timely fashion, reducing the risk of cardiovascular collapse.

IV. RECORDING OF MONITORED PARAMETERS

Patients' ventilatory and oxygenation status and hemodynamic variables should be recorded at a frequency to be determined by the type and amount of medication administered as well as the length of the procedure and the general condition of the patient. At a minimum, this should be: (1) before the beginning of the procedure, (2) after administration of sedative and analgesic agents, (3) on completion of the procedure, (4) during initial recovery, and (5) at the time of discharge. If recording is performed automatically, device alarms should be set to alert the care team to critical changes in patient status.

V. AVAILABILITY OF A STAFF PERSON DEDICATED SOLELY TO PATIENT MONITORING AND SAFETY

A designated individual, other than the practitioner performing the procedure, should be present to monitor the patient throughout procedures performed with sedation and analgesia. This individual may assist with minor, interruptible tasks.

VI. TRAINING OF PERSONNEL

Individuals responsible for patients receiving sedation and analgesia should understand the pharmacology of the agents that are administered, as well as the role of pharmacologic antagonists for opioids and benzodiazepines. Individuals monitoring patients receiving sedation and analgesia should be able to recognize the associated complications. At least one individual capable of establishing a patent airway and positive pressure ventilation, as well as a means for summoning additional assistance, should be present whenever sedation and analgesia is administered. It is recommended that an individual with advanced life-support skills be immediately available.

VII. AVAILABILITY OF EMERGENCY EQUIPMENT

Pharmacologic antagonists as well as appropriately sized equipment for establishing a patent airway and providing positive pressure ventilation with supplemental oxygen should be present whenever sedation and analgesia is administered. Advanced airway equipment and resuscitation medications should be immediately available. A defibrillator should be immediately available when sedation and analgesia is administered to patients with significant cardiovascular disease.

VIII. USE OF SUPPLEMENTAL OXYGEN

Equipment to administer supplemental oxygen should be present when sedation and analgesia is administered. If hypoxemia is anticipated or develops during sedation and analgesia, supplemental oxygen should be administered.

IX. USE OF MULTIPLE SEDATIVE AND ANALGESIC AGENTS

Combinations of sedative and analgesic agents should be administered as appropriate for the procedure being performed and the condition of the patient. Ideally, each component should be administered individually to achieve the desired effect (e.g., additional analgesic medication to relieve pain, additional sedative medication to decrease awareness or anxiety). The propensity for combinations of sedative and analgesic agents to potentiate respiratory depression emphasizes the need to appropriately reduce the dose of each component as well as the need to continually monitor respiratory function.

X. TITRATION OF SEDATIVE AND ANALGESIC MEDICATIONS TO ACHIEVE THE DESIRED EFFECT

Intravenous sedative and analgesic drugs should be given in small, incremental doses that are titrated to the desired endpoints of analgesia and sedation. Sufficient time must elapse between doses to allow the effect of each dose to be assessed before subsequent drug administration. When drugs are administered by non-intravenous routes (e.g., oral, rectal, and intramuscular), allowance should be made for the time required for drug absorption before supplementation is considered.

XI. INTRAVENOUS ACCESS

In patients receiving intravenous medications for sedation and analgesia, vascular access should be maintained throughout the procedure and until the patient is no longer at risk for cardiorespiratory depression.

XII. REVERSAL AGENTS

Specific antagonists should be available whenever opioid analgesics or benzodiazepines are administered for sedation and analgesia. Before or concomitantly with pharmacologic reversal, patients who become hypoxemic or apneic during sedation and analgesia should: (1) be encouraged or stimulated to breathe deeply, (2) receive positive pressure ventilation if spontaneous ventilation is inadequate, and (3) receive supplemental oxygen. After pharmacologic reversal, patients should be observed long enough to ensure that cardiorespiratory depression does not recur.

XIII. RECOVERY CARE

After sedation and analgesia, patients should be observed until they are no longer at increased risk for cardiorespiratory depression. Vital signs and respiratory function should be monitored at regular intervals until patients are suitable for discharge. Discharge criteria should be designed to minimize the risk of central nervous system or cardiorespiratory depression after discharge from observation by trained personnel.

APPENDIX C

Guidelines for Office-Based Anesthesia[4]

QUALITY OF CARE

- The facility should have a medical director or governing body that establishes policy and is responsible for the activities of the facility and its staff. The medical director or governing body is responsible for ensuring that facilities and personnel are adequate and appropriate for the type of procedures performed.

- Policies and procedures should be written for the orderly conduct of the facility and reviewed on an annual basis.
- The medical director or governing body should ensure that all applicable local, state, and federal regulations are observed.
- All health care practitioners and nurses should hold a valid license or certificate to perform their assigned duties.
- All operating room personnel who provide clinical care in the office should be qualified to perform services commensurate with appropriate levels of education, training, and experience.
- The anesthesiologist should participate in ongoing continuous quality improvement and risk management activities.
- The medical director or governing body should recognize the basic human rights of its patients, and a written document that describes this policy should be available for patients to review.

FACILITY AND SAFETY

- Facilities should comply with all applicable federal, state and local laws, codes and regulations pertaining to fire prevention, building construction and occupancy, accommodations for the disabled, occupational safety and health, and disposal of medical waste and hazardous waste.
- Policies and procedures should comply with laws and regulations pertaining to controlled drug supply, storage, and administration.

PATIENT AND PROCEDURE SELECTION

- The anesthesiologist should be satisfied that the procedure to be undertaken is within the scope of practice of the health care practitioners and the capabilities of the facility.
- The procedure should be of a duration and degree of complexity that will permit the patient to recover and be discharged from the facility.
- Patients who by reason of pre-existing medical or other conditions may be at undue risk for complications should be referred to an appropriate facility for performance of the procedure and the administration of anesthesia.

PERIOPERATIVE CARE

- The anesthesiologist should adhere to the "Basic Standards for Preanesthesia Care," "Standards for Basic Anesthetic Monitoring," "Standards for Postanesthesia Care" and "Guidelines for Ambulatory Anesthesia and Surgery" as currently promulgated by the American Society of Anesthesiologists.
- The anesthesiologist should be physically present during the intraoperative period and immediately available until the patient has been discharged from anesthesia care.
- Discharge of the patient is a physician responsibility. This decision should be documented in the medical record.
- Personnel with training in advanced resuscitative techniques (e.g., ACLS, PALS) should be immediately available until all patients are discharged.

MONITORING AND EQUIPMENT

- At a minimum, all facilities should have a reliable source of oxygen, suction, resuscitation equipment, and emergency drugs. Specific reference is made to the ASA "Guidelines for Nonoperating Room Anesthetizing Locations."
- There should be sufficient space to accommodate all necessary equipment and personnel and to allow for expeditious access to the patient, anesthesia machine (when present), and all monitoring equipment.
- All equipment should be maintained, tested, and inspected according to the manufacturer's specifications. Back-up power sufficient to ensure patient protection in the event of an emergency should be available.
- In any location in which anesthesia is administered, there should be appropriate anesthesia apparatus and equipment which allow monitoring consistent with ASA "Standards for Basic Anesthetic Monitoring" and documentation of regular preventive maintenance as recommended by the manufacturer.
- In an office where anesthesia services are to be provided to infants and children, the required equipment, medication, and resuscitative capabilities should be appropriately sized for a pediatric population.

EMERGENCIES AND TRANSFERS

- All facility personnel should be appropriately trained in and regularly review the facility's written emergency protocols.
- There should be written protocols for cardiopulmonary emergencies and other internal and external disasters such as fire.
- The facility should have medications, equipment, and written protocols available to treat malignant hyperthermia when triggering agents are used.
- The facility should have a written protocol in place for the safe and timely transfer of patients to a prespecified alternate care facility when extended or emergency services are needed to protect the health or well-being of the patient.

APPENDIX D

Commonly Utilized Medications for Conscious Sedation and Total Intravenous Anesthesia

FENTANYL

- Narcotic
- IV onset 1 to 2 min, peak 5 to 15 min, and duration 30 to 60 min
- Advantages: great analgesic, rapid onset, and used in morphine-allergic patients
- Disadvantages: chest wall rigidity, and opioid adverse effects
- IV dose for adults: 1 to 2 μg/kg. Repeat doses: half of initial dose

FLUMAZENIL (ROMAZICON)

- Competitive inhibitor of benzodiazipines at the GABA receptor
- IV onset <1 min, peak 2 to 10 min, and duration 45 to 90 min
- Cautions: sudden and complete reversal could cause anxiety, tremors, and seizures
- IV dose: 0.2 mg, wait 30 sec; then 0.3 mg, wait 30 sec; then 0.5 mg, wait 60 sec. May continue to give 0.5 mg to total of 3 mg

KETAMINE

- Nonbarbiturate anesthetic/analgesic agent
- IV onset 30 sec, peak 1 min, and duration 10 to 20 min
- Advantages: minimal respiratory depression, IM dosing, and short-acting
- Disadvantages: produces emergence reactions and central sympathetic stimulation
- IV dose: 0.2 to 0.75 mg/kg (IM 0.5 to 4 mg/kg)

MIDAZOLAM (VERSED)

- Benzodiazipine
- IV onset 1 to 2 min, peak 3 to 5 min, and duration 20 to 60 min
- Advantages: excellent amnestic, rapid onset, short duration, and many routes
- Disadvantages: expense and respiratory depression.
- IV dose for adults: 0.5 to 2 mg. Repeat doses: half initial dose

NALOXONE (NARCAN)

- Competitive inhibitor of opioids at their receptors
- IV onset 1 to 2 min, peak 5 to 15 min, and duration 30 to 90 min
- Cautions: sudden complete reversal of opioids could cause severe hypertension, ventricular dysrhythmias, and pulmonary edema
- IV dose: 0.05 to 0.1 mg every 2 to 3 min

PROPOFOL

- Sedative-hypnotic agent
- IV onset of 40 sec, peak 1 min, and duration 5 to 10 min
- Boluses rapidly produce anesthesia due to lipophilicity
- Potential for adverse effects of profound hypotension and cardiorespiratory depression
- IV dose: 25 to 150 μg/kg/min

APPENDIX E

Total Intravenous Anesthesia Methods*

TRADITIONAL TIVA[16]

1. ASA class I-II adults without gastroesophageal reflux symptoms. ASA Basic Monitoring Standards followed.
2. Equipment available
   a. Oxygen source
   b. Laryngoscope, endotracheal tube, LMA, and face mask
   c. Positive pressure breathing device immediately available
   d. Defibrillator
   e. Suction immediately available
3. Premedication
   a. Glycopyrrolate 0.2 mg IV
   b. Ondansetron 4 mg IV prn
4. Induction
   a. Preoxygenation
   b. Midazolam 2.5-5 mg IV prn
   c. Fentanyl 25-50 μg IV prn
   d. Propofol 2-2.5 mg/kg IV
5. Laryngeal mask airway (LMA) insertion
6. Maintenance
   a. Propofol 50-250 μg/kg/min IV
   b. Fentanyl 25 μg IV prn
7. Remove LMA when awake

DISSOCIATIVE TIVA[17]

1. ASA class I-II adults. Electrocardiogram, noninvasive blood pressure, and pulse oximetry monitored.
2. Equipment available
   a. Oxygen source
   b. Ambu bags
   c. Defibrillator
   d. Bispectral Index Monitor
   e. Suction apparatus
3. Premedication
   a. Glycopyrrolate 0.2 mg IV
   b. Midazolam 2 mg IV prn

*Both techniques are for adult patients and should be conducted by an anesthesiologist.

4. Induction
   a. Propofol (5 mg/ml, diluted 1:1) titrated IV until unconscious, then
   b. Ketamine 50 mg IV
5. LMA insertion for rhinoplasties with osteotomies
6. Maintenance
   a. Propofol infusion IV†
   b. Ketamine 25-50 mg IV prn
   c. Meperidine 20 mg increments prn high risk of postoperative pain

†Average propofol rate of 185 μg/kg/min for females and 118 μg/kg/min for males.

APPENDIX F

Modified Postanesthesia Discharge Scoring System[21]

1. Vital signs
   2 Within 20% of preoperative levels
   1 20% to 40% of preoperative value
   0 40% of preoperative level
2. Activity, mental status
   2 Oriented and steady gait
   1 Oriented or steady gait
   0 Neither
3. Pain, nausea, vomiting
   2 Minimal
   1 Moderate
   0 Severe
4. Surgical bleeding
   2 Minimal
   1 Moderate
   0 Severe
5. Intake and output
   2 PO fluids and voided
   1 PO fluids or voided
   0 Neither

The total score is 10. Patients scoring ≥9 considered fit for discharge to home.

Table 9-2 Selected Opioid Analgesics[46]*

Medication	Oral Dose (mg)	Parenteral Dose (mg)†	Comments	Precautions and Contraindications
Fentanyl	None	0.1	Duragesic patch 25 μg/h roughly equivalent to sustained-release morphine 45 mg/d	12-hour delay in onset and offset of transdermal patch; use short-acting agents when initiating patch.
Hydromorphone	7.5	1.5	Slightly shorter duration than morphine	
Meperidine	300	75	Slightly shorter duration than morphine	Normeperidine (metabolite) accumulates; do not use in children or patients receiving monoamine oxidase inhibitors.
Morphine	30	10	Standard for comparison Long-acting preparations available	
Oxycodone	20	None		

*For all opioids: use caution in patients with asthma, hepatic failure, impaired ventilation.
†Intramuscular doses for acute pain in adults. For single intravenous boluses, use half the intramuscular dose.

Table 9-3 Adjuvant Medications for Analgesics[46]

Medication Class	Indication	Comments
Anticonvulsants	Used for pain associated with peripheral nerve syndromes	Some agents include gabapentin and carbamazepine.
Antihistamines	Analgesic, antiemetic, and sedative activity	Analgesia has been demonstrated only with IM hydroxyzine.
Benzodiazepines	Acute anxiety or muscle spasm associated with pain	No analgesic properties, and sedation may limit ability to escalate opioid doses.
Caffeine	Increase analgesia in uterine cramping, dental pain, and headaches[50]	
Clonidine	Effective with oral, intrathecal, and epidural routes	Sedation and hypotension.
Dextroamphetamine	May produce additive analgesia with opioids; usually used to counteract opioid sedation	
Phenothiazines	May be helpful in agitation	No analgesic effects.
Steroids	Specific and nonspecific effects in cancer pain Useful for spinal cord compression	Chronic use produces weight gain, Cushing's syndrome, myopathy, psychosis, and increased risk for GI bleed; rapid withdrawal may exacerbate pain.
Tricyclic antidepressants	Pain related to diabetic neuropathy and postherpetic neuralgia	Consider anticholinergic side effects; baseline ECG recommended because of conduction side effects.

3. Short-acting opioid analgesics (e.g., fentanyl) should be administered during the operative procedure if needed.
4. Postoperative pain management options should include short-acting opioid analgesics (e.g., fentanyl) and, if not previously utilized, nonopioid analgesics and analgesic adjuvants. For severe pain, longer acting opioids (e.g., morphine and meperidine) and possibly regional analgesia should be considered.

Topical Anesthetics

Topical anesthetics are designed to provide local anesthesia for dermatological procedures. Since these agents have a delayed onset of action, they must be given early in the preoperative period in order to achieve optimal effectiveness during the operative procedure. The most effective topical agents are EMLA and ELA-Max. Both agents have similar efficacy in providing topical anesthesia.[34-36]

EMLA cream is a eutectic mixture of 2.5% lidocaine and 2.5% prilocaine in an oil-in-water emulsion cream. It should be applied to intact skin at least 1 hour before minor procedures, and it reaches maximum effectiveness in 1 to 2 hours. The maximum recommended duration of exposure is 4 hours. The following procedure should be followed when utilizing EMLA cream or patches:

1. For minor dermal procedures, 2.5 g (one-half of a 5 g tube) should be applied over 20 to 25 cm^2 of skin surface, or one anesthetic disk (1 g) over 10 cm^2 for at least 1 hour.
2. For a major dermal procedure such as split thickness skin graft harvesting, apply 2 g cream per 10 cm^2 of skin and allow to remain in contact with the skin for at least 2 hours.
3. If the cream is utilized, a thick layer should be applied and covered with an occlusive dressing.

ELA-Max is a 4% lidocaine cream in a liposomal vehicle. For adults, a thick layer is applied to the operative site and the recommended application time is 15 to 45 minutes. Unlike EMLA, no occlusive dressing is required.

EMLA and ELA-Max should be applied only to intact skin. Neither should be applied to mucous membranes, near eyes, or on open wounds.[37,38] Both products should be actively removed as soon as possible in order to reduce the risk of toxicity. The incidence of systemic adverse effects is directly proportional to the area and time of exposure. The skin at the site of treatment may develop erythema or edema. These reactions are generally mild and transient and resolve spontaneously within 1 to 2 hours. EMLA should not be used in patients with congenital or idiopathic methemoglobinemia and used with caution in patients receiving class I antiarrhythmics (e.g., tocainide and mexiletine).

PROCEDURAL TECHNIQUES

Pain Management

Pharmacologic analgesic therapies can be divided into the following three categories:

1. Nonopioid analgesics (see Table 9-1)
2. Opioid analgesics (see Table 9-2)
3. Analgesic adjuvants (see Table 9-3)

Nonopioid analgesics are usually effective analgesics for acute pain. Most are given orally, and their onset to analgesic effect is around 40 minutes. Unlike opioids, they have a ceiling effect and do not produce tolerance, physical dependence, psychological dependence, respiratory depression, nausea, vomiting, or drowsiness.

Aspirin and acetaminophen are two popular nonopioid analgesics with a vast history of efficacy. Unlike aspirin, acetaminophen does not damage the gastric mucosa or inhibit platelet aggregation; however, acute and chronic overdoses can cause hepatic necrosis.[39]

Tramadol (Ultram) is an analgesic with weak activity on mu opioid receptors, tricyclic antidepressant-like effects on neurotransmitters, and proven effectiveness for postoperative pain compared with opioids.[40-42] Compared with most opioids it has weaker analgesic potency, longer duration, and lower abuse potential. Tramadol's side effects are opioidlike and frequently gastrointestinal. It should not be used in patients with a history of seizures or those at particular risk for seizures.

NSAIDs should always be considered when treating acute pain, especially when inflammation is involved. They work by inhibiting the enzyme cyclooxygenase (Cox). Patients may vary in their relative response to various NSAIDs; therefore, if a patient does not experience an adequate response to one agent, another may be considered. The most common side effects related to NSAIDs are hematological effects (inhibition of platelet aggregation), gastrointestinal effects (dyspepsia, ulcerations, bleeding, or perforation), and renal insufficiency.[43] All NSAIDs should be used cautiously in patients with congestive heart failure, chronic renal insufficiency, cirrhosis with ascites, volume depletion, and multiple myeloma.

NSAIDs refecoxib (Vioxx) and celecoxib (Celebrex) selectively inhibit the Cox-2 enzyme. Two isoforms of Cox have been identified. Cox-1 isoenzyme is normally found in blood vessels, the stomach, and kidneys. Cox-2 is induced in peripheral tissues by inflammation. Since inhibition of Cox-1 is associated with gastric, hematologic, and renal side effects that can occur with NSAID use, Cox-2 inhibitors produce less adverse effects than other NSAIDs.

Opioid analgesics should be added to nonopioids to manage pain that either does not respond or is unlikely to respond to opioids alone. Opioids may be given by many routes of administration including oral, intramuscular, intravenous, transdermal, oral transmucosal, rectal, epidural, or intrathecal. The optimal dose of opioid varies widely among patients.[44,45] Opioid-naïve patients typically require less opioid, and opioid-tolerant patients often utilize relatively large opioid doses. The preoperative assessment may give some indication of the likely individual response.

An adequate trial of opioid analgesics consists of titrating repeated small doses until either adequate analgesia occurs or side effects become intolerable. Repeat dosages should be cautiously administered, particularly when administered before the peak effect of the previous dose (Table 9-4).

The most common side effects of opioids are sedation, constipation, nausea, vomiting, itching, and respiratory depression. Changing the dosing regimen, changing opioids, treating the side effects, or adding an analgesic medication from another class reduces these side effects.

Adjuvant medications include other classes of medications that may enhance the effects of opioids, have independent analgesic effects, or counteract the side effects of analgesics[46] (see Table 9-3). Benzodiazepines are occasionally very effective in patients whose pain is compounded by excessive anxiety. Clonidine may reduce postoperative opioid requirements.[47] Also, some antihistamines, like hydroxyzine, are effective adjuncts to opioids.

Local and regional anesthetics are also important therapies for intraoperative and postoperative pain management, and they are covered in Chapter 7.

Table 9-4 Pharmacokinetic Profiles of Intravenous Agents for Acute Pain[46]

Medication	IV Onset (min)	IV Peak (min)	IV Duration (h)
Fentanyl (Sublimaze)	Within 30 sec	5-15	0.5-1
Hydromorphone (Dilaudid)	<1	5-20	2-4
Meperidine (Demerol)	<1	5-20	2-4
Morphine	<1	5-20	2-4
Ketorolac	<1	60-120	3-6

Nausea Management

General inhalational anesthesia is associated with a significantly higher incidence of PONV compared with all other techniques.[1] Local anesthesia and propofol-based total intravenous anesthesia (TIVA) techniques are associated with a very low incidence of PONV.[1,23,24]

Most therapies for preventing PONV utilize pharmacological antiemetics.[48] These include metoclopramide, droperidol, dexamethasone, and 5-HT_3 antagonists (ondansetron, dolasetron, and granisetron) (Table 9-5). Nonpharmacologic therapies seem promising but are not currently recommended.[49]

Current recommendations regarding prophylactic PONV management are the following[48] (Fig. 9-5):

1. For patients at low risk to develop PONV, routine prophylactic antiemetics are not recommended.
2. Patients at intermediate risk for PONV may receive prophylactic low-dose droperidol.

Table 9-5 Postoperative Nausea and Vomiting Medications[32,46]

Medication	Route	Dose	Onset (min)	Duration of Effect	Comment
Droperidol (Inapsine)	IV	0.625-1.25 mg	3-10	30 min	
Metoclopramide (Reglan)	IV	10-20 mg	1-3	30 min	
Prochlorperazine (Compazine)	PO	5-15 mg	30-40	3-4 h	
	IV	5-10 mg	5-10	3-4 h	
	IM	5-10 mg	10-20	3-4 h	
Promethazine (Phenergan)	PO	25 mg	20	2-8 h	
	IV	12.5-25 mg	3-5	2-8 h	
	IM	12.5-25 mg	20	2-8 h	
Ondansetron (Zofran)	PO	8 mg	60-90	4-6 h	Caution with prolonged QT interval.
	IV	4 mg	5-10	4-6 h	
Granisetron (Kytril)	IV	20-40 μg/kg	5-10	12 h	Caution with prolonged QT interval.
Dolasetron (Anzemet)	PO	100 mg	45-60	6-8 h	Caution with prolonged QT interval.
	IV	12.5 mg	15-30	6-8 h	

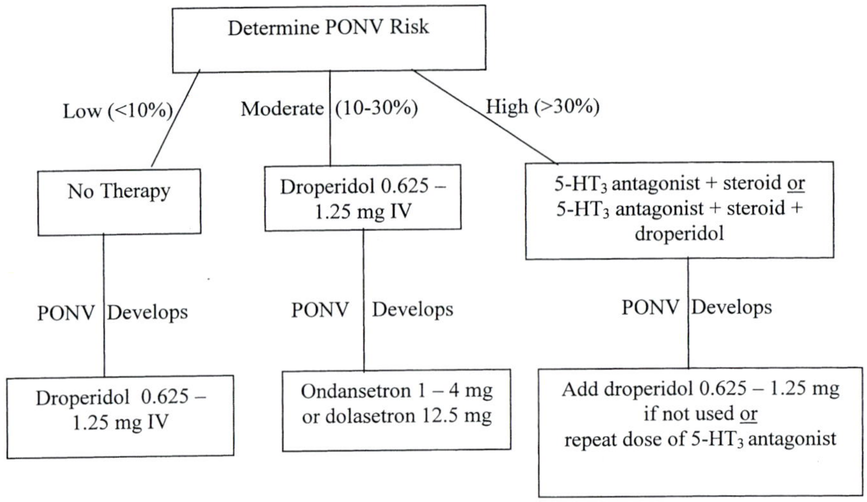

FIG. 9-5
Prevention and treatment of postoperative nausea and vomiting (PONV).[32,48]

3. Patients at high risk may receive a prophylactic combination of a 5-HT_3 antagonist with a steroid (e.g., dexamethasone) or a three-drug regimen (e.g., ondansetron, dexamethasone, and droperidol).
4. When 5-HT_3 antagonists are utilized, they should be administered near the end of the operative procedure.

All these agents are given parenterally, since patients experiencing PONV do not tolerate oral medications.

POSTOPERATIVE CLINICAL CONSIDERATIONS

Pain Management

The single most reliable indicator of the existence and intensity of acute pain is the patient's self-report. Once postoperative pain has occurred, pain assessment should be frequent and simple. Surgical causes of unexplained pain should be considered and excluded. Treatment can then be initiated utilizing the pharmacological analgesic therapies previously discussed. Patients with severe pain that cannot be easily or adequately controlled may need to be admitted to an acute care facility.

Nausea Management

Postoperative PONV should be aggressively managed (see Table 9-5 and Fig. 9-5). The most common antiemetics for the treatment of PONV are droperidol and the 5-HT_3 antagonists.[32] Patients who are given prophylactic antiemetic therapy for PONV and subsequently develop PONV should be treated with an agent from a different pharmacological class than the medication used for prophylaxis.[48]

The side effect profiles of antiemetics differ. Droperidol is associated with a greater incidence of somnolence and rarely can cause akathisia, restlessness, as well as extrapyramidal symptoms. The 5-HT_3 antagonists can cause headache and should be used with caution in patients with prolonged QT interval or those who are on medications that may cause QT prolongation.

CASE 1

A healthy 44-year-old man with androgenetic alopecia was scheduled for hair replacement surgery in the crown area. Two hours before surgery he took diazepam 10 mg PO and celecoxib 200 mg PO. Immediately before the procedure, he received midazolam 10 mg IM. Anesthesia at the donor and recipient sites was achieved with 30 ml 1% lidocaine with 1:100,000 epinephrine and buffered with sodium bicarbonate. In addition, 5 to 10 ml 0.25% bupivacaine with 1:100,000 epinephrine was applied to the donor site for prolonged anesthesia. At the end of the procedure he received prednisone 20 mg PO. About 30 minutes after the procedure, he experienced increasing pain from the donor site that was treated initially with meperidine (Demerol) 75 mg IM. Because of an inadequate response to the meperidine a second dose was administered along with hydroxyzine 25 mg IM. Once his pain was under control, he was discharged home and instructed to take celecoxib 200 mg PO bid for three days and predinsone 20 mg PO once daily for 5 days. He also was given a Tylenol #3 prescription, which he did not use. One week after the surgery he stated that he had minimal discomfort associated with the procedure.

CASE 2

A healthy 55-year-old woman with facial ptosis was scheduled for a face lift. She received no preoperative medications. The procedure was performed with intravenous sedation utilizing fentanyl and propofol. Tumescent anesthesia was achieved with 0.1% lidocaine with 1:250,000 epinephrine. The patient was monitored in recovery for 1 hour after the procedure and received no pain medications. She was discharged home with Tylenol #3; she was instructed to take 1 to 2 tablets every 4 hours as needed. That night she developed a headache, took an extra-strength Bayer aspirin, and fell asleep. The next morning she awoke with increasing facial pain and swelling. Upon removal of the bandaging, her left cheek area was obviously swollen. Under local anesthesia a small portion of the incision was opened to drain the hematoma and closed. She was discharged home with instruction not to take any aspirin products.

CASE 3

A healthy 50-year-old woman with photoaging was scheduled for laser facial resurfacing. Two hours preoperatively she received ibuprofen 800 mg PO. The procedure was performed under total intravenous anesthesia utilizing fentanyl and propofol. Immediately postoperatively, Flexan Extra occlusive dressing was applied to the operative site. Postoperative pain and anxiety were acute and not responsive to 250 μg fentanyl. She was administered 10 mg diazepam in four divided doses, and the pain was dramatically reduced. She was discharged home with Vicodin ES as needed for pain. Four days after surgery she reported that the pain was tolerable with the Vicodin ES and that no other medications were needed.

REFERENCES

1. Chung F, Mezei G. Factors contributing to a prolonged stay after ambulatory surgery. Anesth Analg 1999; 89:1352-1359.
2. Acute pain management guidelines panel. Acute pain management: operative or medical procedures and trauma. Clinical practice guideline. AHCPR Pub. No. 92-0032. Rockville, Md: Agency for Healthcare Policy and Research. Public Health Service, US Dept. of Health and Human Services, Feb. 1992.
3. Practice guidelines for acute pain management in the perioperative setting. ASA task force on pain management. Anesthesiology 1995; 82:1071-1081.
4. White PF, Watcha MF. Postoperative nausea and vomiting: prophylaxis versus treatment. Anesth Analg 1999; 89:1337-1339.
5. Ready N. Acute perioperative pain. In: Miller RD, ed. Anesthesia. Philadelphia: Churchill Livingstone, 2000:2323-2350.
6. Dahl JB, Kellet H. Non-steroidal anti-inflammatory drugs: rationale for use in severe post-operative pain. Br J Anaesth 1991; 66:703-712.
7. Dickenson AH. Mechanisms of the analgesic actions of opiates and opioids. Br Med Bull 1991; 47:690-720.
8. Woolf CJ, Wall PD. Morphine-sensitive and morphine-insensitive actions of C-fiber input on the rat spinal cord. Neurosci Lett 1986; 64:221-225.
9. Basbaum AI. Spinal mechanisms of acute and persistent pain. Reg Anesth Pain Med 1999; 24:59-67.
10. Borison HL. Area postrema: chemoreceptor circumventricular organ of the medulla oblongata. Prog Neurobiol 1989; 32:351-390.
11. Apfel CC, Laara E, Koivuranta M, et al. A simplified risk score for predicting postoperative nausea and vomiting. Anesthesiology 1999; 91:693-700.
12. Seago JA, Weitz S, Walczak S. Factors influencing stay in the postanesthesia care unit: a prospective analysis. J Clin Anesth 1998; 10:579-587.
13. Chung F, Ritchie E, Su J. Postoperative pain in ambulatory surgery. Anesth Analg 1997; 85:808-816.
14. Claxton AR, McGuire G, Chung F, Cruise C. Evaluation of morphine versus fentanyl for postoperative analgesia after ambulatory surgical procedures. Anesth Analg 1997; 84:509-514.
15. Peirce RJ, Fragen RJ, Pemberton DM. Intravenous ketorolac tromethamine versus morphine sulfate in the treatment of immediate postoperative pain. Pharmacotherapy 1990; 10:111S-115S.
16. Powell H, Smallman JM, Morgan M. Comparison of intramuscular ketorolac and morphine in pain control after laparotomy. Anaesthesia 1990; 45:538-542.
17. Sevarino FB, Sinatra RS, Paige D, et al. The efficacy of intramuscular ketorolac in combination with intravenous PCA morphine for postoperative pain relief. J Clin Anesth 1992; 4:285-288.
18. Mixter CG III, Meeker LD, Gavin TJ. Preemptive pain control in patients having laparoscopic hernia repair: a comparison of ketorolac and ibuprofen. Arch Surg 1998; 133:432-437.
19. Wittels B, Faure EA, Chavez R, et al. Effective analgesia after bilateral tubal ligation. Anesth Analg 1998; 87:619-623.
20. Michaloliakou C, Chung F, Sharma S. Preoperative multimodal analgesia facilitates recovery after ambulatory laparoscopic cholecystectomy. Anesth Analg 1996; 82:44-51.
21. Carroll NV, Miederhoff P, Cox FM, Hirsch JD. Postoperative nausea and vomiting after discharge from outpatient surgery centers. Anesth Analg 1995; 80:903-909.
22. Abeles G, Warmuth IP, Sequeira M, et al. The use of conscious sedation for outpatient dermatologic surgical procedures. Dermatol Surg 2000; 26:121-126.
23. Sneyd JR, Carr A, Byrom WD, Bilski AJ. A meta-analysis of nausea and vomiting following maintenance of anesthesia with propofol or inhalational agents. Eur J Anaesth 1998; 15:433-445.
24. Friedberg BL. Propofol-ketamine technique: dissociative anesthesia for office surgery. Anesth Plast Surg 1999; 23:70-75.
25. Gan TJ, Ginsberg B, Grant AP, Glass PS. Double-blind, randomized comparison of ondansetron and intraoperative propofol to prevent postoperative nausea and vomiting. Anesthesiology 1996; 85:1036-1042.
26. Kovac MR, O'Connor T, Duncalf D, et al. Comparison of ondansetron versus placebo to prevent postoperative nausea and vomiting in women undergoing ambulatory gynecologic surgery. Anesthesiology 1993; 78:21-28.
27. Scuderi P, Wetchler B, Sung YF, et al. Treatment of postoperative nausea and vomiting after outpatient surgery with the 5-HT_3 antagonist ondansetron. Anesthesiology 1993; 78:15-20.
28. Domino KB, Anderson EA, Polissar NL, Posner KL. Comparative efficacy and safety of ondansetron, droperidol, and metoclopramide for preventing postoperative nausea and vomiting: a meta-analysis. Anesth Analg 1999; 88:1370-1379.

29. Henzi I, Walder B, Tramer MR. Dexamethasone for the prevention of postoperative nausea and vomiting: a quantitative systematic review. Anesth Analg 2000; 90:186-194.
30. McKenzie R, Tanisira B, Karambelkar DJ. Comparison of ondansetron with ondansetron plus dexamethazone in the prevention of postoperative nausea and vomiting. Anesth Analg 1994; 79: 961-964.
31. Kortilla K, Clergue F, Leeser J, et al. Intravenous dolasetron and ondansetron in prevention of postoperative nausea and vomiting: a multicenter, double-blind, placebo controlled study. Acta Anaesthesiol Scand 1997; 41:914-922.
32. American Society of Health-System Pharmacists. ASHP therapeutic guidelines on the pharmacologic management of nausea and vomiting in adult and pediatric patients receiving chemotherapy or radiation therapy or undergoing surgery. Am J Health Syst Pharm 1999; 56:729-764.
33. Tang J, Wang B, White PF. The effect of timing of ondansetron administration on its efficacy, cost-effectiveness, and cost-benefit as a prophylactic antiemetic in the ambulatory setting. Anesth Analg 1998; 86:274-282.
34. Koppel RA, Coleman KM, Coleman WP. The efficacy of EMLA versus ELA-Max for pain relief in medium-depth chemical peeling: a clinical and histopathologic evaluation. Dermatol Surg 2000; 26:61-64.
35. Friedman PM, Fogelman JP, Nouri K, et al. Comparative study of the efficacy of four topical anesthetics. Dermatol Surg 1999; 25: 950-954.
36. Altman DA, Gildenberg SR. High-energy pulsed light source hair removal device used to evaluate the onset of action of a new topical anesthetic. Dermatol Surg 1999; 25:816-818.
37. Eaglstein NF. Chemical injury to the eye from EMLA cream during erbium laser resurfacing. Dermatol Surg 1999; 25:590-591.
38. McKinlay JR, Hofmeister E, Ross EV, MacAllister W. EMLA cream-induced eye injury. Arch Dermatol 1999; 135:855-856.
39. Whitcomb DC, Block GD. Association of acetaminophen hepatotoxicity with fasting and ethanol use. JAMA 1994; 272:1845-1850.
40. Stamer UM, Maier C, Grond S, et al. Tramadol in the management of post-operative pain: a double-blind, placebo- and active drug-controlled study. Eur J Anaesthesiol 1997; 14:646-654.
41. Vickers MD, Paravicini D. Comparison of tramadol with morphine for post-operative pain following abdominal surgery. Eur J Anaesthesiol 1995; 12:265-271.
42. Lee RC, McTavish D, Sorkin EM. Tramadol: a preliminary review of its pharmacodynamic and pharmacokinetic properties, and therapeutic potential in acute and chronic pain states. Drugs 1993; 46:313-340.
43. Hawkey DJ. Non-steroidal anti-inflammatory drugs and peptic ulcers. Br Med J 1990; 300:278-284.
44. Galer BS, Coyle N, Pasternak GW, et al. Individual variability in the response to different opioids: report of five cases. Pain 1992; 49:87-91.
45. Kaiko RF, Wallenstein SL, Rogers AG, et al. Clinical analgesic studies and sources of variation in analgesic response to morphine. In: Foley KM, Inturrisi CE, eds. Opioid Analgesics in the Management of Clinical Pain. Advances in Pain Research Therapy. New York: Raven Press, 1986; 8:13-23.
46. Omoigui S. The Anesthesia Drugs Handbook, United States. St Louis: Mosby–Year Book, 1995.
47. Park J, Forrest J, Kolesar R, et al. Oral clonidine reduces postoperative PCA morphine requirements. Can J Anaesth 1996; 43:900-906.
48. White PF, Watcha MF. Postoperative nausea and vomiting: prophylaxis versus treatment. Anesth Analg 1999; 89:1337-1339.
49. Lee A, Done ML. The use of nonpharmacologic techniques to prevent postoperative nausea and vomiting: a meta-analysis. Anesth Analg 1999; 88:1362-1369.
50. Laska EM, Sunshine A, Mueller F, et al. Caffeine as an analgesic adjuvant. JAMA 1984; 251:1711-1718.

APPENDIX A

American Society of Anesthesiologists' Practice Guidelines for Acute Pain Management in the Perioperative Setting[3]

- An individualized proactive plan (e.g., a predetermined strategy for postoperative analgesia) should be considered for all surgical patients. Factors that may influence the formulation of a proactive plan include (but are not limited to) type of surgery and expected severity of postoperative pain, underlying medical conditions (e.g., presence of respiratory or cardiac disease, and allergies), the risk-benefit ratio of the techniques available, and patients' preferences and/or previous experience with pain. Proactive planning of perioperative pain should be part of the preoperative evaluation by the anesthesiologist and, in collaboration with others (e.g., nurses, surgeons, and pharmacists), should be part of an institution's general plan for patient care.
- Activities that are commonly encompassed by proactive planning include but are not limited to: (1) obtaining a pain history based on patients' experiences, (2) preoperative pain therapy when appropriate and feasible, (3) intraoperative procedures (e.g., wound infiltration) when appropriate and feasible, and (4) intraoperative or post-incisional preparation of patients for postoperative pain management. Any treatment plan requires regular assessment and refinement based on the changing responses of individual patients.
- Anesthesiologists offering perioperative analgesia services should provide, in collaboration with others as appropriate, ongoing education and training to ensure that hospital personnel are knowledgeable and skilled with regard to the effective and safe use of the available treatment options within the institution. The scope of education should include topics ranging from basic bedside skills for evaluation of acute pain to an understanding of sophisticated pharmacologic techniques and nonpharmacologic techniques (e.g., relaxation, imagery, hypnotic methods). The need for education and training is ongoing as new personnel enter an institution and as modifications in therapeutic approaches are made.
- Anesthesiologists offering perioperative analgesia services should provide, in collaboration with others as appropriate, education to patients and families regarding their roles in achieving comfort, reporting pain, and using the recommended analgesic methods to optimal benefit. Common misconceptions about the risk of side effects and addiction should be dispelled.

- Anesthesiologists offering perioperative analgesia services should use, in collaboration with others as appropriate, pain assessment instruments to facilitate the regular evaluation and documentation of pain, the effects of pain therapy, and side effects caused by the therapy.
- Most analgesic techniques place patients at some risk for side effects or complications that require prompt medical evaluation. Anesthesiologists responsible for perioperative analgesia, in collaboration with others as appropriate, should be available at all times to consult with ward nurses, surgeons, or other involved physicians and assist in evaluating patients who are experiencing problems with any aspect of postoperative pain relief.
- Anesthesiologists offering perioperative analgesia services should participate in developing, in collaboration with others as appropriate (especially nurses), standardized institutional policies and procedures for ordering, administering, discontinuing, and transferring responsibility for postoperative pain management.
- Anesthesiologists managing perioperative pain should make available as appropriate a variety of analgesic techniques and should consider their use in combination under appropriate circumstances.
- Anesthesiologists who manage perioperative pain should develop (in collaboration with nurses, surgeons, pharmacists, and others) an organized, interdisciplinary approach to perioperative pain management within their institutions.
- Anesthesiologists who treat perioperative pain in pediatric patients should be familiar with the special features of this group. Based on that knowledge, pharmacologic and nonpharmacologic strategies for perioperative analgesia appropriate for the age of the child should be offered in a manner that promotes efficacy and safety.
- Anesthesiologists who treat perioperative pain in geriatric patients should be familiar with the special features of this group. In particular, dose reduction for drugs that may cause central nervous system depression should be considered.
- Anesthesiologists who care for ambulatory surgery patients should proactively plan therapeutic strategies appropriate for them, recognizing that they are expected to leave the surgical facility within a few hours after the completion of surgery.

PART III

COSMETIC SURGERY PROCEDURES AND TECHNIQUES

CHAPTER 10

Topical Skin Care

ZOE DIANA DRAELOS

BASIC SCIENCE AND CLINICAL STUDIES

Topical skin care is an important part of the complete surgical equation when considering skin preparation prior to surgery, skin care during wound healing, and skin care maintenance. Many new technologies are entering the market, claiming to be of value as part of the antiaging armamentarium. Since this aspect of skin care is a hybrid of science and aesthetics, products must be carefully evaluated to assess efficacy in terms of performance criteria and benefits in terms of consumer perceptions. Interestingly enough, products with poor actual scientific performance may be enthusiastically received by consumers. Herein lies the confusion surrounding the cosmetics that fall into this category. This chapter presents the current science and information necessary to evaluate the use of hydroxy acids, vitamins, and botanicals in dermatology and the surgical setting.

The Hydroxy Acids

Physicians and consumers alike have become fascinated by an interesting group of substances known as hydroxy acids, which provide antiaging and skin-smoothing effects. Hydroxy acids, which are incorporated into a seemingly infinite array of skin care products, can be subdivided into the following categories based on chemical composition: alpha hydroxy acids, beta hydroxy acid, combination hydroxy acids, and polyhydroxy acids.

All of the hydroxy acids are intended to induce exfoliation, or removal of desquamating corneocytes on the skin surface. It is the removal of these dead skin cells that improves skin surface smoothness and skin color. The most important issues regarding hydroxy acid performance can be evaluated in terms of type, concentration, and pH of the hydroxy acid, combined with the vehicle effects.

Alpha Hydroxy Acids. The alpha hydroxy group of organic carboxylic acids is distinguished by a substituted hydroxy group (–OH) covalently bonded to the alpha carbon of a carboxylic acid. The linear, aliphatic nature of the alpha hydroxy acid (AHA) structure accounts for its water soluble or hydrophilic properties (Fig. 10-1). The three subcategories of AHAs are

1. Monocarboxylic acids: glycolic acid (2-hydroxyethanoic acid), lactic acid (2-hydroxy-propanoic acid), and mandelic acid (2-hydroxy-2-phenylethanoic acid)
2. Dicarboxylic acids: malic acid (2-hydroxy-1,4-butanedioic acid) and tartaric acid (2,3-dihydroxy-1,4-butanedioic acid)
3. Tricarboxylic acid: citric acid (2-hydroxy-1,2,3-propanetricarboxylic acid)

The intricacies of the formulation are more important than the nature of the AHA in terms of efficacy.[1]

AHAs induce immediate epidermal effects through corneocyte disadhesion, which is thought to be operative by disruption of ionic bonding.[2] Several mechanisms that have been proposed for this ionic bonding alteration are summarized in Box 10-1.[3] This corneocyte disadhesion occurs histologically in the stratum corneum at the level of the stratum granulosum, until the cutaneous barrier has been disrupted, followed by dermal penetration.[4] The epidermal effects of AHAs are a thinned stratum corneum with epidermal acanthosis.

The dermal effects of AHAs are delayed and include decreased melanogenesis, unaltered angiogenesis, increased synthesis of glycosaminoglycans, prevention of topical corticosteroid atrophy, and increased dermal thickness, possibly due to the production of collagen through fibroblast proliferation, in a dose dependent manner.[5,6] AHAs have also been shown by Griffin et al. to induce factor XIIIa transglutaminase expression in dermal dendrocytes, which may account for some of the dermal changes seen in photoaged skin.[7] This proliferative effect is more pronounced with glycolic acid than with lactic or malic acid.[8] Penetration of the AHA into the deeper dermis can cause burning and stinging, as well as inflammation. It is currently unknown whether the antiaging dermal effects observed are due

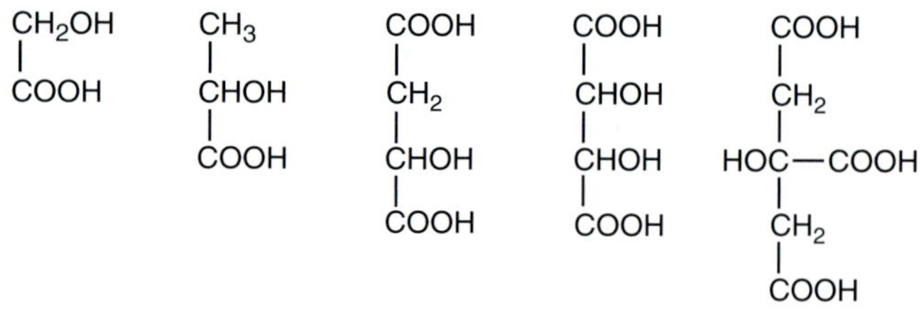

1 2 3 4 5

FIG. 10-1
Chemistry of the alpha hydroxy acids. *1,* Glycolic acid; *2,* lactic acid; *3,* malic acid; *4,* tartaric acid; *5,* citric acid.

BOX 10-1 Alpha Hydroxy Acid Proposed Mechanisms for Corneocyte Disadhesion Through Disruption of Ionic Bonding

Mechanism 1: Increased distance between corneocytes due to hydration reducing cell cohesion.
Mechanism 2: Enzymatic inhibition of transferases and kinases resulting in decreased electronegative sulfate and phosphate groups on the outer walls of the corneocytes reducing cell cohesion.
Mechanism 3: Decreased pH leading to dissolution of desmosomes and reduced corneocyte adhesion.

BOX 10-2 Aesthetic Benefits of Glycolic Acid Peels

1. Improved skin color
2. Enhanced skin brightness
3. Smoother surface texture
4. Better skin tone
5. Increased skin firmness
6. Decreased wrinkling
7. Decreased dyspigmentation
8. More even facial cosmetic application
9. Enhanced benefits from the use of topical retinoids

BOX 10-3 Dermatologic Uses of Alpha Hydroxy Acids

Skin Conditions
1. Photodamaged skin
2. Ichthyosis
3. Xerotic eczema
4. Acne
5. Rosacea
6. Seborrheic keratoses
7. Actinic keratoses
8. Lentigenes
9. Verruca

Cutaneous Effects
1. Moisturizing exfoliant
2. Skin peeling agent
3. Penetration enhancer
4. Preventative for corticosteroid induced skin atrophy

to this inflammation or a direct effect on cellular metabolism through actively or passively changing the ionic structure of various molecules in various pathways.

AHAs are widely used in dermatology as peeling agents. Glycolic acid is the most common AHA used for this purpose in concentrations varying from 10% to a fully saturated solution of 70%. Peel concentrations up to but not including 20% can be performed by an unsupervised esthetician, but 20% and above concentration glycolic acid peels must be performed under the supervision of a physician. The danger from the use of glycolic acid peels arises from the fact that the material must be neutralized or removed from the skin surface to prevent further cutaneous effects. Chemical burns can result from prolonged exposure to high concentrations of glycolic acid. Moy et al. demonstrated the benefit of 50% to 70% glycolic acid peeling solutions left on the skin for 3 to 7 minutes at 4-week intervals in patients with wrinkles and photoaging.[9] Enhanced peeling benefit was demonstrated by Elson when glycolic acid peels were combined with topical retinoids.[10] Box 10-2 lists the aesthetic benefits attributed to the use of glycolic acid peels.

There are other uses for AHA technology, besides its antiaging benefits previously discussed, as elucidated by Van Scott and Yu (Box 10-3). Lactic acid, at the concentration of 12% and pH of 4.4, has been investigated for its ability to enhance skin moisturization, especially of the lower legs where xerosis and ichthyosis are common.[11] A study conducted by DiNardo et al. demonstrated an 82% decrease in skin roughness and a 333% increase in skin hydration, as measured by electrical conductance.[12] Interestingly, they also found a 24% increase in transepidermal water loss, which they felt was not substantiated histologically, since no defect in barrier function was observed. It is the author's opinion that removal of the stratum corneum does result in increased transepidermal water loss, which must be compensated by the moisturizing capabilities of the vehicle carrying the lactic acid, or enhanced xerosis may occur with long-term use. There is benefit, however, to the use of lactic acid in a moisturizing, emollient vehicle for removing rough unexfoliated skin that may be mistakenly perceived as dry skin by the patient.[13]

Disruption of corneocyte adhesion is ultimately valuable in a large variety of dermatologic conditions.[14] For example, AHAs can be incorporated into an acne treatment regimen for their ability to induce epidermolysis and dislodge comedones; however, AHAs cannot enter the milieu of the pore.[15] Benefit has also been shown by Briden et al. in the treatment of rosacea with

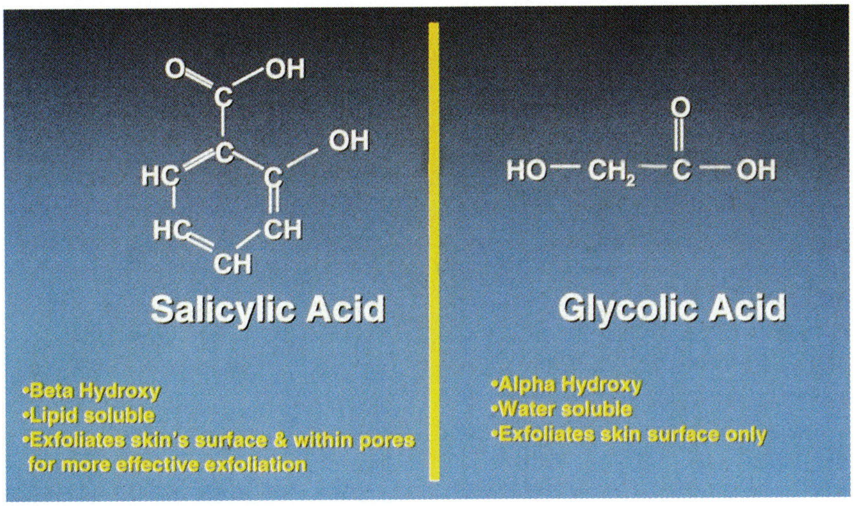

FIG. 10-2
The aliphatic structure of the alpha hydroxy acids is demonstrated with glycolic acid as compared to the aromatic structure of salicylic acid, somewhat loosely characterized as beta hydroxy acid.

monthly glycolic acid peels.[16] Sloughing of corneocytes and smoothing of seborrheic keratoses, verruca, and calluses can also be achieved.[17,18] Glycolic acid preparations, formulated as either topicals or short-contact peels, appear to be appropriate for fair and darkly complected individuals.[19]

Last, alpha hydroxy acids have been purported to function as anti-inflammatories and antioxidants by alleviating the erythema associated with cutaneous ultraviolet exposure.[20] Glycolic acid appears to confer an SPF of 2.4 to the skin.[21]

Beta Hydroxy Acid. The previously discussed alpha hydroxy acids form only one component of the hydroxy acid family, which have been demonstrated to enhance cutaneous functioning. A similar but chemically different hydroxy acid is salicylic acid (orthohydrobenzoic acid), the only beta hydroxy acid (BHA). Salicylic acid is an organic aromatic carboxylic acid with a hydroxy group in the beta position (Fig. 10-2). This phenolic, hydrophobic, lipophilic compound is a white crystalline powder chemically unrelated to the alpha hydroxy acids. Perhaps even labeling it as a hydroxy acid is somewhat of a marketing misnomer.

Salicylic acid is unique among the hydroxy acids, since it can enter the milieu of the sebaceous unit, inducing exfoliation in the oily areas of the face.[22] For this reason, it has been used for years by dermatologists as a comedolytic in over-the-counter (OTC) preparations designed to improve comedonal acne.[23,24] Salicylic acid is approved in the treatment of acne as an OTC drug monographed by the FDA at a level of 2% or less. It is also an excellent keratolytic, inducing exfoliation of calluses, corns, and warts.[25] Salicylic acid is incorporated into many shampoos designed to remove undesquamated corneocytes from the scalp in patients with seborrheic dermatitis and psoriasis.[26]

Salicylic acid is thought to function through solubilization of intercellular cement, thereby reducing corneocyte adhesion. It appears to eliminate the stratum corneum layer by layer from the outermost level downward.[27] This is in contrast to the alpha hydroxy acids that appear to diminish cellular cohesion between the corneocytes at the lowest levels of the stratum corneum. This is probably due in part to the water soluble characteristics of the alpha hydroxy acids that readily penetrate into the stratum corneum and the oil soluble characteristics of salicylic acid that remains on the stratum corneum. Differences in penetration also explain the decreased stinging and burning experienced with topical salicylic acid compared with glycolic acid, since the salicylic acid does not readily penetrate to the dermis.

Topical application of salicylic acid can also take the form of short-contact cutaneous peels. Salicylic acid can be used alone in concentrations of 10% to 50% or combined with the alpha hydroxy acid lactic acid in Jessner's solution. Salicylic acid will remain in solution in concentrations of 20% or less in 95% ethyl alcohol; however, at concentrations of 30% and above it precipitates, necessitating shaking of the peels prior to use. In contrast to glycolic acid peels, salicylic acid is a self-neutralizing peel that ends with the formation of white salicylic acid crystals on the skin.[28] The crystals are easily rinsed from the skin surface with water, but remain in the follicular ostia providing a prolonged keratolytic effect. Thus, salicylic acid peels are useful for general exfoliation in patients with photoaging, for comedolysis in acne patients, and in sensitive skin patients, such as rosacea patients, where dermal penetration should be minimized.

Combination Hydroxy Acids. Combination hydroxy acid (CHA) formulations combine an AHA and the BHA salicylic acid intending to retain the cutaneous benefits of both exfoliants, previously discussed. Thus, CHAs are not new chemical entities, but rather combination products that are difficult if not impossible to optimally formulate. This is due to the fact that only the free acid component of the hydroxy acid can provide antiaging benefit to the skin, an important clinically relevant concept. The hydroxy acid that exists in the acid form is biologically active, while the hydroxy acid that exists in the salt form is not biologically active. Most hydroxy acid formulations contain both free acid and salt forms, since the products have been partially neutralized to prevent a low pH product from inducing a chemical burn. The amount of free acid and salt can be readily determined by considering the pK_a of alpha and beta hydroxy acids.

The pK_a for the alpha hydroxy acids is 3.83, while the pK_a for beta hydroxy acid is 2.98 (Fig. 10-3). Products must be formulated at a pH close to the pK_a for optimal free acid concentration and optimal efficacy. Thus, when a CHA is formulated, it must be either AHA or BHA dominant, due to the inherently different pK_as of the hydroxy acids. At this time, CHA moisturizers designed for antiaging benefits are more of a marketing success than a clinical success.

Polyhydroxy Acids. The stinging and burning induced by the rapid penetration of alpha hydroxy acids into the dermis has led to the search for equally effective chemicals with perhaps less dermal irritation. It is chemically known that substances with larger molecular weight traverse the epidermis more slowly than substances with smaller molecular weight. This had resulted in the development of polyhydroxy acid (PHA) exfoliant products that are chemically similar to AHAs, but their larger molecular weight limits dermal penetration. The decreased dermal penetration theoretically means that there will be less stinging, burning, and irritation, possibly allowing sensitive skin patients with rosacea or atopic dermatitis to find the products acceptable. PHAs, such as gluconolactone, are water soluble like the AHAs and exfoliate on the skin surface, not within the sebaceous unit. Their benefit depends solely on the formulation selected, and the decrease in dermal penetration may be only 1% to 2%.[29] Most cosmetic companies are now utilizing sophisticated polyhydroxy acids in their exfoliant products to decrease consumer complaints of stinging, burning, and itching.

Hydroxy Acid Formulation Issues. The extensive preceding discussion of the various types of hydroxy acids and their dermatologic effects would not be complete without an understanding of the formulation issues key to their efficacy. The basis of their efficacy lies in the chemistry of the formulation. Hydroxy acids can induce exfoliation only at an acidic pH and at a sufficient concentration to induce a biologic effect. The hydroxy acid must also be placed in a vehicle that delivers the desired clinical benefit with minimal irritation. It is only through consideration of these factors that a dermatologist can recommend effective hydroxy acid preparations to patients.

All hydroxy acids perform better at low pH, but the optimal pH for formulation is determined by the pK_a of

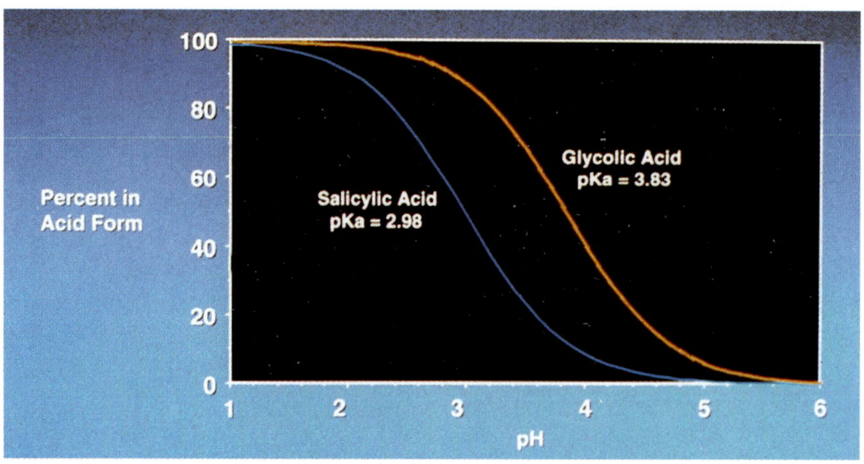

FIG. 10-3
The different pK_as of glycolic acid and salicylic acid make combination exfoliant lotions difficult to optimally formulate.

the active ingredient, as discussed previously. One method of controlling pH is by altering the concentration of the hydroxy acid.[30] For example, 10% glycolic acid is 4 times more acidic than 1% glycolic acid. The acidity is chemically determined by electrostatic, inductive, and steric effects. In general, higher hydroxy acid concentration yields a lower pH and a greater biologic effect. This concept is demonstrated in Figure 10-4, where the relationship between salicylic acid concentration, pH, and exfoliation can be observed. Notice that completely neutralized antiaging BHA creams produce little increase in exfoliation. Thus the exposure of the skin to an acidic pH is key to inducing exfoliation.

There is a lower limit, however, to the acidity of a chemical that can be safely placed on the skin surface without inducing a chemical burn. Pure glycolic acid at 70% may be appropriate for peeling purposes with a short exposure time, but it is not appropriate for use in leave-on moisturizers and toners. For these preparations, it is recommended by the Cosmetic Ingredient Review (CIR) that the concentration of glycolic acid should be limited to 8%. The improved efficacy of higher concentration AHAs has been demonstrated by Smith, who showed only surface and epidermal effects with 5% lactic acid and both epidermal and dermal effects with 12% lactic acid.[31] The CIR is currently studying other issues regarding the safety of glycolic acid preparations, including the substantiation of preliminary observations that skin treated with glycolic acid prior to sun exposure demonstrates an increase in apoptotic cells. It is anticipated that a recommendation will be forthcoming from the US Food and Drug Administration, in response to the CIR inquiry, that alpha hydroxy acids should be used in combination with a sunscreen on a daily basis.

Formulating hydroxy acid products means balancing efficacy with skin compatibility. To accomplish this end, neutralization and buffering are used to adjust the pH and free acid content of AHA preparations.[32] Hydroxy acids can be neutralized with an inorganic alkali or organic base to raise the product pH. Glycolic acid preparations are frequently neutralized with sodium hydroxide, allowing for less cutaneous irritation. Completely neutralized glycolic acid, however, with a pH above 4.8, contains largely sodium glycolate, which has no antiaging properties. Thus, hydroxy acid products designed to induce cutaneous exfoliation may undergo only partial neutralization.

Hydroxy acid preparations can also be buffered to create a solution that resists pH change when an acid or alkali is added. This is important because the pH of the product may change when it encounters eccrine and sebaceous secretions or the intercellular compartments of the skin. Buffered formulations are not necessarily less irritating than their unbuffered counterparts. Buffering is strictly a method of ensuring that some free acid is available to induce exfoliation once the product reaches the skin.

Properly formulated hydroxy acid products have a profound effect on the skin. Stratum corneum pH changes may persist for up to 2 hours. The extent of these pH changes depends on concentration: low 1% hydroxy acid concentrations can alter the pH of the outer 3 layers of the stratum corneum, while higher 10% hydroxy acid concentrations can affect the stratum corneum pH 10 to 20 layers deep. Thus, higher concentration hydroxy acids yield greater dermal penetration. For example, following glycolic acid application to the skin, 2.4% remains on the stratum corneum, 11.6% reaches the epidermis, and 8.6% resides in the dermis.[33] It is possible to enhance this dermal penetration through

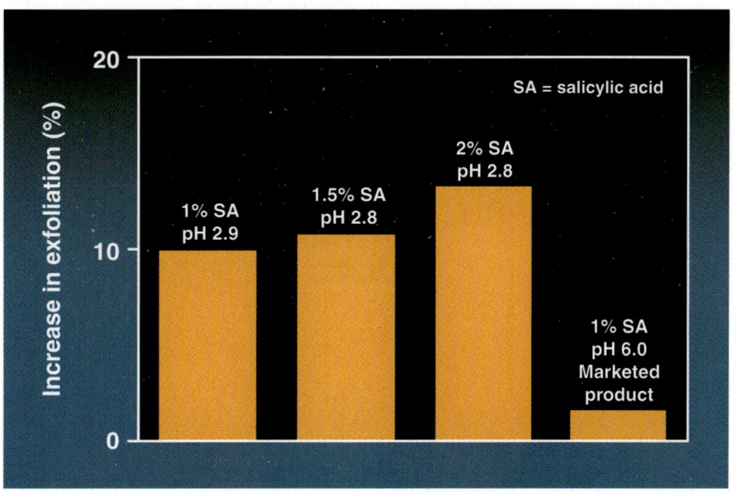

FIG. 10-4
The relationship between pH and exfoliation is demonstrated for salicylic acid.

the use of substances that increase epidermal permeability, such as propylene glycol.[34]

In addition to considering the hydroxy acid concentration and free acid amount, the effects of the vehicle on the skin must also be considered. Vehicle considerations are particularly important, especially when evaluating hydroxy acid moisturizers. The vehicle of delivery can increase the in-use aesthetics, resulting in better patient compliance, and decrease the transepidermal water loss that may increase due to cutaneous exfoliation. It can also soothe any irritation that may occur from higher concentration products; however, it is important to discern which skin benefits are due to the vehicle and which are due to the active agent. Figure 10-5 demonstrates that regular moisturizer application alone results in an increase in exfoliation. Notice that the high-concentration glycolic acid preparations formulated at a pH above 4 produce no greater exfoliation than a bland moisturizer. Thus, the vehicle, not the glycolic acid, may be accounting for the therapeutic benefit. Formulations must be critically evaluated in clinical testing to determine that the active agent is truly active.

Vitamins

Another area of rapid growth in cutaneous research is topical vitamin preparations. The value of oral vitamins in terms of wound healing and skin health is not disputed, but the usefulness of topical vitamin application remains controversial. This discussion examines what is currently known about vitamins commonly used in over-the-counter preparations designed to enhance skin functioning. Several vitamins have been implicated in the health of the skin: vitamin A, vitamin C, vitamin E, panthenol, niacin, niacinamide, essential fatty acids, biotin, and ubiquinone.

Vitamin A. Vitamin A is of primary importance to the survival of human and plant life in an environment rich in oxygen.[35] Vitamin A, and its precursor beta-carotene, are found in yellow, orange, and green vegetables, egg yolk, liver, butter, and fish oils. Plants especially high in vitamin A include spinach, carrots, sweet potatoes, squash, and cantaloupe. In the plant kingdom, vitamin A (retinol) functions as a free radical scavenger, protecting plants from UV radiation damage. To humans, vitamin A is one of a family of natural and synthetic related derivatives collectively known as retinoids.[36] Retinoids are biologic modifiers that produce receptor-specific effects within the body. The naturally occurring retinoids will be discussed first.

Vitamin A is a component of all multivitamins sold for both children and adults. Current recommendations from the US Department of Agriculture and the National Cancer Institute call for a beta-carotene intake of 5.6 to 6 mg per day, either from natural or supplemental sources.[37] This minimum daily oral intake was determined after the review of human studies demonstrating an increased risk of lung cancer in persons with low beta-carotene consumption.[38,39] Vitamin A reservoirs are maintained in the liver; however, systemic toxicity can occur with excessive oral intake. Vitamin A is a known teratogen, but it remains a component of prenatal vitamins in low concentration. High intake of vitamin A should be avoided during pregnancy.

As mentioned previously, oral vitamin A is an important endogenous antioxidant.[40] Oxidation occurs due to formation of oxygen radical species, such as hydrogen peroxide, superoxide anion, and hydroxy radicals that transfer their energy to living human cells, resulting in damage. Cellular proteins, enzymes, DNA, and RNA are damaged, but oxidative damage to the unsaturated fatty acid component of cell membranes is

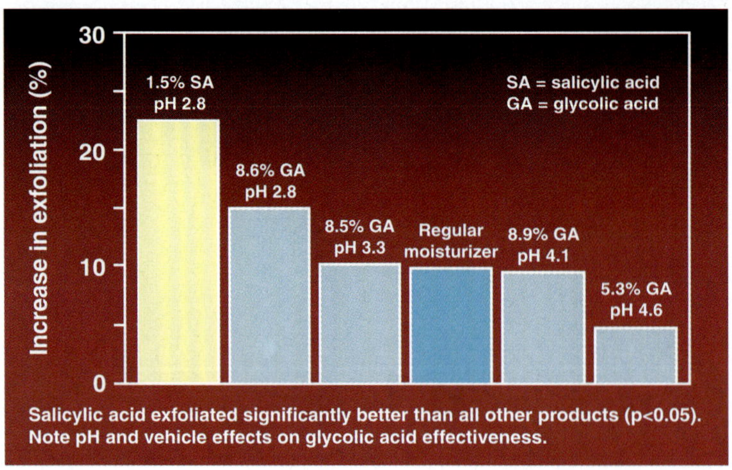

FIG. 10-5
Moisturizers without an active agent can induce exfoliation.

of primary importance. Hydroxy radicals initiate lipid peroxidation in cell membranes to form lipid peroxides that are responsible for accelerated cutaneous aging. One of the primary oxidation products thought to induce aging is malondialdehyde (MDA).[41] Interestingly, MDA is also increased in cells that have undergone carcinogenesis. Oral vitamin A appears to have an effect on this process.

Recently, the use of topical forms of naturally occurring vitamin A in skin care products has been popularized. Vitamin A can perform several different functions when topically applied. It is a known humectant, meaning that it can attract water from the dermis and viable epidermis to the stratum corneum. This aids in skin hydration when the humectant vitamin A is combined with an occlusive agent, such as petrolatum or mineral oil, to prevent water evaporation. Vitamin A (in the form of retinyl palmitate) can also function as a preservative by preventing oxidation of the lipids in the moisturizer. However, this naturally occurring form of vitamin A has no biologic activity.

There is some evidence that naturally occurring forms of vitamin A, such as retinyl palmitate and retinol, can function as topical antioxidants, enhancing functioning of the skin. It is now well recognized that the skin is an enzymatically active organ capable of metabolic alteration of topically applied substances. Retinyl palmitate can become biologically active following cutaneous enzymatic cleavage of the ester bond and subsequent conversion of retinol to retinoic acid. It is this cutaneous conversion of retinol to retinoic acid that is responsible for the biologic activity of some of the new stabilized over-the-counter vitamin A preparations.[42] Unfortunately, only small amounts of retinyl palmitate and retinol can be converted by the skin, accounting for the increased efficacy seen with prescription preparations containing retinoic acid, to be discussed next.

The vitamin A derivatives that have been discussed up to this point are considered nutritional supplements and thus are found in cosmetic preparations. Synthetic vitamin A derivatives, designed to alter the structure and function of the skin, include tretinoin (Retin-A, Ortho), 13-cis-retinoic acid (Accutane, Roche), acitretin (Soritane, Roche), adapalene (Differin, Galderma), and tazarotene (Tazorac, Allergan). The synthetic retinoids, as well as the naturally occurring forms of vitamin A, are difficult to formulate because of their inherent photoinstability. As antioxidants, they degrade immediately upon light exposure to biologically inactive forms. For this reason, oral forms of synthetic and natural vitamin A are packaged in amber bottles to prevent UV radiation exposure, and prescription topical retinoids are packaged in opaque metal or plastic tubes. Topical preparations where the retinoid has oxidized turn yellow, an indication that some degradation has occurred.[43]

The remainder of this discussion focuses on the use of topical synthetic retinoids for purposes of decreasing and reversing the signs of cutaneous aging.[44] The use of retinoids in the reversal and prevention of photoaging was discovered by Albert Kligman, MD, PhD, who noted that topical tretinoin improved wrinkling, lentigines, roughness, and precancerous actinic keratoses.[45] The list of observed retinoid effects is summarized in Box 10-4.[46,47]

The initial effect observed following the first few weeks of topical tretinoin treatment is improvement in tactile smoothness. This is felt to be due to a stratum corneum with a more compact pattern with increased epidermal thickness due to spongiosis.[48] Increased hyaluronic acid is also produced, allowing the water-holding capacity of the skin to increase, also contributing to the early improvement in skin smoothness.[49] Thickening also occurs in the epidermal granular cell layer.[50] The effects of topical tretinoin following 4 months of use are improvement in fine wrinkles, representing a dermal effect. This improvement is due to an increase in collagen production.[51] Furthermore, it has been demonstrated that tretinoin decreases UVB-induced collagenase activity, thus preventing photoaging.[52] Topical tretinoin does not prevent photoaging by acting as a sunscreen, since it does not reduce UVB-induced erythema. The improvement in skin condition continues

BOX 10-4 Cutaneous Effects of Vitamin A

Gross Dermatologic Effects

1. Improvement in fine and coarse facial wrinkling
2. Decreased tactile roughness
3. Reduction of actinic keratoses
4. Lightening of solar lentigenes

Histologic Dermatologic Effects

1. Reduction in stratum corneum cohesion
2. Decreased epidermal hyperplasia
3. Increased production of collagen, elastin, and fibronectin
4. Reduction in tonofilaments, desmosomes, melanosomes
5. More numerous Langerhans cells
6. Angiogenesis
7. Decreased glycosaminoglycans
8. Reduced activity of collagenase and gelatinase
9. Normalization of keratinization of the pilosebaceous unit

Dermatologic Disease

1. Enhanced wound healing
2. Reduction in open and closed comedones
3. Improved appearance of striae distensae
4. Healing of inflammatory cystic acne
5. Improvement in disorders of keratinization
6. Normalization of skin in psoriasis

with prolonged use and may be seen in both sun-exposed and sun-protected skin.[53,54] Side effects are consistent with hypervitaminosis A of the skin and include mild skin irritation (erythema, peeling, burning) and a clinically insignificant burning sensation in the eyes.[55]

Topical tretinoin also appears to have an effect on skin pigmentation as seen by a decrease in cutaneous freckling and lentigines.[56] It is the irregular grouping and activation of melanocytes that accounts for the dyspigmentation associated with photoaging,[57] but normalization of this change has been histologically demonstrated by Bhawan et al.[58] Improvement in dyspigmentation with tretinoin has also been demonstrated in Asian and black skin.[59,60]

Initial studies also demonstrate that topical tretinoin may improve the appearance of early stretch marks, although the mechanism of action has not yet been elucidated.[61] Topical tretinoin has been anecdotally used on a variety of dermatoses ranging from keratosis pilaris to oral lichen planus to actinic cheilitis. It has been utilized as a penetration enhancer in combination with topical corticosteroids. Large-scale scientific studies have not been performed for these indications. It is certain that the role of topical retinoids in dermatology will become increasingly important as new synthetic derivatives are developed.

Vitamin C. Vitamin C, another of the antioxidant vitamin family, is vitally important to the proper functioning of the skin. The biologically active form of vitamin C is L-ascorbic acid, which functions as an antioxidant by scavenging and quenching free radicals and by regenerating vitamin E from its radical form (see Fig. 10-3).[62,63] However, vitamin C can also act as an oxidant when in the presence of transition metal ions, such as iron. Thus, its function is dependent on the hydrophilic cellular milieu in which it resides.

Vitamin C is a water-soluble vitamin found in vegetables and citrus fruits. Due to its water solubility, no toxic effects have been observed in populations taking more than 100 times the recommended daily dose of 60 mg/d. Oral consumption of vitamin C is necessary for wound healing, since it is a necessary cofactor for lysyl and prolyl hydroxylase, which stabilize the triple helical structure of collagen. Deficiency of endogenous vitamin C, known as scurvy, results in fragile tissues, bleeding gums, and the characteristic corkscrew hairs. While the necessity of oral vitamin C ingestion is undisputed, the value of topical supplementation remains controversial.

The dermatology literature contains a few published reports of the topical effects of vitamin C, which are worth reviewing. Darr et al. demonstrated enhanced cutaneous vitamin C levels following topical application of 10% L-ascorbic acid.[64] This work was completed in a porcine model, and corresponding human data have not been published. Further work by Murray et al. demonstrated a decrease in the minimal erythema dose and less erythema following UVB exposure in human subjects treated with topical 10% L-ascorbic acid.[65] At this writing, vitamin C is not an approved photoprotectant in the United States.

Even though the preliminary research on topical vitamin C has shown promise, this vitamin has been slow to enter the mass cosmetic market. This is due to the inherent instability of vitamin C when exposed to light, oxygen, and moisture. Products containing vitamin C readily discolor on the shelf due to autooxidation, rendering them biologically inactive (Fig. 10-6). One attempt to stabilize vitamin C is the development of magnesium L-ascorbyl-2-phosphate, which has enhanced stability and can be enzymatically converted by the skin to active L-ascorbic acid. Kameyama et al. have reported lightening of skin dyspigmentation with magnesium L-ascorbyl-2-phosphate.[66]

Current vitamin C research has focused on methods of enhancing cutaneous reservoirs of vitamin C that are rapidly depleted upon exposure to sunlight. Once the stores are depleted, the body's ability to protect the skin from oxidative damage and ultimate photodamage is decreased. At this writing the best way to deliver vitamin C to the skin is through oral ingestion. Body stores of vitamin C are only 1500 mg, which means that vitamin C deficiency can occur rapidly. Steady, regular consumption of fruits and vegetables is necessary to maintain a constant body reservoir, rather than the use of topical vitamin C preparations.

Vitamin E. Vitamin E is a broad group of chemicals that includes the tocopherols and tocotrienols. The only biologically active forms are alpha and gamma tocopherol, with alpha tocopherol possessing greater biologic activity than gamma tocopherol. Vitamin E is

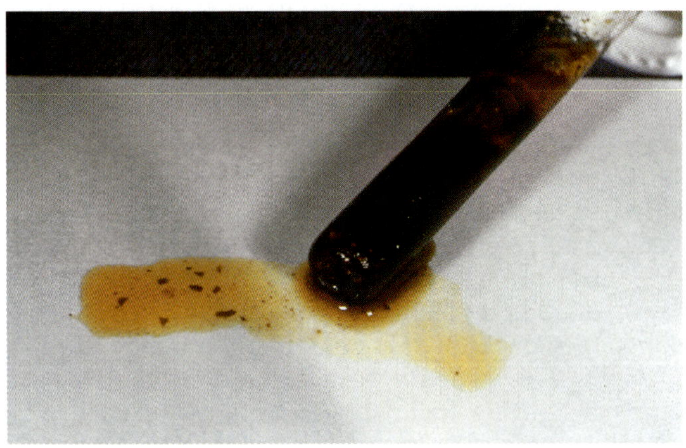

FIG. 10-6
Discoloration of vitamin C products indicates that oxidation has occurred.

naturally found in the membranes of cells and organelles. It prevents oxidation of the polyunsaturated fatty acids of the phospholipids in the membranes by capturing singlet oxygen species.[67] It also stabilizes the membranes against damage by phospholipase A, free fatty acids, and lysophospholipids.[68]

Vitamin E is present in vegetables, oils, seeds, corn, soy, whole wheat flour, margarine, nuts, and some meats and dairy products. It is felt to be safe in doses of up to 3000 mg/d for extended periods of time, but oral supplementation in the range of 400 to 1000 mg/d is generally recommended in patients with a history of coronary artery disease. In this instance, vitamin E is used to decrease clotting of the blood and minimize athlerosclerotic plaques through its antioxidant effect. Patients who are undergoing surgery must stop oral vitamin E supplements, since it is a potent anticoagulant and can increase postoperative bleeding. It may also cause increased bruising.

The antioxidant capabilities of alpha-tocopherol are due to its ability to function as a lipid radical scavenger able to terminate lipid radical chain reactions. In this reaction, a low-energy tocopheroxyl radical is formed; however, this radical cannot function further as an antioxidant. Regeneration can occur in the presence of vitamin C to again allow the vitamin E to function as a radical scavenger.[69] It may also protect membrane proteins containing selenium or sulfur. The vitamin E concentration in the epidermis is about 1 nmol/g.[70] Even though its concentration in the body is relatively low, it is the most important lipid-soluble membrane-bound antioxidant in the body.

A variety of claims have been made regarding the topical effects of vitamin E on the skin, including improved moisturization, increased softness, and better smoothness. These are cosmetic claims that do not require scientific validation. Medical photoprotective effects have been evaluated for both topical preparations. Topically applied alpha-tocopherol has been shown to inhibit UVB-induced edema and erythema, conferring an SPF of 3.[71] This is thought to be due to its ability to marginally absorb light and function as a free-radical-quenching, lipid-soluble antioxidant.[72] Oral vitamin E was shown to confer no photoprotective effects.[73]

Vitamin E may also have an anti-inflammatory effect on the skin, due to the inhibition of the production and release of chemical mediators, such as histamine. It may also stabilize the membranes of lysosomes by interacting with eicosanoids to reduce prostaglandin E_2 synthesis and increase IL-2 production.[74] This produces both anti-inflammatory and immunostimulatory effects.[75] A survey of elderly individuals found that high plasma tocopherol levels predisposed to a lower incidence of both infection and cancer.[76]

Vitamin E is lipophilic and can be incorporated into products for both the skin and hair in the form of vitamin E acetate, the stable esterified form of vitamin E, and vitamin E linoleate. One report lists vitamin E linoleate as a source of allergic contact dermatitis in a body lotion, probably due to improper formulation.[77] Vitamin E linoleate can enter into the epidermal lipids, providing enhanced moisturization. It should be formulated at a pH between 4.5 and 8.0 to enhance stability, in the presence of ascorbyl palmitate, BHA, and BHT.

Alpha tocopherol is used as an antioxidant preservative in formulations to prevent the rancidity of fats, particularly unsaturated fatty acids and their derivatives. It is a more potent antioxidant when combined with ascorbyl palmitate, inhibiting the production of nitrosamines. There is some preliminary data, however, that alpha tocopherol may be enzymatically metabolized during skin permeation, negating any antioxidant activity.[78]

Panthenol. The prior discussion has focused on the antioxidant vitamins A, C, and E, which are biologically active in skin physiology. There are other vitamins that are incorporated into topical formulations for their ability to function as actives, without biologic relevance. An important topical vitamin in this regard is panthenol. Panthenol is the biologically active alcohol form of pantothenic acid, also known as vitamin B_5, and is enzymatically converted to pantothenic acid in the skin. It is widely used topically as a skin and hair conditioning agent in moisturizers, shampoos, hair sprays, hair styling aids, and so forth. Its function is best characterized as a humectant, since it can both hold and attract water. This is important, since water is the plasticizing agent naturally found in both skin and hair.

There are four forms of panthenol utilized in hair and skin care products: *d*-panthenol (the dextrorotatory isomer), *dl*-panthenol (the racemic form), *d*-calcium pantothenate, and ethyl panthenol. The physiologic activity of the racemic form is 50% less than the dextrorotatory isomer.[79] Although *d*-panthenol is a colorless liquid and *dl*-panthenol is white crystalline powder, both are oil insoluble. Aqueous solutions are most stable between pH 4 and 7. Panthenol can be used to control viscosity, maintain water content in formulation, increase spreadability, act as a plasticizer, impart better glide, and improve the clarity of gel formulations. In skin preparations, it is usually found at a concentration of 5%.

Many vitamin-enriched moisturizing creams and lotions contain panthenol in a concentration of 5%, which has been shown to enhance wound healing. As a humectant ingredient, it is able to attract water from the viable epidermis and dermis to the stratum corneum where it must be trapped by an occlusive ingredient, if the barrier to transepidermal water loss is impaired. Under conditions where the ambient humidity exceeds 70%, panthenol could also draw water from the environment. Pathenol is an important ingredient in many moisturizer formulations, since water that is applied to the skin in the absence of a humectant is rapidly lost to the atmosphere.[80] Humectants may also allow the skin to feel smoother by filling voids between the corneocytes through swelling.[81] Thus, panthenol functions not only to enhance the water-holding capacity of the skin but also to improve the tactile attributes of rough skin.

Panthenol functions similarly in hair care products, where humectancy is also important to increase the water content of the hair shaft, thus increasing elasticity. Elasticity prevents hair shaft breakage by increasing its resistance to trauma. Panthenol functions well in rinse-off products, since it is substantive for hair keratin and can actually penetrate the hair shaft through voids where the cuticle has been disrupted. Panthenol is used in concentrations of 0.75% to 1% for rinse-off products, such as shampoos, 0.5% to 0.75% for leave-on products such as styling gels, and 0.25% for hair sprays. Thus, panthenol imparts increased manageability, better shine, less static electricity, and improved softness to damaged hair.

Niacin. Niacin is one component of the B vitamin complex; however, it can be synthesized in the human body as nicotinic acid. It is an important part of two coenzymes of intermediate metabolism, nicotinamide adenine dinucleotide (NAD) and nicotinamide adenine dinucleotide phosphate (NADP). Severe deficiencies are characterized by dermatitis, diarrhea, and dementia. Nicotinic acid produces flushing, due to a transient increase in cutaneous blood flow. It is not a vitamin additive commonly used in skin preparations, but it is useful for assessing the vascular stasis of the skin and is mentioned for this reason. Methyl nicotinate is applied topically in noninvasive testing to assess the effect of test formulations with laser Doppler flowmetry. However, its amide form, niacinamide, is incorporated into moisturizer formulations.

Niacinamide. Niacinamide, also known as nicotinamide, is the pyridine-3-carboxylic acid amide form of niacin. It is a white crystalline solid that is soluble in water and stable to both heat and oxygen. It is found in the body in all metabolically active tissues, including the skin.[82] Niacinamide does not produce the flushing experienced with niacin, nor is it valuable in the treatment of hyperlipidemias. It has no effect on blood pressure, pulse, or body temperature.[83]

Topical niacinamide is an interesting topical vitamin with some rather diverse reported cutaneous effects. Niacinamide has been shown to be of dermatologic benefit in the treatment of papular and pustular acne in a 4% gel.[84] It has also been reported to aid in the treatment of bullous pemphigoid[85,86] and necrobiosis lipoidica.[87] Interestingly, niacinamide may be valuable in the antiaging armamentarium of the dermatologist. The antiaging cutaneous effects of niacinamide include the promotion of antitumor characteristics in keratinocytes[88] and the suppression of UVB photocarcinogenesis.[89]

The beneficial cutaneous effects from the topical application of niacinamide, especially the improvement in photocarcinogenesis and its antitumor characteristics, have led to further research as to the usefulness of niacinamide as a moisturizer additive. It is easy to formulate due to its water solubility and stability in the presence of light and oxygen. Niacinamide has appeared in several newly marketed antiaging moisturizers.

Essential Fatty Acids. Other substances that are traditionally ingested have also found their way into antiaging moisturizers. For example, essential fatty acids (EFAs), sometimes referred to as vitamin F in the skin care industry, are composed of unsaturated linoleic, linolenic and arachidonic acid. These fatty acids are termed essential since they cannot be synthesized by the body, thus requiring oral ingestion. Rodents that are fed diets missing EFAs develop skin that is rough and dry appearing, due to hyperkeratinization.[90] Rubbing sunflower oil on the skin surface reduces the hyperkeratinization, since this oil is high in EFAs, but dietary intake of the EFAs is the recommended treatment. It is difficult for humans to eat a modern diet completely deficient in EFAs.

The EFAs are very important in maintenance of the barrier function of the stratum corneum. Linoleic acid is found in high concentration in ceramides, which are a major component of the intercellular lipids filling the spaces between the corneocytes. Topical application of pure linoleic acid is not desirable, since it is a strong cutaneous irritant and unstable. Vitamin E linoleate is a better choice for topical supplementation of EFAs. For this reason, many barrier repair creams contain vitamin E linoleate.

Biotin. Biotin is an oral supplement that has gained modest scientific acceptance in dermatology, although it is technically not a vitamin. Biotin is a monocarboxylic acid functioning as a coenzyme in carboxylation reactions of fat, carbohydrates, and protein. It is considered a conditional B vitamin. It is synthesized by intestinal bacteria. It is mentioned in the context of vitamins, since it has been used as a supplement for preventing cracking in the hoofs of thoroughbred race horses. Human oral supplementation has been shown to be effective in improving nail brittleness and nail peeling.[91] The beneficial nail effects of topical biotin have not been demonstrated, however. No standard accepted dose for oral biotin supplementation for nail splitting has been identified.

Ubiquinone. Ubiquinone, also known as coenzyme Q_{10}, is a fat-soluble vitaminlike substance synthesized in all tissues of the body. It is not a true vitamin, since it can be manufactured endogenously from tyrosine. It is available, however, as an oral supplement and is finding its way into topical antiaging moisturizers. It is the "ubiquitous" nature of this quinone family coenzyme that led Morton in 1957 to name the substance he isolated from rat liver as ubiquinone. Folker and coworkers at Merck defined its chemical structure, but the first human application for oral ubiquinone was developed by Yamamura to aid in the treatment of congestive heart failure. Ubiquinone is found in mitochondria as part of the electron transport chain and is felt to aid in heart muscle contractility.[92] Medications such as lovastatin, used to lower cholesterol, are HMG-CoA reductase inhibitors and also block ubiquinone synthesis.[93] Ubiquinone supplementation orally is also used in Japan for patients with periodontal disease and cancer.

Ubiquinone may also function as an antioxidant by providing electrons to oxygen radicals. For this reason, it is becoming an additive in many therapeutic dermatologic moisturizers. Since it is an endogenous antioxidant synthesized by the body when a normal solid food diet is consumed, it is unclear how topical supplementation affects the skin.

Dermatologic Issues Regarding Topical Vitamins. The prior discussion concerning vitamins has presented the best science that is currently available regarding their usefulness in topical preparations. It is rather amazing that so little is known about the dermatologic benefits of vitamins, despite their large presence in the marketplace. Remember that vitamins are currently unregulated and considered a food supplement. This means that they can be easily added to a variety of skin preparations, without making any specific claim attributed to their functioning or effects. Once claims are made in this manner, the product becomes a drug and not a cosmetic. Thus, few manufacturers really wish to determine the implications of topical vitamin application. Rather, most companies simply state on the label that the product "contains" a given vitamin, which technically is not a claim, but a statement of fact. Nevertheless, the physician needs to carefully assess the value of topical vitamin formulations. This discussion is aimed at providing a logical framework for product analysis.

Proper formulation of topical vitamins is the key to preparing a product with true skin benefit. The requirements for proper formulation are listed in Box 10-5. First, it is of primary importance that the vitamin additive meet the requirements for cosmetic grade ingredients. This means that the raw material is without contaminants, with verified concentration and purity. Cosmetic grade vitamins are less likely to cause allergic and irritant contact dermatitis. Second, the amount of the vitamin in the product must be sufficient to allow for adequate bioavailability. Also, the vehicle must be carefully selected to maintain the biologic activity of the vitamin and promote cutaneous bioavailability. Third, the vitamin must remain biologically active until it is applied to the skin surface. This means that the vehicle must prevent chelation, inactivation, and degradation of the vitamin. Table 10-1 details the oxygen, light, temperature, acid, and base stability of some of the vitamins discussed previously. Notice for example, that vitamin A and vitamin C cannot be combined in their biologically active forms in a moisturizer. This is due to the fact that vitamin C is an acid and vitamin A is unstable in the presence of acids. Last, the vitamin must enter the skin, escape enzymatic degradation, and reach the target tissue in a biologically active form. In some cases this may be the epidermis, which is the active site for the humectant panthenol. In other cases this may be the dermis, which is the site of oxygen radical formation where antioxidants must reside in order to be biologically effective and protect collagen and elastin.

In summary, much research remains to be conducted on topical vitamins and their value as part of the cutaneous antiaging armamentarium. New formulations that are forthcoming should provide enhanced efficacy with scientifically documented results.

BOX 10-5 Considerations for Formulating Topical Vitamin Preparations

1. The vitamin must be nontoxic and of cosmetic grade.
2. The vitamin must be bioavailable in the vehicle selected with substantivity for the skin.
3. The vitamin must remain in its biologically active form during manufacture, in its final packaging, and under consumer use conditions.
4. The vitamin must reach the target tissue in its biologically active form.

Table 10-1 Vitamin Stability

Vitamin	Oxygen	Light	100° C	Acids	Bases
A	U	U	S	U	S
E	U	U	S	S	S
Niacinamide	S	S	S	S	S
Panthenol	S	S	U	U	U
C	U	U	U	S	U

U, Unstable; S, stable.

Botanicals

Another source of additives to skin care products, aside from the vitamins previously discussed, are plant extracts, also known as botanicals. Botanicals formed the basis of all medical treatments at the time European settlers were first coming to America. These Europeans learned that the American Indians had an extensive pharmacopeia, based on native plants, that was passed from generation to generation through the wisdom of the medicine man in each community. These plant concoctions were mastered by the settlers, transported back to England, and incorporated into some of the earliest books on medical treatment. Increased understanding of human physiology, disease processes, and chemistry led to the extraction and synthesis of many medically important substances from these early botanical remedies. Recently, there has been a resurgence in botanicals in the form of additives found in many skin care products. These botanically based skin care products are nonprescription, unregulated remedies that appeal to the current popular trend of natural healing.

This section discusses some of the botanical extracts of current popularity to acquaint the physician with their purported value, chemical constituents, and interesting details. Botanical pharmacopeias contain thousands of plants with anecdotal purported skin benefits, unfortunately lacking scientific validation. Some of the botanical extracts used with supposed anti-inflammatory and soothing skin benefits are presented here. This information is presented for interest only, since clinical data is scarce.

Botanical Anti-inflammatories. Botanical anti-inflammatory additives are used in many different skin preparations, since inflammation is the final common pathway of numerous dermatoses. The extracts discussed include Ginkgo biloba, green tea, Echinacea, Thuja, and Sarsaparilla.

Ginkgo Biloba. Ginkgo biloba is a plant with numerous purported benefits that is a common part of homeopathic medicine in the Orient. The plant leaves are said to contain unique polyphenols such as terpenoids (ginkgolides, bilobalides), flavinoids, and flavonol glycosides that have anti-inflammatory effects. These anti-inflammatory effects have been linked to antiradical and antilipoperoxidant effects in experimental fibroblast models.[94] Ginkgo flavonoid fractions containing quercetin, kaempferol, sciadopitysin, ginkgetin, and isoginkgetin have been demonstrated to induce human skin fibroblast proliferation in vitro. Increased collagen and extracellular fibronectin were also demonstrated by radioisotope assay.[95]

Various unknown Ginkgo fractions are added to skin moisturizers for antiaging benefits, even though no controlled trials exist regarding cutaneous benefits. Since Ginkgo is added to products considered cosmetics, no antiaging claims can be made. Generally, Ginkgo is claimed to "enhance the skin appearance," which is a cosmetic claim not requiring validation, because appearance is a subjective assessment.

Green Tea. Green tea is another botanical popular in the Orient for both topical application and oral ingestion. Orally, green tea is said to contain beneficial flavonoids that act as potent antioxidants. Green tea packaging currently claims that the product enhances energy levels, not that it reverses aging. Again, the claims made must be of a cosmetic or nutritional nature, rather than scientific drug claims.

A study by Katiyar et al. demonstrated the anti-inflammatory effects of topical green tea application on C3H mice. A topically applied green tea extract containing GTP (epigallocatechin-3-gallate) was found to reduce UVB-induced inflammation as measured by double skinfold swelling.[96] At present, green tea remains a nutritional supplement and not an approved sun protective agent.

Echinacea. Echinacea, also known as black-eyed Susans or American cone flower, is native to Kansas, Nebraska, and Missouri but can be propagated as an annual in any environment with ample water. It was a common botanical homeopathic remedy used by the American Indians that is currently seeing renewed topical popularity. The American Indians used every part of the plant for medicinal purposes. The fresh leaves were ground to produce an antiseptic and pain reliever for wounds and bites. The juice of the roots was used to bathe burns.

Echinacea purpurea species is currently advocated for its value in treating psoriasis and reducing the inflammation associated with a variety of dermatologic conditions. An oral Echinacea purpurea extract is sold as a homeopathic remedy for psoriasis, but the mechanism of action is unknown. Echinacea is listed as a botanical additive in many moisturizers designed for sensitive skin. At this point, Echinacea has to be regarded as a botanical with a rich medicinal history, but little supporting data.

Thuja. Thuja, also known as cedarwood or arborvitae, is another American Indian homeopathic remedy for psoriasis. It too is found in moisturizing preparations for skin that is sensitive or easily irritated. Interestingly, Thuja is also incorporated into homeopathic salves used in the treatment of warts. Other homeopathic uses include the treatment of tinea corporis and oral candidiasis, but the antifungal effects of Thuja have never been demonstrated clinically.

Sarsaparilla. Many botanical extracts that were once considered medications are still used as modern flavorings, perhaps with some additional homeopathic benefits. An example of such a botanical is Sarsaparilla. Sarsaparilla was used as a flavoring in sodas sold in pharmacies to children and adults. It is still possible to purchase sarsaparilla candy and sodas in gourmet food establishments.

Sarsaparilla is also claimed to possess topical benefits due to the presence of plant sterols and saponins. It is said to have both antiseptic and antipruritic properties. For this reason, it is incorporated into homeopathic topical preparations to treat both eczema and psoriasis.

Botanical Skin Soothing Agents. Another common dermatologic use of botanical extracts is to provide skin-soothing benefits. Many products that claim to calm, normalize, replenish, or relax the skin incorporate botanical ingredients such as prickly pear, sagebrush, jojoba, aloe vera, or allantoin. These plants have been selected for discussion due to their current novelty and popularity.

Prickly Pear. Prickly pear, a plant native to the Southwestern desert, is a cactus also known as cactus pear, Indian pear, or tuna fig. It was imported to Europe in the sixteenth century and became a part of a salve designed to soothe cutaneous wounds and burns. The fleshy pad of the prickly pear contains 83% water and 10% sucrose with small amounts of tartaric acid, citric acid, and other mucopolysaccharides. American Indians would rub the mucilage from the broken pad over the skin surface to act as a sunscreen and moisturizer.

Mucilages in general have a soothing, cooling effect on the skin, due to evaporation of water, when the plant juice is rubbed over the skin. Additionally, the mucopolysaccharides dry to form a protective coating over wounds or dermatitis. An extract of prickly pear is found in some moisturizer formulations; however, the extract is added as a dried powder and not as a mucilage. This defeats the skin-soothing benefits for the most part. Nevertheless, prickly pear juice is found in a variety of skin care products.

Sagebrush. Sagebrush is another desert plant that was used widely by the Indians of the southwestern United States, such as the Navajo, as a powder to sprinkle onto cuts and wounds. The powder was felt to have both antibiotic and skin-soothing effects. Ground sagebrush leaves cooked and mixed with olive oil are still applied to irritated skin by homeopathic healers in Mexico and the southwestern United States. This is the rationale behind the incorporation of sagebrush extract into night creams designed to soothe irritated skin.

Jojoba. Jojoba is currently a protected endangered plant in the southwestern United States. The plant is valued for the light-weight oil obtained from its fruit that is highly desirable in the skin care industry. Jojoba is difficult to domesticate; thus it is an expensive botanical additive. Jojoba oil was first used by the American Indians and Mexicans for its ability to soothe and heal wounds. The oil is now finding its way into botanical moisturizers as a specialty additive, an ingredient designed to capture consumer attention.

Aloe Vera. Probably the most widely used botanical additive to soothe the skin is aloe vera. The mucilage is released from the plant leaves as a colorless gel and contains 99.5% water and a complex mixture of mucopolysaccharides, amino acids, hydroxy quinone glycosides, and minerals. Compounds isolated from aloe vera juice include aloin, aloe emodin, aletinic acid, choline, and choline salicylate.[97] The reported cutaneous effects of aloe vera include increased blood flow, reduced inflammation, decreased skin bacterial colonization, and enhanced wound healing.[98]

In most skin preparations, aloe vera is added as a powder, not as a mucilage. The composition of aloe vera powder may not be the same as aloe vera juice that oozes from the freshly broken plant leaf. Aloe vera extract is found in soaps, hair shampoos, hand lotions, body moisturizers, and so forth. It is estimated that aloe vera must be present at a concentration of 10% to have a moisturizing effect in products designed to remain on the skin for extended periods of time. Concentration and formulation are important considerations when determining whether a botanical additive has a skin benefit.

Allantoin. Allantoin is a currently popular botanical extract that is obtained from common comfrey root. It is the basis for sensitive skin claims made for a number of moisturizers marketed to dermatologists. Most allantoin currently used in skin care products is not botanically derived, but rather manufactured by the alkaline oxidation of uric acid in a cold environment. It is a white crystalline powder that is readily soluble in hot water, making it easy to formulate in a variety of products. Allantoin is felt to induce cell proliferation and is also incorporated into botanical healing salves.

FUTURE TRENDS IN COSMETICS AND COSMECEUTICALS

This discussion will conclude by taking a closer look at the broad categories of skin care products we have been considering. Alpha hydroxy acids are nonmonographed ingredients, designed to induce cutaneous exfoliation, yet they are categorized as cosmetics. Salicylic acid is a cutaneous exfoliant, monographed ingredient, currently classified in some formulations as an OTC drug. Tretinoin was discussed for its antiaging benefits, but it is classified as a drug and available only by prescription. The other vitamin additives and botanicals discussed are classified as unregulated nutritional supplements, and products containing these ingredients are cosmetics. This system of regulating cosmetics, OTC drugs, and prescription drugs is confusing, antiquated, and cumbersome.

This problem has arisen out of the rapid technological developments that have been achieved in the realm of topical formulation, without similar advancements in the rules and regulations governing such products in the United States. At present, in the United States and Europe, a drug is defined as "an article intended for the use in the diagnosis, mitigation, treatment or prevention of disease or intended to affect the structure or any function of the body." Conversely, a cosmetic is defined by the federal Food, Drug and Cosmetic Act, written in 1938, as "articles intended to be rubbed, poured, sprinkled, or sprayed on, introduced into, or otherwise applied to the human body or any part thereof for cleansing, beautifying, promoting attractiveness, or altering the appearance" without affecting structure or function.[99]

In between drugs and cosmetics there lies an undefined arena of formulations that do not fit neatly into any current FDA classification. To more accurately describe biologically active skin formulations that are available to the consumer for direct purchase, Albert M. Kligman, MD, developed the concept of cosmeceuticals. He defined cosmeceuticals as products that are cosmetics, yet have documented and intended pharmaceutical activity. Cosmeceuticals are now a reality due to the expanding dermatologic knowledge base that has rendered obsolete the prior outdated clear distinction between cosmetics and drugs.[100] The concept of cosmeceuticals was embraced by the cosmetics industry in 1961 when Reed published the guidelines for cosmeceuticals presented in Box 10-6.[101]

Failure to create a new category for cosmeceuticals in the United States has prevented scientific advancement in the realm of cutaneous actives.[102] Japan has created a category of products defined and regulated as cosmeceuticals. This has allowed tremendous advancement in the quality of new skin care product development, since the claims made regarding such products must be scientifically supported. This has partially eliminated the opportunity to make low-level cosmetic claims concerning ineffective formulations that currently dominate much of the pseudocosmeceutical market in the United States. Japan has now technologically progressed ahead of the United States in product formulation. In summary, a new category defined as cosmeceuticals would increase the ability of the government to ensure that marketed products are safe and efficacious. It would also officially recognize this active arena of skin research.

BOX 10-6 Reed Concept of Cosmeceuticals

1. A cosmeceutical is a scientifically designed product intended for external application to the human body.
2. A cosmeceutical produces a useful, desired product.
3. A cosmeceutical has desirable aesthetic characteristics.
4. A cosmeceutical meets rigid chemical, physical, and medical standards.

It is clear from reading the material presented in this chapter that all the substances discussed could easily be considered cosmeceuticals; however, it is somewhat bewildering to realize that water is also a cosmeceutical. Water profoundly influences the structure and function of the viable epidermis, which is now known to be a biologically active organ. Many substances can function as cosmeceuticals if entry into and through the stratum corneum is facilitated through the use of penetration enhancers, such as propylene glycol, isopropyl myristate, and pyrrolidone derivatives. Propylene glycol profoundly alters the barrier characteristics of the stratum corneum while isopropyl myristate is capable of penetrating into the liposomal bilayers of cell membranes. Pyrrolidone derivatives interact with both keratin and the stratum corneum lipids to drive substances into the skin. These substances are commonly found in cosmetic formulations, but new understanding of skin physiology allows recognition of their profound effects on the skin, which were previously unknown.

The science of skin formulation in the realm of cosmeceuticals is moving forward at an extremely rapid rate due to the high-quality dermatologic research currently under way. It is only through a better understanding of skin physiology that new products can be conceived, studied, and brought to the marketplace.

REFERENCES

1. Stiller MJ, Bartolone J, Stern R, et al. Topical 8% glycolic acid and 8% l-lactic acid creams for the treatment of photodamaged skin. Arch Dermatol 1996; 132:631-636.
2. Dietre CM, Griffin TD, Murphy GF, et al. Effects of alpha-hydroxy acids on photoaged skin. J Am Acad Dermatol 1996; 34:187-195.
3. Berardesca E, Maibach H. AHA mechanism of action. Cosmet Toilet 1995; 110:30-31.
4. Van Scott EJ, Yu RJ. Hyperkeratinization, corneocyte cohesion and alpha hydroxy acids. J Am Acad Dermatol 1984; 11:867-879.
5. Bernstein EF, Uitto J. Connective tissue alterations in photoaged skin and the effects of alpha hydroxy acids. J Geriatr Dermatol 1995; 3(suppl):7A-18A.

6. Lavker RM, Kaidbey K, Leyden JJ. Effects of topical ammonium lactate on cutaneous atrophy from a potent topical corticosteroid. J Am Acad Dermatol 1992; 26:535-544.
7. Griffin TD, Murphy GF, Sueki H, et al. Increased factor XIIIa transglutaminase expression in dermal dendrocytes after treatment with alpha-hydroxy acids: potential physiologic significance. J Am Acad Dermatol 1996; 34:196-203.
8. Kim SJ, Park JH, Kim DH, et al. Increased in vivo collagen synthesis and in vitro cell proliferative effect of glycolic acid. Am J Dermatol Surg 1998; 24:1054-1058.
9. Moy LS, Murad H, Moy RL. Glycolic acid peels for the treatment of wrinkles and photoaging. J Dermatol Surg Oncol 1993; 19:243-246.
10. Elson ML. Treatment of photoaging—a personal comment and open study of the use of glycolic acid. J Dermatol Treat 1993; 4: 215-218.
11. Van Scott EJ, Yu RJ. Control of keratinization with alpha hydroxy acids and related compounds; I: topical treatment of ichthyotic disorders. Arch Dermatol 1974; 110:586-590.
12. DiNardo JC, Grove GL, Moy LW. 12% ammonium lactate versus 8% glycolic acid. J Geriatr Dermatol 1995; 3:144-147.
13. Wehr RF, Kantor I, Jones EL, et al. A controlled comparative efficacy study of 5% ammonium lactate lotion versus an emolient control in the treatment of moderate xerosis. J Am Acad Dermatol 1991; 25:849-851.
14. Van Scott EJ, Yu RJ. Alpha hydroxy acids: procedures for use in clinical practice. Cutis 1989; 43:222-228.
15. Van Scott EJ, Yu RJ. Alpha hydroxy acids: therapeutic potentials. Can J Dermatol 1989; 1:108-112.
16. Briden ME, Rendon-Pellerano MI. Treatment of rosacea with glycolic acid. J Geriatr Dermatol 1996; 4(SB):17B-21B.
17. Klaus MV, Wehr RF, Rogers RS, et al. Evaluation of ammonium lactate in the treatment of seborrheic keratoses. J Am Acad Dermatol 1990; 22:199-203.
18. Siskin SB, Quinlan PJ, Finkelstein MS, et al. The effects of ammonium lactate 12% lotion versus no therapy in the treatment of dry skin of the heels. Int J Dermatol 1993; 32:905-907.
19. Kakita LS, Petratos MA. The use of glycolic acid in Asian and darker skin types. J Geriatr Dermatol 1996; 4(SB):8B-11B.
20. Perricone NV. An alpha hydroxy acid acts as an antioxidant. J Geriatr Dermatol 1993; 1:101-104.
21. Perricone NV, DiNardo JC. Photoprotective and antiinflammatory effects of topical glycolic acid. Dermatol Surg 1996; 22:435-437.
22. Davies M, Marks R. Studies on the effect of salicylic acid on the normal stratum corneum. Br J Dermatol 1980; 103:191-196.
23. DiNardo JC. A comparison of salicylic acid, salicylic acid with glycolic acid and benzoyl peroxide in the treatment of acne. Cosmet Dermatol 1995; 8.
24. Kligman A, Kligman AM. Salicylic acid as a peeling agent for the treatment of acne. Cosmet Dermatol 1997; 10:44-47.
25. Huber C, Christopher E. Keratolytic effect of salicylic acid. Arch Dermatol Res 1977; 257:293-297.
26. Draelos ZD. Salicylic acid in the dermatologic armamentarium. Cosmet Dermatol 1997; September suppl:7-8.
27. Roberts DL, Marshall R, Marks R. Detection of the action of salicylic acid on the normal stratum corneum. Br J Dermatol 1980; 103:191-196.
28. Kligman D, Kligman AM. Salicylic acid peels for the treatment of photoaging. Dermatol Surg 1998; 24:325-328.
29. Kraeling ME, Bronaugh RL. In vitro percutaneous absorption of alpha hydroxy acids in human skin. J Soc Cosmet Chem 1997; 48:187-197.
30. DiNardo JC, Grove GL, Moy L. Clinical and histological effects of glycolic acid at different concentrations and pH levels. Dermatol Surg 1996; 22:421-424.
31. Smith WP. Epidermal and dermal effects of topical lactic acid. J Am Acad Dermatol 1996; 35:388-391.
32. Yu RJ, Van Scott EJ. Bioavailability of alpha-hydroxy acids in topical formulations. Cosmet Dermatol 1996; 9:54-62.
33. Smith WP. Hydroxy acids and skin aging. Cosmet Toilet 1994; 109:41-48.
34. Sah A, Mukherjee S, Wickett RR. An in vitro study of the effects of formulation variables and product structure on percutaneous absorption of lactic acid. J Cosmet Sci 1998; 49:257-273.
35. Goodman DS. Vitamin A and retinoids in health and disease. N Engl J Med 1984; 310(16):1023-1031.
36. Garmyn M, Ribaya-Mercado JD, Russel RM, Gilchrest BA. Effect of beta-carotene supplementation on the human sunburn reaction. Exp Dermatol 1995; 4:104-111.
37. Lachance P. Dietary intake of carotenes and the carotene gap. Clin Nutr 1988; 7:118-122.
38. Ziegler RG. Vegetables, fruits, and carotenoids and the risk of cancer. Am J Clin Nutr 1991; 53(suppl):251S-259S.
39. Shekelle RB, Lepper M, Liu S, et al. Dietary vitamin A and the risk of cancer in the Western Electric Study. Lancet 1981; 2:1185-1190.
40. Noy N. Interactions of retinoids with lipid bilayers and with membranes. In: Livrea MA, Packer L, eds. Retinoids. New York: Marcel Dekker, 1993:17-27.
41. Osawa T. Plant antioxidants: protective role against oxygen radical species. Cosmet Toilet 1994; 109:77-81.
42. Duell EA, Derguini F, Kang S, et al. Extraction of human epidermis treated with retinol yields retro-retinoids in addition to free retinol and retinyl esters. J Invest Dermatol 1996; 107:178-182.
43. Tsunoda T, Takabayashi K. Stability of all-trans-retinol in cream. J Soc Cosmet Chem 1995; 46:191-198.
44. Kligman LH, Do CH, Kligman AM. Topical retinoic acid enhances the repair of ultraviolet damaged dermal connective tissue. Connect Tissue Res 1984; 12:139-150.
45. Kligman AM, Grove GL, Hirose R, Leyden JJ. Topical tretinoin for photoaged skin. J Am Acad Dermatol 1986; 15:836-859.
46. Goodman DS. Vitamin A and retinoids in health and disease. N Engl J Med 1984; 310(16):1023-1031.
47. Noy N. Interactions of retinoids with lipid bilayers and with membranes. In: Livrea MA, Packer L, eds. Retinoids. New York: Marcel Dekker, 1993:17-27.
48. Weiss JS, Ellis CN, Headington JT, et al. Topical tretinoin improves photoaged skin: a double-blind, vehicle controlled study. JAMA 1988; 259:527-532.
49. Fisher GJ, Tavakkol A, Griffiths CEM, et al. Differential modulation of transforming growth factor-beta one expression and mucin deposition by retinoic acid and sodium lauryl sulfate in human skin. J Invest Dermatol 1992; 98:102-108.
50. Olsen EA, Katz I, Levine N, et al. Tretinoin emollient cream: a new therapy for photodamaged skin. J Am Acad Dermatol 1992; 26:215-224.
51. Woodley DT, Zelickson AS, Briggaman RA, et al. Treatment of photoaged skin with topical tretinoin increases epidermal-dermal anchoring fibrils: a preliminary report. JAMA 1990; 263: 3057-3059.
52. Fisher GJ, Datta SC, Talwar HS, et al. Molecular basis of sun-induced premature skin ageing and retinoid antagonism. Nature 1996; 379:335-339.
53. Goldfarb MT, Ellis CE, Weiss JS, Voorhees JJ. Topical tretinoin therapy: its use in photoaged skin. J Am Acad Dermatol 1989; 21:645-650.
54. Kligman AM, Dogadkina D, Lavker RM. Effects of topical tretinoin on non-sun-exposed protected skin of the elderly. J Am Acad Dermatol 1993; 29:25-33.
55. Weiss JS, Ellis CE, Headington JT, Voorhees JJ. Topical tretinoin in the treatment of aging skin. J Am Acad Dermatol 1988; 19: 169-175.
56. Weinstein GD, Nigra TP, Pochi PE, et al. Topical tretinoin for treatment of photodamaged skin. Arch Dermatol 1991; 127:659-665.

57. Gilchrest BA, Blog FB, Szabo G. Effects of aging and chronic sun exposure on melanocytes in human skin. J Invest Dermatol 1979; 73:141-143.
58. Bhawan J, Serva AG, Nehal K, et al. Effects of tretinoin on photodamaged skin: a histologic study. Arch Dermatol 1991; 127:666-672.
59. Griffiths CEM, Goldfarb MT, Finkel LJ, et al. Topical tretinoin (retinoic acid) treatment of hyperpigmented lesions associated with photoaging in Chinese and Japanese patients. J Am Acad Dermatol 1994; 30:76-84.
60. Green CK, Griffiths CEM, Finkel LJ, et al. Topical retinoic acid (tretinoin) for melasma in black patients. Arch Dermatol 1994; 130:727-733.
61. Kang S, Kim KJ, Griffiths CEM, et al. Topical tretinoin (retinoic acid) improves early stretch marks. Arch Dermatol 1996; 132: 519-526.
62. Chan AC. Partners in defense, vitamin E, and vitamin C. Can J Physiol Pharmacol 1993; 71:725-731.
63. Beyer RE. The role of ascorbate in antioxidant protection of biomembranes: interaction with vitamin E and coenzyme Q. Arch Bioeng Biomem 1994; 26:349-358.
64. Darr D, Combs S, Dunston S, Manning T, Pinnell SR. Topical vitamin C protects porcine shin from ultraviolet radiation-induced damage. Br J Dermatol 1992; 127:247-253.
65. Murray J, Darr D, Reich J, Pinnell S. Topical vitamin C treatment reduces ultraviolet B radiation-induced erythema in human skin. Abstract. J Invest Dermatol 1991; 96:587.
66. Kameyama K, Sakai C, Kondoh S, et al. Inhibitory effects of magnesium L-ascorbyl-2-phosphate on melanogenesis in vitro and in vivo. J Am Acad Dermatol 1996; 34:29-33.
67. Burton GW, Joyce A, Ingold KU. Is vitamin E the only lipid-soluble, chain-breaking antioxidant in human blood plasma and erythrocyte membranes? Arch Biochem Biophys 1983; 221:281-290.
68. Kagan VE. Tocopherol stabilizes membrane against phospholipase A, free fatty acids, and lysophospholipids. Ann NY Acad Sci 1989; 570:121-135.
69. Kagan V, Witt E, Goldman R, Scita G, Packer L. Ultraviolet light-induced generation of vitamin E radicals and their recycling. A possible photosensitizing effect of vitamin E in skin. Free Rad Res Comms 1992; 16:51-64.
70. Fuchs J, Hufleijt ME, Rothfuss LM, et al. Acute effects of near ultraviolet and visible light on the cutaneous antioxidant defense system. Photochem Photobiol 1989; 50:739-744.
71. Idson B. Vitamins and the skin. Cosmet Toilet 1993; 108:79-92.
72. Mayer P, Pittermann W, Wallat S. The effects of vitamin E on the skin. Cosmet Toilet 1993; 108:99-109.
73. Werninghaus K, Meydani M, Bhawan J, et al. Evaluation of the photoprotective effect of oral vitamin E supplementation. Arch Dermatol 1994; 130:1257-1261.
74. Diplock AT, Xu G, Yeow C, Okikiola M. Relationship of tocopherol structure to biological activity, tissue uptake, and prostaglandin synthesis. In: Diplock AT, Machlin LJ, Paker L, Pryor WA, eds. Vitamin E: Biochemistry and Health Implications. New York: New York Academy of Sciences, 1989:72-84.
75. Meydani SN, Barklund MP, Liu S, et al. Vitamin E supplementation enhances cell-mediated immunity in healthy elderly subjects. Am J Clin Nutr 1990; 52:557-563.
76. Knekt P, Aromaa A, Maatela J, et al. Vitamin E and cancer prevention. Am J Clin Nutr 1991; 53:283S-286S.
77. Perrenoud D, Homberger HP, Auderset PC, et al. An epidemic outbreak of papular and follicular contact dermatitis to tocopheryl linoleate in cosmetics. Dermatology 1994; 189:225-233.
78. Lee AC, Tojo K. Metabolism of vitamin E during skin permeation. J Soc Cosmet Chem 1996; 47:85-95.
79. Idson B. Vitamins and the skin. Cosmet Toilet 1993; 108:79-94.
80. Rieger MM, Deem DE. Skin moisturizers; II: the effects of cosmetic ingredients on human stratum corneum. J Soc Cosmet Chem 1974; 25:253-262.
81. Robbins CR, Fernee KM. Some observations on the swelling of human epidermal membrane. J Soc Cosmet Chem 1983; 37:21-34.
82. Hankes LV. Nicotinic acid and nicotinamide. In: Machlin LJ, ed. Handbook of Vitamins. New York: Marcel Dekker, 1984:329-377.
83. Stratford MRL, Rojas A, Hall DW, et al. Pharmacokinetics of nicotinamide and its effect on blood pressure, pulse and body temperature in normal human volunteers. Radiother Oncol 1992; 25:37-42.
84. Ellis CN, article in Skin and Allergy News 1988; 19(8):3.
85. Honl BA, Elston DM. Autoimmune bullous eruption localized to a breast reconstruction site: response to niacinamide. Cutis 1998; 62:85-86.
86. Fiverson DP, Breneman DL, Rosen GB, Hersh CS, Cardone S, Mutasim D. Nicotinamide and tetracycline therapy of bullous pemphigoid. Arch Dermatol 1994; 13:753-758.
87. Handfield-Jones S, Jones S, Peachey R. High dose nicotinamide in the treatment of necrobiosis lipoidica. Br J Dermatol 1988; 118:693-696.
88. Ludwig A, Dietel M, Schafer G, Muller K, Hilz H. Nicotinamide and nicotinamide analogues as antitumor promoters in mouse skin. Cancer Res 1990; 50:2470-2475.
89. Gensler HL. Prevention of photoimmunosupression and photocarcinogenesis by topical nicotinamide. Nutrition and Cancer 1997; 29:157-162.
90. Elias PM, Brown BE, Ziboh VA. The permeability barrier in essential fatty acid deficiency: evidence for a direct role for linoleic acid in barrier function. J Invest Dermatol 1980; 75:230-233.
91. Hochman LG, Scher RK, Meyerson MS. Brittle nails: response to daily biotin supplementation. Cutis 1993; 51:303-305.
92. Mortensen SA, Vadhanavikit S, Folkers K. Deficiency of coenzyme Q_{10} in myocardial failure. Drugs Exp Clin Res 1984; 7:497-502.
93. Folkers K, Langsjoen PH, Willis R, et al. Lovastatin decreases coenzyme Q levels in humans. Proc Natl Acad Sci 1990; 87:8931-8934.
94. Joyeux M, Lobstein A, Anton R, Mortier F. Comparative antilipoperoxidant, antinecrotic and scavenging properties of terpenes and biflavones from Ginkgo and some flavonoids. Plant Med 1995; 61:126-129.
95. Kim SJ, Lim MH, Chun IK, Won YH. Effects of flavonoids of Ginkgo biloba on proliferation of human skin fibroblast. Skin Pharmacol 1997; 10:200-205.
96. Katiyar SK, Elmets CA, Agarwal R, et al. Protection against ultraviolet-B radiation-induced local and systemic suppression of contact hypersensitivity and edema responses in C3H/HeN mice by green tea polyphenols. Photochem Photobiol 1995; 62: 855-861.
97. McKeown E. Aloe vera. Cosmet Toilet 1987; 102:64-65.
98. Waller T. Aloe vera. Cosmet Toilet 1992; 107:53-54.
99. 21 USC §§301-392.
100. Vermeer BJ, Gilchrest BA. Cosmeceuticals. Arch Dermatol 1996; 132:337-340.
101. Epstein H. Factors in formulating cosmeceutical vehicles. Cosmet Toilet 1997; 112:91-99.
102. Lavrijsen APM, Vermeer BJ. Cosmetics and drugs: is there a need for a third group: cosmeceutics. Br J Dermatol 1991; 124: 503-504.

CHAPTER 11

Lasers in the Treatment of Vascular Lesions

RICHARD J. ORT
KENNETH A. ARNDT
JEFFREY S. DOVER

SECTION ONE

History and Scientific Review

BACKGROUND AND HISTORY

Vascular lesions are a common occurrence in all age groups. Most vascular anomalies can be classified into three primary categories: malformations, benign neoplasms, and dilatations of preexisting vessels[1] (Table 11-1). Vascular malformations are categorized according to the predominant vessel type: venous, venular, capillary, lymphatic, arterial, arteriovenous, or a combination thereof.[2,3] Malformations are congenital lesions that are always present at birth and never regress. Although malformations do not exhibit cellular proliferation, they expand as patients age because of change in body contour and size and progressive ectasia of preexisting vessels. Port wine stains (PWS) are a type of vascular malformation, consisting of ectatic venules within the dermis.

Benign vascular neoplasms are classified according to their cellular differentiation and the characteristics of the involved vessels. Hemangiomas are the most common benign vascular neoplasm in infancy and childhood. These lesions usually appear several weeks after birth, grow rapidly during the first year of life, and then usually spontaneously involute over years as fibrous tissue replaces vascular parenchyma. Whereas the rate of endothelial turnover is normal in malformations, it is increased in hemangiomas during the proliferative phase. The category of benign vascular neoplasms includes the common cherry angioma as well as rarer lesions such as kaposiform hemangioendothelioma and glomus tumor.

Vascular dilatations have normal endothelial turnover but demonstrate ectasia of preexisting vessels. This category includes telangiectases, which represent permanent dilatations of end vessels, primarily venules. Telangiectases may be seen in numerous conditions, including rosacea, collagen vascular diseases, and cutaneous mastocytosis, or may appear secondary to trauma, radiation therapy, sun damage, endocrine factors, or high venous pressure. Other vascular dilatations include venous lakes, spider angiomas, angiokeratomas, and lymphangiectases.

Prior to the advent of laser technology, treatment options for vascular lesions were limited to surgical excision, electrosurgery, cryosurgery, radiation therapy, dermabrasion, or overtattooing. These techniques were largely ineffective and carried an unacceptably high risk of scarring and pigmentary change. The introduction of the argon laser in the 1960s heralded a new era in the treatment of vascular lesions. By targeting hemoglobin within blood vessels with blue-green light, the argon laser could effectively treat many vascular anomalies. However, high expectations were soon tempered by the realization that use of the argon laser was associated with possible adverse effects, including hypertrophic scarring and permanent hypopigmentation.

In the early 1980s, investigators postulated a more sophisticated understanding of laser-tissue interaction known as the principle of selective photothermolysis.[4,5] The flashlamp-pumped pulsed dye laser was developed based on this principle to specifically target blood vessels within pediatric PWS. The pulsed dye laser quickly replaced the argon and other continuous wave lasers as the treatment of choice for most PWS and other vascular lesions. The pulsed dye laser has since undergone modifications in wavelength, beam size, and pulse duration and it remains the most widely used laser to treat vascular lesions. A number of other devices have been utilized to treat vascular lesions, including a variety of continuous wave and pulsed lasers as well as a high intensity, pulsed flashlamp (Table 11-2). While some of these devices are no longer widely used, many of them continue to play an important role in current practice.

Table 11-1 Classification of Cutaneous Vascular Lesions[1]

Category	Examples	Age at Onset	Endothelial Turnover Rate	Spontaneous Involution
Malformations	Port wine stains, venous arterial, and lymphatic malformations	Always present at birth	Normal	No
Benign neoplasms	Hemangiomas	Variable; often arise in first year of life	Increased	Often
Dilatations	Telangiectases, venous lakes, spider angiomas	Variable; often arise in adulthood	Normal	No

Table 11-2 Lasers and Light Sources for Treatment of Vascular Lesions (by Increasing Wavelength)

Laser Type, Brand (Manufacturer)	Wavelength (nm)
Copper Bromide	511, 578
ProYellow+ (Aesculap Meditec)	
Krypton	521, 530, 568
Spectrum K1 (HGM)	
Pulsed KTP	532
Aura/Orion (Laserscope)	
VersaPulse (Lumenis)	
Diolite (Iriderm)	
Illustra (Cynosure)	
Pulsed Dye	585
SPTL-1b (Candela)	
Erasure (Cynosure)	
Long-Pulse Pulsed Dye	585, 590, 595, 600
ScleroPLUS (Candela)	
PhotoGenica VLS (Cynosure)	
Variable-Pulse Pulsed Dye Laser	595
Vbeam (Candela)	
PhotoGenica V-Star (Cynosure)	
Long-Pulsed Alexandrite	755
GentleLASE (Candela)	
LPIR/Apogee (Cynosure)	
EpiTouch Alex (Lumenis)	
Diodes	
LightSheer (Lumenis)	800
Diomed (LaserLite)	810
SLP 1000 (Palomar)	810
Medilas D SkinPulse (Dornier MedTech)	940
Long-Pulsed Nd:YAG	1064
CoolGlide (Altus)	
VascuLite (Lumenis)	
VeinLase (HGM)	
Orion (Laserscope)	
Pulsed Light Source	515-1200
Photoderm (Lumenis)	
Ellipse (Danish Dermatologic Development)	550-950

Laser Technology

Continuous and Quasi-Continuous Wave Lasers

Argon Laser. The argon laser emits blue-green light at six different wavelengths from 457.9 to 514.5 nm. Eighty percent of the total emissions occur at 488 and 514 nm. In most argon laser systems, all six wavelengths can be delivered or a cutoff filter can be used that allows emission of only green (514 nm) light. The active medium is pressurized argon gas that has had an electron removed to form a positive ion. The positive ions are excited by a high current discharge. Although light is delivered through a fiberoptic cable as a continuous beam, the laser can be manually or mechanically shuttered to deliver pulses as short as approximately 200 ms duration (Table 11-3).

The argon laser may be used to treat both vascular and pigmented lesions, as blue-green light is absorbed by both hemoglobin and melanin. Absorption of laser energy by hemoglobin within blood vessels results in thermal damage to the vessels. However, competitive absorption by epidermal melanin interferes with pene-

Table 11-3 Laser Types

Laser Type	Examples	Pulse Duration
Continuous wave	Argon, krypton lasers	Continuous beam or shuttered as short as 200 ms
Quasi-continuous wave	Copper vapor laser	Beam appears continuous because of extremely rapid repetition rate; can be shuttered
Pulsed		
Q-switched (QS)	QS ruby, QS Nd:YAG, QS alexandrite lasers	Nanosecond domain
Grouped Q-switched pulses	532 nm KTP laser (e.g., Aura)	Millisecond domain
Pulsed	Pulsed dye laser	450 μs
Pulsed ("long" pulse)	Pulsed dye laser	Millisecond domain (1.5 ms)
Pulsed ("variable" pulse)	Pulsed dye laser	Millisecond domain (1.5-40 ms)

A

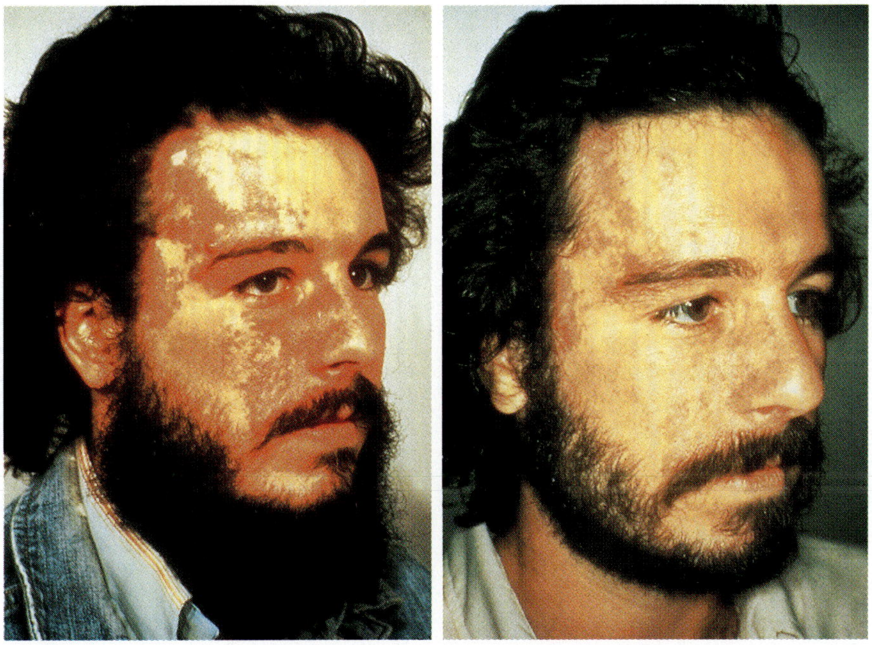

B

FIG. 11-1
A, Extensive facial port wine stain prior to treatment. (Courtesy Bard Cosman, MD.) **B,** After treatment with the argon laser, there is breakup of the solid color mass and lightening of the port wine stain.

tration of light into the dermis. In darkly pigmented individuals the overlying epidermis may suffer thermal damage while blood vessels are shielded from laser light. Because light is delivered as a continuous beam, heat diffuses from blood vessels within vascular malformations into adjacent tissues, which may result in nonselective thermal damage. The result is nonspecific thermal necrosis of epidermis and superficial dermis, the depth of which correlates with exposure dose.[6] The thermally denatured tissue forms a crust that heals by reepithelialization and fibrosis over several months. Ectatic blood vessels are replaced by smaller vessels, resulting in clinical lightening of vascular lesions.

In the treatment of PWS, good to excellent results are achieved in 70% to 80% of patients,[7] but outcome is highly operator dependent (Fig. 11-1). Best results are achieved in older patients with mature, purple lesions that contain ectatic blood vessels. Flat, pink lesions respond poorly to argon laser treatment. The primary limitation of argon laser treatment is the potential for hypertrophic scarring, atrophy, and permanent hypopigmentation. Scarring occurs in approximately 6% of patients, although the risk is higher in children with immature PWS and in certain anatomic areas such as the lip and neck.[8,9] To a large extent, the argon laser has been supplanted by pulsed lasers capable of selective photothermolysis.

Copper Vapor and Copper Bromide Lasers. Copper lasers emit yellow light at 578 nm, alone or in combination with green light at 511 nm (Table 11-4). The laser cavity consists of a neon gas–filled tube that contains copper pellets near each end. Copper vapor is created by heating the laser tube to very high temperatures with a pulsed electronic discharge. The laser tube must be heated for 45 minutes before the laser can be fired. The overall electrical efficiency of the copper vapor laser is low, requiring high-input power. Currently, only one copper laser (ProYellow+, Aesculap Meditec, Germany) is commercially available.

The copper vapor laser produces a 6 kHz (6000 pulses per second) train of extremely short (15 to 50 ns), low energy (0.2 mJ) pulses that appears continuous to the human eye (see Table 11-3). Although the 578 nm wavelength is well absorbed by oxyhemoglobin, the quasi-continuous wave beam results in thermal diffusion from the target vessel and nonselective thermal damage. A robotized scanning device (e.g., Hexascan[10]) has been used with continuous wave sources such as the copper vapor laser to place pulses of laser energy in a uniform, precise, nonadjacent pattern. Neumann and colleagues have demonstrated that when the copper vapor laser is used with the Hexascan (pulsewidth 50 to 74 ms, fluence 8 to 12 J/cm^2) to treat PWS, thermal damage is confined to blood vessels and a perivascular cuff of collagen, and the epidermis is spared.[11] This is in contrast to the argon laser, which causes nonspecific epidermal injury when used at identical fluences and pulsewidths.

There are few clinical studies that evaluate the use of copper lasers in the treatment of PWS. The copper vapor laser is probably best suited for the treatment of dark purple lesions, using the freehand technique for smaller lesions and the robotized scanning device for larger lesions.[12] Histologic studies have shown that treatment of small vessels with the copper vapor laser causes thermal injury which extends to a cuff of perivascular collagen.[11] Treatment of small vessel disorders such as childhood PWS would be expected to have a higher risk of nonspecific injury and scarring. The copper vapor laser has been shown to be an effective treatment modality for facial telangiectases.[13] Mild crusting usually occurs following copper vapor laser treatment, but wound healing generally occurs within two weeks when proper wound care is followed.

Continuous Wave Dye Laser. The continuous wave (CW) dye laser utilizes an argon laser to pump an organic dye solution to produce an adjustable band of wavelengths from 488 to 638 nm. Light is emitted in a continuous fashion, but can be mechanically or electronically shuttered to produce pulses as short as 20 ms. With rhodamine as the dye, wavelengths of 577 nm and 585 nm are produced, which are at or near the 577 nm absorption peak of oxyhemoglobin. In theory, these wavelengths produce more selective thermal damage to ectatic blood vessels than do the wavelengths of the argon laser. The CW dye laser has been reported to safely and effectively treat a variety of vascular lesions, including spider nevi, facial telangiectases, pyogenic granulomas, and PWS.[14,15] However, several studies have shown that CW dye laser treatment of PWS is no better than argon laser treatment in terms of efficacy and side effects.[16,17] The long exposure times used in the treatment of vascular lesions create the potential for significant thermal diffusion and nonspecific tissue injury.

As with the copper vapor laser, robotized scanning devices have been used with the CW dye laser in an attempt to convert the continuous beam to a pulsed beam. The scanning devices do decrease the risk of scarring without sacrificing efficacy. However, the pulsed dye laser has still been shown to be slightly superior than the CW dye laser with Hexascan in the treatment of PWS.[18]

A novel technique with the 577 nm CW dye laser has been reported, in which a 0.1 mm beam is used to trace individual blood vessels within PWS viewed under ×8 magnification.[19] Because PWS are composed of a network of dilated vessels with intervening normal skin, if only the individual vessels are treated, injury to adjacent normal skin is minimized. In 82 adult patients, 46% had an excellent response while 43% had good

Table 11-4 Continuous and Quasi-Continuous Wave Lasers

Device (Company)	Laser Type	Wavelength (nm)	Pulse Duration	Spot Size (mm)	Maximum Speed	Comments
ProYellow+ (Aesculap Meditec)	Copper bromide	511, 578	Shuttered from 5-950 ms	0.6, 1.5	1 Hz	511 nm for pigmented lesions
Spectrum K1 (HGM)	Krypton	568, 521, 530	CW or shuttered from 0.02 to 5 s	0.1	1 Hz or CW	521 or 530 nm for pigmented lesions

tures such as hair follicles or leg veins. One device (LightSheer, Lumenis, Santa Clara, CA) is now widely used for hair removal. While the 800 nm wavelength is poorly absorbed by melanin, it is absorbed to a small extent by hemoglobin and penetrates deeply into the dermis. Preliminary reports have shown encouraging results in the treatment of medium-sized leg veins (0.4 to 1 mm diameter).[39,40]

A variety of diode lasers that deliver wavelengths in the 900 to 980 nm range are under development and becoming available (Table 11-9). Compared with the 800 nm diodes, these devices penetrate even deeper. Preliminary reports have shown effective treatment of vessels from 0.3 to 1 mm diameter.[41,42] These devices may also offer some capability for hair removal.

Millisecond-Pulsed Nd:YAG Laser. New pulsed 1064 nm Nd:YAG lasers delivering high-powered, 1 to 100 ms pulses are now available (Table 11-10). On some systems, single pulses or multiple synchronized sequential pulses may be selected. Because there is slight hemoglobin absorption at the 1064 nm wavelength, the Nd:YAG laser can produce selective vessel damage provided that sufficient fluence is delivered. Incomplete absorption by hemoglobin may allow penetration of laser light into the entire vessel, including the posterior wall. The 1064 nm wavelength is poorly absorbed by melanin, which reduces the risk of epidermal injury in patients with darker skin types. Reduced scattering by dermal collagen allows 1064 nm light to penetrate deeply into the skin.

Table 11-8 800-810 nm Diode Lasers

Device (Company)	Laser Type	Wavelength (nm)	Pulse Duration (ms)	Spot Size (mm)	Maximum Speed (Hz)	Comments
LightSheer (Lumenis)	Diode	800	5-30	9 × 9	2	Sapphire contact cooling; also for hair removal
LightSheer XC (Lumenis)	Diode	800	5-100	12 × 12	2	Sapphire contact cooling; also for hair removal
Diomed (LaserLite)	Diode	810	50-250	2, 4	10	Scanner available; also for hair removal
SLP 1000 (Palomar)	Diode	810	100-1000+	10	1-3	Integrated contact cooling; also for hair removal

Table 11-9 940 nm Diode Laser

Device (Company)	Laser Type	Wavelength	Pulse Duration	Spot Size	Maximum Speed	Comments
Medilas D SkinPulse (Dornier MedTech)	Diode	940 nm	10 ms-1 s or continuous	0.5-1.5 mm	10 Hz	Contact cooling available

Table 11-10 1064 nm Long-Pulsed Nd:YAG Lasers

Device (Company)	Laser Type	Wavelength (nm)	Pulse Duration (ms)	Spot Size (mm)	Maximum Speed (Hz)	Comments
VascuLite (Lumenis)	Nd:YAG	1064	1-16	6	0.33	Single, double, or triple pulse
VeinLase (HGM)	Nd:YAG	1064	0.5-50	0.6-4	1	Dual wavelength: 532 and 1064 nm
Orion (Laserscope)	Nd:YAG	532, 1064	1-50	0.25-4	10	Scanner available
CoolGlide (Altus)	Nd:YAG	1064	10-100	9 × 9	2	Copper contact precooling

Table 11-11 Non-coherent Intense Pulsed Light Source

Device (Company)	Laser Type	Wavelength	Pulse Duration	Spot Size (mm)	Maximum Speed	Comments
Photoderm (Lumenis)	Flashlamp	Variable from 515 to 1200 nm	0.5-25 ms	8 × 15, 8 × 35	1 pulse every 8 s	Single, double, or triple pulse
Ellipse (Danish Development Corporation)	Flashlamp	Broad spectrum 550-950 nm	0.5-88.5 ms	10 × 48 or 8 mm round		Available worldwide except in U.S. and Canada

Pulsed Nd:YAG lasers are potentially useful for treating larger, deeper vessels such as blue periorbital veins and reticular leg veins. In a preliminary study of leg vessels from 0.5 to 3 mm diameter (50 sites treated on 30 patients), most vessels improved by 75% 12 weeks after a single treatment.[43] While epidermal injury was not observed, posttreatment hyperpigmentation developed in 42% of patients, which resolved in 83% at the 3-month follow-up. Additional studies are necessary to clarify the precise role of pulsed Nd:YAG lasers in the treatment of vascular lesions. An additional application of millisecond pulsed Nd:YAG lasers is in laser hair removal, where several systems are currently under investigation.

Intense Pulsed Light (IPL) Source. The Photoderm VL/PL (Lumenis, Santa Clara, CA) is an intense, nonlaser flashlamp device that produces incoherent, multiwavelength light from 515 to 1200 nm (visible to infrared light) (Table 11-11). A series of filters is used to cut off the output below a predetermined wavelength (515, 550, 570, or 590 nm), depending on patient skin type and lesion depth. Light is delivered through a large rectangular handpiece measuring 8 × 15 mm or 8 × 35 mm. Pulses of 0.5 to 25 ms duration are produced via a sequence of single, double, or triple pulses separated by a variable delay (1 to 300 ms). A thin layer of cold aqueous gel is applied to the skin to protect the epidermis and improve light coupling to the skin. In addition, a cooling bracket can be used to circulate chilled water (1° to 4°C) around the 8 × 35 mm handpiece, which is in contact with the skin. Use of the cooling bracket permits delivery of higher fluences, improves patient comfort, and lowers the risk of thermal injury to the epidermis.[44] A second generation intense pulsed light source (Ellipse, Danish Dermatologic Development, Denmark) has been developed but is currently not available in North America.

The intense pulsed light source has been used to successfully treat a variety of vascular lesions, including PWS,[45-47] hemangiomas, venous malformations,[48] poikiloderma of Civatte,[49] telangiectases,[49] and leg veins.[50] In general, an increased number of sessions is required to clear vascular lesions compared with the PDL. The primary advantage of the IPL is its versatility given its wide range of wavelengths, pulse durations, and pulse sequences. In addition, the large spot size permits deeper penetration of light because of reduced scattering. Although purpura is not produced in most instances, it may occur with use of high fluences and short pulse durations.

The IPL delivers a broad range of wavelengths, which may allow targeting of deeper structures but includes wavelengths that are preferentially absorbed by melanin. This may account for the increased incidence of adverse effects such as pigmentary change, blistering, and scarring in some reports.[51] Use of the IPL may be bewildering to the novice given the multitude of treatment parameters that must be selected by the operator. However, recent software upgrades have helped to reduce the risk of adverse events and lower the learning curve. Studies to date with the IPL have been small and retrospective and have not consistently used uniform treatment parameters. Large, prospective clinical trials are needed to refine treatment parameters and clarify the benefits and risks of this device.

Cooling. Epidermal melanin functions as a competing chromophore for absorption of laser light, particularly when shorter wavelengths are used. Thermal injury to the epidermis raises the risk of pain, blistering, hyperpigmentation, hypopigmentation, and scarring. Cooling of the epidermis has been designed as a means to protect the epidermis from thermal damage and permit the safe use of higher fluences and the treatment of patients with darker skin types. Epidermal cooling is generally accomplished through one of two methods, contact (conductive) cooling or evaporative (cryogen spray) cooling (Table 11-12).

In contact cooling, a cold object is directly applied to the skin surface just before the laser is fired, and the laser pulse is usually delivered through the cooling medium. In this way, cooling of the skin can occur before, during, and after the laser pulse. Passive contact methods utilize ice or refrigerated aqueous gel, but these substances warm rapidly and are messy to use. More sophisticated, active methods utilize a glass or sapphire window through which chilled water (about

Table 11-12 Types of Cooling

	Advantages	Disadvantages
Passive		
Refrigerated aqueous gel	Low cost; provides index matching	Least effective cooling; messy
Active		
Conductive cooling (chilled glass or sapphire window)	Cooling before, during, and after the laser pulse; provides index matching	Higher risk of dermal cooling; may require separate cooling window and water chiller
Evaporative cooling (cryogen spray cooling)	Intrinsically efficient cooling with large temperature gradients; low risk of dermal cooling	Cryogen cost; no index matching; cryogen may interfere with penetration of laser light
Chilled air cooling	No interference with laser light; no disposables cost	Air is a poor thermal conductor; requires bulky cooling device

4°C) circulates in a closed loop with an electrostatic chiller. The cooling window is placed directly in contact with the skin and laser light is fired through it. Because of its high thermal conductivity, sapphire provides more rapid heat extraction from the surface than glass.

In some systems, the cooling window slides onto the end of the laser handpiece (e.g., VersaPulse, Lumenis, Santa Clara, CA) or it is permanently integrated within the handpiece. The cooling window may also be entirely independent of the laser handpiece, allowing use with a variety of laser systems (e.g., Slim Pack and Cool Wand, Cool Laser Optics, Westborough, MA).[52] Another variation is the cooling bracket that fits around and cools the quartz handpiece of the intense pulsed light source. An advantage to most contact cooling methods is that index matching optimizes coupling of laser light into the skin and reduces backscatter.[53] On the downside, conductive cooling may cause inadvertent cooling of dermal structures (such as targeted blood vessels) if the application time is too long.

In evaporative cooling, a brief pulse of cryogen is sprayed onto the skin just before delivery of the laser pulse. Evaporative cooling is intrinsically more efficient than conductive cooling, creating larger gradients between the epidermis and dermis and lowering the risk of inadvertent dermal cooling.[53,54] The device that is commercially available, the dynamic cooling device (DCD), is used in conjunction with a pulsed dye laser (ScleroPLUS or Vbeam, Candela Corporation, Wayland, MA). The cryogen is 1,1,1,2-tetrafluoroethane, which is a nontoxic, nonflammable Freon substitute (boiling point: –26.2°C). The duration of the cryogen spurt (20 to 100 ms) and the time delay between the spurt and the laser pulse (10 ms to 1 s) are programmed by the operator. If sufficient time does not elapse for cryogen evaporation before the laser is fired, cryogen remaining on the skin surface may interfere with penetration of light into the skin. In the treatment of PWS, it has been shown that use of the DCD (50 ms spray, 10 ms delay) permits the use of higher fluences, leading to improved clearance without producing complications such as scarring or dyspigmentation.[55]

A novel cooling method employing chilled air has recently become available (SmartCool, Cynosure, Chelmsford, MA). A continuous flow of chilled air is directed at the skin during laser treatment. Different rates of airflow may be selected for greater degrees of cooling. Controlled studies comparing chilled air to other cooling devices have not yet been reported.

Clinical Applications

Port Wine Stains

Pulsed dye laser. Port wine stains are benign vascular lesions consisting of dilated dermal vessels. Originally classified as capillary malformations,[2] they consist of postcapillary venules and are actually venular malformations.[3] Unlike hemangiomas, PWS are always present at birth and are nonproliferative. However, as patients age, PWS characteristically deepen in color from pink to purple and develop raised or nodular areas.[56] Histologically, PWS are characterized by an increase in vessel number and vessel ectasia.[56] Although vessel dilatation is often not seen histologically in the first decade of life, vessels become progressively dilated thereafter.[57] Unlike vessel ectasia, vessel number and mean vessel depth (approximately 0.46 mm) increase little with age.[56,57] The diameter of PWS vessels varies from approximately 20 to 150 μm.[4] In contrast, the diameter of normal blood vessels in the papillary dermis ranges from 10 to 35 μm, while those in the deepest dermis measure 40 to 50 μm in diameter.[58] PWS may occur in association with other disorders, including Sturge-Weber syndrome and Klippel-Trénaunay-Weber syndrome.

The pulsed dye laser is currently the treatment of choice for most PWS, especially those that are macular, mildly hypertrophic, or present in children (Fig. 11-4). Most studies have demonstrated that at least 80% of PWS treated with the PDL achieve 50% or greater clearance.[59-63] Multiple treatment sessions are required for maximum clearing. In a study of 76 patients, overall 79% lightening was achieved after an average of 9 treatments.[64] It has been shown that up to 25 repetitive treatments may be necessary to achieve maximum lightening.[65] However, complete clearing of PWS is infrequent, occurring in less than 20% of cases.[60,61,65]

Macular, pink PWS respond more favorably to PDL surgery than darker, nodular, or hypertrophic lesions. An early study reported complete clearing of macular, pink to red PWS in 35 children after an average of 6.5 laser treatments.[59] In contrast, Garden et al. found that 6 out of 52 patients (12%), all of whom had purple, nodular lesions, failed to achieve at least 50% lightening after multiple treatments.[28] The larger red cell content within ectatic vessels of hypertrophic PWS may shield deeper vessels from laser light. Deeper vessels may also be present that are beyond the effective penetration depth of the PDL.

Many studies report that young children require fewer treatments for clearance and achieve more lightening per treatment than older patients.[59,60,64,66,67] Pediatric PWS are thought to respond more favorably to treatment because of their smaller vessel diameter, their more superficial vessel location, and their smaller overall size. However, in a recent prospective study of 100 patients, no significant difference was found among age groups in the average lightening of PWS, and in no patient was complete clearing of PWS noted.[68]

Anatomic location is a useful predictor of response to laser treatment.[61,69] PWS located on the face and neck respond most favorably.[63] Centrofacial regions (medial aspect of cheek, upper cutaneous lip, and nose) respond less favorably than other regions on the face (periorbital, forehead/temple, lateral aspect of cheek, neck, and chin). Lesions localized to dermatome V2 are more resistant than those in dermatomes V1, V3, and C2/C3. PWS located exclusively in the midline of the face are very amenable to treatment. Lesions located on the upper and lower extremities respond poorly.[61,63,70] In addition to location, initial lesion size is another predictor of response to laser therapy.[71,72] For all age groups, the smaller the lesion, the greater the final maximal response.

Morphological characteristics such as vessel depth, number, and diameter also determine response of PWS to laser treatment.[63,73] PWS with superficial vessels respond more favorably. The critical mean depth of vessels for favorable prognosis has been estimated to be 930 μm. Conflicting data have been reported regarding the role of vessel size and number. In one report, poor responders had significantly smaller vessels (mean vessel diameter 19 μm) than moderate and good responders (mean vessel diameter around 40 μm), as well as a significantly higher vessel number.[73]

Patients with darker skin often do not respond favorably to PDL treatment. Use of higher fluences is required to overcome competitive absorption by epidermal melanin. Temporary hypopigmentation with little or no lesional lightening often results. Therefore, treatment of PWS in darkly pigmented patients may not always be warranted.

There is insufficient experience with the 1.5 to 40 ms pulse duration PDL to make any definitive comments. The long pulse duration, however, may allow greater clearing of PWS per treatment without purpura, and may be more effective in the treatment of nodular PWS.

A

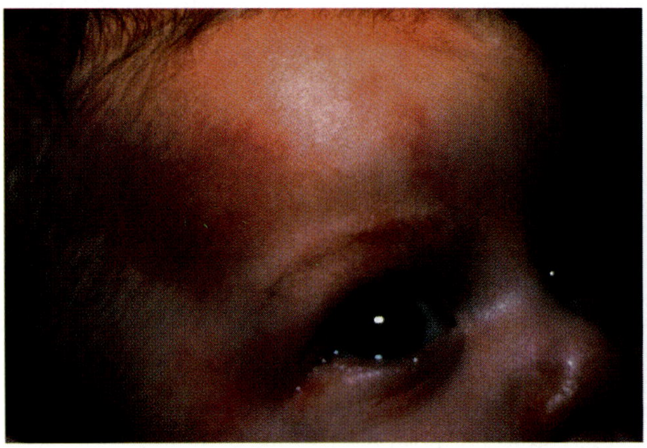

B

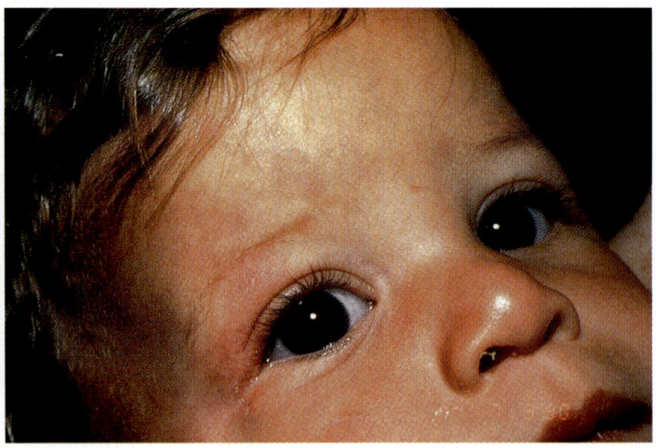

FIG. 11-4
A, A 3-month old with an extensive upper facial port wine stain prior to treatment. **B,** At 1 year of age after six treatments, there is significant lightening of the port wine stain in all treated areas. Note that the upper eyelid was not treated.

Alternative lasers and light sources. Alternative devices such as pulsed 532 nm lasers and intense pulsed light sources may be beneficial in the treatment of PWS. By delivering longer pulsewidths and shorter or longer wavelengths, these devices may be particularly useful in the treatment of hypertrophic lesions. Dierickx and colleagues used a pulsed, 532 nm laser to treat 11 patients with nonfacial, pink to purple PWS.[36] The laser was used with a computer-driven scanner that placed 127 spots of 1 mm diameter in a hexagonal pattern. Pulse durations of 3, 5, 10, and 15 ms were compared. Best results were obtained with a 3 or 5 ms pulsewidth at a fluence of 15 or 20 J/cm^2. The immediate clinical response was transient blanching without purpura, but delayed purpura occurred at all sites within several days. Additional studies are needed to establish the exact role of pulsed 532 nm lasers in the treatment of PWS.

The intense pulsed light source has been reported to effectively treat both previously untreated[45,47] and nonresponding PWS.[46] In a retrospective study, good to complete (70% to 100%) clearance was achieved in 28 of 40 PWS treated with the IPL.[45] Although better results were seen with pink and red PWS, good clearance (70% to 99%) was achieved in 6 of 11 purple lesions. Treatment parameters were not standardized, but the most frequently used parameters were 515 and 550 nm cutoff filters, pulse durations of 2.5 to 5 ms, and fluences of 24 to 60 J/cm^2. Purpura developed in most patients, while crusting was seen in 20% and superficial blistering in 8%. No scarring was observed.

Continuous wave or quasi-continuous wave lasers such as the argon or copper vapor lasers may also be used to shrink nodules or smooth out cobblestoned areas. However, use of the PDL in mildly hypertrophic PWS carries a much lower risk of textural change or permanent pigmentary alteration.

Facial Telangiectases and Other Small Vessel Disorders. The most appropriate treatment modality for telangiectases depends on the diameter of the vessel, its anatomic location, and the age of the patient. Small-diameter vessels on the face usually respond favorably to any of the lasers previously discussed. The PDL represents an excellent treatment modality for facial telangiectases[74] (Fig. 11-5*A* and *B*). Its large spot size (up to 10 mm) allows confluent treatment of large areas at once. Alternatively, larger telangiectases may be treated individually along their length with an elliptical spot (Fig. 11-5C). The PDL provides the greatest amount of clearance per treatment session. Its primary disadvantage is the occurrence of purpura immediately after treatment, which may last up to 2 weeks. The recently developed 10 to 40 ms PDL induces considerably less purpura, but few reports yet exist about its efficacy in the treatment of vascular lesions.

Continuous and quasi-continuous wave lasers such as the krypton, argon, and CW dye lasers may be used to trace out individual telangiectases, often leaving a thin, linear crust over the vessel but no purpura. The spot size is chosen to match the diameter of individual ectatic vessels. The vessel is traced out, and the heat zippers the vessel shut. By tracing the vessel at the correct speed, physically directed spatial thermal confinement is produced, thus limiting damage to the surrounding skin. Slight postoperative crusting may be more cosmetically acceptable to patients than purpura.[13] However, the risk of cutaneous depressions or scarring is higher with continuous wave devices, especially in paranasal areas.

Facial telangiectases also respond very favorably to millisecond pulsed 532 nm green light lasers[35] (Fig. 11-5*D-F*). Pulsed green light lasers coagulate small- and medium-diameter vessels without producing purpura. The target vessel is traced with the laser beam at a spot size that approximates the diameter of the vessel. Because these lasers are pulsed, nonspecific thermal damage is minimized. Treatment may be safely performed even on higher-risk areas such as the ala and the alar grooves. Recanalization may follow treatment, necessitating retreatment of some vessels.

The intense pulsed light source is another effective treatment modality for facial telangiectases. It does not leave purpura, and its large handpiece allows confluent treatment of large areas. In a small study, Raulin and colleagues reported good to excellent clearing of telangiectases (mostly facial) after an average of 4.4 treatments.[49]

Spider and cherry angiomas typically respond after one or two treatments with the PDL.[75] One pulse with the 3 or 5 mm spot size usually treats the entire lesion. Pulsed 532 nm lasers are also effective, but higher fluences may be necessary for large cherry angiomas and high-flow spider angiomas. The raised central feeding vessel within spider angiomas must be coagulated before the "legs of the spider" are traced. Spider and cherry angiomas also respond well to the intense pulsed light source, but the spot size cannot be matched to the size of the lesion (minimum handpiece size 8 × 15 mm). CW and quasi-CW lasers are also effective, but the risks of pigmentary and textural changes are higher with these devices. The PDL is preferable for the treatment of either telangiectases or spider angiomas in young children, given its high therapeutic safety index.

Larger blue vessels are often present in the periorbital area. Due to their large size and greater depth, these vessels respond least well to the PDL. They may respond to treatment with long-pulsed infrared devices such as the long-pulsed alexandrite laser, long-pulsed Nd:YAG laser, or the intense pulsed light source. The effective treatment of these vessels often depends on the skill of the physician.

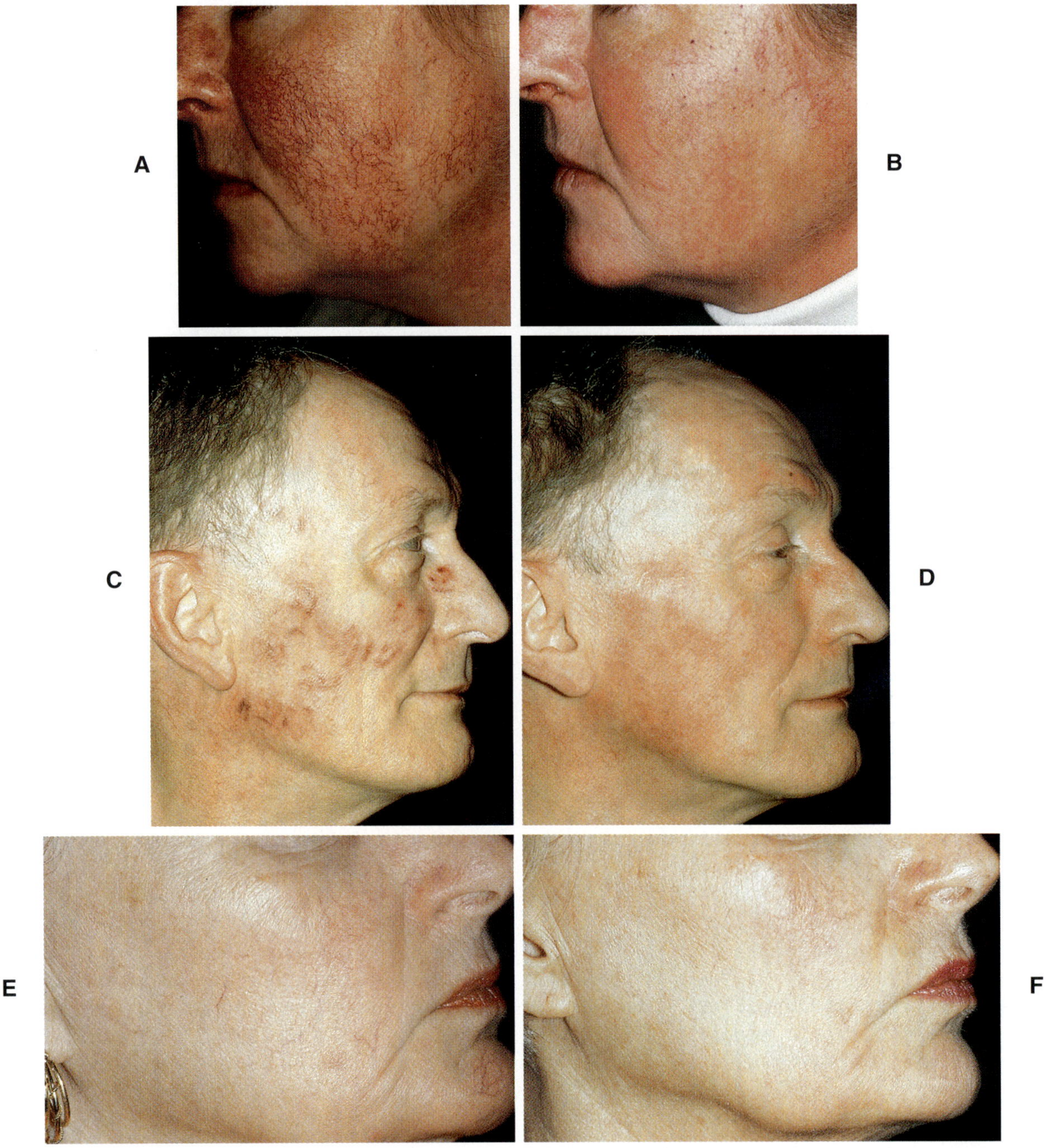

FIG. 11-5

A, Extensive telangiectasia of the face prior to treatment. **B,** After two treatments with the pulsed dye laser, there is dramatic lightening of the telangiectasia. The lateral face under the sideburn area was not treated. **C,** Immediately after pulsed dye laser treatment with a 2 × 7 mm spot, there is linear purpura. **D,** On the contralateral side, the cheek was treated with a long pulsed 532 nm KTP laser. There is erythema, but no purpura posttreatment. **E,** Telangiectasia of the cheek prior to treatment. **F,** After one single treatment with a 532 nm long pulsed KTP laser, there is dramatic improvement of the vessels. There was no posttreatment purpura, but there was crusting that lasted a full week after treatment.

Hemangiomas. Hemangiomas are the most common benign neoplasms of infancy. They may appear anywhere on the skin but affect the head and neck most commonly.[76] Unlike PWS, hemangiomas are rarely present at birth but appear soon thereafter as a pink or blanched macule. They characteristically undergo a proliferative period in which they grow rapidly, becoming raised and bright red. Enlargement of hemangiomas occurs by rapid cellular proliferation of endothelial cells.[76] Most hemangiomas undergo an involutional phase after a period of months to years, in which endothelial proliferation decreases and fibrous tissue separates vascular spaces.[76] Involuted lesions frequently leave sequelae such as residual fibrofatty tissue, telangiectases, and atrophic skin.

Cutaneous hemangiomas may be superficial (capillary) or deep (cavernous). Superficial lesions are located in the papillary dermis, while deep lesions involve the reticular dermis and subcutaneous fat.[76] Whereas superficial hemangiomas usually exhibit a bright red color, deeper lesions typically appear as subcutaneous nodules with normal overlying skin or with an overlying blue hue. Hemangiomas often exhibit combined superficial and deep components.

Treatment of hemangiomas has long been a source of controversy. In the past, most hemangiomas were left untreated because of their natural history of involution. However, increased sensitivity to the psychosocial trauma suffered by children, as well as the availability of newer treatment modalities, have forced a reevaluation of traditional dogma. Modern management options for hemangiomas include nonintervention, pulsed dye laser treatment, surgical excision, cryosurgery, intralesional corticosteroids, systemic corticosteroids, and subcutaneous interferon alpha injections. Radiation, embolization, and cytotoxic medication are reserved for exceptional cases failing other therapies.[77]

Choice of treatment modality depends on many factors, including anatomic location, type of hemangioma (superficial vs. deep), size and extent of lesion, phase of the lesion (preproliferation, growth, plateau, or involution), whether functional impairment is present, and level of parental concern.[77] Certain hemangiomas always require treatment, such as those causing life- or function-threatening complications such as consumptive coagulopathy, congestive heart failure, gastrointestinal bleeding, or ocular compromise.[78] Treatment is generally indicated for hemangiomas on the nose, lip, or ear, as these areas if untreated are more likely to heal with scarring or permanent anatomic distortion.[78] Many physicians will consider treatment for any cosmetically significant hemangioma, including any lesion on the head and neck that is conspicuous and not easily hidden.[79]

The pulsed dye laser is the treatment of choice for almost all superficial hemangiomas and many mixed lesions.[80,81] Small, superficial lesions and some large, plaquelike lesions respond well, provided that treatment is started early enough[78] (Fig. 11-6). Because of the laser's limited penetration depth (about 1.2 mm),[25] best results are obtained with hemangiomas in the preproliferative or early proliferative stage before significant thickening has occurred. Typically the laser produces lightening and flattening of hemangiomas as well as a slowing of their proliferation. Multiple treatment sessions are usually required to achieve the maximum benefit. Treatment of lesions that are not rapidly proliferating should be repeated at 4- to 6-week intervals. On occasion, treatment of a superficial hemangioma will not prevent development of a deep component, presumably because of continued proliferation within the deep component, which is beyond the penetration depth of the laser.[78,82]

PDL treatment is less effective for proliferating hemangiomas that have acquired significant thickness or

A 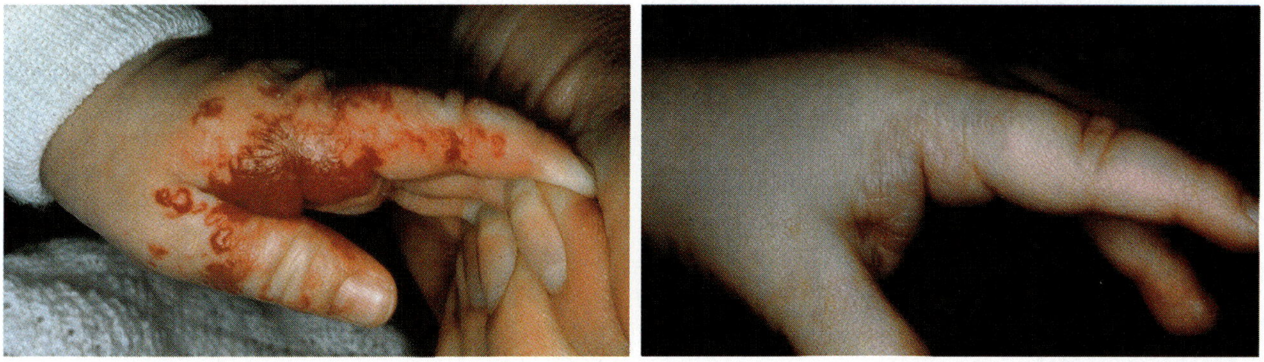 B

FIG. 11-6
A, A hemangioma of the left thumb and first finger prior to treatment. **B,** After a series of four treatments with the pulsed dye laser, the hemangioma cleared completely. (Courtesy Jerome Garden, MD.)

depth. Whereas lesions that are raised 3 mm or less off the skin surface resolve almost completely, those raised more than 4 mm may lighten with therapy but show less diminution in thickness.[83] Use of a PDL with longer wavelength (595 nm) and pulse duration (1.5 ms or longer) may be more effective for thicker hemangiomas. In general, thicker lesions require the use of higher fluences. Because proliferating hemangiomas may grow rapidly, they should be treated at more frequent intervals (2 to 3 weeks).

Combined lesions with a superficial and deep component may be treated with the PDL, but the deep component will not benefit from laser treatment because of the laser's limited penetration depth. The deeper component may require an alternative form of therapy such as intralesional or systemic corticosteroids. Interferon alfa-2a is generally reserved for complicated or life-threatening hemangiomas that have failed steroid therapy.[84] The PDL has no role in the treatment of predominantly deep hemangiomas.[80] Nonselective treatment with the CW Nd:YAG laser may be considered for large, tumorlike hemangiomas, particularly those located on mucosal surfaces.

Superficial hemangiomas in the involutional phase respond well to laser treatment.[85] Although these lesions are in a stage of regression, they are often slow to resolve and may persist beyond school age. The response is usually rapid (within two to four treatment sessions). Involuting superficial hemangiomas should be treated every 1 to 2 months. The PDL is less useful for deep hemangiomas in the involutional phase. The superficial portion of mixed lesions may benefit from PDL treatment, but deep lesions in the involutional phase may require surgical excision.

Ulceration is seen in approximately 5% to 10% of hemangiomas during the rapid growth phase.[86] Lesions located in the perineum or on the digits have a higher likelihood of ulceration. Treatment of ulcerated hemangiomas with the PDL leads to rapid healing (within one to three treatment sessions).[80] Laser treatment decreases the associated pain, minimizes the risk of infection and bleeding, and reduces the risk of scarring.[80] Biocclusive dressings such as Duoderm are a useful adjunct to laser therapy.

SECTION TWO

Atlas of Surgical Procedures

PREOPERATIVE CLINICAL CONSIDERATIONS

Anesthesia

Most patients experience only a transient stinging sensation during laser or intense pulsed light source treatment that is well tolerated, thus limiting the need for anesthesia. However, cumulative pulses may produce increasing and intolerable discomfort. Anesthesia is often required in young children or individuals with large lesions. In many instances, use of topical anesthetics such as EMLA or ELA-MAX cream alone is sufficient. Application of a thick layer of cream under occlusion for 60 minutes followed by removal 10 to 30 minutes before treatment is necessary for maximal effectiveness. If needed, local infiltration or regional nerve block may be performed with lidocaine. Epinephrine should generally not be used during local infiltration because it may constrict the targeted vessels. Premedication with hypnotics, sedatives, or analgesics may be required in anxious patients. Children who require immobilization may need intravenous sedation or general anesthesia.

Laser Safety

Safety goggles covering the appropriate wavelength of light must be worn by all personnel in the treatment room. When treatment is in the periorbital area, the patient's eyes should be protected with handheld gauze folded into small triangles, or eye shields should be inserted after numbing of the ocular surface with anesthetic drops.

The PDL has been reported to cause flash fires at the site of laser impact as well as in areas distant from the site of laser pulsing in certain circumstances.[87] Other lasers, light sources, and electrosurgical devices also pose an incendiary risk. The risk of fire is greatest when oxygen is present. All potentially combustible materials in the treatment field such as hair or gauze must be moistened with water, saline, or a water-based lubricant (e.g., Surgilube). All makeup should be removed prior to treatment. If alcohol is used to clean the skin or the laser handpiece, it should be allowed to dry completely before treatment. Whenever possible, lasers should be used with room air only. If oxygen use is required, a closed airway system should be used to avoid oxygen leakage. Water and a fire extinguisher should be immediately available.

PROCEDURAL TECHNIQUES

Pulsed Dye Laser

Port Wine Stains

Test Areas. For practitioners with limited experience, it may be useful to perform test areas prior to treatment of an entire PWS. The test area helps determine the optimal fluence for treatment and prepares the patient for the expected postoperative course, especially with regard to posttreatment purpura. An area should be chosen that is representative of the entire lesion. Several test spots may be treated using different fluences to determine the best therapeutic response. The desired endpoint is immediate ashen-gray discoloration, which is due to the formation of an intravascular coagulum. The discolored area becomes purpuric over the next several hours and fades over the next 5 to 14 days.

Macular and mildly hypertrophic PWS, especially in children, respond best to the traditional 585 nm PDL (450 μs), whereas nodular or hypertrophic lesions, or adult patients, respond most favorably to the 595 nm PDL (1.5 ms). The intensity of purpura is less with the 595 nm, 1.5 ms PDL than with the 585 nm, 450 μs PDL. There is also significantly less discoloration when the cryogen spray is used. It should be noted that, due to differences in beam profiles from one PDL to another, different fluences may be required to achieve equivalent tissue responses.[88] When the Cynosure PDL is used, fluence should be decreased by approximately 30% from settings used with the Candela PDL. Because of competitive absorption by epidermal melanin, patients with tan or darker skin require the use of higher fluences to produce lightening than light-skinned individuals. Cryogen spray cooling helps protect the epidermis in these patients. In patients with a significant tan, it is usually prudent to delay treatment until the tan has faded.

Test areas should be evaluated in 4 to 6 weeks for degree of lightening as well as for any undesired textural or pigmentary sequelae. If noticeable lightening has occurred, treatment can proceed using the fluence that produced the best results. Absence of lightening indicates that higher fluences, longer wavelengths, or longer pulsewidths may be required. If necessary, repeat test areas may be performed with fluences increased at increments of 0.25 J/cm^2. If the initial test area was treated with the 450 μs PDL at 585 nm, it may be beneficial to switch to the 595 nm, 1.5 ms PDL. If the lesion is still unresponsive, consideration should be given to one of the millisecond pulsed green light lasers used with scanners, the intense pulsed light source, or the PDL used at supercooled temperatures, higher fluences, and longer pulse durations.

Treatment. The laser handpiece should be held perpendicular to the skin, with the attached spacer resting on the skin. It is important that "skip areas" not be left behind during treatment. This is accomplished by moving the laser handpiece in a methodical fashion across the skin such that adjacent areas are treated consecutively. In order to avoid leaving a reticulate pattern of residual PWS, pulses should be overlapped by up to 18% and larger spot sizes should be used (7 or 10 mm).[89] Any reticulate patterning that occurs after treatment can be improved by retreating the PWS in subsequent treatment sessions. During treatment, an erythematous flare often develops that obscures the margins of the PWS. To avoid this problem, one should treat the edges of the PWS first (resulting purpura will outline the margins) or use a skin marking pen to delineate the border prior to treatment. If the dynamic cooling device is used, fluences should be increased by 10% to 15%. To avoid singeing eyebrows and hairlines, these areas should be protected with a water-based lubricant such as Surgilube or K-Y Jelly prior to treatment. The extent of PWS treated per session depends on patient tolerance and type of anesthesia used.

Complete clearing of PWS after one treatment is very rare. More commonly, multiple treatment sessions are required to obtain maximal clearing. Repeat treatment sessions may be performed as early as 1 month after the previous treatment without additional risk. True 100% clearing may never be attained. If there is significant postinflammatory hyperpigmentation, retreatment should be delayed until the hyperpigmentation has faded, since it will block penetration of laser light to dermal blood vessels.

Postoperative Clinical Considerations. Postoperative purpura is most intense several hours after treatment. It then fades over the next 7 to 14 days. Transient swelling and erythema are common after treatment, especially in the periorbital area. Immediate postoperative discomfort may be treated by application of cold tap water soaked gauze, ice packs, or a hydroocclusive dressing such as Spenco Second Skin or Vigilon. Oral analgesics are rarely necessary. Patients should wash the treated area gently with soap and water and apply an ointment such as Aquaphor Healing Ointment twice a day. Mild crusting, which develops in approximately 20% of patients, should be treated with an antibacterial ointment after soap and water washing twice a day until crusting resolves. Vesiculation and thick crusting does not occur.

The use of makeup is acceptable provided that crusting is not present. Skin discoloration is often difficult to conceal completely except with opaque makeup. An undercoat with a green base may be useful. When makeup is removed, the skin should not be wiped and astringents or irritants should be avoided. Instead, an emollient such as Lubriderm or Cetaphil can be used to remove makeup by patting it off. Patients should avoid excessive sun exposure and wear sunscreen with SPF 15 or higher for several months after treatment to reduce the risk of hyperpigmentation.

When PDL treatment is performed with appropriate fluences and correct technique, serious postoperative complications are very rare. Treated skin usually maintains the ability to tan and retain normal skin mobility, elasticity, hair growth, and skin markings. Cutaneous depressions or atrophic scarring, which have been reported in up to 4% of patients,[90,91] may be due to excessive fluences, spot overlap, or trauma. Hypertrophic scarring is distinctly uncommon but has been reported to occur on the face,[92] neck,[91] and chest[93] and in patients taking isotretinoin.[94] In most cases, textural changes are transient and resolve spontaneously within 1 year. Transient hyperpigmentation, which occurs in about 25% of patients,[90,95] is associated with sun exposure and darker skin type. Hypopigmentation is uncommon and usually resolves within 3 to 6 months. The risk of hypopigmentation is highest in patients with actinic bronzing and skin types III or higher.

Facial Telangiectases and Spider Angiomas

Treatment. Experienced operators are usually able to predict the optimal fluence based on the location and type of vessel and the patient's background pigmentation, thus avoiding the need for test areas. The traditional 585 nm, 450 μs PDL works well for most telangiectases, although the 595 nm, 1.5 ms PDL is often more effective for deeper vessels and larger-diameter vessels such as those frequently present on the nasal dorsum, nasal ala, and lateral cheeks. Treatment technique is similar to that used for PWS treatment. The elliptical spot is particularly useful for treatment of linear telangiectases. The handpiece should be positioned at one end of the vessel and moved progressively along its length so that the entire vessel is treated without overlapping pulses. The direction of treatment, either in or against the direction of blood flow, is unimportant. Reactive erythema often develops in the irradiated areas during treatment, making it difficult to see residual vessels. Patients should be informed that multiple treatments will be necessary for optimal results.

When treating spider angiomas, a spot size large enough to cover the entire lesion should be used, if possible. The radiating "legs" should be treated even if they appear to blanch after treatment of the central papule. Treatment may be performed through a glass slide compressed against the skin to target the deeper component. If significant blood flow persists within the angioma after irradiation, it may be necessary to repeat treatment immediately using higher fluence.

Postoperative Clinical Considerations. Postoperative care is similar to that used after treatment of PWS. Purpura is often limited to a linear array of circular or elliptical gray spots around vessels. Most telangiectases and spider angiomas respond very well to PDL treatment. Smaller telangiectases resolve almost completely after one treatment. Larger vessels and those located in the nasal folds may require several treatments. High-flow spider angiomas may require repeated treatments, may benefit from CW laser or electrocoagulation of the central feeding vessel, and may even prove resistant to treatment.

Hemangiomas

Treatment. Anesthesia is usually not required, although larger lesions may require topical, intralesional, or even general anesthesia. Test treatments may help determine whether a hemangioma will respond to laser treatment. However, performing a test treatment delays treatment of the entire lesion by at least 2 weeks. In addition, some hemangiomas appear to respond only when they are treated in their entirety. Typical fluences are much higher than those used in the treatment of PWS and telangiectases, especially in the treatment of proliferating hemangiomas (7.5 to 9 J/cm^2 with a 5 mm spot, 7 to 8 J/cm^2 with a 7 mm spot, and 4.5 to 5 J/cm^2 with a 10 mm spot with the Candela PDL). The PDLs with longer wavelengths (595 nm) and pulse durations (1.5 ms or longer) may be effective even for thicker lesions. Unlike with PWS or telangiectases, significant overlapping of pulses, or even stacking of pulses over the same area, may be necessary. The number of pulses required in a given site is correlated directly with the thickness of the lesion. Generally four to six treatments are required for adequate clinical response. Treatments are usually repeated at 2- to 8-week intervals, with the shorter intervals used for proliferating lesions.

Postoperative Clinical Considerations. Postoperative care is similar to that described for PWS and telangiectases. Ulcerative hemangiomas may respond to application of biocclusive dressings such as Duoderm. When appropriate technique is used, complications are rare and similar to that for PWS, except that the hypopigmentation that sometimes occurs after spontaneous involution may also occur following PDL treatment.

Pulsed 532 nm Lasers

Port Wine Stains

Treatment. Because of the large treatment area, anesthesia is usually required. Topical anesthesia applied under occlusion usually suffices, but local infiltration and regional blocks can be employed if necessary. Because reactive erythema often develops around the treated site, which obscures the edge of the PWS, it may be helpful to outline the margins with a marking pen prior to treatment. Treatment may be accomplished via the freehand or scanning technique. For the freehand method, the largest laser beam spot size that delivers sufficient fluence should be used. The handpiece should be held perpendicularly to the skin surface and the handpiece spacer should be placed on the skin surface. Magnification of at least ×5 to ×10 is needed to visualize the individual vessels that make up PWS. The most effective device for visualizing intradermal vessels is a polarized magnified light source (Syris Scientific v600, Gray, ME).

The vessels should be traced at a speed that heat seals the vessel without causing overlying epidermal coagulation. If the vessel does not disappear, the handpiece should be moved more slowly or the fluence should be slowly increased until threshold fluence for vessel disappearance is reached. It may also be necessary to adjust the pulsewidth independently of the fluence (not possible with all systems), depending on the caliber of the vessel being treated. Optimal clearing of PWS has been reported at a pulsewidth of 3 or 5 ms.[36] Larger-diameter vessels may require the use of longer pulsewidth for vessel coagulation.

If epidermal whitening is noted, either the fluence is too high, the vessel is being traced too slowly, or excessive overlapping is occurring. Once the optimal fluence, pulse duration, and tracing speed have been determined, the rest of the vessels of that caliber, depth, and color can be treated with these parameters. Repeated tracing is required to coagulate some vessels, especially large-caliber deep vessels, but any one area should be treated only once with each pass.

The scanning technique is performed with a scanning device that is attached with fiberoptics to the laser. When using the Aura (Laserscope, San Jose, CA) laser and the Smartscan, fluences used are 15 to 20 J/cm^2 at a pulse duration of 3 to 10 ms. The scanning handpiece should be held directly perpendicular to the skin surface. The fluence should be slowly raised until the threshold fluence, defined as subtle blanching of the skin, is reached. The scanner should not be moved until the entire scanning pattern has been delivered. The handpiece should then be moved in methodical fashion to an adjacent area, taking care not to overlap previously treated areas.

Postoperative Clinical Considerations. Posttreatment discomfort can be lessened with application of cold tap water–soaked gauze, ice packs, or hydroocclusive dressings (e.g., Second Skin or Vigilon). Erythema usually subsides within 24 hours. Crusting may develop within 1 to 2 days and last for 7 to 14 days. Crusting occurs more commonly when patients with darker skin phototypes are treated. Although purpura generally does not occur with pulsed 532 nm lasers, mild purpura may develop with the use of high fluences and short pulse durations.

Patients should wash the treated area gently with a mild soap and water twice a day and then apply an occlusive ointment such as Aquaphor Healing Ointment. Bandages are not needed. Patients should avoid sun exposure and wear broad spectrum sunscreen for at least 6 weeks after treatment. Repeat treatments should be delayed by at least 6 weeks to allow maximal lightening and to ensure that complete healing has occurred and that any postinflammatory hyperpigmentation has faded.

Facial Telangiectases and Spider Angiomas

Treatment. Anesthesia is usually not required. Topical anesthetics applied under occlusion 1 hour prior to treatment may be utilized in sensitive patients. The spot size, pulse duration, and fluence are determined by vessel size and depth. The spot size should be slightly wider than the vessel diameter and the pulse duration slightly longer than the thermal relaxation time of the vessel. The laser handpiece should be held perpendicular to the skin surface, with the handpiece spacer in contact with the skin. Use of a polarized magnifying device greatly improves visualization of dermal vessels.

Vessels should be traced at a speed just slow enough to cause heat sealing and vessel disappearance without producing epidermal damage such as whitening. Using too high a repetition rate increases the risk for double-pulsing sites, raising the risk of side effects such as epidermal necrosis and scarring. Particular caution should be used when treating the nasal ala and alar creases, as these sites are prone to atrophic scarring. If vessel disappearance does not occur during treatment, the fluence and pulse duration should be increased incrementally or the handpiece should be moved more slowly.

When using a laser with a sapphire or quartz cooling tip (e.g., VersaPulse, Lumenis, Santa Clara, CA), the handpiece should be held perpendicularly to the skin surface with the cooling tip flat and in direct contact with the skin. A thin layer of aqueous gel applied to the skin will facilitate moving the tip and prevent it from fogging up. Very little pressure should be applied with the cooling tip so that vessels remain patent. If too much pressure is applied, the vessel may be blanched, making treatment less effective.

When treating spider and cherry angiomas, the spot size should be selected to match the diameter of the target lesion. The technique used is similar to that for telangiectases. With spider angiomas the radiating vessels must also be treated. When large cherry angiomas or high-flow spider angiomas are treated, it may be necessary to use higher fluences that coagulate the epidermis to ensure sufficient thermal damage to the target vessels. Occasionally the central feeder vessel must be treated through a glass slide that is applied with moderate pressure over the skin. The immediate endpoint of treatment is disappearance of the lesion or superficial whitening.

Postoperative Clinical Considerations. Postoperative care is similar to that described for treatment of PWS. Application of cold tap water–soaked gauze, ice packs, or hydroocclusive dressings will ameliorate posttreatment burning or stinging. The treated area should be gently washed twice a day and an emollient such as Aquaphor Healing Ointment should then be applied. Reactive erythema that develops around the treated area usually fades within 24 hours. Crusting occurs rarely, but can appear 1 day after treatment and last 3 to 14 days. Crusting is usually a sign of overly aggressive treatment, except in the case of deep or wide-caliber vessels that respond only if treated aggressively. Crusting is much more common if darker patients or patients with a "suntan" are treated.

Although facial telangiectases generally respond extremely well to treatment, two or more treatment sessions may be required to achieve optimal clearing. Occasionally, recanalization occurs after treatment, causing recurrence of the vessel. Retreatment may be safely performed 6 weeks after the original treatment.

Intense Pulsed Light Source

Treatment. The intense pulsed light source requires that the user select a number of treatment parameters, including filter, pulse mode (single, double, or triple), pulse duration, pulse delay, and fluence. The software provides suggested treatment parameters based on lesion type, skin type, and predicted vessel depth. These parameters may be changed based on individual experience.

The cutoff filter should be chosen according to the patient's skin type and lesion depth. A shorter wavelength filter (e.g., 515 nm) should be used for superficial and smaller vessels on skin type I only. A longer wavelength (e.g., 570 nm) should be used for deeper and larger vessels. Patients with darker skin phototypes should be treated with a longer wavelength filter and a longer pulse delay. Theoretically, use of a longer pulse delay allows the epidermis to cool down between pulses, reducing the risk of epidermal coagulation. Single pulses should be used for small vessels, double pulses for medium vessels, and triple pulses for larger vessels. The theoretical advantage of multiple pulses is the ability to damage larger and deeper vessels through additive heating.[45] Pulse delays should be longer for larger vessels to allow uniform heating of the entire vessel. Conversely, pulse delays should be very short for small vessels.

Lower fluences (20% below those recommended by the manufacturer) should be used initially until the skin response has been observed. If the targeted lesion appears unchanged and there are no epidermal changes, the fluence may be increased by 10% and an adjacent area treated. If no response is observed, the fluence can again be increased by 10%. If the desired tissue change is not seen, the pulse width should be increased by 10% to 15%, leaving fluence the same.

Before commencing treatment, a thick layer of cooling gel should be applied on the area to be treated. If available, the cooling crystal collar may be placed around the quartz handpiece. The handpiece should be placed directly perpendicular to the skin surface, floating in the layer of gel approximately 1 to 2 mm from tissue. After the pulse is delivered, the gel should be wiped off to allow inspection of the tissue response.

Postoperative Clinical Considerations. Reactive erythema usually develops around the treated area but typically subsides within 24 hours. Cold water–soaked gauze or biologic dressings (e.g., Second Skin) may be applied to reduce immediate posttreatment discomfort. The treated area should be washed gently twice a day with soap and water and should be covered with an emollient (e.g., Aquaphor Healing Ointment). Bandages are not required. Crusting is an uncommon occurrence. It is seen most commonly in patients with darker skin types and is associated with the use of excessive fluence or short wavelength filter. Patients should be instructed to avoid excessive sun exposure and use broad spectrum sunscreens for 3 to 4 weeks prior to treatment and at least 4 weeks after treatment.

REFERENCES

1. Requena L, Sangueza OP. Cutaneous vascular anomalies, part I: hamartomas, malformations, and dilatation of preexisting vessels. J Am Acad Dermatol 1997; 37:523-549.
2. Mulliken JB, Glowacki J. Hemangiomas and vascular malformations in infants and children: a classification based on endothelial characteristics. Plast Reconstr Surg 1982; 69:412-422.
3. Waner M, Suen JY. A classification of congenital vascular lesions. In: Waner M, Suen JY, eds. Hemangiomas and Vascular Malformations of the Head and Neck. New York: Wiley-Liss, 1999:1-12.
4. Anderson RR, Parrish JA. Microvasculature can be selectively damaged using dye lasers: a basic theory and experimental evidence in human skin. Laser Surg Med 1981; 1:263-276.
5. Anderson RR, Parrish JA. Selective photothermolysis: precise microsurgery by selective absorption of pulsed radiation. Science 1983; 220:524-527.
6. Greenwald J, Rosen S, Anderson RR, et al. Comparative histological studies of the tunable dye (at 577 nm) laser and argon laser: the specific vascular effects of the dye laser. J Invest Dermatol 1981; 77:305-310.
7. Noe JM, Barsky SH, Geer DE, Rosen S. Port wine stains and the response to argon laser therapy: successful treatment and the predictive role of color, age, and biopsy. Plast Reconstr Surg 1980; 65:130-139.
8. Dixon JA, Huether S, Rotering R. Hypertrophic scarring in argon laser treatment of port-wine stains. Plast Reconstr Surg 1984; 73: 771-777.
9. McBurney EI. Clinical usefulness of the argon laser for the 1990s. J Dermatol Surg Oncol 1993; 19:358-362.
10. McDaniel D, Mordon S. Hexascan: a new robotic scanning laser handpiece. Cutis 1990; 45:300-305.
11. Neumann RA, Knobler RM, Leonhartsberger H, Gebhart W. Comparative histochemistry of port-wine stains after copper vapor laser (578 nm) and argon laser treatment. J Invest Dermatol 1992; 99:160-167.
12. Dinehart SM, Waner M, Flock S. The copper vapor laser for treatment of cutaneous vascular and pigmented lesions. J Dermatol Surg Oncol 1993; 19:370-375.
13. Waner M, Dinehart SM, Wilson MB, Flock ST. A comparison of copper vapor and flashlamp pumped dye lasers in the treatment of facial telangiectasia. J Dermatol Surg Oncol 1993; 19:992-998.
14. Cotterill JA. Preliminary results following treatment of vascular lesions of the skin using a continuous wave dye laser which emits at 577 nm. Clin Exp Dermatol 1986; 11:628-635.
15. Orenstein A, Nelson JS. Treatment of facial vascular lesions with a 100-micron spot 577-nm pulsed continuous wave dye laser. Ann Plast Surg 1989; 23:310.

16. Lanigan SW, Carwright P, Cotterill JA. Continuous wave dye laser therapy of port-wine stains. Br J Dermatol 1989; 121:343-352.
17. Malm M, Rigler R, Jurell G. Continuous wave (CW) dye laser vs. CW argon laser treatment of port-wine stain (PWS). Scand J Plast Reconstr Surg 1988; 22:241-244.
18. Dover JS, Geronemus R, Stern RS, et al. Dye laser treatment of port wine stains: comparison of the continuous wave dye laser with a robotized scanning device and the pulsed dye laser. J Am Acad Dermatol 1995; 32:237-240.
19. Scheibner A, Wheeland RG. Argon-pumped tunable dye laser therapy for facial port-wine stain hemangiomas in adults—a new technique using small spot size and minimal power. J Dermatol Surg Oncol 1989; 15:277-282.
20. Scheibner A, Wheeland R. Use of the argon-pumped tunable dye laser for port-wine stains in children. J Dermatol Surg Oncol 1991; 17:735-739.
21. Anderson RR, Parrish JA. The optics of human skin. J Invest Dermatol 1981; 77:13-19.
22. Landthaler M, Hohenleutner U. The Nd:YAG laser in cutaneous surgery. In: Arndt KA, Dover JS, Olbricht, eds. Lasers in Cutaneous and Aesthetic Surgery. Philadelphia: Lippincott-Raven, 1997:124-149.
23. Landthaler M, Haina D, Brunner R, et al. Neodymium-YAG laser therapy of vascular lesions. J Am Acad Dermatol 1986; 14:197-217.
24. Dixon JA, Davis RK, Gilbertson JJ. Laser photocoagulation of vascular malformations of the tongue. Laryngoscope 1986; 96: 537-541.
25. Tan OT, Murray S, Kurban AK. Action spectrum of vascular specific injury using pulsed irradiation. J Invest Dermatol 1989; 92: 868-871.
26. van Gemert MJC, Welch AJ, Amin AP. Is there an optimal laser treatment for port wine stains? Laser Surg Med 1986; 6:76-83.
27. Dierickx CC, Casparian JM, Venugopalan V, et al. Thermal relaxation of port-wine stain vessels probed in vivo: the need for 1-10-millisecond laser pulse treatment. J Invest Dermatol 1995; 105: 709-714.
28. Garden JM, Polla LL, Tan OT. The treatment of port-wine stains by the pulsed dye laser: analysis of pulse duration and long-term therapy. Arch Dermatol 1988; 124:889-896.
29. Garden JM, Tan OT, Kerschmann R, et al. Effect of dye laser pulse duration on selective cutaneous vascular injury. J Invest Dermatol 1986; 87:653-657.
30. Edstrom DW, Ros AM. The treatment of port-wine stains with the pulsed dye laser at 600 nm. Br J Dermatol 1997; 136:360-363.
31. Paul BS, Anderson RR, Jarve J, Parrish JA. The effect of temperature and other factors on selective microvascular damage caused by pulsed dye laser. J Invest Dermatol 1983; 81:333-336.
32. Goldberg DJ, Marcus J. The use of the frequency-doubled Q-switched Nd:YAG laser in the treatment of small cutaneous vascular lesions. Dermatol Surg 1996; 22:841-844.
33. Dierickx CC, Farinelli WA, Anderson RR. Clinical and histological responses of blood vessels to long (msec) 532 nm laser pulses. Laser Surg Med 1996; 18(suppl 8):48.
34. van Gemert MJC, Welch AJ, Pickering JW, et al. Wavelengths for laser treatment of port wine stains and telangiectasia. Laser Surg Med 1995; 16:147-155.
35. Goldberg DJ, Meine JG. A comparison of four frequency-doubled Nd:YAG (532 nm) laser systems for treatment of facial telangiectases. Dermatol Surg 1999; 25:463-467.
36. Dierickx CC, Farinelli WA, Flotte T, Anderson RR. Effect of long-pulsed 532 nm Nd-YAG laser on portwine stains (PWS). Laser Surg Med 1996; 18(suppl 8):33.
37. McDaniel DH, Ash K, Lord J, et al. Laser therapy of spider veins: clinical evaluation of a new long pulsed alexandrite laser. Dermatol Surg 1999; 25:52-58.
38. Kauvar ANB, Lou WW, Quintana AT. Effect of cryogen spray cooling on treatment of leg telangiectasia with 585 nm, 1.5 msec and 755 nm, 3 msec lasers. Laser Surg Med 1999; 11(suppl):19.
39. Dierickx CC, Duque V, Anderson RR. Treatment of leg telangiectasia by a pulsed, infrared laser system. Laser Surg Med 1998; 10(suppl):40.
40. Garden JM, Bakus AD, Miller ID. Diode laser treatment of leg veins. Laser Surg Med 1998; 10(suppl):32.
41. Campos VB, Lucchina LC, Dierickx CC, Anderson RR. Treatment of leg telangiectasia by a pulsed, 915 nm infrared laser system. Laser Surg Med 1999; 11(suppl):20-21.
42. Kaudewitz P, Rother W. Pulsed diode laser 940 nm: first experience on the treatment of leg veins. Laser Surg Med 2000; 12(suppl):29-30.
43. Weiss RA, Weiss MA. Initial results with a new synchronized pulsed 1064 nm laser for larger leg telangiectasias. Laser Surg Med 1999; (suppl 11):21.
44. Weiss RA, Weiss MA. Epidermal cooling crystal collar (E3C) device for improved results on leg veins using intense pulsed light. Laser Surg Med 1999; (suppl 11):20.
45. Raulin C, Schroeter CA, Weiss RA, et al. Treatment of port-wine stains with a noncoherent pulsed light source: a retrospective study. Arch Dermatol 1999; 135:679-683.
46. Raulin C, Hellwig S, Schonermark MP. Treatment of a nonresponding port-wine stain with a new pulsed light source (Photoderm VL). Laser Surg Med 1997; 21:203-208.
47. Cliff S, Misch K. Treatment of mature port wine stains with the Photoderm VL. J Cutan Laser Ther 1999; 1:101-104.
48. Raulin C, Werner S. Treatment of venous malformations with an intense pulsed light source (IPLS) technology: a retrospective study. Laser Surg Med 1999; 25:170-177.
49. Raulin C, Weiss RA, Schonermark MP. Treatment of essential telangiectasias with an intense pulsed light source (Photoderm VL). Dermatol Surg 1997; 23:941-946.
50. Goldman MP, Eckhouse S. Photothermal sclerosis of leg veins. Dermatol Surg 1996; 22:323-330.
51. Green D. Photothermal removal of telangiectases of the lower extremities with the Photoderm VL. J Am Acad Dermatol 1998; 38: 61-68.
52. Chess C. Fire and ice: current methods of simultaneous lasing and cooling. Cosmet Dermatol 1999; 42-44.
53. Ross EV, Ladin Z, Kreindel M, Dierickx C. Theoretical considerations in laser hair removal. Dermatol Clin 1999; 17:333-355.
54. Nelson JS, Milner TE, Anvari B, et al. Dynamic epidermal cooling in conjunction with laser-induced photothermolysis of port wine stain blood vessels. Laser Surg Med 1996; 19:224-229.
55. Chang CJ, Nelson JS. Cryogen spray cooling and higher fluence pulsed dye laser treatment improve port-wine stain clearance while minimizing epidermal damage. Dermatol Surg 1999; 25: 767-772.
56. Barsky SH, Rosen S, Geer DE, Noe JM. The nature and evolution of port wine stains: a computer assisted study. J Invest Dermatol 1980; 74:154-157.
57. Finley JL, Noe JM, Arndt KA, Rosen S. Port-wine stains: morphologic variations and developmental lesions. Arch Dermatol 1984; 120:1453-1455.
58. Braverman IM. Ultrastructure and organization of the cutaneous microvasculature in normal and pathologic states. J Invest Dermatol 1989; 93:2S-9S.
59. Tan OT, Sherwood K, Gilchrest BA. Treatment of children with port-wine stains using the flashlamp-pulsed tunable dye laser. N Engl J Med 1989; 320:416-421.
60. Reyes BA, Geronemus R. Treatment of port-wine stains during childhood with the flashlamp-pumped pulsed dye laser. J Am Acad Dermatol 1990; 23:1142-1148.
61. Orten SS, Waner M, Flock S, et al. Port-wine stains: an assessment of 5 years of treatment. Arch Otolaryngol Head Neck Surg 1996; 122:1174-1179.

62. Fitzpatrick RE, Lowe NJ, Goldman MP, et al. Flashlamp-pumped pulsed dye laser treatment of port-wine stains. J Dermatol Surg Oncol 1994; 20:743-748.
63. Onizuka K, Tsuneda K, Shibata Y, et al. Efficacy of flashlamp-pumped pulsed dye laser therapy for port wine stains: clinical assessment and histopathological characteristics. Br J Plast Surg 1995; 48:271-279.
64. Alster TS, Wilson F. Treatment of port-wine stains with the flashlamp-pumped pulsed dye laser: extended clinical experience in children and adults. Ann Plast Surg 1994; 32:478-484.
65. Kauvar ANB, Geronemus RG. Repetitive pulse dye laser treatments improve persistent port-wine stains. Dermatol Surg 1995; 21:515-521.
66. Goldman MP, Fitzpatrick RE, Ruiz-Esparza J. Treatment of port-wine stains (capillary malformation) with the flashlamp-pumped pulsed dye laser. J Pediatr 1993; 122:71-77.
67. Ashinoff R, Geronemus RG. Flashlamp-pumped pulsed dye laser for port-wine stains in infancy: earlier versus later treatment. J Am Acad Dermatol 1991; 24:467-472.
68. Van der Horst CMAM, Koster PHL, de Borgie AJM, et al. Effect of the timing of treatment of port-wine stains with the flash-lamp-pumped pulsed-dye laser. N Engl J Med 1998; 338:1028-1033.
69. Renfro L, Geronemus RG. Anatomical differences of PWS in response to treatment with the pulsed dye laser. Arch Dermatol 1993; 129:182-188.
70. Lanigan SW. Port wine stains on the lower limb: response to pulsed dye laser therapy. Clin Exper Dermatol 1996; 21:88-92.
71. Morelli JG, Weston WL, Huff C, Yohn JJ. Initial lesion size as a predictive factor in determining the response of port-wine stains in children treated with the pulsed dye laser. Arch Pediatr Adolesc Med 1995; 149:1142-1144.
72. Yohn JJ, Huff JC, Aeling JL, et al. Lesion size is a factor for determining the rate of port-wine stain clearing following pulsed dye laser treatment in adults. Cutis 1997; 59:267-270.
73. Fiskerstrand EJ, Svaasand LO, Kopstad G, et al. Laser treatment of port wine stains: therapeutic outcome in relation to morphological parameters. Br J Dermatol 1996; 134:1039-1043.
74. Ruiz-Esparza J, Goldman MP, Fitzpatrick RE, et al. Flashlamp-pumped dye laser treatment of telangiectasia. J Dermatol Surg Oncol 1993; 19:1000-1003.
75. Geronemus RG. Treatment of spider telangiectases in children using the flashlamp-pumped pulsed dye laser. Pediatr Dermatol 1991; 8:61-63.
76. Requena L, Sangueza OP. Cutaneous vascular proliferations, part II: hyperplasias and benign neoplasms. J Am Acad Dermatol 1997; 37:887-920.
77. Frieden IJ, Eichenfeld LF, Esterly NB, et al. Guidelines of care for hemangiomas of infancy. J Am Acad Dermatol 1997; 37:631-637.
78. Frieden IJ. Which hemangiomas to treat—and how? Arch Dermatol 1997; 133:1593-1595.
79. Waner M, Suen JY. Special symposium: management of hemangiomas. Pediatr Dermatol 1997; 14:79-81.
80. Morelli JG. Special symposium: management of hemangiomas. Pediatr Dermatol 1997; 14:68-69.
81. Sherwood KA, Tan OT. Treatment of a capillary hemangioma with the flashlamp pumped-dye laser. J Am Acad Dermatol 1990; 22:136-137.
82. Ashinoff R, Geronemus RG. Failure of the flashlamp-pumped pulsed dye laser to prevent progression to deep hemangioma. Pediatr Dermatol 1993; 10:77-80.
83. Garden JM, Bakus AD, Paller AS. Treatment of cutaneous hemangiomas by the flashlamp-pumped pulsed dye laser: prospective analysis. J Pediatr 1992; 120:555-560.
84. Tamayo L, Ortiz DM, Orozco-Covarrubias L, et al. Therapeutic efficacy of interferon alfa-2b in infants with life-threatening giant hemangiomas. Arch Dermatol 1997; 133:1567-1571.
85. Ashinoff R, Geronemus RG. Capillary hemangiomas and treatment with the flashlamp-pumped pulsed dye laser. Arch Dermatol 1991; 127:202-205.
86. Morelli JG, Tan OT, Weston WL. Treatment of ulcerated hemangiomas with the pulsed tunable dye laser. Am J Dis Child 1991; 145:1062-1064.
87. Waldorf HA, Kauvar ANB, Geronemus RG, Leffell DJ. Remote fire with the pulsed dye laser: risk and prevention. J Am Acad Dermatol 1996; 34:503-506.
88. Jackson BA, Arndt KA, Dover JS. Are all 585 nm pulsed dye lasers equivalent? J Am Acad Dermatol 1996; 34:1000-1004.
89. Dinehart SM, Flock S, Waner M. Beam profile of the flashlamp-pumped pulsed dye laser: support for overlap of exposure spots. Laser Surg Med 1994; 15:277-280.
90. Wlotzke U, Hohenleutner U, Abd-el-raheem TA, et al. Side-effects and complications of flashlamp-pumped pulsed dye laser therapy of port-wine stains: a prospective study. Br J Dermatol 1996; 134:475-480.
91. Seukeran DC, Collins P, Sheehan-Dare RA. Adverse reactions following pulsed tunable dye laser treatment of port wine stains in 701 patients. Br J Dermatol 1997; 136:725-729.
92. Gaston DA, Clark DP. Facial hypertrophic scarring from pulsed dye laser. Dermatol Surg 1998; 24:523-525.
93. Swinehart JM. Hypertrophic scarring resulting from flashlamp-pumped pulsed dye laser surgery. J Am Acad Dermatol 1991; 25:845-846.
94. Bernestein LJ, Geronemus RG. Keloid formation with the 585-nm pulsed dye laser during isotretinoin treatment. Arch Dermatol 1997; 133:111-112.
95. Fiskerstrand EJ, Svaasand LO, Volden G. Pigmentary changes after pulsed dye laser treatment in 125 northern European patients with port wine stains. Br J Dermatol 1998; 138:477-479.

CHAPTER 12

Lasers in the Treatment of Pigmented Lesions

RICHARD J. ORT
KENNETH A. ARNDT
JEFFREY S. DOVER

SECTION ONE

History and Scientific Review

BACKGROUND AND HISTORY

In 1963, Goldman and colleagues first demonstrated that ruby laser radiation with a 0.5 ms pulse duration was selectively absorbed by pigmented skin.[1] These same investigators demonstrated that the threshold radiant exposure for epidermal damage was 10 to 100 times lower for a Q-switched ruby laser (QSRL) with pulse width of 50 ns.[2] Despite these initial reports, the ability of the QSRL to selectively target pigment was not appreciated, and pigmented lesions for many years were treated with nonselective continuous wave sources such as the argon[3] and carbon dioxide lasers.[4] Over the last decade, on the basis of a large amount of basic and clinical investigation performed with pulsed lasers, Q-switched lasers have become the treatment of choice for both epidermal and dermal pigmented lesions, including tattoos.

BASIC SCIENCE

Laser-Tissue Interactions in Pigmented Skin

In 1983, Anderson and Parrish described the principle of selective photothermolysis,[5] which predicted that selective thermal damage to an absorbing target could be achieved using suitable laser parameters. This concept requires the use of a wavelength well absorbed by the target, a pulse duration shorter than the thermal relaxation time of the target (defined as the time required for a heated target to cool by 50%), and sufficiently high energy density to achieve the desired tissue effect. This principle was first applied to the treatment of port wine stains with oxyhemoglobin as the target chromophore. Soon thereafter it was applied to the treatment of pigmented lesions where either endogenous melanin or an exogenous chromophore such as carbon particles served as the target.

Melanin has a broad absorption spectrum within the ultraviolet, visible, and near-infrared range, but absorption decreases steadily with longer wavelengths[6] (Fig. 12-1). It is the primary absorber between 600 and 1100 nm, the "optical window" where light penetrates deeply into the dermis.[6] Microscopically, melanin consists of melanosome granules that evolve through four stages of increasing melanization before being transferred from melanocytes to keratinocytes. With a diameter of 1 μm, melanosomes are predicted to have a thermal relaxation time of 50 to 500 ns.[5,7] Depending on coloration, individual tattoo pigments can be characterized by their own absorption spectra.[8] For example, black pigment absorbs broadly from 600 nm to near infrared while red pigment has maximum absorption from 505 to 560 nm.[8] With a diameter of approximately 40 nm, the most common type of tattoo pigment particle has a predicted thermal relaxation time of less than 10 ns.[9,10]

The principle of selective photothermolysis predicts that thermal confinement to the melanosome or tattoo particle will occur over a range of wavelengths if the laser pulsewidth is less than 1 μs. The delivery of an extremely high energy laser pulse within this time span results in rapid heating of the target particle (estimated at 10 million degrees per second), causing it to explode.[11] Selective damage to melanosomes in human skin was first demonstrated with a 351 nm XeF excimer laser delivering 20 ns pulses.[12] Although light at 351 nm is well absorbed by melanin, it penetrates less than 100 μm into the skin because of pronounced dermal scattering at shorter wavelengths.[6] Longer wavelengths penetrate progressively deeper into the skin, such that wavelengths of 694 nm or greater penetrate at least 1 mm.[6] It was subsequently demonstrated that selective damage to melanosomes could be produced by

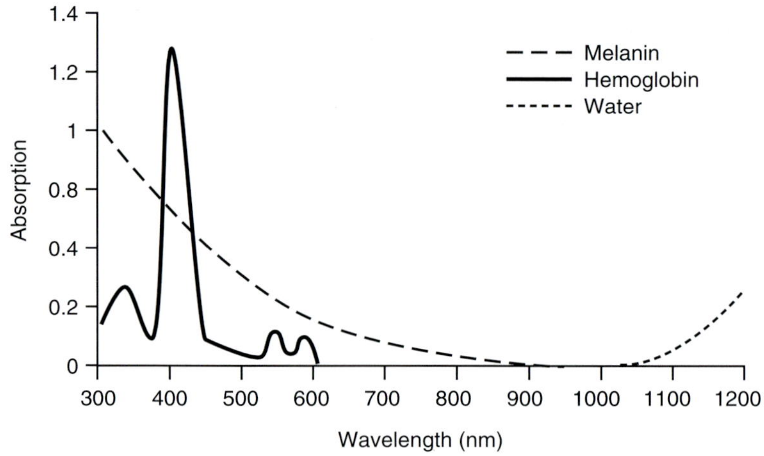

FIG. 12-1
Absorption spectrum of melanin.

the pulsed tunable dye laser[13,14] (wavelength 435 to 750 nm, pulsewidth 300 to 750 ns), Q-switched ruby laser[7] (wavelength 694 nm, pulsewidth 40 ns) and the Q-switched neodymium:YAG laser[15] (wavelength 355, 532, and 1064 nm, pulsewidth 10 to 12 ns). Electron microscopy confirmed highly selective, dose-dependent disruption of melanosomes within melanocytes and melanized keratinocytes.

It is believed that destruction of pigment-containing cells is due to mechanical damage from acoustic waves that emanate from the absorbing melanosome or tattoo particle.[9,16] Damage to these cells results in vacuolization, condensation of pigment and nuclear material at the cellular periphery, and subepidermal vesiculation at the level of the lamina lucida. In both guinea pig[17] and human skin[18] treated with the QSRL, necrotic pigmented cells slough in a fine scale or crust over several weeks, followed by transient hypopigmentation and gradual repigmentation without textural change. Repigmentation results from migration of residual melanocytes within adnexal structures or within unirradiated adjacent skin.

Q-switched lasers produce an immediate ash-white color at the site of impact. Although the exact cause of this tissue response is unknown, it is most likely due to scattering of visible light by steam cavities formed within melanosomes.[17] The threshold exposure dose for melanosome damage correlates well with the clinical threshold for immediate skin whitening. Darker skin has a lower threshold whitening dose due to higher epidermal melanin content.[18] The required threshold dose increases progressively with longer wavelength, grossly consistent with the melanin absorption spectrum.[14,15] Longer wavelengths up to 1064 nm penetrate more deeply into the dermis, causing melanosome alterations within follicles at a depth of over 1 mm.[15] Subthreshold fluences appear to actually stimulate melanogenesis because of activation of epidermal melanocytes after nonlethal injury.[18]

Q-switched and Pulsed Lasers and Light Sources

A variety of lasers can be used to treat pigmented lesions of the skin (Table 12-1). These can be categorized into lasers that are pigment nonselective, those that are somewhat pigment selective, and those that are highly selective for pigment removal. Pigment nonselective lasers such as the carbon dioxide[4,19] (10,600 nm) and erbium:YAG (2940 nm) lasers can be used to eliminate epidermal pigment because of their ability to target water and remove the entire epidermis, including melanocytes and melanized keratinocytes, in atraumatic fashion. Pigment is removed as a secondary event. Continuous wave (CW) and quasi-CW visible light lasers, such as argon laser (488, 514 nm), copper vapor laser (511 nm), and krypton laser (521, 530 nm), can be used to selectively remove epidermal pigmented lesions, although reproducible spatial thermal injury confinement is not possible. The risk/benefit ratio is higher with these devices than with pulsed lasers. To date, only pulsed lasers have been shown to treat both epidermal and dermal pigmented lesions effectively in a safe, reproducible manner (Table 12-2).

There are four principal short-pulsed, pigment-selective lasers that are widely used today: the Q-switched ruby laser (QSRL), the Q-switched alexandrite laser, the Q-switched neodymium:YAG (Nd:YAG) laser, and the pigmented lesion pulsed dye laser. These lasers specifically target melanosomes or tattoo particles by delivering high-intensity, short-pulsed radiation at appropriate wavelengths. The term *Q-switched* is short for "quality-switched," which refers to the ability to store large amounts of energy in the laser cavity through the use of an optical shutter. When the laser fires, the shutter releases an extremely high powered pulse (10^9 W) with an ultra-short pulse duration (nanosecond range).

Table 12-1 Lasers in the Treatment of Pigmented Lesions

Device	Manufacturer	Laser Type	Wave-length (nm)	Pulse Duration	Spot Size (mm)	Maximum Repetition Rate (Hz)	Comments
Spectrum RD-1200	Spectrum (Palomar)	QS ruby	694	28 ns	5, 6.5	0.8	Large spot size promotes deeper penetration
EpiTouch	Lumenis	QS ruby	694	25 ns	5	0.8	Long pulse mode available for hair removal
RubyStar	Aesculap Meditec	QS ruby	694	40 ns	1.5, 3, 4	1	Long pulse mode available for hair removal
AlexLAZR	Candela	QS alexandrite	755	50 ns	2, 3, 4	5	Fiberoptic delivery system
HT 10	Cynosure	QS alexandrite	755	45-75 ns	2.4	10	Fiberoptic delivery system
VersaPulse VPC	Lumenis	FD Nd:YAG	532	2-50 ms	2-10	6	Four lasers within one box
		QS FD Nd:YAG	532	4 ns	2-6	10	
		QS Nd:YAG	1064	5 ns	2-6	10	
		QS alexandrite	755	45 ns	2-6	10	
Medlite IV	Continuum Biomedical	QS FD Nd:YAG	532	5-7 ns	2, 3, 4, 6	10	Handpiece converts λ to 585 and 650 nm
		QS Nd:YAG	1064	5-7 ns	3, 4, 6, 8	10	
TatuLAZR	Candela	Pulsed dye	510	400 ns	3-5	1	Fiberoptic delivery system

FD, Frequency doubled; QS, Q-switched

Table 12-2 Treatment of Pigmented Lesions and Tattoos

Laser	Epidermal Lesions	Dermal Lesions	Mixed Lesions	Amateur Tattoos (Blue or Black)	Professional Tattoos (Primary Colors)
Q-switched ruby (694 nm)	++++	++++	+	++++	++++ (black, blue, green)
Q-switched Nd:YAG (1064 nm)	++	++++	+	++++	++++ (black, blue)
Q-switched Nd:YAG (532 nm)	++++	+ to ++	+	++	+++ (red and other bright colors)
Q-switched Nd:YAG (585 nm)	+++	+ to ++	+	++	+++ (light blue)
Q-switched Nd:YAG (650 nm)	+++	+ to ++	+	++	+++ (green)
Q-switched alexandrite (755 nm)	+++	+++	+	+++	+++ (black, blue, green)
Pulsed dye (510 nm)	++++	++	+	+	++++ (red, yellow)

+, Poor; ++, fair; +++, good; ++++, excellent.

The QSRL emits red light at a wavelength of 694 nm and pulse duration of 28 to 40 ns. Light is delivered through a mirrored articulated arm at a spot size of 5 or 6.5 mm and repetition rate of 1 Hz. The Q-switched Nd:YAG laser emits infrared light at 1064 nm. By placing a frequency-doubling KTP (potassium-titanyl-phosphate) crystal in the laser beam's path, the wavelength may be halved to 532 nm (green light). Recently introduced dye-impregnated handpieces can convert the 532 nm wavelength to either 585 nm (yellow) or 650 nm (red) light. Pulses of 5 to 10 ns duration are delivered through an articulated arm at a spot size of 1.5 to 4 mm and repetition rate of up to 10 Hz. The Q-switched alexandrite laser has a wavelength of 755 nm (infrared), pulse duration of 50 to 100 ns, spot size of 2 to 4 mm, and repetition rate of up to 10 Hz. Light is delivered through an articulated arm or through a semiflexible fiberoptic cable. The pigmented lesion pulsed dye laser (non-Q-switched) utilizes a xenon flashlamp to pump a coumarin-containing dye that emits pulses of laser energy at 510 nm (green light). It has a somewhat longer pulse duration of 400 ns, spot size of 3 to 5 mm, firing rate of 1 Hz, and a fiberoptic delivery system.

Long-pulsed (millisecond domain) 532 nm (KTP) Nd:YAG lasers, which are commonly used to treat vascular lesions, can be used to treat superficial pigmented lesions. However, the long pulsewidth of these lasers approximates the thermal relaxation time of the entire epidermis (about 10 ms)[20] and does not allow for selective damage to subcellular organelles such as melanosomes. The small spot size (2 mm or less) of many systems necessitates the use of a "painting technique" to treat larger lesions, which raises the risk of double pulsing. Because of the limited penetration depth of the 532 nm wavelength, these lasers are not effective for treatment of dermal pigmented lesions.

Long-pulsed ruby, alexandrite, and Nd:YAG lasers, widely used for laser hair removal, share the same wavelengths as their Q-switched counterparts but operate in a normal (non-Q-switched) mode and deliver high-energy pulses in the millisecond rather than nanosecond domain. Because of their higher fluences and longer pulse duration, these lasers can target large pigmented structures such as hair follicles or nests of cells rather than individual melanosomes or pigmented cells. The role of these long-pulsed lasers in the treatment of congenital and acquired nevi is currently being investigated.[21,22]

Pigment removal can also be accomplished with a noncoherent light source that emits polychromatic light ranging from 515 to 1200 nm (visible to infrared). Filters are used to cut off the light below a predetermined wavelength. Light is emitted as a sequence of single, double, or triple pulses (millisecond domain), which are separated by variable time intervals. This laserlike device has been primarily used for treatment of vascular lesions and hair removal, and aside from anecdotal reports, there are no studies addressing its efficacy in the treatment of pigmented lesions of the skin.[23]

CLINICAL STUDIES AND DISCUSSION

Epidermal Pigmented Lesions

Numerous clinical studies have confirmed the efficacy and safety of Q-switched lasers[24-26] and the 510 nm pulsed dye laser[27] in the treatment of various epidermal pigmented lesions, including ephelides, lentigines, café au lait macules, seborrheic keratoses, nevi spilus, and Becker's nevi. Pigment in epidermal lesions is located superficially, so shorter-wavelength devices can be used effectively despite their limited penetration depth. For example, the 510 nm wavelength of the pulsed dye laser penetrates only about 250 μm into the skin but is highly absorbed by melanin.[6] The Q-switched ruby and alexandrite lasers effectively treat both epidermal and dermal lesions, since their wavelengths are well absorbed by melanin and penetrate deeply into the dermis. The 1064 nm wavelength of the Nd:YAG laser penetrates deeply but is poorly absorbed by melanin, making the 532 nm wavelength a better choice when treating epidermal lesions. At the 510 nm and 532 nm (green) wavelengths, hemoglobin competes with melanin for absorption of light. Ultrashort (nanosecond range) pulses at these wavelengths cause rupture of superficial blood vessels, which is evident clinically as purpura.[14]

Lentigines. Lentigines are extremely common hyperpigmented macules that most often result from chronic sun exposure. Histologically, melanocytes in the basal layer are increased in number without nesting and rete ridges are elongated. Lentigines can be classified into several categories, including those due to chronic sun exposure (solar lentigines), those associated with a syndrome (e.g., Peutz-Jeghers [Fig. 12-2]), and the labial melanotic macule. All three Q-switched

A B

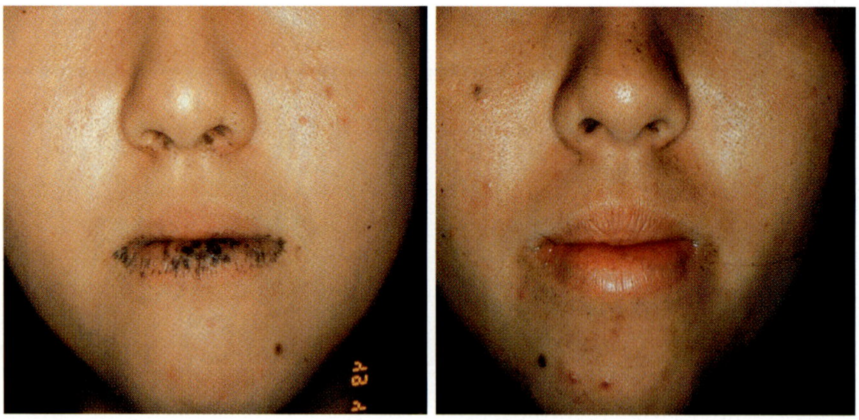

FIG. 12-2

A, A patient with Peutz-Jeghers syndrome with extensive macular pigmented lesions over the lip prior to treatment. **B,** After two treatments with the Q-switched ruby laser, the lesions are completely cleared. (Courtesy Tadashi Tezuka, MD.)

lasers and the 510 nm pulsed dye laser are highly effective in the treatment of lentigines. After one treatment, at least 50% clearing is expected, although additional treatments may be required to remove residual pigment (Fig. 12-3). Labial melanotic macules respond equally well to laser treatment.[28,29] One study determined that treatment of facial lentigines with the 532 nm Q-switched Nd:YAG laser was more effective than application of 35% trichloroacetic acid.[30] In another study, blinded observers found that the 532 nm Q-switched Nd:YAG laser was superior to cryotherapy with liquid nitrogen in efficacy, healing time, and patient preference.[31]

Café au Lait Macules. Café au lait macules (CALMs) are well circumscribed, light brown macules that may occur as isolated lesions in the general population or as multiple lesions in association with a syndrome (e.g., neurofibromatosis and Albright's syndrome). Histologically, one sees an increase in the number of melanocytes, hypermelanosis of melanocytes and keratinocytes, and giant melanin granules. The efficacy of lasers in the removal of CALMs is variable, and results are often unpredictable.[32] Short-term lightening or clearing is frequently achieved after multiple treatments (Fig. 12-4). However, recurrences are common, seen in up to 50% of treated lesions, even when complete clearing has occurred initially. Transient postinflammatory hyperpigmentation is frequent following laser treatment of CALMs, especially in patients with skin phototypes III and higher. Alster reported complete elimination of most CALMs after an average of 8.4 treatment sessions with the 510 nm pulsed dye laser, indicating that multiple treatments may be necessary to achieve optimal results.[33] Complete clearing of a dark facial CALM previously resistant to Q-switched ruby and Nd:YAG laser treatment has been reported after erbium:YAG laser resurfacing.[34]

Other Epidermal Lesions. Ephelides (freckles) are small hyperpigmented macules located on sun-exposed skin. Histologically, there is hyperpigmentation of the basal layer but no increase in the concentration of melanocytes. These lesions uniformly respond well to Q-switched and 510 nm pulsed dye laser treatment (Fig. 12-5). Flat seborrheic keratoses also respond well to laser treatment,[27] but thicker lesions are resistant and should be treated with cryosurgery. Nevi spilus and Becker's nevi, which may have combined epidermal and dermal components, respond variably to laser treatment. Results are unpredictable, and incomplete clearing or recurrences are not uncommon. Successful clearing of the darker nevocellular component of nevus spilus has been reported with the QSRL, but the background café au lait component tends to recur.[24] Becker's nevus is a large, hyperpigmented, slightly verrucous plaque that occurs most commonly on the shoulder area of males. These lesions are reported to be similar to café au lait macules in their response to laser treatment, with a high incidence of posttreatment hyperpigmentation and recurrence within 6 to 12 months.[35]

Dermal Pigmented Lesions and Tattoos

Q-switched lasers have revolutionized the treatment of dermal pigmented lesions, including melanocytoses, some melanocytic nevi, and tattoos. Prior to the use of Q-switched lasers, treatment of these lesions was limited to nonspecific destructive methods such as excision,[36,37] dermabrasion,[38] salabrasion,[39] liquid nitrogen,[40] solid carbon dioxide ice,[41] or continuous wave laser ablation.[42] Treatment was relatively ineffec-

A

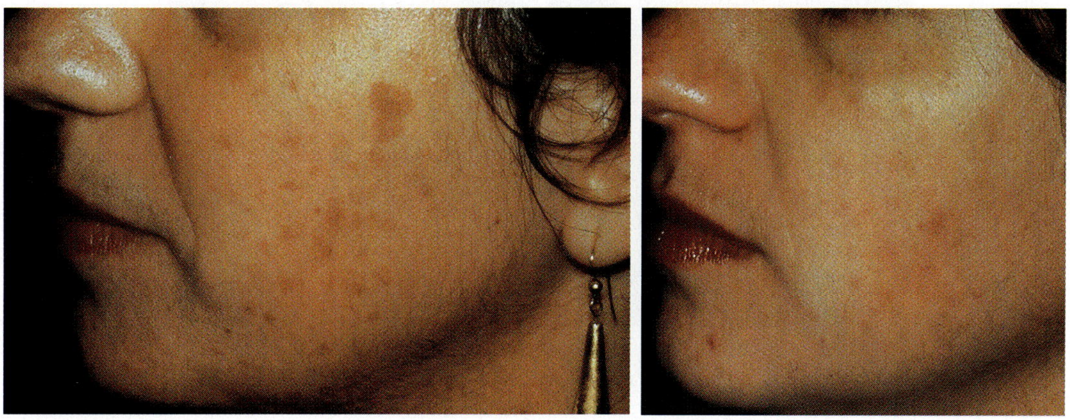

B

FIG. 12-3
A, A woman in her early 40s with significant photoaging and numerous lentigines prior to treatment. **B,** Six weeks after one single treatment with a Q-switched ruby laser. There is about 70% improvement of the lesion. No further treatments were requested by the patient.

tive and almost always resulted in scarring or pigmentary changes. By selectively targeting dermal pigment, Q-switched lasers provide highly effective treatment of these lesions while dramatically reducing the risk of textural or permanent pigmentary change. The Q-switched ruby, alexandrite, and 1064 nm Nd:YAG lasers are most commonly used. The wavelength range of these lasers falls within the optical window that transmits light deeply into the dermis. Shorter wavelengths such as 510 or 532 nm are highly scattered by dermal collagen and penetrate poorly into the dermis (about 300 μm),[6] making them inappropriate sources for the treatment of dermal pigment. Because they are so well absorbed by the color red, however, they are effective for treating red tattoo pigment.

Nevus of Ota. Nevus of Ota is a mottled, bluish or gray-brown patch that is usually located unilaterally within the distribution of the first and second branches of the trigeminal nerve. It is classified into four types, depending on extent and distribution of pigmentation (I—small, II—moderate, III—extensive, IV—bilateral). Nevus of Ota may affect mucosal surfaces such as cornea, sclera, nasal and buccal mucosa, and tympanic membrane. The lesion is present at birth in about 50% of cases, while the remainder usually appear by the second decade of life. Asians are most commonly affected, with an incidence of 1 in 500 reported in Japan.[43] The incidence in Caucasians is significantly lower. Women are five times more likely to be affected than men. The occurrence of melanoma within nevus of Ota

A B C D

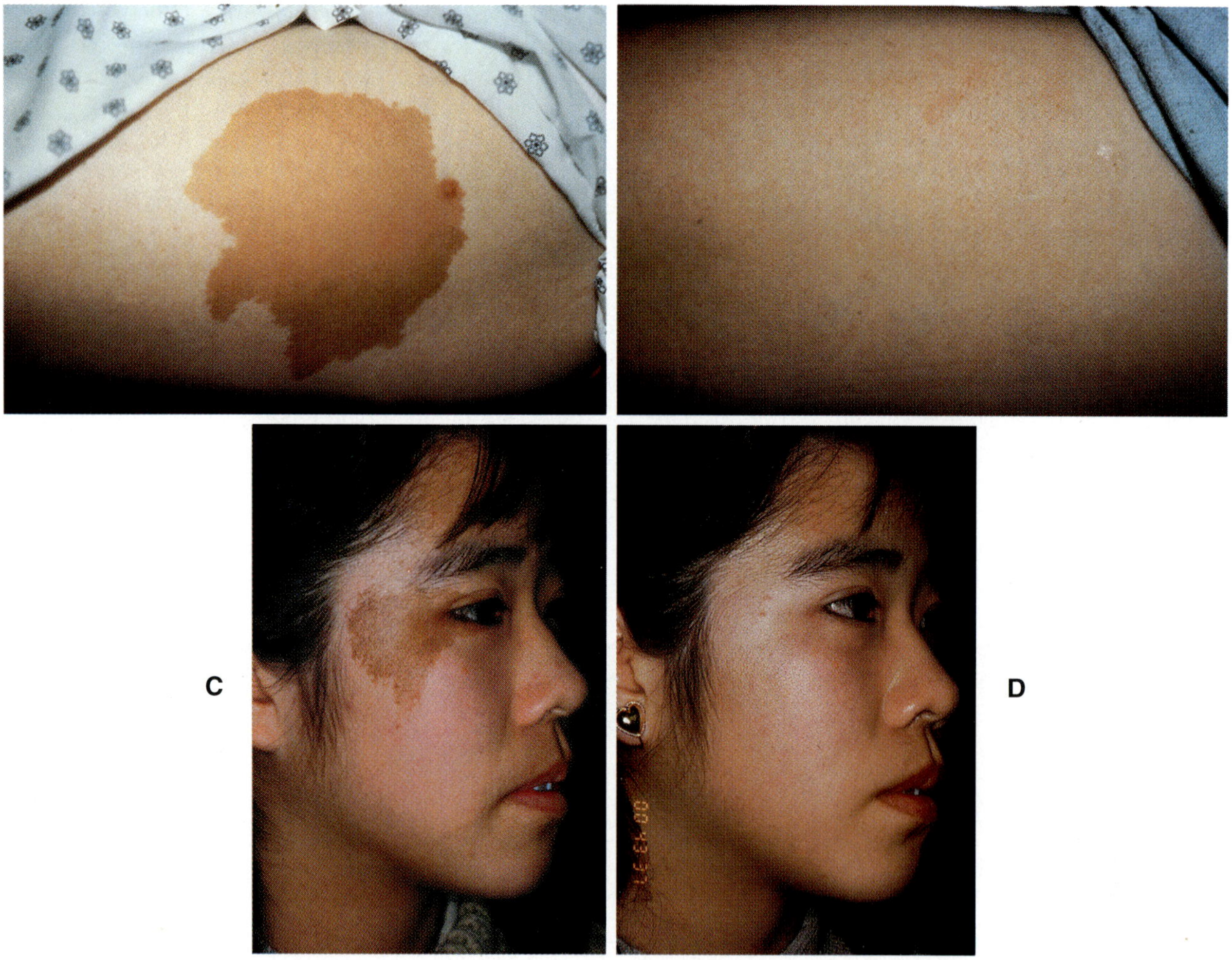

FIG. 12-4
A, Café au lait macule of the thigh. (Courtesy Karen Wiss, MD.) **B,** Café au lait macule after four treatments with a Q-switched ruby laser, showing near complete clearing of the lesion. There is one small focal scar that is the result of a skin biopsy. (Courtesy Karen Wiss, MD.) **C,** A young woman with a café au lait macule of the right temple prior to treatment. (Courtesy Tadashi Tezuka, MD.) **D,** After four treatments with the Q-switched ruby laser, there is dramatic lightening of the lesion.

has been reported[44] but is rare. Histologically, dendritic melanocytes are scattered within the papillary and reticular dermis.

Q-switched lasers provide an extremely effective means of treating this condition. The degree of lightening is usually directly proportional to the number of treatments performed. Lightening of 70% or more has been reported in the vast majority of patients treated four or five times with the QSRL[45] (Fig. 12-6). Although pigmentary change such as hyperpigmentation or hypopigmentation occurs occasionally, textural change has not been reported. Posttreatment biopsies have revealed degeneration of melanocytes up to a depth of 1.5 mm from the skin surface.[45] Although the QSRL has been most widely used,[45-49] the Q-switched alexandrite[50] and Nd:YAG[25] lasers appear as effective. Large-

A

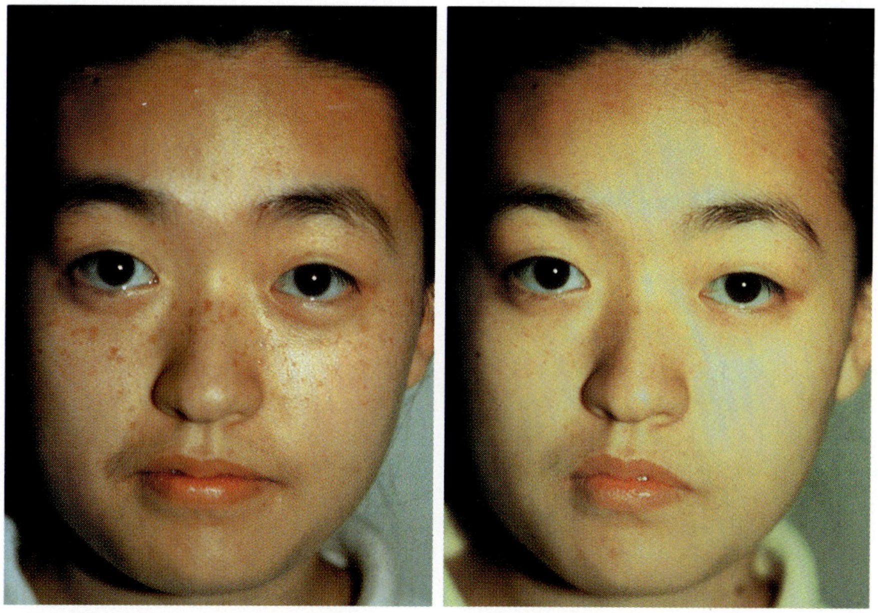

B

FIG. 12-5
A, Japanese male with extensive numbers of freckles prior to treatment. **B,** After treatment with a Q-switched ruby laser, the freckles are entirely clear. (Courtesy T.K. Lee, MD.)

A

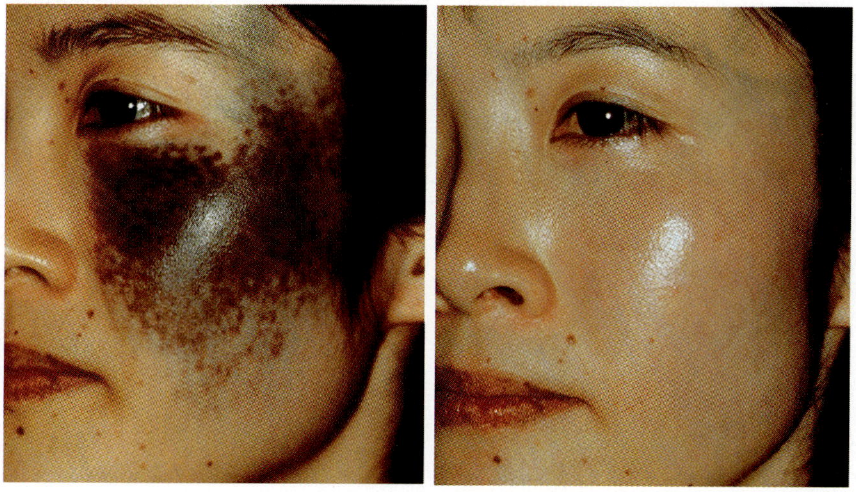

B

FIG. 12-6
A, A young girl with a nevus of Ota extending over a significant portion of the face prior to treatment. **B,** After a series of treatments with the Q-switched ruby laser, there is impressive lightening of the lesion with no textural change. (Courtesy S. Ueda, MD.)

scale comparative trials between these lasers have not been performed.

Melanocytic Nevi. Laser treatment of nevomelanocytic lesions is controversial, as it is unclear whether nonlethal laser irradiation has any potential to induce malignant change in nevomelanocytic cells. In vitro studies of melanoma cells treated with Q-switched lasers have found changes in cell surface integrin expression, with subsequent alteration of such cellular behavior as migration.[51] In addition, benign lesions that recur following treatment may show clinical and histologic atypia, a condition termed pseudomelanoma.[52] However, true malignant transformation of a benign pigmented lesion following laser treatment has never been reported.[53] Theoretically, laser treatment of melanocytic lesions might decrease the risk of malignant transformation by reducing the population of available premalignant cells.[54] Additional study is required to assess the effects of Q-switched laser irradiation on nevomelanocytic cells. For the time being, it is recommended that Q-switched laser treatment be reserved for benign nevomelanocytic lesions exhibiting little to no atypia. If any doubt exists about the clinical diagnosis, a biopsy should be performed prior to laser treatment. Laser treatment should not be performed in patients with a personal or family history of malignant melanoma.

Studies indicate that the Q-switched ruby, alexandrite, and 1064 nm Nd:YAG lasers all have some degree of effectiveness in the removal of flat or slightly raised, junctional or compound, acquired nevi.[55-57] Lighter nevi often respond best to shorter wavelengths that maximize melanin absorption, while darker nevi typically respond to any wavelength. Multiple treatments are usually necessary for maximal lightening. It is often not possible to achieve complete clearing of nevi,[57] and recurrence after laser treatment is not uncommon. There may be persistence of nevomelanocytes containing little or no pigment or located within deeper layers that are shielded from laser radiation by pigmented superficial cells.[55] Q-switched laser radiation does not penetrate sufficiently to effectively treat thicker lesions such as papillated or dome-shaped dermal nevi. The QSRL has been reported to successfully eliminate flat blue nevi.[58]

Although Q-switched lasers may effectively lighten congenital nevi, there is a high rate of repigmentation due to persistence of nevomelanocytes within the deeper reticular dermis and within adnexae.[53,54] In theory, millisecond-domain pulses are more appropriate than Q-switched pulses for treating thick lesions such as congenital nevi because they produce less selective thermal damage, destroying entire nests of cells rather than individual pigmented cells. Japanese investigators have reported impressive long-term clearing of congenital nevi treated with the millisecond-domain normal-mode ruby laser[21,22] (Fig. 12-7). Clinical lightening is associated with the development of a subtle microscopic scar up to 1 mm thick that obscures residual nevus cells. Long-pulse ruby lasers also offer the potential to reduce the amount of hair within congenital nevi. Because congenital nevi have the potential to transform into malignant melanoma, and residual nevus cells persist in the dermis after laser treatment, cautious long-term follow-up of nevi treated with lasers is required. In Japanese studies, no histological or clinical evidence of malignancy has been demonstrated up to 8 years after normal-mode ruby laser treatment.[21,22]

Both continuous wave lasers[59,60] and the QSRL[61] have been used to treat lentigo maligna. However, there are several reports of lentigo maligna recurring following

A

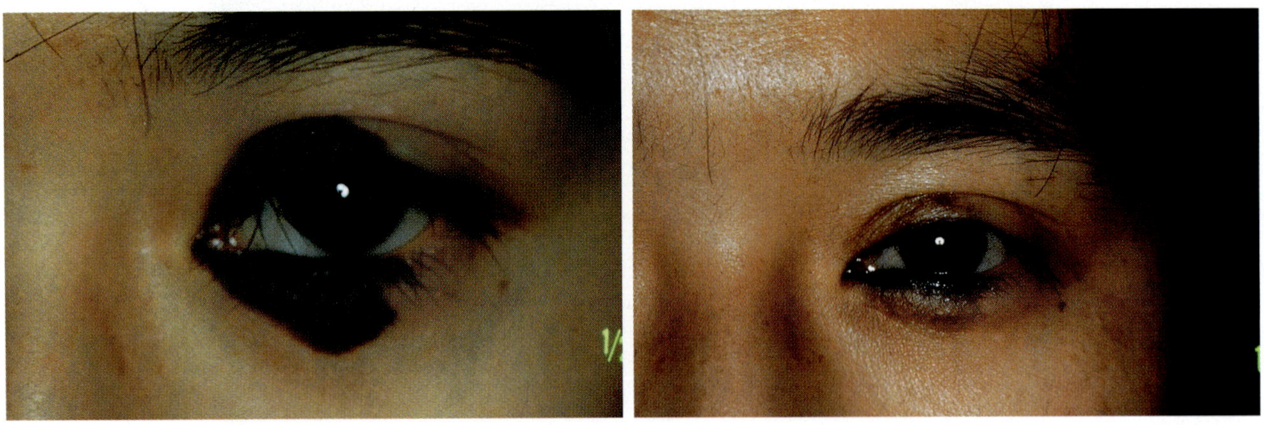

B

FIG. 12-7
A, A congenital nevus of the upper and lower eyelid prior to treatment. **B,** After a series of treatments with a long-pulsed ruby laser, there is significant lightening but incomplete clearing of the nevus. (Courtesy S. Ueda, MD.)

laser treatment, most likely due to persistence of melanocytes within deeper adnexal structures.[62,63] Laser treatment of lentigo maligna should be considered only in situations where surgical excision is not feasible due to large lesion size, advanced patient age, or underlying medical condition. Close follow-up to detect any early recurrence is essential.

Other Dermal Pigmented Lesions. Melasma is a common acquired facial hypermelanosis, occurring most commonly on the cheeks, forehead, upper lip, nose, and chin and varying in color from brown to blue-gray. It is particularly common in women of childbearing age and in individuals with skin phototypes III or higher. It is associated with sun exposure, pregnancy, and use of oral contraceptives, although its presence often cannot be ascribed to any known cause. Postinflammatory hyperpigmentation is another type of acquired hypermelanosis that may develop following nearly any cutaneous injury or inflammatory process. Histologically, three types of pigmentation occur in these two conditions: (1) the epidermal type in which there is increased melanin in the epidermis; (2) the dermal type in which melanophages are found in the superficial and mid-dermis; and (3) a combination of epidermal and dermal types.

Traditional treatment of these disorders includes cessation of offending medication such as oral contraceptives, sun protection, and use of topical steroids, hydroquinone, retinoids, azelaic acid, and superficial chemical peels. While the epidermal component often responds to this regimen, dermal pigmentation is generally resistant. Studies have shown that Q-switched lasers are for the most part ineffective in the treatment of melasma and postinflammatory hyperpigmentation.[25,64] Q-switched laser treatment may actually cause an increase in dermal melanophages and worsening of hyperpigmentation. Carbon dioxide[65] or erbium:YAG[66] laser resurfacing provides an alternative treatment modality for melasma, but postinflammatory hyperpigmentation is an almost universal occurrence in the postoperative period. Aggressive topical therapy should be initiated promptly following laser resurfacing. The use of these lasers should be reserved only for refractory melasma not responsive to conventional therapy.

Infraorbital hyperpigmentation (dark circles) may result from a variety of causes, including dermal melanin deposition, postinflammatory hyperpigmentation from atopic or allergic contact dermatitis, prominent superficial blood vessels, and shadowing from skin laxity and infraorbital swelling.[67] The QSRL has been reported to effectively treat infraorbital hyperpigmentation when due to deposition of dermal melanin.[67] Improvement of this condition has also been reported following carbon dioxide laser resurfacing.[68] Blepharoplasty may be indicated when infraorbital darkening is due to excessive skin laxity.

Minocycline therapy may cause localized or diffuse mucocutaneous pigmentation. Minocycline-induced pigmentation occurs in approximately 5% of acne vulgaris patients treated with the drug after prolonged use.[69] Two patterns of pigmentation have been reported. In type I, focal blue-gray pigmentation occurs in inflamed or scarred skin, or in previously normal skin. Histologic studies show pigment within dermal macrophages that stains positively for melanin and iron.[70] Type II consists of generalized blue to brown discoloration that is more prominent on sun-exposed areas. Histologically, epidermal and superficial dermal pigment is present that stains only for melanin.[70] Although pigmentation typically fades after discontinuation of the drug, it may persist for years following cessation of therapy. The Q-switched ruby laser is highly effective in treating minocycline-induced pigmentation, with clearing occurring after one to four treatment sessions without untoward sequelae.[71-73] Successful treatment has also been reported with the Q-switched 532 nm and 1064 nm Nd:YAG laser,[74,75] although the latter wavelength has not proved effective in several reports.[73,74] Similar results have been reported with amiodarone-induced hyperpigmentation treated with the Q-switched ruby laser.[76] In order to prevent recurrences, laser treatment of these conditions should be deferred until the offending medication has been discontinued and sufficient time has elapsed to allow most of the pigmentation to resolve spontaneously.

Q-switched laser treatment may cause paradoxical hyperpigmentation in patients receiving certain medications. In one report, localized chrysiasis developed in a patient on parenteral gold therapy who underwent treatment with a Q-switched ruby laser for postinflammatory hyperpigmentation.[77] This phenomenon is due to a laser-induced alteration in the physiochemical properties of dermal gold deposits and resembles the pigment darkening that may occur following Q-switched laser treatment of tattoos containing iron oxide or titanium dioxide (see the next section).

Tattoos. Tattoos are produced when an exogenous pigment is implanted traumatically or intentionally into the dermis. In most amateur tattoos, a crude instrument is used to drive a carbon-based pigment such as india ink into the skin. Pigment is usually lightly concentrated within various levels of the dermis. In contrast, professional tattoos are made with an electric tattoo machine that uses rapidly vibrating needles to repeatedly puncture the skin. Pigment is densely concentrated primarily at the junction of the papillary and reticular dermis.[9] Professional tattoo pigments are composed of mixtures of metallic salts and organic dyes. Common pigments include mercuric oxide (red), cadmium sulfide (yellow), chromium salts (green), cobalt salts (dark blue), titanium dioxide (white), and iron oxide (red-brown). Although tattooing is widely practiced, there is virtually no federal and inconsistent state regulation of the industry. The FDA does not regulate the manufacture or use of tattoo pigment, despite the potential for infection, allergic reaction, and metal toxicity.[78]

After a tattoo is placed, an initial inflammatory healing phase occurs in which ink is internalized by a variety of cells, including keratinocytes, fibroblasts, and macrophages.[79] Clinically, slight erythema, induration, crusting, and tenderness occur at the tattoo site, lasting about 10 days.[80] Although tattoo needles deposit pigment within both epidermis and dermis, only dermal pigment remains permanently, as the epidermis typically sloughs within 1 week after tattoo placement. During this time, inflammatory cells carry some dermal pigment to the skin surface through the disrupted epidermis. The epidermis and basement membrane regenerate within 1 month, preventing further loss of pigment via this route. Thereafter, tattoos evolve in a slowly progressive manner over the course of the bearer's lifetime. Some pigment is gradually carried

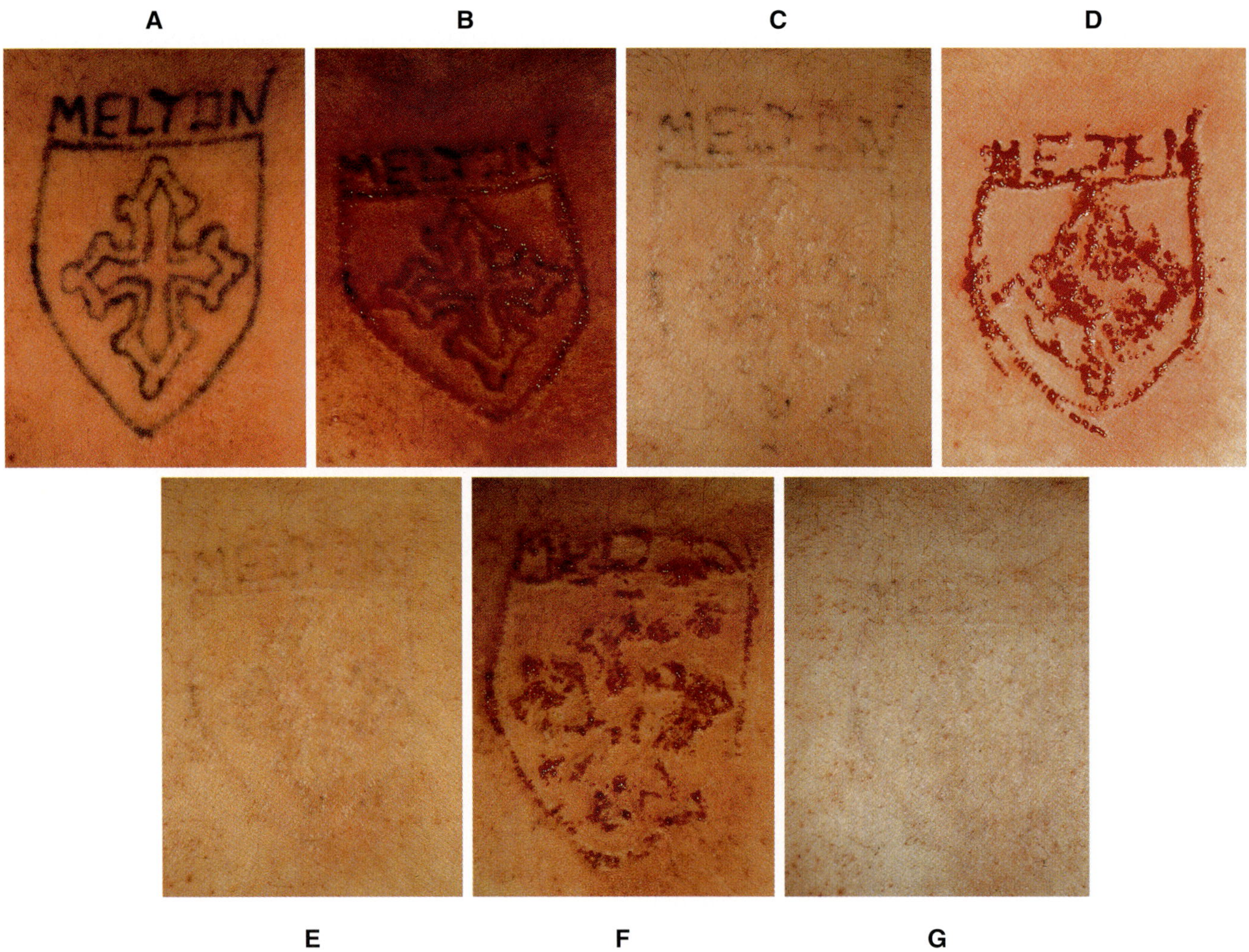

FIG. 12-8
A, An amateur tattoo of the back of a young man prior to treatment. **B,** Immediately after Q-switched Nd:YAG laser treatment, there is some epidermal disruption and hemorrhage. **C,** Six weeks after the first treatment, there is dramatic lightening of the tattoo. **D,** Immediately after the second treatment, there is an epidermal disruption and hemorrhage. **E,** Six weeks after the second treatment, there is improved lightening of the tattoo. **F,** Immediately after the third treatment with the Q-switched Nd:YAG laser, there is some epidermal disruption but less hemorrhage. This is accounted for by the decreasing amount of pigment after two treatments. **G,** The tattoo 6 weeks after the third treatment.

out of the skin into the lymphatic system by macrophages. Older tattoos contain only a fraction of the original pigment, which is contained primarily within dermal fibroblasts surrounded by a prominent connective tissue network.[79]

Q-switched lasers can lighten almost all tattoos, but the degree of clearing depends on pigment density, color, and composition. Black amateur tattoos generally respond well, typically clearing within 3 to 6 treatment sessions (Fig. 12-8). The response of densely pigmented, multicolored professional tattoos is far more variable. These tattoos typically require 6 to 12 treatment sessions for clearing but may require up to 20 sessions.[81] Although most tattoos can be lightened significantly, it is often not possible to achieve true 100% clearing, as small pockets of ink may persist in the skin despite repeated treatments[81] (Fig. 12-9). Tattoos located on the distal extremities may be more resistant to treatment, possibly because of decreased lymphatic drainage from these areas.[81] Because they contain less pigment, older tattoos may require fewer treatment sessions than fresh tattoos containing dense deposits of ink.

No single laser can remove all tattoo colors. The Q-switched ruby[82-84] and alexandrite[85-87] lasers are most useful for the treatment of black, blue, and green colors, while the Q-switched 1064 nm Nd:YAG laser[88] effectively treats black and blue pigment (not green). The 510 nm pulsed dye[89] and Q-switched 532 nm Nd:YAG[81] lasers are most effective for treatment of red and yellow colors. In vitro agarose gel assays have revealed that the newer 585 nm and 650 nm wavelengths of the Nd:YAG laser are absorbed by sky blue and green pigment, respectively.[90]

There are few well-controlled studies comparing different Q-switched lasers. Zelickson et al. compared the efficacy of various Q-switched lasers on a spectrum of tattoo colors in hairless guinea pigs.[91] They found that black pigment responded best to the alexandrite and Nd:YAG lasers (1064 and 532 nm), while purple pigment responded best to the QSRL. In addition, they found that the alexandrite laser was most effective for removing blue and green pigment, the 1064 nm Nd:YAG laser was best for removing red-brown, dark brown, and orange pigment, and the 532 nm Nd:YAG laser was best for treating red pigment. In contrast, several studies in humans found that the QSRL was more effective than other lasers in the treatment of black ink.[92-94] The enhanced efficacy of the QSRL in these reports may have been the result of its larger spot size (6.5 mm) rather than its precise wavelength. Indeed, DeCoste and Anderson found that, when the QSRL and Nd:YAG lasers were used at the same fluence and spot size, there was no difference in the lightening of blue-black tattoos.[95]

Tattoos showing signs of allergic reaction such as erythema, induration, or pruritus should not be treated with Q-switched lasers to avoid triggering a generalized allergic reaction.[96] Q-switched laser treatment releases pigment into the extracellular space, where it may be recognized by the immune system as a foreign body. Tattoos with localized reactions can be treated nonselectively with a continuous wave carbon dioxide laser, but textural change will result inevitably.[97] Extreme caution is advised when treating cosmetic tattoos that commonly exhibit shades of white, red, orange, tan, or brown.[98] These tattoos are at risk for immediate, irreversible pigment darkening after laser exposure because of reduction of pigment containing iron oxide or titanium dioxide. Should this paradoxical darkening occur, there are limited therapeutic options available.

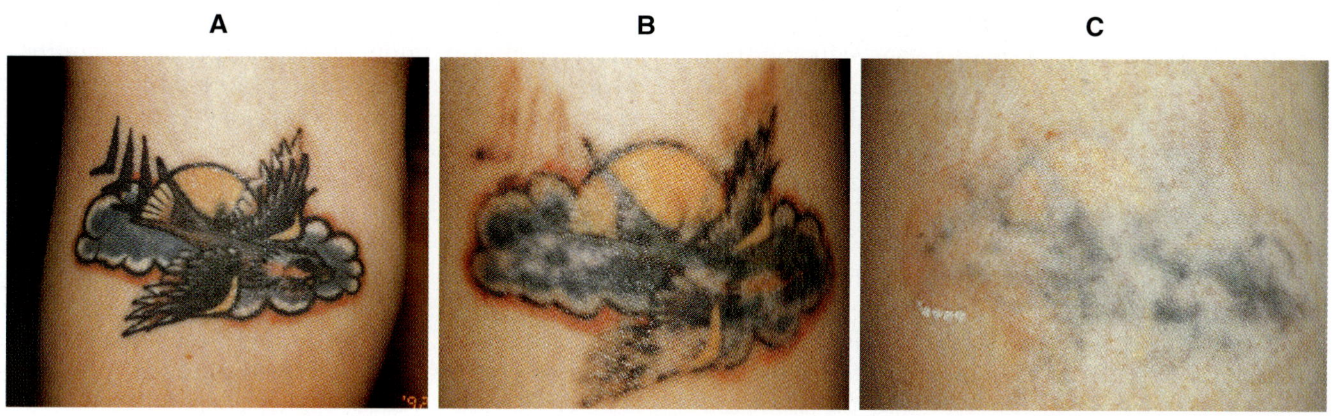

FIG. 12-9
A, Multicolored tattoo of the arm prior to treatment. **B,** The tattoo after three treatments with both the Q-switched ruby and Q-switched Nd:YAG laser. **C,** Tattoo after six treatments shows dramatic lightening of all colors of the tattoo but some residual tattoo ink. Incomplete clearing of tattoos is not uncommon with Q-switched laser treatment.

The darkened pigment may respond to further treatment with Q-switched lasers. Alternatively, it can be excised. To minimize the risk of pigment darkening, test spots should be performed prior to treating any cosmetic tattoo. The test site should be evaluated about 10 minutes after exposure, since immediate skin whitening may temporarily obscure the color change.

SECTION TWO

Atlas of Surgical Procedures

PREOPERATIVE CLINICAL CONSIDERATIONS

Safety Procedures

The primary hazard of Q-switched laser treatment is retinal injury, which can occur from direct exposure or reflection from a shiny surface such as the face of a watch. Infrared wavelengths such as 1064 nm are particularly insidious because they are invisible. The retina does not sense pain and the first symptom of ocular injury may be blindness. Protective goggles covering the appropriate wavelength must be worn by all personnel in the treatment room. In the treatment of a multicolored tattoo, the use of two or more lasers may be necessary, each requiring the use of different goggles. If treatment is in the immediate periocular area, protective metal eye shields should be inserted over the conjunctiva after the application of a topical ophthalmic anesthetic agent. A nonflammable, water-based lubricant such as Surgilube or K-Y Jelly should be applied to the eyebrows to avoid singeing the hair. The room should be designed in such a way that all reflective surfaces and windows are covered, the door is locked from the inside, appropriate signs are posted, and no flammable materials or anesthetics are present.

Q-switched laser pulses may produce a significant amount of blood and tissue splatter, especially the 1064 nm Nd:YAG laser. Use of universal precautions is mandatory, including use of gloves, goggles, and laser masks. The protective plastic cone provided with most Q-switched lasers should always be attached to the handpiece before use to minimize tissue splatter and keep tissue debris off the handpiece lens. The plastic cone must be placed in direct contact with the skin to efficiently trap tissue debris. To minimize tissue splatter, pulses may be delivered through a clear hydrogel dressing (e.g., Tegaderm) placed on the skin, although this reduces transmission of light into the skin and raises the risk of ocular injury from reflection of light off the dressing surface. Vacuum suction is useless at capturing tissue splatter because it leaves the surface of the skin far too rapidly.

All makeup and sunblock should be removed from the area to be treated, as these products will prevent transmission of light to the skin surface. Furthermore, many of these products contain metal-based salts and oxides (such as titanium dioxide) that may ignite following exposure to Q-switched laser pulses.

Anesthesia

The need for anesthesia when treating pigmented lesions and tattoos depends on the location and size of the lesion as well as the pain threshold of the patient. The sensation of a laser pulse at low fluences has been likened to a rubber band snapping against the skin surface. The higher fluences used in the treatment of dermal pigmented lesions such as nevus of Ota or tattoos produce more discomfort and are more likely to require some type of anesthesia. When limited areas are treated, such as small tattoos or scattered lentigines, many patients require no anesthesia at all. For the treatment of larger tattoos or pigmented lesions, one or more of the following anesthetic techniques may be required: topical anesthesia (e.g., EMLA or ELA-Max cream), local infiltration of lidocaine with or without epinephrine, regional nerve block, or oral or intramuscular sedation. In many children and rarely in adults, intravenous sedation or general anesthesia may be necessary. Following treatment, the use of ice packs is helpful to reduce postoperative discomfort and swelling.

Patient Evaluation

A general medical history should be obtained prior to treatment, including information on wound healing, any bleeding diatheses, or history of infectious diseases, particularly hepatitis and HIV infection. The presence of HIV proviral DNA has been demonstrated in the laser plume generated by carbon dioxide laser irradiation of HIV-infected tissue culture.[99] Patients with a history of isotretinoin use within the last 6 months or history of hypertrophic scarring should be treated with caution because they may have a higher risk of scarring after laser treatment.

Before treating any pigmented lesion, it is imperative to correctly diagnose the lesion in question. A pretreatment biopsy should be performed if there is any question of atypia in a pigmented lesion or if the diagnosis is at all unsure. Once the correct diagnosis has been established, the appropriate laser can be selected based on the probable depth of pigment in the skin (i.e., epidermal vs. dermal), its type, and the way it is packaged.

Many patients are ill-informed and harbor unrealistic expectations about the benefits of laser surgery. Patients should be fully informed of what to expect from each treatment, potential side effects, and that there is no guarantee that the lesion will clear entirely.

PROCEDURAL TECHNIQUES

Epidermal Pigmented Lesions

Technique. Anesthesia is usually not required for treatment of epidermal lesions. When needed, a topical anesthetic may be sufficient (e.g., EMLA or ELA-Max cream under occlusion applied for at least 1 hour). Infiltration of lidocaine into the skin, although effective in providing anesthesia, often causes as much discomfort as the treatment itself.

The laser should always be calibrated prior to treatment. The laser handpiece should be held perpendicular to the skin with the attached plastic cone or guide resting on the skin to ensure that the laser beam is focused on the area to be treated. Exact parameters vary depending on the particular laser, the patient's Fitzpatrick skin type, and the type of lesion (Table 12-3). In general, lower fluence is used for dark lesions that contain larger amounts of absorbing chromophore. One or two laser pulses should be fired at the lesion to ensure that a threshold response occurs, which is defined as immediate whitening of the skin. The optimal tissue end point is uniform but faint immediate whitening without epidermal disruption.

If the fluence is too low, the whitening will be barely perceptible. If the fluence is too high, whitening is bright white and solid, and epidermal damage with bleeding may occur. When fluences less than threshold are used, hyperpigmentation due to stimulation of melanogenesis can result. Use of excessive fluences may cause tissue sloughing, prolonged healing, and a greater likelihood of postinflammatory hyperpigmentation or hypopigmentation or textural changes. After the optimal fluence is determined, pulses can be delivered rapidly (up to 10 Hz, depending on the laser), with overlapping of about 10% to ensure confluent whitening.

Patients with darker skin (phototypes IV and V) should be treated with caution at lower fluences, since their threshold response will likely occur at lower fluences than patients with lighter skin. Patients with "suntans" should not be treated because they are at risk of spotty hypopigmentation, which can last for weeks to months after treatment.

In most cases, additional treatment sessions may be safely performed 6 weeks after the original treatment. While some pigmented lesions (e.g., lentigines) may require only one to two treatments, other lesions (e.g., café au lait macules) may need multiple treatments.

Table 12-3 Standard Treatment Parameters for Pigmented Lesions and Tattoos

Lesion	Laser	Spot Size (mm)	Fluence (J/cm^2)	Retreatment Interval
Lentigines	QS ruby	6.5	2.0-4.0	4-8 weeks
	QS Nd:YAG (532 nm)	3	0.7-1.0	
	QS alexandrite	3	4.0-6.0	
	Pulsed dye (510 nm)	3	2.5	
Café au lait macules	QS ruby	6.5	3.0-4.5	4-8 weeks
	QS Nd:YAG (532 nm)	3	1.0-1.5	
	QS alexandrite	3	2.5-3.5	
	Pulsed dye (510 nm)	5	2.0-3.5	
Becker's nevus	QS ruby	6.5	3.0-4.5	4-8 weeks
	QS Nd:YAG (532 nm)	3	1.5-1.8	
	QS Nd:YAG (1064 nm)	3	4.0-5.0	
	QS alexandrite	3	5.0-6.0	
Nevus spilus	QS ruby	6.5	3.0-4.5	4-8 weeks
	QS Nd:YAG (532 nm)	3	1.5-2.0	
	QS Nd:YAG (1064 nm)	3	4.0-4.4	
	QS alexandrite	3	4.0-6.0	
Nevus of Ota	QS ruby	6.5	5.0-6.0	6-12 weeks
	QS Nd:YAG (1064 nm)	3	4.0-5.0	
	QS alexandrite	3	5.5-6.5	
Tattoos	QS ruby	5	7.0-10.0	6-12 weeks
		6.5	3.0-6.0	
	QS Nd:YAG (532 nm)	3	2.0-3.5	
	QS Nd:YAG (1064 nm)	3	4.0-8.0	
	QS alexandrite	3	6.0-6.5	
	Pulsed dye (510 nm)	3-5	2.5-3.5	

QS, Q-switched.

Postoperative Changes. The white tissue response that develops immediately after treatment fades within 20 minutes. An urticarial reaction, causing erythema, edema, itching, and stinging, may develop in and around the treated area. This may last for several hours and can be treated, but not prevented, by taking an antihistamine preoperatively. The treated area may actually appear darker for several days before developing a crust that falls off in 7 to 10 days, depending on the site and aggressiveness of treatment. Following treatment with the Q-switched 532 nm Nd:YAG or 510 nm pulsed dye lasers, purpura usually develops after skin whitening has faded. This occurs because, in addition to being absorbed by melanin, these wavelengths are well absorbed by hemoglobin, causing rupture of blood vessels. Purpura persists for 5 to 7 days, and its occurrence is a distinct disadvantage of treatment with the above devices.

Postoperative Care. Postoperative discomfort may be treated with application of cold water–soaked gauze, ice packs, or a hydroocclusive dressing such as Second Skin or Vigilon. Analgesics are usually not needed. Patients should be instructed to gently wash the treated area with mild soap and apply an occlusive ointment (e.g., Aquaphor Healing Ointment) twice a day. Any crusting should be allowed to slough spontaneously. In order to minimize the risk of hyperpigmentation, patients should avoid excessive sun exposure and use a broad-spectrum sunscreen of SPF 30 or higher for at least several months after treatment.

Dermal Pigmented Lesions

Technique. Anesthesia is rarely required for small lesions. For larger lesions, use of topical anesthetics, local infiltration of lidocaine, or regional nerve blocks may be required. In the treatment of nevus of Ota, nerve blocks plus supplemental infiltration of lidocaine usually provide excellent anesthesia. Nerve blocks are performed with 1% or 2% lidocaine with 1:100,000 or 1:200,000 epinephrine. The forehead may be anesthetized by blocking the supraorbital and supratrochlear nerves, branches of the ophthalmic division of the trigeminal nerve. The supraorbital nerve exits from the supraorbital notch, located in the midpupillary line in the supraorbital ridge, while the supratrochlear nerve exits from the supratrochlear notch at the medial edge of the eyebrow. The lower eyelid, medial cheek, upper lip, and part of the medial nose may be anesthetized by blocking the infraorbital nerve, which exits in the midpupillary line 1 cm below the infraorbital ridge. Although infraorbital blocks can be performed transcutaneously, it is often preferable to inject through the mouth after numbing the buccal mucosa with topical benzocaine or tetracaine. For local tissue infiltration, especially around the eyes, a mixture of equal parts of 2% lidocaine with 1:100,000 epinephrine and 0.5% bupivacaine, plus 75 U of hyaluronidase (Wydase), provides effective and long-lasting anesthesia. The hyaluronidase facilitates tissue diffusion of anesthetic.

The laser should always be calibrated prior to treatment. Actual treatment technique is similar to that used for treatment of epidermal lesions, with the handpiece held perpendicular to the skin, the protective cone held flush with the skin surface, and pulses delivered with approximately 10% overlap. Exact parameters vary depending on type of lesion, choice of laser, and patient skin phototype (see Table 12-3). In general, dermal lesions require higher fluences than epidermal lesions. Treatment should start with just one or two laser pulses fired onto the lesion to ensure that the threshold whitening response occurs. An end point of uniform whitening of the irradiated site is desirable. Use of subthreshold fluences may result in poor efficacy and postinflammatory hyperpigmentation. Suprathreshold fluences may produce excessive epidermal injury and bleeding, resulting in increased patient discomfort and prolonged wound healing, as well as an increased risk of postoperative pigmentary and textural change.

Lower fluences should be used in the treatment of patients with darker skin types, since the threshold response will likely occur at a lower fluence. Patients with darker skin are at greater risk for postoperative hyperpigmentation or hypopigmentation. It may be preferable to utilize a longer wavelength device, such as the 1064 nm Nd:YAG laser, since longer wavelengths are less absorbed by melanin and produce less epidermal damage.

In general, dermal pigmented lesions require multiple treatment sessions for maximal clearing. Treatment is usually performed at 4- to 6-week intervals or longer. Lesions such as nevus of Ota will continue to gradually lighten for several months after each treatment session.

Postoperative Changes. Because dermal lesions typically require the use of higher fluences, postoperative changes are more apparent. The whitening response that occurs immediately after treatment fades within 20 minutes. Erythema and swelling are usually seen in the immediate postoperative period, especially in the periorbital area of the face. The amount of crusting that occurs depends on the aggressiveness of treatment. Crust generally falls off spontaneously within 10 days. The treated area will appear darker for up to 10 days until the superficial scale/crust sloughs. Overly aggressive treatment may result in vesiculation or frank blistering. The risk of blistering is highest when shorter wavelength devices (e.g., QSRL) are used to treat patients with dark skin phototypes.

Postoperative Care. Ice packs, cold water–soaked gauze, or hydroocclusive dressings (e.g., Second Skin,

Vigilon) help reduce immediate postoperative discomfort and swelling. Patients should wash the treated area gently and apply an occlusive ointment (e.g., Aquaphor Healing Ointment) at least twice a day. Analgesics more potent than acetaminophen are rarely required. To reduce the risk of hyperpigmentation, patients should avoid excessive sun exposure and wear a broad-spectrum sunscreen for at least several months after treatment.

Tattoos

Technique. Patients must be counseled appropriately based on tattoo type (amateur or professional), color, ink density, age, body location, and patient skin phototype. In appropriately selected tattoos (e.g., blue or black amateur tattoos), dramatic lightening can be expected. On the other hand, patients with multicolored, intensely pigmented, professional tattoos should be informed that 100% clearing of pigment is unlikely. Tattoo treatment typically requires multiple treatment sessions for maximal lightening. Traditional treatment modalities such as excision or CW carbon dioxide laser may be less costly in time and expense because fewer treatment sessions are required,[100] but only Q-switched lasers offer the potential for tattoo clearing without scarring. Preoperative photographs should be taken to provide objective evidence of treatment response. Patients with cosmetic tattoos should be informed of the risk of immediate pigment darkening.

Anesthesia is often not required for small tattoos, but larger tattoos usually require the use of topical anesthetics or local infiltration of lidocaine. For infiltrating lidocaine, a 30-gauge needle should be used to minimize patient discomfort. Use of a 1-inch needle permits infiltration of anesthetic into large areas via a fanning motion, minimizing the number of needle insertions into the skin.

Treatment technique is similar to that outlined for treatment of dermal lesions. The laser handpiece should be held perpendicular to the skin and pulses delivered in a slightly overlapping manner to avoid leaving untreated fragments of tattoo. Exact parameters vary based on tattoo color, ink density, laser chosen, and patient skin phototype (see Table 12-3). Generally, high-energy fluences are required for the optimal removal of tattoos. The desired clinical end point is immediate, bright tissue whitening. At the start of treatment, one or two laser pulses should be fired at the tattoo to determine the tissue response, with fluence adjusted accordingly. The presence of significant epidermal disruption or bleeding indicates use of excessive fluence, although pinpoint bleeding is acceptable with the 1064 nm Nd:YAG laser. In general, lower fluence is used for dark tattoos that contain large amounts of absorbing chromophore. In subsequent treatment sessions, the fluence may need to be increased as the amount of pigmentation decreases. Fluences should be decreased when treating patients with darker skin phototypes, since the threshold for skin whitening is lower. The 1064 nm Nd:YAG laser is the treatment of choice for blue or black tattoos in darkly pigmented patients, since its longer wavelength largely spares epidermal melanocytes.[101]

Multicolored tattoos require the use of multiple-wavelength devices. When switching between lasers, extreme caution is required to ensure that correct goggles are worn. If adequate energy is available from the laser, it is best to use the largest spot size because it promotes deeper penetration of light and shortens the treatment time. Treatment duration depends on tattoo size as well as on the available spot size and repetition rate of the given machine. Treatment sessions should be performed at intervals of 1 month or longer. Some patients will notice that the tattoo ink continues to lighten for several months following treatment.

Postoperative Changes. Skin whitening fades within 20 minutes of treatment. Some erythema and swelling usually develop around the tattoo, although edema is generally insignificant unless the periorbital area or an extended area is treated. Patients can expect a surface crust that falls off within 10 to 14 days. True vesiculation is not uncommon for the first day or two after treatment, particularly when shorter-wavelength devices are used (e.g., QSRL). In the vast majority of cases, tattoos heal without any permanent alteration in skin texture.

Postoperative Care. Postoperative stinging, which usually lasts less than 6 hours, may be treated with ice packs, cold water–soaked gauze, or hydroocclusive dressings (e.g., Second Skin, Vigilon). If swelling develops, keep the area elevated. Wash the treated site gently with mild soap and cover with an occlusive ointment (e.g., Aquaphor Healing Ointment or bacitracin) at least twice a day. Any crusting should be allowed to slough spontaneously. Alternatively, oxygen-permeable dressings (e.g., Opsite, Tegaderm) can be used for several days to promote moist wound healing. Acetaminophen is generally sufficient to control postoperative discomfort. Patients should avoid sun exposure in the postoperative period because resultant hyperpigmentation will interfere with subsequent treatment sessions and raise the risk of hypopigmentation.

Complications

Although Q-switched lasers are far safer than traditional treatment modalities, treatment is not without some risk. In general, because treatment of dermal lesions and tattoos is more aggressive, it is associated with a higher risk of side effects than treatment of epidermal lesions. The most common side effect is the occurrence of pigmentary change. Hyperpigmentation is commonly seen in patients with darker skin phototypes but almost always resolves with time. Use of topical hydroquinone creams may help speed resolution. Patients at risk for hyperpigmentation should avoid sun exposure and use a UVA/UVB sunblock of SPF 30 or higher for at least several months after treatment. Transient hypopigmentation is also common, but true depigmentation is extremely rare. The risk of hypopigmentation is wavelength dependent, with shorter-wavelength devices such as the QSRL posing higher risk due to greater injury to epidermal melanocytes.

The risk of scarring with pigment-specific lasers is extremely low. When appropriate parameters are used, the risk of scarring from treatment of epidermal lesions is negligible. In the treatment of tattoos, the risk is reported to be less than 5%.[81] Scarring is associated with the use of excessive fluences or very small spot sizes that cause a greater degree of tissue damage. Tattoos located on the chest, deltoid, or ankle as well as those with dense deposits of ink (e.g., "double tattoos") have a higher risk of scarring.[102] The act of tattooing may itself produce subtle textural change that remains unnoticed by the patient until after the pigment has cleared. Preoperative photographs provide essential documentation.

REFERENCES

1. Goldman L, Blaney DJ, Kindel DJ, Franke EK. Effect of the laser beam on the skin: preliminary report. J Invest Dermatol 1963; 40:121-122.
2. Goldman L, Wilson RG, Hornby P, Meyer RG. Radiation from a Q-switched ruby laser: effect of repeated impacts of power output of 10 megawatts on a tattoo of man. J Invest Dermatol 1965; 44:69-71.
3. Ohshiro T, Maruyama Y. The ruby and argon lasers in the treatment of naevi. Ann Acad Med 1983; 12:388-395.
4. Dover JS, Smoller BR, Stein RS, et al. Low-fluence carbon dioxide laser irradiation of lentigines. Arch Dermatol 1988; 124:1219-1224.
5. Anderson RR, Parrish JA. Selective photothermolysis: precise microsurgery by selective absorption of pulsed radiation. Science 1983; 220:524-527.
6. Anderson RR, Parrish JA. The optics of human skin. J Invest Dermatol 1981; 77:13-19.
7. Polla LL, Margolis RJ, Dover JS, et al. Melanosomes are a primary target of Q-switched ruby laser irradiation in guinea pig skin. J Invest Dermatol 1987; 89:281-286.
8. Hodersdal M, Bech-Thomsen N, Wulf HC. Skin reflectance-guided laser selections for treatment of decorative tattoos. Arch Dermatol 1996; 132:403-407.
9. Taylor CR, Anderson RR, Gange RW, et al. Light and electron microscopic analysis of tattoos treated by Q-switched ruby laser. J Invest Dermatol 1991; 97:131-136.
10. Ross EV, Naseef G, Lin C, et al. Comparison of responses of tattoos to picosecond and nanosecond Q-switched neodymium: YAG lasers. Arch Dermatol 1998; 134:167-171.
11. Levins PC, Anderson RR. Q-switched ruby laser for the treatment of pigmented lesions and tattoos. Clin Dermatol 1995; 13: 75-79.
12. Murphy GF, Shepard RS, Paul BS, et al. Organelle-specific injury to melanin-containing cells in human skin by pulsed laser irradiation. Lab Invest 1983; 49:680-685.
13. Sherwood KA, Murray S, Kurban AK, Tan OT. Effect of wavelength on cutaneous pigment using pulsed irradiation. J Invest Dermatol 1989; 92:717-720.
14. Margolis RJ, Dover JS, Polla LL, et al. Visible action spectrum for melanin-specific selective photothermolysis. Laser Surg Med 1989; 9:389-397.
15. Anderson RR, Margolis RJ, Watenabe S, et al. Selective photothermolysis of cutaneous pigmentation by Q-switched Nd:YAG laser pulses at 1064, 532, and 355 nm. J Invest Dermatol 1989; 93:28-32.
16. Ara G, Anderson RR, Mandel KG, et al. Irradiation of pigmented melanoma cells with high intensity pulsed radiation generates acoustic waves and kills cells. Laser Surg Med 1990; 10:52-59.
17. Dover JS, Margolis RJ, Polla LL, et al. Pigmented guinea pig skin irradiated with Q-switched ruby laser pulses. Arch Dermatol 1989; 125:43-49.
18. Hruza GJ, Dover JS, Flotte TJ, et al. Q-switched ruby laser irradiation of normal human skin. Arch Dermatol 1991; 127:1799-1805.
19. Nakamura Y, Hossain M, Hirayama K, Matsumoto K. A clinical study on the removal of gingival melanin pigmentation with the CO_2 laser. Laser Surg Med 1999; 25:140-147.
20. Ross EV, Ladin Z, Kreindel M, Dierickx C. Theoretical considerations in laser hair removal. Dermatol Clin 1999; 17:333-355.
21. Ueda S, Imayama S. Normal-mode ruby laser for treating congenital nevi. Arch Dermatol 1997; 133:355-359.
22. Imayama S, Ueda S. Long- and short-term histological observations of congenital nevi treated with the normal-mode ruby laser. Arch Dermatol 1999; 135:1211-1218.
23. Gold MH, Foster TD, Bell MW. Nevus spilus successfully treated with an intense pulsed light source. Dermatol Surg 1999; 25:254-255.
24. Taylor CR, Anderson RR. Treatment of benign pigmented epidermal lesions by Q-switched ruby laser. Int J Dermatol 1993; 32:908-912.
25. Tse Y, Levine VJ, McClain SA, Ashinoff R. The removal of cutaneous pigmented lesions with the Q-switched ruby laser and the Q-switched neodymium:yttrium-aluminum-garnet laser. J Dermatol Surg Oncol 1994; 20:795-800.
26. Kilmer SL, Wheeland RG, Goldberg DJ, Anderson RR. Treatment of epidermal pigmented lesions with the frequency-doubled Q-switched Nd:YAG laser. Arch Dermatol 1994; 130:1515-1519.
27. Fitzpatrick RE, Goldman MP, Ruiz-Esparza J. Laser treatment of benign pigmented epidermal lesions using a 300 nsecond pulse and 510 nm wavelength. J Dermatol Surg Oncol 1993; 18:341-347.
28. Ashinoff R, Geronemus RG. Q-switched ruby laser treatment of labial lentigos. J Am Acad Dermatol 1992; 27:809-811.
29. Gupta G, MacKay IR, MacKie RM. Q-switched ruby laser in the treatment of labial melanotic macules. Laser Surg Med 1999; 25:219-222.
30. Yung-Tsai L, Kao-Chia Y. Comparison of the frequency-doubled Q-switched Nd:YAG laser and 35% trichloroacetic acid for the treatment of face lentigines. Dermatol Surg 1999; 25:202-204.
31. Todd M, Rallis T, Hata T. A comparison of three lasers and liquid nitrogen in the treatment of solar lentigines: a randomized, controlled, comparative trial. Arch Dermatol 2000; 50:536-540.
32. Grossman MC, Anderson RR, Farinelli W, et al. Treatment of cafe au lait macules with lasers: a clinicopathologic correlation. Arch Dermatol 1995; 131:1416-1420.
33. Alster TS. Complete elimination of large cafe-au-lait birthmarks by the 510-nm pulsed dye laser. Plast Reconstr Surg 1995; 96: 1660.

34. Alora MB, Arndt KA. Successful treatment of a cafe-au-lait macule with the erbium:YAG laser. J Am Acad Dermatol 2000. In press.
35. Goldberg DJ. Benign pigmented lesions of the skin. J Dermatol Surg Oncol 1993; 19:376-379.
36. Rosio TJ. Techniques for tattoo removal. In: Wheeland RG, ed. Cutaneous Surgery. Philadelphia: WB Saunders; 1994:982-997.
37. Kobayashi T. Microsurgical treatment of nevus of Ota. J Dermatol Surg Oncol 1991; 17:936-941.
38. Clabaugh WA. Tattoo removal by superficial dermabrasion: five year experience. Plast Reconstr Surg 1975; 55:401-405.
39. Koerber WA, Price NM. Salabrasion of tattoos: a correlation of the clinical and histological results. Arch Dermatol 1978; 114:884-888.
40. Dvir E, Hirshowitz B. Tattoo removal by cryosurgery. Plast Reconstr Surg 1980; 66:373-378.
41. Cosman B, Apfelberg DB, Drucker D. An effective cosmetic treatment for Ota's nevus. Ann Plast Surg 1989; 22:36-42.
42. Reid R, Muller S. Tattoo removal by CO_2 laser dermabrasion. Plast Reconstr Surg 1980; 65:717-728.
43. Hidano A, Kajama H, Ikeda S, et al. Natural history of nevus of Ota. Arch Dermatol 1967; 95:187-195.
44. Jay B. Malignant melanoma of the orbit in a case of oculodermal melanocytosis (nevus of Ota). Br J Ophthalmol 1965; 49:359.
45. Watanabe S, Takahashi H. Treatment of nevus of Ota with the Q-switched ruby laser. N Engl J Med 1994; 331:1745-1750.
46. Geronemus RG. Q-switched ruby laser therapy of nevus of Ota. Arch Dermatol 1992; 128:1618-1622.
47. Lowe NJ, Wieder JM, Sawcer D, et al. Nevus of Ota: treatment with high energy fluences of the Q-switched ruby laser. J Am Acad Dermatol 1993; 29:997-1001.
48. Taylor CR, Flotte TJ, Gange W, Anderson RR. Treatment of nevus of Ota by Q-switched ruby laser. J Am Acad Dermatol 1994; 30:743-751.
49. Chang CJ, Nelson JS, Achauer BM. Q-switched ruby laser treatment of oculodermal melanosis (nevus of Ota). Plast Reconstr Surg 1996; 98:784-790.
50. Alster TS, Williams CM. Treatment of nevus of Ota by the Q-switched alexandrite laser. Dermatol Surg 1995; 21:592-596.
51. van Leeuwen RL, Dekker SW, Byers HR, et al. Modulation of $\alpha 4\beta 1$ and $\alpha 5\beta 1$ integrin expression: heterogenous effects of Q-switched ruby, Nd:YAG, and alexandrite lasers on melanoma cells in vitro. Laser Surg Med 1996; 18:63-71.
52. Dummer R, Kempf W, Burg G. Pseudo-melanoma after laser therapy. Dermatology 1998; 197:71-73.
53. Grevelink JM, van Leeuwen RL, Anderson RR, Byers R. Clinical and histological responses of congenital melanocytic nevi after single treatment with Q-switched lasers. Arch Dermatol 1997; 133:349-353.
54. Waldorf HA, Kauvar ANB, Geronemus RG. Treatment of small and medium congenital nevi with the Q-switched ruby laser. Arch Dermatol 1996; 132:301-304.
55. Vibhagool C, Byers R, Grevelink JM. Treatment of small nevomelanocytic nevi with a Q-switched ruby laser. J Am Acad Dermatol 1997; 36:738-741.
56. Rosenbach A, Williams CM, Alster TS. Comparison of the Q-switched alexandrite (755 nm) and Q-switched Nd:YAG (1064 nm) lasers in the treatment of benign melanocytic nevi. Dermatol Surg 1997; 23:239-245.
57. Duke D, Byers R, Sober AJ, et al. Treatment of benign and atypical nevi with the normal-mode ruby laser and the Q-switched ruby laser: clinical improvement but failure to completely eliminate nevomelanocytes. Arch Dermatol 1999; 135:290-296.
58. Milgraum SS, Cohen ME, Auletta MJ. Treatment of blue nevi with the Q-switched ruby laser. J Am Acad Dermatol 1995; 32: 307-310.
59. Arndt KA. Argon laser treatment of lentigo maligna. J Am Acad Dermatol 1984; 10:953-957.
60. Kopera D. Treatment of lentigo maligna with the carbon dioxide laser. Arch Dermatol 1995; 131:735-736.
61. Thissen M, Westerhof W. Lentigo maligna treated with ruby laser. Acta Derm Venereol 1997; 77:163.
62. Arndt KA. New pigmented macule appearing 4 years after argon laser treatment of lentigo maligna. J Am Acad Dermatol 1986; 14:1092.
63. Lee PK, Rosenberg CN, Tsao H, Sober AJ. Failure of Q-switched ruby laser to eradicate atypical-appearing solar lentigo: report of two cases. J Am Acad Dermatol 1998; 38:314-317.
64. Taylor CR, Anderson RR. Ineffective treatment of refractory melasma and postinflammatory hyperpigmentation by Q-switched ruby laser. J Dermatol Surg Oncol 1994; 20:592-597.
65. Nouri K, Bowes L, Chartier T, et al. Combination treatment of melasma with pulsed CO_2 laser followed by Q-switched alexandrite laser: a pilot study. Dermatol Surg 1999; 25:494-497.
66. Manaloto RMP, Alster T. Erbium:YAG laser resurfacing for refractory melasma. Dermatol Surg 1999; 25:121-123.
67. Lowe NJ, Wieder JM, Shorr N, et al. Infraorbital pigmented skin: preliminary observations of laser therapy. Dermatol Surg 1995; 21:767-770.
68. West TB, Alster TS. Improvement of infraorbital hyperpigmentation following carbon dioxide laser resurfacing. Dermatol Surg 1998; 24:615-616.
69. Dwyer CM, Cuddihy AM, Kerr REI, et al. Skin pigmentation due to minocycline treatment of facial dermatoses. Br J Dermatol 1993; 129:158-162.
70. Argenyi ZB, Finelli L, Bergfeld WF, et al. Minocycline-related cutaneous hyperpigmentation as demonstrated by light microscopy, electron microscopy and X-ray energy spectroscopy. J Cutan Pathol 1987; 14:176-180.
71. Collins P, Cotterill JA. Minocycline-induced pigmentation resolves after treatment with the Q-switched ruby laser. Br J Dermatol 1996; 135:317-319.
72. Knoell KA, Milgraum SS, Kutenplon M. Q-switched ruby laser treatment of minocycline-induced cutaneous hyperpigmentation. Arch Dermatol 1996; 132:1251-1253.
73. Tsao H, Dover JS. Treatment of minocycline-induced hyperpigmentation with the Q-switched ruby laser. Arch Dermatol 1996; 132:1250-1251.
74. Wilde JL, English JC, Finley EM. Minocycline-induced hyperpigmentation: treatment with the neodymium:YAG laser. Arch Dermatol 1997; 133:1344-1346.
75. Greve B, Schonermark MP, Raulin C. Minocycline-induced hyperpigmentation: treatment with the Q-switched Nd:YAG laser. Laser Surg Med 1998; 22:223-227.
76. Karrer S, Hohenleutner U, Szeimies RM, Landthaler M. Amiodarone-induced pigmentation resolves after treatment with the Q-switched ruby laser. Arch Dermatol 1999; 135:251-253.
77. Trotter MJ, Tron VA, Hollingdale J, Rivers JK. Localized chrysiasis induced by laser therapy. Arch Dermatol 1995; 131:1411-1414.
78. Tope WD. State and territorial regulation of tattooing in the United States. J Am Acad Dermatol 1995; 32:791-799.
79. Lea PJ, Pawlowski A. Human tattoo: electron microscopic assessment of epidermis, epidermal-dermal junction, and dermis. Int J Dermatol 1987; 26:453-458.
80. Sperry K. Tattoos and tattooing, part II: gross pathology, histopathology, medical complications, and applications. Am J Foren Med Pathol 1992; 13:7-17.
81. Kilmer SL, Anderson RR. Clinical use of the Q-switched ruby and the Q-switched Nd:YAG (1064 nm and 532 nm) lasers for treatment of tattoos. J Dermatol Surg Oncol 1993; 19:330-338.
82. Reid WH, Miller ID, Murphy MJ, et al. Q-switched ruby laser treatment of tattoos: a 9-year experience. Br J Plast Surg 1990; 43: 663-669.
83. Scheibner A, Kenny G, White W, Wheeland RG. A superior

method of tattoo removal using the Q-switched ruby laser. J Dermatol Surg Oncol 1990; 16:1091-1098.
84. Taylor CR, Gange RW, Dover JS, et al. Treatment of tattoos by Q-switched ruby laser: a dose-response study. Arch Dermatol 1990; 126:893-899.
85. Fitzpatrick RE, Goldman MP. Tattoo removal using the alexandrite laser. Arch Dermatol 1994; 130:1508-1514.
86. Stafford TJ, Lizek R, Tan OT. Role of the alexandrite laser for removal of tattoos. Laser Surg Med 1995; 17:32-38.
87. Alster TS. Q-switched alexandrite laser treatment (755 nm) of professional and amateur tattoos. J Am Acad Dermatol 1995; 33:69-73.
88. Kilmer SL, Lee MS, Grevelink JM, et al. The Q-switched Nd:YAG laser effectively treats tattoos: a controlled, dose-response study. Arch Dermatol 1993; 129:971-978.
89. Grekin RC, Shelton RM, Geisse JK, Frieden I. 510-nm pigmented lesion dye laser: its characteristics and clinical uses. J Dermatol Surg Oncol 1993; 19:380-387.
90. Kauvar ANB, Bigelman J, Geronemus RG. In-vitro analysis of tattoo pigment response to Q-switched and long pulsed lasers. Laser Surg Med 1999; 11(suppl):31.
91. Zelickson BD, Mehregan DA, Zarrin AA, et al. Clinical, histologic, and ultrastructural evaluation of tattoos treated with three laser systems. Laser Surg Med 1994; 15:364-372.
92. Levine VJ, Geronemus RG. Tattoo removal with the Q-switched ruby laser and the Q-switched Nd:YAG laser: a comparative study. Cutis 1995; 55:291-296.
93. Goyal S, Arndt KA, Stern RS, et al. Laser treatment of tattoos: a prospective, paired, comparison study of the Q-switched Nd:YAG (1064 nm), frequency-doubled Q-switched Nd:YAG (532 nm), and Q-switched ruby lasers. J Am Acad Dermatol 1997; 36:122-125.
94. Leuenberger ML, Mulas MW, Hata TR, et al. Comparison of the Q-switched alexandrite, Nd:YAG, and ruby lasers in treating blue-black tattoos. Dermatol Surg 1999; 25:10-14.
95. DeCoste SD, Anderson RR. Comparison of Q-switched ruby and Q-switched Nd:YAG laser treatment of tattoos. Laser Surg Med 1991; 3(suppl):64.
96. Ashinoff R, Levine VJ, Soter NA. Allergic reactions to tattoo pigment after laser treatment. Dermatol Surg 1995; 21:291-294.
97. Kyanko ME, Pontasch MJ, Brodell RT. Red tattoo reactions: treatment with the carbon dioxide laser. J Dermatol Surg Oncol 1989; 15:652-656.
98. Anderson RR, Geronemus R, Kilmer SL, et al. Cosmetic tattoo ink darkening: a complication of Q-switched and pulsed-laser treatment. Arch Dermatol 1993; 129:1010-1014.
99. Baggish MS, Poiesz BJ, Joret D, et al. Presence of human immunodeficiency virus DNA in laser smoke. Laser Surg Med 1991; 11:197-203.
100. Ort RJ, Arndt KA. Tattoos and their treatment: traditional treatments. Med Surg Dermatol 1999; 6:1-5.
101. Grevelink JM, Duke D, van Leeuwen RL, et al. Laser treatment of tattoos in darkly pigmented patients: efficacy and side effects. J Am Acad Dermatol 1996; 34:653-656.
102. Alora MBT, Arndt KA, Taylor CR. Scarring following Q-switched laser treatment of "double tattoos." Arch Dermatol 2000; 136:269-270.

CHAPTER 13

Laser Hair Removal

RICHARD J. ORT
CHRISTINE DIERICKX

SECTION ONE

History and Scientific Review

BACKGROUND AND HISTORY

Modern culture has created unwritten standards for acceptable levels of facial and body hair. In order to conform to society's expectations, millions of individuals either hide areas of excessive hair or attempt to reduce the amount of visible hair. Traditional methods of hair removal have included shaving, bleaching, plucking, waxing, use of chemical depilatories, and electrolysis. These techniques have been limited by their pain, inconvenience, and poor long-term efficacy. Only electrolysis has offered the potential for permanent hair removal, but the technique is tedious, highly operator dependent, and impractical for the treatment of large numbers of hairs. Recently, a number of lasers and other light sources have been developed specifically to target hair follicles. These devices offer the potential for rapid treatment of large areas and long-lasting hair removal. Physicians and patients alike have embraced this technology, although published studies assessing the permanency of hair removal have emerged only recently. With the proliferation of devices targeting hair and unsubstantiated claims by manufacturers, significant confusion exists in this field. This chapter will attempt to sort through the muddle by exploring hair follicle biology as well as the scientific underpinnings of hair removal by light before examining the attributes of specific laser systems. A detailed discussion of treatment guidelines as well as preoperative and postoperative considerations follows.

BASIC SCIENCE

Anatomy and Growth Cycle of the Hair Follicle

The hair follicle consists of three regions in vertical sections: the infundibulum, isthmus, and inferior segment (Fig. 13-1). The infundibulum is the uppermost portion of the follicle, extending from the skin surface to the sebaceous duct entrance. The isthmus is a short section that extends from the entrance of the sebaceous duct to the insertion of the arrector pili muscle. The inferior segment of the follicle lies below the arrector pili muscle insertion and includes the hair bulb and dermal papilla. The hair bulb represents an expansion of the lowermost portion of the follicle during its growing, or anagen, phase. It is made up of germinative matrix cells along with interspersed melanocytes. The hair bulb surrounds a core of richly vascularized connective tissue known as the dermal papilla.

Hair follicles show a cyclical pattern of growth, progressing from the growing (anagen) phase to the resting (telogen) phase via the intermediary (catagen) phase (Fig. 13-2). During anagen, matrix cells proliferate and move upward, giving rise to the hair shaft and inner root sheath. Anagen follicles of terminal hair extend deeply into the subcutaneous fat, lying 2 to 7 mm below the skin surface, depending on body site.[1] During catagen, cell division and melanin production in the bulb cease and the entire lower portion of the hair follicle undergoes apoptosis.[2] Only a thin cord of epithelial cells remains; it shrinks and retracts upward to become the secondary germ. The ensuing telogen phase represents a stage of follicular quiescence. When a new anagen phase begins, a burst of epithelial cell division occurs near the insertion of the arrector pili muscle and hair growth resumes as the secondary hair germ grows downward to form a new bulb.

Initially it was thought that follicular stem cells resided within or near the matrix of the hair bulb.[3,4] In mouse follicles, however, a population of slow-cycling stem cells has been found in a bulge coming off the outer root sheath.[5] The bulge is located at the site of attachment of the arrector pili muscle, approximately 1 mm below the skin surface. This represents the lower end of the "permanent" portion of the hair follicle.[5] Recently, follicular stem cells expressing cytokeratin 15

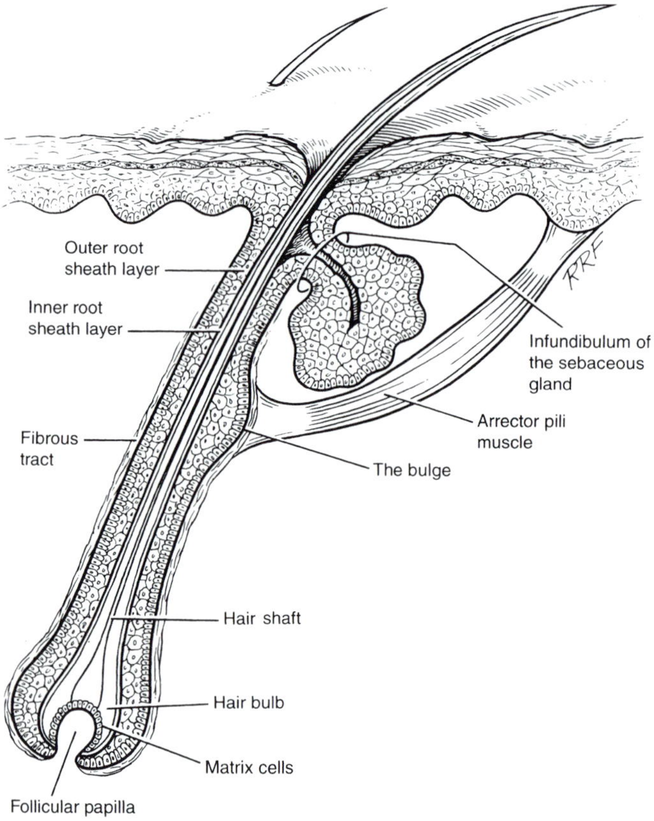

FIG. 13-1
Hair follicle anatomy. (From McDaniel DH, Lord J, Ash K, et al. Laser hair removal: a review and report on the use of the long-pulsed alexandrite laser for hair reduction of the upper lip, leg, back, and bikini region. Dermatol Surg 1999; 25:426-430.)

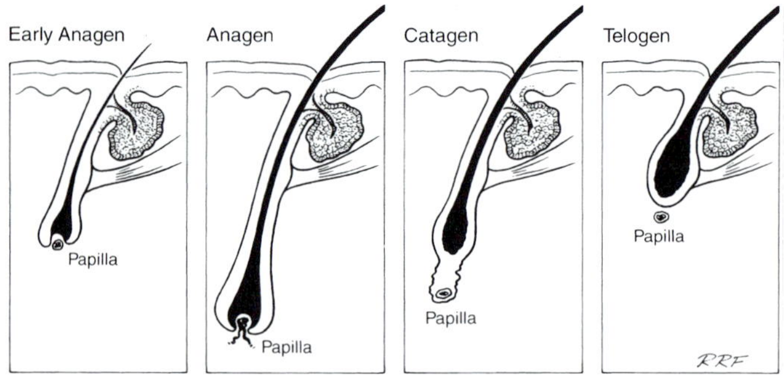

FIG. 13-2
The hair growth cycle. (From McDaniel DH, Lord J, Ash K, et al. Laser hair removal: a review and report on the use of the long-pulsed alexandrite laser for hair reduction of the upper lip, leg, back, and bikini region. Dermatol Surg 1999; 25:426-430.)

Table 13-1 Hair Cycle Estimates[7,8,18]

Body Area	Anagen Duration	Telogen Duration	Telogen Percentage
Scalp	2-6 years	3 months	15%
Face (beard, mustache)	2 months-1 year	1-3 months	33%
Extremities	1-6 months	2-6 months	75%

and β_1 integrin have been identified. It is now believed that, during late telogen or early anagen, the bulge stem cells are activated by dermal papilla cells and proliferate briefly to form the epithelial downgrowth before returning to their normally dormant state.

The duration of anagen and telogen phases, as well as the ratio of anagen to telogen hairs, depends on body location (Table 13-1). At any given time, about 84% of scalp hairs are in anagen phase, 2% in catagen phase, and 14% in telogen phase.[7] In contrast, over 50% of leg or arm hair is in telogen at any given time.[8] Since duration of anagen is the primary determinant of hair length, body sites with long hair have a prolonged anagen phase, whereas sites with shorter hair have a shorter anagen phase and a somewhat longer telogen phase. The anagen phase of scalp hair lasts up to 6 years, and the telogen phase lasts about 3 months.[1] In contrast, hairs on other body sites such as the extremities or trunk have anagen phases lasting from 1 to 6 months and telogen phases lasting up to 9 months.[1,8] This implies that long-lasting hair loss can be achieved by any method of hair removal that can induce telogen. To assess permanency of hair removal, it is necessary to follow patients for at least the duration of one complete hair cycle.

Hair color is dependent upon the type and amount of melanin within the hair shaft. Melanin is produced by melanocytes within the bulb, which transfer melanin granules to matrix cells. Melanin production occurs only during anagen, as melanocytes within the bulb degenerate during catagen. Follicular melanocytes produce two distinct types of melanin, eumelanin and pheomelanin. Dark hair contains abundant, heavily melanized eumelanin granules while red hair contains primarily pheomelanin granules. In gray hair, melanocytes show degenerative changes such as vacuolization and poorly melanized melanosomes, while in white hair melanocytes are greatly reduced in number or absent.[9]

The diameter and length of hair is variable, ranging from fine, nonpigmented vellus hairs to coarse terminal hairs. Hair shaft diameter is determined by the size of the dermal papilla and hair bulb.[10] In cross section, the diameter of the bulb from terminal hairs varies from 200 to 300 μm,[1] while the diameter of terminal hair shafts ranges from 40 to 120 μm.[11] Vellus hair is arbitrarily defined as having a cross-sectional diameter of 30 μm or less.[12] The type of hair produced by a given follicle can change, as evidenced by the follicular miniaturization that occurs in androgenetic alopecia. In individuals with excessive hair, it is generally the terminal hairs that are of cosmetic concern.

Causes of Excessive Hair

Excessive hair is termed hypertrichosis or hirsutism. Hypertrichosis is defined as an increase in hair growth that is not androgen dependent.[13] It may result from intake of certain medications such as phenytoin, cyclosporine, cortisone, and penicillamine, or the topical use of minoxidil.[14] It may also be seen in a variety of diseases such as porphyria cutanea tarda, thyroid disorders, metastatic carcinoma, and malnutrition/anorexia nervosa.[14] Hirsutism is characterized by the growth of terminal hair in women on androgen-dependent areas of the body such as the upper lip, chin, or chest. Often the result of androgen excess, hirsutism may be accompanied by acne, androgenetic alopecia, and acanthosis nigricans. The most common hormonal cause of hirsutism is polycystic ovary disease, estimated to occur in 1% to 4% of the female population of reproductive age.[14] Rapid onset of hirsutism or other signs of androgen excess should prompt a hormonal evaluation, including levels of free testosterone and dehydroepiandrosterone-sulfate (DHEA-S), to rule out the presence of an androgen-secreting neoplasm.

Myocutaneous flaps may contain unwanted hair that interferes with proper function. For example, hair growth from skin flaps used in urethral reconstruction may cause urinary obstruction, calcification, or infection.[15,16] In addition, patients who have had wounds reconstructed with hair-bearing flaps may seek hair removal for cosmetic reasons.

Traditional Treatment Methods

Many different methods have been used to treat unwanted hair, including shaving, plucking, waxing, bleaching, and the use of chemical depilatories.[17] Although shaving is effective, simple, and inexpensive, it is a frequent chore that is unacceptable to many women with facial hair. Hair removal by plucking and waxing can last up to several months but treatment is painful and may be complicated by hyperpigmentation, ingrown hairs, folliculitis, or scarring. Chemical depilatories most commonly contain thioglycolates mixed with either NaOH or CaOH and dissolve hair structure by hydrolyzing disulfide bonds. Although they can provide results that last up to 2 weeks by dissolving part of the hair shaft below the skin surface, they are messy and commonly cause irritant dermatitis.[18] Antiandrogenic medications such as oral contraceptives, spironolactone, cyproterone acetate, and flutamide may provide modest improvement of hirsutism. However, results are temporary as treatment is suppressive rather than curative,[14] and undesirable side effects are not uncommon.

Until recently, electrolysis was the only method capable of producing permanent hair removal. There are several types of electrolysis, although all utilize a needle to carry current deep into the follicle. In galvanic electrolysis, direct electric current acts on tissue saline to produce sodium hydroxide, which chemically destroys the follicle. In contrast, thermolysis passes a high-frequency alternating current down the needle to thermally destroy the follicle.[19] Although it is generally accepted that electrolysis can provide permanent hair removal, there is little scientific data on which to base efficacy.[18] Potential side effects include pain, hyperpigmentation, hypopigmentation, and scarring. Both efficacy and side effects are highly operator dependent. The technique is most useful for epilation of a few stubborn hairs but is impractical for the treatment of large areas or large amounts of excessive hair.

LASER HAIR REMOVAL

Basic Mechanisms

In the past, lasers were used to remove hair from skin grafts and flaps[15,16,20] as well as to treat trichiasis,[21-23] but these devices did not target hair follicles selectively. Recently, a number of lasers and light sources have been developed to remove hair based on the principle of selective photothermolysis.[24] According to this principle, selective thermal destruction of a target will occur if sufficient energy is delivered at a wavelength well absorbed by the target within a time period less than or equal to the thermal relaxation time of the target. Under these conditions, it is possible to selectively target structures such as hair follicles.

To damage hair follicles, laser light must be absorbed by a chromophore within the follicle. Most lasers target the endogenous chromophore melanin within the pigmented hair shaft by delivering red or near-infrared wavelengths. Melanin is the primary light absorber in the optical window between 600 and 1100 nm.[25] Wavelengths in this range are poorly absorbed by competing chromophores such as hemoglobin and penetrate deeply into the dermis. The ability of these wavelengths to damage hair correlates directly with the amount and type of melanin within the follicle.[26] Dark hair that contains large amounts of eumelanin readily absorbs these wavelengths and is most susceptible to laser-induced damage. As an alternative to melanin, various exogenous chromophores can be targeted by laser light. For example, Q-switched Nd:YAG lasers have been used to target topically applied carbon particles massaged into hair follicles. This was the first FDA-cleared method of laser hair removal, but it appears to be impermanent. Light can also be used to photochemically activate an exogenously administered photosensitizer within hair follicles, a technique known as photodynamic therapy.

To confine thermal damage to the hair follicle, the pulse duration must not exceed the thermal relaxation time of the follicle, which is estimated to be 40 to 100 ms for terminal follicle diameters of 200 to 300 μm.[27] By confining the pulse duration to the millisecond range, diffusion of heat away from the hair follicle during the pulse is minimized. However, it is not desirable if the pulse duration is much shorter than the millisecond range because some thermal conduction from the hair shaft is necessary to damage vital structures such as the bulge and dermal papilla. This concept is well illustrated by the Q-switched ruby laser (QSRL), which delivers pulses in the nanosecond (10^{-9} s) range and is widely used to treat pigmented lesions. The QSRL induces leukotrichia and causes a temporary hair growth delay, but it does not inactivate the follicle itself.[28] On the other hand, the normal mode ruby laser, with pulses in the millisecond (10^{-3} s) range, targets the entire follicular epithelium by allowing thermal conduction from the hair shaft to the entire follicular structure.

Longer pulse durations are predicted to limit thermal damage to the epidermis. If the pulse duration exceeds the thermal relaxation time of the basal cell layer (about 0.1 ms) or entire epidermis (about 10 ms),[1] these structures will cool as they are heated during the laser pulse. This concept has been termed thermokinetic selectivity. The ideal pulse duration is in the 3 to 50 ms range, between the thermal relaxation times of epidermis and hair follicle. However, pulse durations longer than 30 ms should probably not be used in densely haired areas such as the beard. In these areas, long pulse durations may exceed the time for conduction of heat *between* adjacent hair follicles, raising the likelihood of nonspecific thermal injury.

Studies with the long-pulsed ruby laser have shown that hair loss is fluence dependent, with the greatest loss achieved by the highest fluence (60 J/cm^2 with 6 mm spot).[27] It has been predicted that the threshold surface fluence for bulb destruction at 700 nm is roughly 25 J/cm^2.[1] Larger spot sizes lower the threshold fluence, since there is substantially greater penetration of light into the depths of the dermis. With small spot sizes, sideways scattering of light by dermal collagen rapidly reduces the effective tissue fluence. Use of longer wavelengths such as 800 nm and above necessitates the use of higher fluences (up to 50 to 100 J/cm^2) to compensate for decreased melanin absorption.

It is widely held that anagen hair follicles are more sensitive to laser treatment than telogen follicles. In part, this belief has been based on studies in mice that showed that hair loss after ruby laser treatment is strongly dependent on the phase of the growth cycle, with anagen hairs being most sensitive.[29] However, this finding may not be applicable to humans as there are significant differences between murine and human follicles. In mice, the intradermal portion of telogen hair has essentially no melanin, while human telogen hair follicles retain a pigmented shaft within the dermis. A human study that mapped individual follicles before and after laser treatment found that the probability of hair loss did not differ for anagen and telogen hairs.[30] In humans, it appears that the most essential variable is the presence of a pigmented hair shaft within the skin to function as a light absorber. It is therefore likely that both anagen and telogen follicles are sensitive to laser treatment.[31]

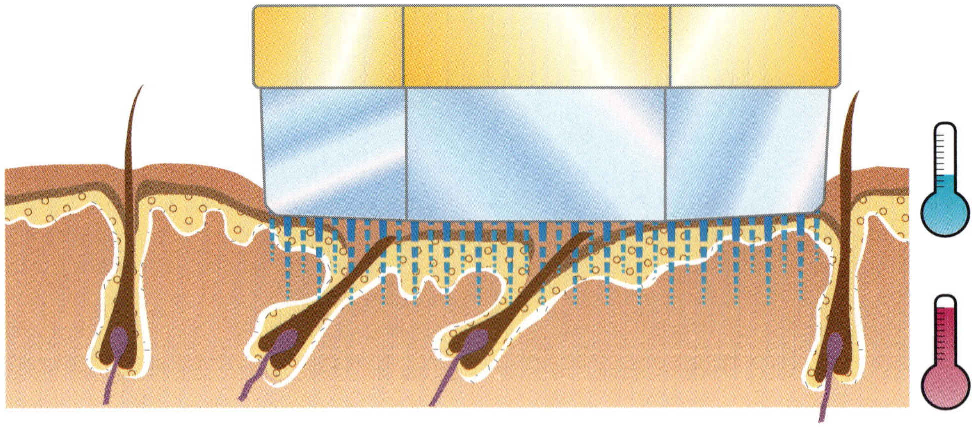

FIG. 13-3
Contact cooling handpiece of the E2000 ruby laser. (Courtesy Palomar Medical Technologies, Lexington, MA.)

Cooling

Melanin within the overlying epidermis functions as a competing absorber for laser light. Risk of epidermal injury increases with increasing skin pigmentation, whether constitutive or the result of a "tan." Various methods can be used to protect the epidermis from thermal damage, including longer pulse duration and longer wavelength. An alternative is to externally cool the skin surface either before, during, or after the laser pulse. The simplest, least expensive, and least effective method of skin cooling is to apply ice or refrigerated aqueous gel to the skin. A more sophisticated method is to utilize conductive contact cooling by circulating cold water (2° to 6°C) through a glass housing or sapphire window placed on the skin surface (Fig. 13-3). Sapphire has a higher thermal conductivity than glass, providing more rapid extraction of heat from the skin. When a 0°C sapphire window is applied for 0.5 s to the skin, the temperature of the basal layer drops 20°C.[1] Sapphire also provides index matching with the stratum corneum, optimizing coupling of laser light into the skin and decreasing backscattered light into the epidermis. In addition, when the glass or sapphire window is pressed into the skin with moderate pressure, the dermis is compacted, decreasing the relative depth of the bulb and bulge by up to 30% relative to the skin surface.[1] A recently introduced device (SmartCool, Cynosure, Chelmsford, MA) uses a forced flow of chilled air as the cooling medium. The efficacy of this device relative to glass or sapphire window cooling has not been evaluated. Theoretically, air cooling is less optimal because air is a good insulator with a thermal conductivity of only 1/50 that of sapphire.[1]

An alternative technique utilizes evaporative cooling by delivering a cryogen spray just prior to the laser pulse. Because evaporative cooling is more efficient than conductive cooling, larger temperature gradients can be created between epidermis and dermis, with less risk of inadvertent dermal cooling.[1] The commercially available device (dynamic cooling device or DCD, Candela Corporation, Wayland, MA) utilizes tetrafluoroethane as the cryogen (Fig. 13-4). The duration of the cryogen spray and the time interval between the spray and the laser pulse can be programmed by the operator. A longer spray duration provides a greater degree of cooling. The time delay between cryogen spray and laser pulse must be long enough to allow complete evaporation of cryogen, because any cryogen remaining on the skin surface will tend to disperse incident laser light. Cryogen is a consumable that must be purchased and replaced periodically.

Clinical comparisons of cooling methods have not yet been reported. However, it is clear that all of them provide some protection against epidermal injury in pigmented skin and that actively cooled sapphire and cryogen spray cooling is more protective than passive methods.

Specific Laser Systems

A summary of different commercially available hair removal devices is presented in Table 13-2. The FDA initially used electrolysis as a benchmark to evaluate laser treatment efficacy, despite the lack of scientific data on electrolysis. To receive FDA clearance, lasers must demonstrate a 30% decrease in hair growth 3 months after a single treatment.[32] As noted above, this criterion clearly does not equate with permanent hair loss, because the duration of telogen can easily exceed 3 months. A more functional definition of permanent hair removal has been proposed, based on the cyclic

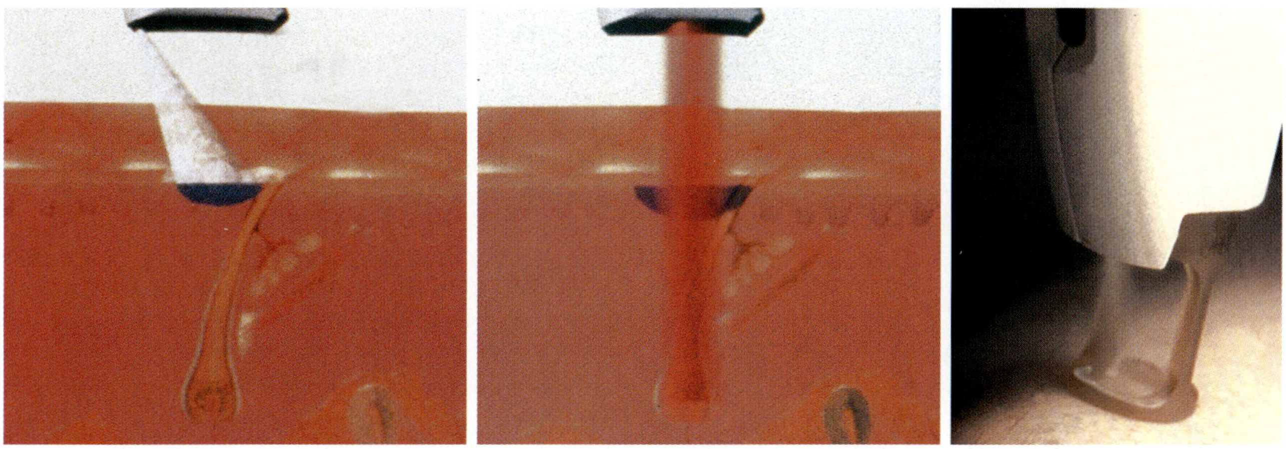

FIG. 13-4
Dynamic Cooling Device. (Courtesy Candela Corporation, Wayland, MA.)

Table 13-2 Laser Hair Removal

Device (Company)	Wavelength (nm)	Pulse Duration (ms)	Spot Size (mm)	Maximum Fluence (J/cm²)	Maximum Speed (Hz)	Cooling Device	Comments
E2000 (Palomar/ConBio)	694	3 or 100	10 mm hexagon, 20 mm square	50	1	Sapphire contact	Employs photon recycling
EpiTouch Ruby (Lumenis)	694	1.2	4-6	40	1.2	Gel	Q-switched mode available
RubyStar (Aesculap Meditec)	694	2	3-14	35	1	Contact plate precooling	Q-switched mode available
GentleLASE (Candela)	755	3	7-18	100	1	Dynamic cooling device (DCD)	2 × 7 mm spot for leg veins
EpiTouch Plus Alex (Lumenis)	755	2-40	5-10	50	5	Gel	Scanner available
LPIR/Apogee (Cynosure)	755	5-40	7-16	50	1	Cold air flow	Scanner available
LightSheer (Lumenis)	800	5-30	9 × 9	60	1	Sapphire contact	Diode array in handpiece
CoolGlide (Altus Medical)	1064	10-100	9 × 9	100	2	Copper contact precooling	FDA approval pending
Lyra (Laserscope)	1064	10-50	3-5	100	4	Contact cooling	FDA approval pending; scanner
Softlight (Thermolase)	1064	10-20	7	2-3	10	Not needed	Carbon makes no difference
Flashlamp (Lumenis)	Variable from 550-1200	Variable	8 × 33 or 10 × 45	30-65	<1	Circulating cooling device	Sequence of multiple pulses

growth phases for hair follicles. Permanent hair loss can be defined as a significant reduction in the number of terminal hairs, which is stable for a period longer than the complete growth cycle of hair follicles at a given body site.[33] There are currently four laser systems that have received FDA approval for hair removal: the Q-switched Nd:YAG (plus topical carbon), long-pulse (millisecond domain) ruby, alexandrite, and diode lasers. In addition, a pulsed flashlamp has been cleared by the FDA for hair removal. A particular ruby (Palomar Medical Technologies, Burlington, MA) laser and diode laser (Lumenis, Santa Clara, CA) have been cleared by FDA for permanent hair reduction.

Q-switched Nd:YAG Laser

In 1996 the FDA approved a patented laser process for hair removal that utilized a Q-switched Nd:YAG laser after pretreatment wax epilation and application of carbon-based solution (Softlight, Thermolase, La Jolla, CA). The QS Nd:YAG laser delivers light at 1064 nm (near infrared range) with a pulse duration of 10 to 20 ns. It is utilized at relatively low fluences (2 to 3 J/cm²) with a 7 mm spot size and repetition rate of 10 Hz. The Softlight technique utilizes a proprietary carbon suspension similar to india ink as an exogenous chromophore. The carbon solution is briefly massaged onto the skin to facilitate penetration down hair follicles and is wiped off prior to laser treatment. Absorption of a QS Nd:YAG laser pulse by a carbon particle produces a rapid temperature rise, cavitation (sudden vaporization of water), and local shock waves, causing thermal and mechanical damage to the follicle.[34] However, it is unlikely that the carbon penetrates deeply into follicles, since the solution is applied for only a few seconds before being wiped off.

The Softlight system was marketed aggressively through a national network of hair removal salons, despite a lack of any evidence showing long-term efficacy. In a well-controlled study, Nanni and Alster demonstrated that the Softlight technique produces only a temporary hair growth delay that lasts less than 6 months.[35] Use of the carbon solution is not necessary to induce hair growth delay[36] as melanin within the follicle functions as an alternative chromophore.[37] A modified approach has been described, in which smaller carbon particles are applied to the skin followed by a low-fluence treatment with the Nd:YAG

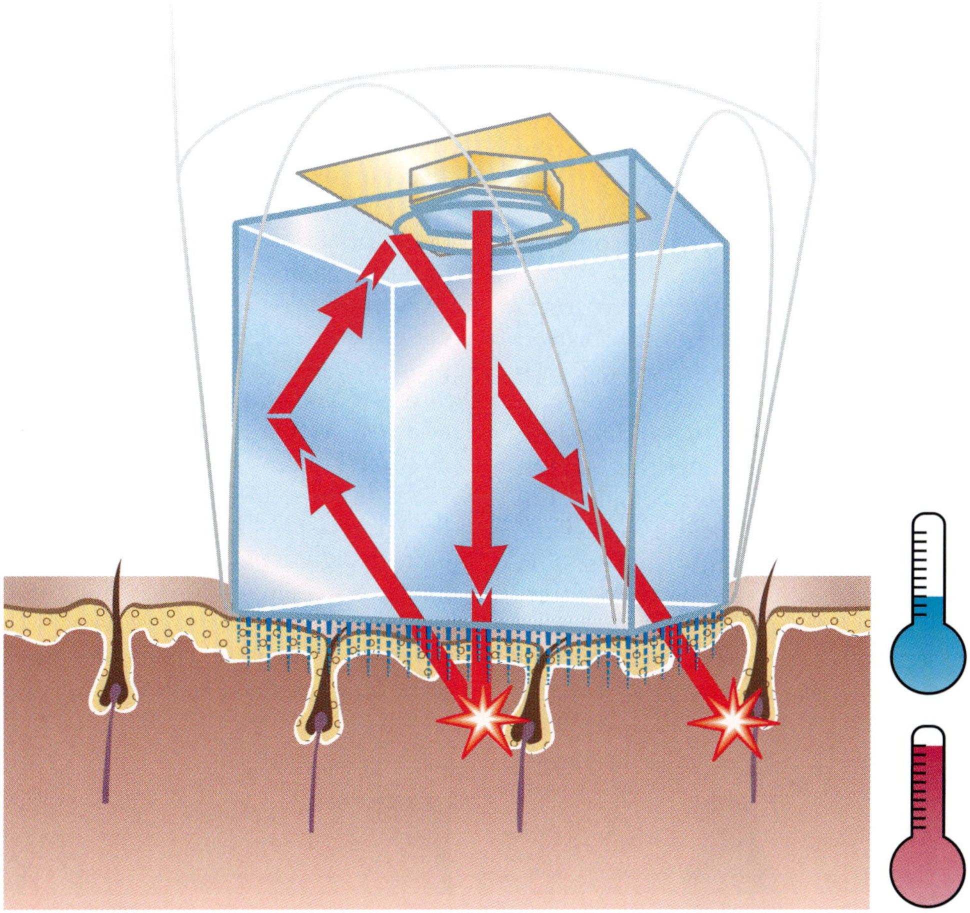

FIG. 13-5
Photon recycling with E2000 ruby laser. (Courtesy Palomar Medical Technologies, Lexington, MA.)

laser to propel the particles into the follicle.[38] A second laser pass is then performed using higher fluences to target the carbon particles within the follicle. It is unknown whether this modification has any advantages over the original technique. In current practice, conventional Q-switched Nd:YAG lasers can be used to provide temporary hair reduction, but hair loss is not expected to be permanent.

Long-Pulsed (Millisecond Domain) Ruby Laser

Use of the ruby laser for dermatologic purposes was first reported by Dr. Leon Goldman in the 1960s. The ruby laser delivers red light at a wavelength of 694 nm. In the Q-switched mode the ruby laser has been widely used over the last decade to treat pigmented lesions and tattoos. More recently, the long-pulsed ruby laser has been utilized in the treatment of excessive hair. At least three ruby lasers are FDA approved for hair removal: the Epilaser/E2000 (Palomar/Continuum Biomedical, Ridgewood, NJ), the EpiTouch Ruby (Lumenis, Santa Clara, CA), and the RubyStar (Aesculap Meditec, Germany).

The Epilaser has been the most widely used but has been supplanted by the second generation E2000. The E2000 delivers either a 3 ms or a 100 ms pulse, in which the laser energy is split into two 3 ms pulses separated by a 100 ms delay (twin pulse mode). A spot size of 10 mm (hexagon) or 20 mm (square) provides fluences of up to 50 J/cm^2 and 8 J/cm^2, respectively. The E2000 also employs photon recycling, in which backscattered light is reflected back toward the skin, thereby increasing the effective fluence (Fig. 13-5). Pulses are delivered at 1 Hz through a flexible optical fiber. An actively cooled sapphire handpiece (0°C or –10°C) is pressed firmly against the skin during treatment (Figs. 13-3 and 13-6).

The EpiTouch and RubyStar are both dual-mode ruby lasers that can operate in either Q-switched mode or in long-pulsed normal mode to target hair follicles. In the long-pulsed mode, EpiTouch delivers a 1.2 ms pulse at a spot size of 4 to 6 mm and repetition rate of

1.2 Hz. It can achieve a fluence of 40 J/cm^2 at the smaller spot size. A cooling gel is utilized to help protect the epidermis from thermal damage. A thin, patented, laser beam aligning sheet can be placed over the gel to help ensure homogenous coverage of the skin.[39] RubyStar delivers a 2 ms pulse with a spot size of up to 12 mm, repetition rate of 1 Hz, and fluence of up to 35 J/cm^2. An optional contact handpiece cools the skin prior to delivery of the laser pulse.

Grossman et al initially reported selective injury to hair follicles by the long-pulsed ruby laser.[27] Thirteen patients with fair skin and dark hair were treated once on the thighs or back at fluences of 20 to 60 J/cm^2 with spot size of 6 mm. Hair growth delay was induced for 1 to 3 months in all subjects at all fluences, at both shaved and wax-epilated sites. Biopsies obtained immediately after treatment showed selective thermal damage to pigmented hair follicles, with vaporization of the hair shafts, large patches of necrosis in the follicular epithelium, and occasional rupture with perifollicular dermal injury suggestive of steam vents. Transient pigmentary changes occurred in several patients but scarring was not observed. At 1 to 2 years follow-up, four of seven recalled patients had persistent hair loss, which was greatest in sites treated at the highest fluence.[33] Biopsies from one patient showed a reduced number of terminal hairs with a reciprocal increase in small velluslike hairs, but no evidence of fibrosis or destruction of hair follicles. It was suggested that permanent hair loss after ruby laser treatment results from miniaturization of the follicular bulb and papilla, akin to the mechanism of androgenetic alopecia.[40]

Additional studies with larger numbers of patients have confirmed that hair counts are reduced by approximately 30% after a single treatment with the ruby laser.[41-44] The effects of multiple treatment sessions are additive, as hair counts are reduced by approximately 60% after three or four treatment sessions[41,42,44] (Fig. 13-7). Because of its comparatively short wavelength, the ruby laser is best suited for the treatment of dark hair in light skin. It may be more efficacious than longer wavelength devices for the treatment of light hair or red to red-brown hair.[1,45] Because of a high melanin absorption coefficient at 694 nm, the ruby laser must be used with caution in darkly pigmented or tan patients.[46]

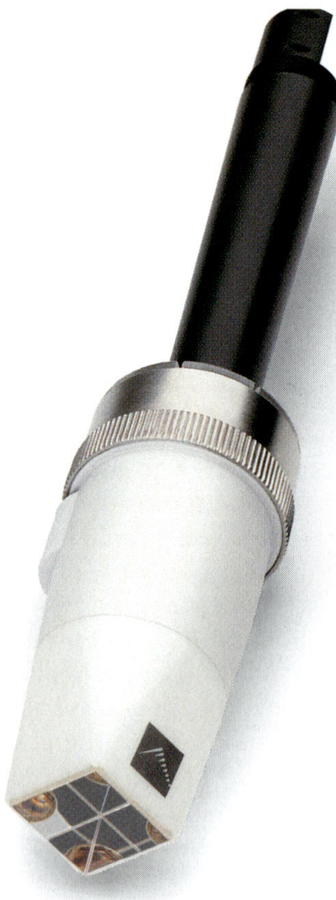

FIG. 13-6
20 × 20 mm handpiece adapter for E2000 ruby laser. (Courtesy Palomar Medical Technologies, Lexington, MA.)

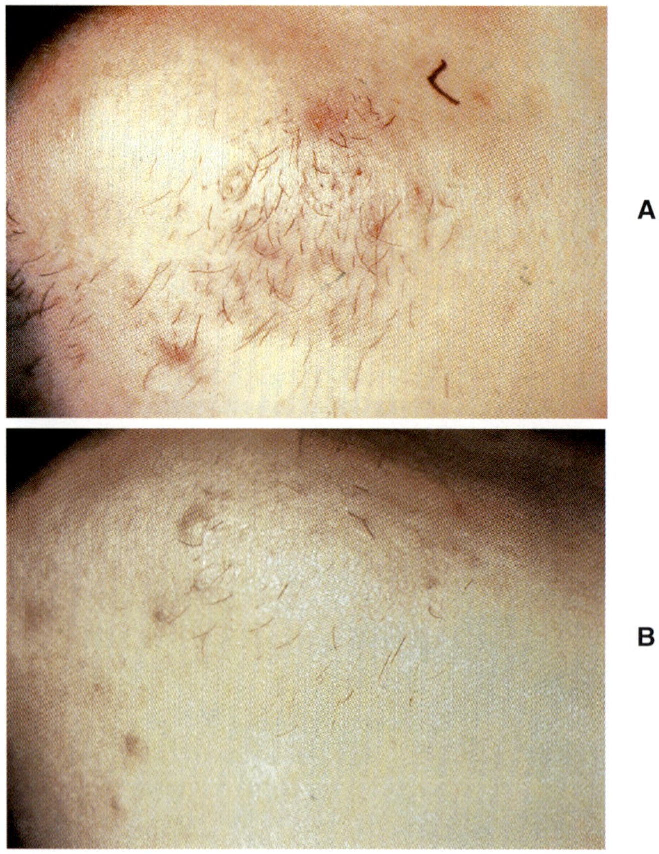

FIG. 13-7
Hirsutism and folliculitis on chin of female. **A,** Pretreatment. **B,** 12 months after four treatments with long-pulsed ruby laser.

Alexandrite Lasers

There are currently three alexandrite laser systems that have been approved by the FDA for hair removal: the GentleLASE (Candela, Wayland, MA), the EpiTouch Alex (Lumenis, Santa Clara, CA), and the Apogee, formerly called PhotoGenica LPIR (Cynosure, Chelmsford, MA). All deliver near-infrared light at 755 nm through a fiberoptic cable. The GentleLASE utilizes a fixed pulse duration of 3 ms, spot size of 7 to 18 mm, fluence of 10 to 100 J/cm^2, and repetition rate up to 1 Hz. It delivers a pulse of cryogen (tetrafluoroethane) spray to the skin just prior to the laser pulse (see Fig. 13-4). The EpiTouch has a pulse duration of 2 to 40 ms, fluence up to 50 J/cm^2, spot size of 5 to 10 mm, repetition rate of up to 5 Hz, and an accompanying scanner (Fig. 13-8). The Apogee features a variable split-pulse duration of up to 40 ms, spot size of 7 to 16 mm, fluence of 5 to 50 J/cm^2, and repetition rate of 1 Hz. The EpiTouch is used with refrigerated gel to cool the skin while the Apogee is used with either cold gel or with forced air cooling. The longer pulse durations (up to 40 ms) of the EpiTouch and Apogee are the result of multiple synchronized pulses rather than true single pulses. They are intended to protect the epidermis by allowing more time for heat extraction compared with single, shorter pulses.

The 755 nm wavelength is absorbed about 20% less strongly by melanin compared with the ruby laser wavelength of 694 nm. Because dermal scattering decreases with increasing wavelength, 755 nm light penetrates deeper into tissue than shorter wavelengths. In theory, the use of longer wavelengths increases the ratio of energy deposited in the dermis to the epidermis, which results in relative bulb heating and epidermal sparing.[1] A recent study found that one treatment with a variable pulse alexandrite laser produced maximum hair growth reduction at 6 months of 40% to 56% for the lip, leg, and back.[47] Sites treated with a 10 ms pulse duration were found to have significantly better hair reduction rates than those treated with 5 ms or 20 ms pulsewidths. However, the optimal pulse duration for efficacy is unclear, as other studies have found no differences in response when comparing pulse durations between 2 ms and 20 ms.[48-50] Some studies have shown that the 20 ms pulse duration reduces the risk of epidermal damage and pigmentary alteration, but treatment is more painful when longer pulse durations are used.[48,51]

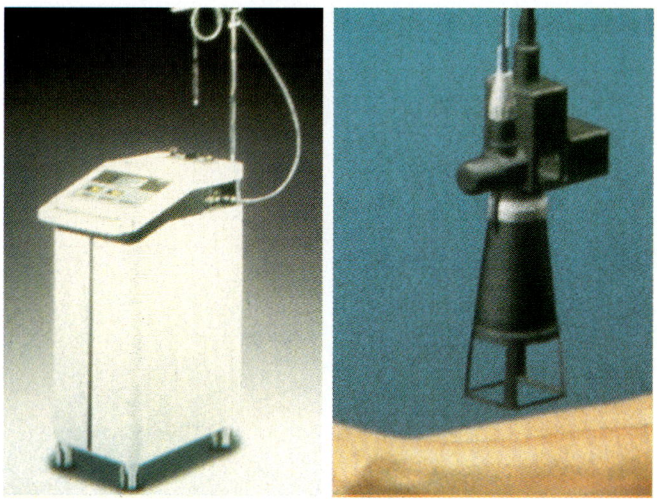

FIG. 13-8
EpiTouch Alex Laser with scanner. (Courtesy Lumenis, Santa Clara, CA.)

Diode Laser

Semiconductor diode lasers are setting a new standard for efficiency, reliability, and portability. The LightSheer laser (Lumenis, Santa Clara, CA) is a high-powered (1600 watt) diode array that has been FDA approved for permanent hair removal (Fig. 13-9). It emits 800 nm light (infrared range) with a pulse duration of 5 to 30 ms, fixed spot size of 9 × 9 mm, and fluence of 10 to 60 J/cm^2. The pulse duration is automatically set at half the fluence or manually set at 30 ms. The LightSheer provides cooling via a sapphire handpiece that is placed directly in contact with the skin. Because of reduced scattering at longer wavelengths, light from the diode laser penetrates deeply into the skin. At 800 nm, 24% of incident fluence remains at a depth of 3 mm (the bulb), whereas only 5% remains for 700 nm light.[1] The long wavelength and pulse duration as well as the presence of active cooling helps protect the epidermis in darkly pigmented patients.

Several studies have demonstrated the efficacy of the diode laser for hair removal.[52-54] In one study of 50 patients, quantitative hair counts performed for 9 months after treatment showed long-lasting and possibly permanent hair loss.[52] In other studies, the diode laser showed fewer pigmentary side effects and greater efficacy than the long-pulsed ruby laser for the treatment of thick, coarse hair.[45,53] Several other diode lasers emitting at 800 nm are under investigation and are expected to enter the marketplace in the near future.

Flashlamp

An intense, pulsed flashlamp called the EpiLight (Lumenis, Santa Clara, CA) has received FDA approval for hair removal. It delivers noncoherent, multi-wavelength (nonlaser) light from 500 to 1200 nm. One of four filters (590 nm, 615 nm, 645 nm, or 695 nm) is used to eliminate shorter wavelengths (Fig. 13-10*A*).

A B

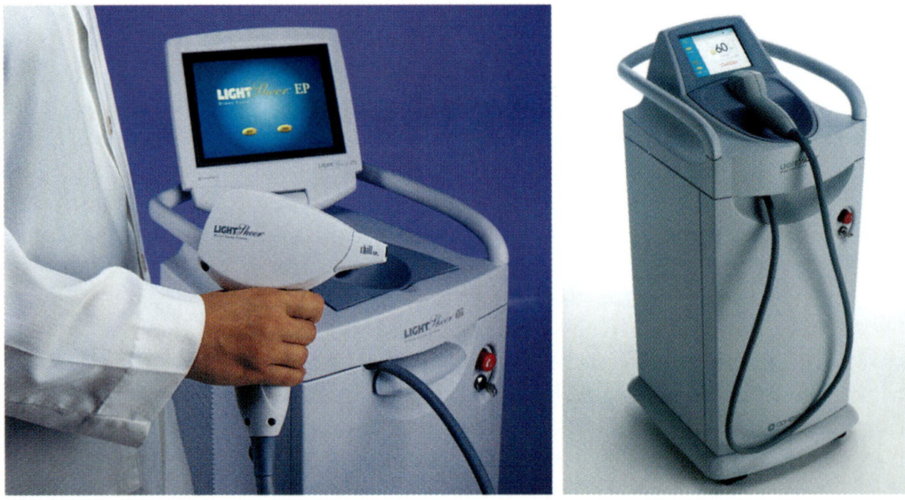

FIG. 13-9
A, LightSheer diode laser with handpiece. (Courtesy Lumenis, Santa Clara, CA.) **B,** LightSheer XC. (Courtesy Lumenis, Santa Clara, CA.)

A

B

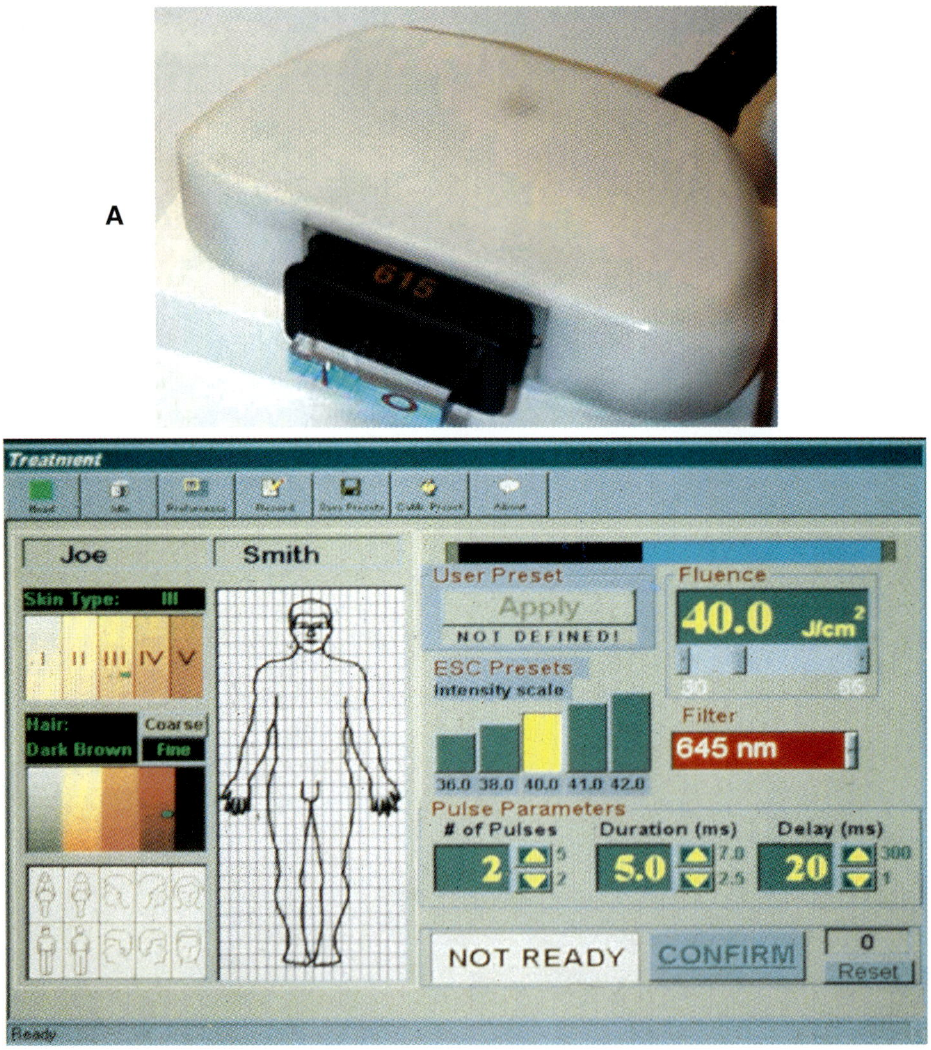

FIG. 13-10
A, EpiLight handpiece with 615 nm filter. (Courtesy Lumenis, Santa Clara, CA.) **B,** EpiLight treatment screen. (Courtesy Lumenis, Santa Clara, CA.)

Light is delivered through a large rectangular handpiece measuring either 10 × 45 mm or 8 × 35 mm. The device produces a fluence of 30 to 65 J/cm^2 that is spread over a sequence of two to five pulses, each of 2.5 to 5 ms duration. The delay between pulses ranges from 1 to 300 ms and the series of pulses is delivered once every few seconds (Fig. 13-10*B*). In the past, a refrigerated, transparent gel was used to cool the skin, but a water-cooled handpiece now available can be cooled down to 4°C. The software within the EpiLight device provides suggested treatment parameters based on patient skin type and hair color and caliber. However, most practitioners familiar with the device adjust the output individually according to their experience.

Although the EpiLight has been a source of controversy among clinicians, several studies have demonstrated the long-term efficacy of the device.[55-57] In a study of 67 subjects of Fitzpatrick type I to IV, mean hair loss was 48% at 6 months or more after a single treatment.[57] There were no statistically significant differences in hair counts after single vs. multiple treatments. Side effects were limited to localized erythema with no scarring or pigmentary change. In biopsy samples taken from 2 weeks to 20 months after treatment, damage was confined exclusively to hair follicles, which showed apoptotic keratinocytes, perifollicular fibrosis, and perifollicular melanophages. There were no differences detected in terminal/vellus ratios, anagen/telogen ratios, or hair shaft diameter. The authors theorized that photoepilation induced by the flashlamp is due to thermal damage to hair follicles rather than follicular miniaturization.

The broad range of wavelengths delivered by the EpiLight has some advantages. The presence of longer wavelengths provides better penetration depth into dermis than ruby or alexandrite lasers. While the shorter wavelengths can be filtered out for darker patients to protect the epidermis, they can be used in lighter patients with dark hair to maximally exploit the contrast between skin and hair color.[1] The shorter wavelengths may also be useful to target red-brown hair.[1] Although the company claims that the device removes all hair colors, histologic studies have shown that hypopigmented hair shafts are spared after treatment.[57] The device does include wavelengths absorbed by water, which may increase the risk of adverse effects.

Successful use of the EpiLight requires a certain level of experience, since the large number of variable parameters can be bewildering to the novice. Probably the greatest technical advantage of the EpiLight is the large exposure area that improves damage of deep follicles. However, the slow pulse repetition rate makes the device equivalent in speed to other lasers. Unlike most lasers, the optical pulse energy is not calibrated with each use, such that treatment dose may need to be arbitrarily reduced when the flashlamp is replaced. Another disadvantage is that the rectangular spot size prevents treatment of areas with marked convexities or concavities.[1]

Long-Pulsed Nd:YAG Laser

Several Nd:YAG lasers with millisecond domain pulses have been designed to target hair, including Lyra (Laserscope, San Jose, CA) and CoolGlide (Altus Medical, Burlingame, CA). However, these devices are still awaiting FDA approval for hair removal. With a wavelength of 1064 nm, these Nd:YAG lasers penetrate deeper into skin than shorter-wavelength devices. Theoretically, this should allow more effective targeting of the bulb, which is located deep within the dermis. The Nd:YAG laser may allow safer treatment of darkly pigmented patients (up to skin type V) because of reduced melanin absorption at 1064 nm. However, because of reduced absorption by follicular melanin, very high fluences (50 to 100 J/cm^2) are required to damage pigmented hair follicles. Such high fluences increase the level of pain during treatment and may raise the risk of epidermal damage. Preliminary studies suggest that the long-pulsed Nd:YAG laser provides hair loss comparable to other devices.[58,59] The long-term efficacy and precise role of the long-pulsed Nd:YAG laser remain to be established.

Photodynamic Therapy (PDT)

Photodynamic therapy is defined as the use of light to activate a chemical photosensitizer to induce a specific tissue effect. Although most experience with PDT has been in the treatment of cutaneous neoplasms using intravenous porphyrins, recent studies have investigated the use of topical photosensitizers such as δ-aminolevulinic acid (ALA). ALA is the first intermediate in heme synthesis and, when present in excess, is converted to protoporphyrin IX, a potent photosensitizer. Topically applied 20% ALA is absorbed by hair follicles and converted to protoporphyrin IX over a period of several hours. Subsequent exposure of the skin to red light near 635 nm activates protoporphyrin IX, leading to the formation of singlet oxygen that damages follicular cell membranes. In a small human study, ALA-PDT was reported to selectively damage hair follicles.[60] Partial hair loss was induced for at least 3 months and was dependent on ALA concentration and light dose. A potential advantage of PDT is that hair and skin color are not expected to be important variables, and light sources as simple as a slide projector can potentially be used. Although the technique is still experimental, ongoing studies should help define its role in hair removal.

SECTION TWO

Atlas of Surgical Procedures

PREOPERATIVE CLINICAL CONSIDERATIONS

Treatment of hair with lasers or flashlamps almost always results in temporary hair loss, regardless of hair color. Growth delay lasts for several months and is due to induction of telogen.[61] The ability to achieve persistent hair removal that lasts beyond the growth cycle of a given follicle depends largely on hair color. Dark hair with ample amounts of eumelanin can be effectively treated by multiple devices, provided that appropriate fluence and spot size are used. Under these conditions, the average long-term hair loss per treatment is about 20% to 30%, based on studies performed with ruby lasers. Multiple treatment sessions are usually required to achieve the maximal level of hair reduction, although this has not been confirmed in all studies.[57] It should be stressed to the patient that the true permanence of hair removal is unknown and that removal of *all* hair is unlikely. In individuals with blonde, red, gray, or white hair, it is unlikely that laser treatment will produce long-lasting hair removal. However, such patients may be willing to undergo treatments spaced about 2 to 4 months apart as necessary to maintain temporary hair loss.

The ideal candidate for laser hair removal is fair skinned with little melanin within the overlying epidermis. Such patients tolerate the use of higher fluences, resulting in more effective treatment. While treatment can be safely performed with a shorter wavelength device (e.g., ruby laser) in fair patients, it may be preferable to utilize a longer-wavelength device in darker patients. Epidermal protection is also afforded by utilizing longer pulse durations and active cooling. Patients with darker skin who are at risk for postinflammatory hyperpigmentation can be treated with a hydroquinone bleaching cream (e.g., Solaquin Forte) twice daily for 4 to 6 weeks prior to treatment. Individuals with a suntan have a significantly higher risk of epidermal damage from laser treatment. Treatment should be delayed by several months until the tan has faded. All patients should be instructed preoperatively to avoid sun exposure and wear a broad spectrum sunscreen of SPF 30 or higher on exposed areas. Patients with a history of hypertrophic or keloidal scarring should be treated more conservatively, using test spots and lower fluences. Likewise, patients with a history of recent isotretinoin use (within the last 6 to 12 months) should be treated less aggressively.

Laser treatment is much more effective when the pigmented hair shaft is present within the follicle. Patients should not pluck, wax, or undergo electrolysis for at least 1 month prior to treatment. Shaving, bleaching, or use of chemical depilatories are acceptable alternatives for patients awaiting laser treatment. The skin should always be shaved immediately prior to treatment to remove all visible external hair. This minimizes the production of noxious plume during treatment, which results from the vaporization of external hair. Shaving also reduces the risk of skin damage due to heat transfer from coagulated surface hair that has adhered to the skin. Since close shaving may obscure the border of the treatment area, a red marking pen can be used to mark the border prior to shaving.

PROCEDURAL TECHNIQUES

Topical anesthetics such as EMLA cream help reduce the discomfort of treatment. The cream should be applied liberally and occluded with plastic wrap at least 1 hour before treatment. Local infiltration of lidocaine or regional nerve blocks may be utilized, but these techniques are rarely necessary. The laser should always be calibrated before treatment and after changing fluence, spot size, or any other parameter. The laser handpiece should be held perpendicularly to the skin and the skin should be stretched taut. Pulses should be delivered in a slightly overlapping pattern to ensure confluent skin coverage. A grid may be utilized to facilitate placement of laser pulses and minimize skip areas or doubly pulsed areas. Routine use of a grid is usually not required provided that the operator is attentive during treatment. Skin cooling should always be utilized, whether it consists of contact cooling, cryogen spray cooling, forced air cooling, or application of refrigerated aqueous gel.

Before performing a full treatment, it may be helpful to perform test spots in inconspicuous areas using varying fluences, especially in patients with darker skin phototypes. For such patients, it may be prudent to use a more conservative fluence for the initial treatment session and to increase the fluence in subsequent sessions if treatment has been well tolerated. Because efficacy is fluence dependent, most patients should be treated at the highest tolerated fluence (based on pain and evidence of epidermal injury). The desired clinical end point is perifollicular erythema, which usually develops within several minutes of treatment. Marked or confluent erythema, whitening, blistering, or purpura indicates acute epidermal injury from overly aggressive treatment. Fluence should be reduced by 20% to 30% if any of these signs are noted.

A large spot size should be used to promote deeper penetration of light and provide more rapid treatment. For ruby and alexandrite lasers, best results are achieved with a spot size of at least 7 mm and a fluence of at least 30 J/cm^2. It may be necessary to reduce the fluence as spot size is increased to 10 mm or more, since an equivalent tissue response will occur at lower fluences due to greater penetration of light into the dermis. Devices emitting at longer wavelengths (e.g., 1064 nm) require the use of higher fluences to compensate for reduced melanin absorption.

POSTOPERATIVE CLINICAL CONSIDERATIONS

Most patients develop mild edema and erythema after treatment, which generally lasts no more than 1 to 2 days. Postoperative pain is mild and transient, rarely requiring the use of oral analgesics. The use of ice packs and a short course (1 to 2 days) of high-potency topical steroids may lessen posttreatment erythema and discomfort. Patients should apply bland emollients to the treated area twice a day, particularly if any crusting or blistering has occurred. Treated hairs may be shed over the course of several weeks and should not be confused with actual hair regrowth.

Side effects following laser hair removal are generally minor and transient. The most common side effects are postinflammatory hyperpigmentation[62] and hypopigmentation. The overall incidence of these pigmentary changes is approximately 10% to 20%.[63] Hyperpigmentation typically lasts for approximately 2 months, whereas hypopigmentation lasts an average of 3.5 months.[63] To reduce the risk of hyperpigmentation, patients should be instructed to avoid sun exposure and wear a UVA/UVB sunscreen with SPF 30 or higher for at least 2 months after treatment. Other less common side effects include crusting, purpura, blistering, and erosions. Scarring after laser hair removal is rare but is more likely to occur when excessive fluences are used. Reactivation of perioral or genital HSV is distinctly uncommon, and antiviral prophylaxis is not necessary prior to treatment unless there is a very strong history of HSV reactivation.[63]

Side effects after laser treatment are directly correlated with skin type, with darker-skinned and tanned patients experiencing a much higher rate of complications. Complication rates also vary according to the anatomic location treated. Sun-exposed areas such as the extensor extremities have a higher rate of side effects than sites protected from the sun, such as axillary and inguinal areas.[63] All lasers and light sources that target melanin have the potential to produce epidermal damage through competitive absorption by epidermal melanin. However, the risk of side effects is probably higher with shorter-wavelength devices (e.g., ruby laser). The use of lower fluences, active cooling, longer pulse durations, and minimal overlap of pulses can help to spare the epidermis from injury.

Although the optimal schedule for repeat treatments is unknown, most practitioners recommend repeat treatments every 4 to 8 weeks, or when the first signs of regrowing hair are present. Regrowing hairs are often more lightly pigmented and of decreased caliber, which contributes to patient satisfaction with treatment.

SAFETY WITH HAIR REMOVAL DEVICES

The devices used for hair removal all target melanin deep within the skin. The highest concentration of melanin in the body is in the retina and choroid, which extend all the way to the front of the eye. Consequently, it is imperative that both patient and physician wear protective eyewear with sideguards that covers the emission wavelength of the device being used. Extreme caution must be used when treating around the eye, as ocular injury may occur even when light is delivered through the intact eyelid and sclera combined. Even the insertion of laser-protective eye shields over the cornea does not provide complete safety because they cover only the anterior surface of the globe. The flashlamp device presents less risk of ocular injury at a great distance than laser devices because it delivers incoherent light. However, at close (treatment) range, it is at least as hazardous as true lasers.

When hair-bearing skin is treated with lasers or flashlamps, hair vaporization produces a noxious plume with an unpleasant, sulfurous odor. It is not known whether the plume poses any health risks. Hair should be closely shaved prior to treatment to minimize the vaporization of external hairs. The use of smoke evacuators and adequate ventilation is essential.

Summary

The presence of unwanted hair continues to plague many individuals for whom traditional methods of hair removal remain unsatisfactory. Laser and flashlamp technology now offers the potential for rapid, safe, and effective treatment of unwanted hair. An ever-increasing number of published studies have confirmed the long-term efficacy of laser and flashlamp treatment. For the most part, however, the benefits of this technology have been limited to individuals with dark hair and relatively fair skin. The remaining challenge is to develop the means to eliminate light-colored hair as well as the capability to safely treat individuals with darker skin. The rapid pace of technological advancement as well as continued studies of hair follicle biology promise to improve this field over the years to come.

REFERENCES

1. Ross EV, Ladin Z, Kreindel M, Dierickx C. Theoretical considerations in laser hair removal. Dermatol Clin 1999; 17:333-355.
2. Seiberg M, Marthinuss J, Stenn KS. Changes in expression of apoptosis-associated genes in skin mark early catagen. J Invest Dermatol 1995; 104:78-82.
3. Van Scott EJ, Ekel TM, Auerbach R, et al. Determinants of rate and kinetics of cell division in scalp hair. J Invest Dermatol 1963; 41:269-273.

4. Kligman AM. The human hair cycle. J Invest Dermatol 1959; 33: 307-316.
5. Cotsarelis G, Sun TT, Lavker RM. Label-retaining cells reside in the bulge area of pilosebaceous unit: implications for follicular stem cells, hair cycle, and skin carcinogenesis. Cell 1990; 61:1329-1337.
6. Lyle S, Christofidou-Solomidou M, Liu Y, et al. The C8/144B monoclonal antibody recognizes cytokeratin 15 and defines the location of human hair follicle stem cells. J Cell Sci 1998; 111:3179-3188.
7. Murphy GF. Histology of the skin. In: Elder D, Elenitsas R, Jaworsky C, Johnson B, eds. Lever's Histopathology of the Skin. Philadelphia: Lippincott-Raven, 1997:5-50.
8. Seago SV, Ebling FJG. The hair cycle on the human thigh and upper arm. Br J Dermatol 1985; 113:9-16.
9. Hertzberg J, Gusck W. Das Ergrauen des Kapfhaares. Eine histo- und fermentschemische sowie elektronen-mikroskopische Studie. Arch Klin Exp Dermatol 1970; 236:368-375.
10. Van Scott E, Ekel T. Geometric relationships between the matrix of the hair bulb and its dermal papilla in normal and alopecic scalp. J Invest Dermatol 1958; 29:281-287.
11. Hayashi A. Trichogram. J Invest Dermatol 1975; 60:70.
12. Headington JT. Transverse microscopic anatomy of the human scalp: a basis for a morphometric approach to disorders of the hair follicle. Arch Dermatol 1984; 120:449-456.
13. Kvedar JC, Gibson M, Krusinski PA. Hirsutism: evaluation and treatment. J Am Acad Dermatol 1985; 12:215-225.
14. Liew SH. Unwanted body hair and its removal: a review. Dermatol Surg 1999; 25:431-439.
15. Finkelstein LH, Blatstein LM. Epilation of hair-bearing urethral grafts using the Neodymium:YAG surgical laser. J Urol 1991; 146: 840-842.
16. Durwood DE, Orihuela E, Crotty K, et al. Laser ablation of urethral hair. Lasers Surg Med 1999; 24:261-263.
17. Richards RN, Uy M, Meharg G. Temporary hair removal in patients with hirsutism: a clinical study. Cutis 1990; 45:199-202.
18. Olsen EA. Methods of hair removal. J Am Acad Dermatol 1999; 40:143-155.
19. Richards RN, Meharg GE. Electrolysis: observations from 13 years and 140,000 hours of experience. J Am Acad Dermatol 1995; 33:662-666.
20. Kuriloff DB, Finn DG, Kimmelman CP. Pharyngoesophageal hair growth: the role of laser epilation. Otolaryngol Head Neck Surg 1988; 98:342-345.
21. Gossman MD, Brightwell JR, Huntington AC. Experimental comparison of laser and cryosurgical cilia destruction. Ophthalmol Surg 1992; 23:179-183.
22. Bartley GB, Bullock JD, Olsen TG, Lutz PD. An experimental study to compare methods of eyelash ablation. Ophthalmology 1987; 94:1286-1289.
23. Gossman MD, Yung R, Berlin AJ. Prospective evaluation of the argon laser in the treatment of trichiasis. Ophthalmol Surg 1992; 23:183-187.
24. Anderson RR, Parrish JA. Selective photothermolysis: precise microsurgery by selective absorption of pulsed radiation. Science 1983; 220:524-527.
25. Anderson RR, Parrish JA. The optics of human skin. J Invest Dermatol 1981; 77:13-19.
26. Liew SH, Ladhani K, Grobbelaar AO, et al. Ruby laser-assisted hair removal success in relation to anatomic factors and melanin content of hair follicles. Plast Reconstr Surg 1999; 103:1736-1743.
27. Grossman MC, Dierickx C, Farinelli W, et al. Damage to hair follicles by normal-mode ruby laser pulses. J Am Acad Dermatol 1996; 35:889-894.
28. Dover JS, Margolis RJ, Polla LL, et al. Pigmented guinea pig skin irradiated with Q-switched ruby laser pulses. Arch Dermatol 1989; 125:43-49.
29. Lin TYD, Manuskiatti W, Dierickx C, et al. Hair growth cycle affects hair follicle destruction by ruby laser pulses. J Invest Dermatol 1998; 111:107-113.
30. Dierickx CC, Campos VB, Lin D, et al. Influence of hair growth cycle on efficacy of laser hair removal. Lasers Surg Med 1999; 11(suppl):21.
31. Liew SH, Grobbelaar AO, Gault D, et al. A preliminary report of the correlation between efficacy of treatment and melanin content of hair and the growth phases of hair at a specific site. Ann Plast Surg 1999; 42:255-258.
32. Tope WD, Hordinsky MK. A hair's breadth closer? Arch Dermatol 1998; 134:867-869.
33. Dierickx CC, Grossman MC, Farinelli WA, Anderson RR. Permanent hair removal by normal-mode ruby laser. Arch Dermatol 1998; 134:837-842.
34. Goldberg DJ, Littler CM, Wheeland RG. Topical suspension-assisted Q-switched Nd:YAG laser hair removal. Dermatol Surg 1997; 23:741-745.
35. Nanni CA, Alster TS. Optimizing treatment parameters for hair removal using a topical carbon-based solution and 1064-nm Q-switched neodymium:YAG laser energy. Arch Dermatol 1997; 133:1546-1549.
36. Kilmer SL, Chotzen VA. Q-switched Nd:YAG laser (1064 nm) hair removal without adjuvant topical preparation. Lasers Surg Med 1997; 9(suppl):31.
37. Anderson RR, Margolis RJ, Watenabe S, et al. Selective photothermolysis of cutaneous pigmentation by Q-switched Nd:YAG laser pulses at 1064, 532, and 355 nm. J Invest Dermatol 1989; 93:28-32.
38. Littler CM. Topical suspension assisted Q-switched Nd:YAG laser hair removal: evaluation of a modified technique. Lasers Surg Med 1998; 10(suppl):43.
39. Lask G, Elman M, Slatkine M, et al. Laser-assisted hair removal by selective photothermolysis: preliminary results. Dermatol Surg 1997; 23:737-739.
40. Abell E. Pathology of male pattern alopecia. Arch Dermatol 1984; 120:1607-1608.
41. Sommer S, Render C, Burd R, Sheehan-Dare R. Ruby laser treatment for hirsutism: clinical response and patient tolerance. Br J Dermatol 1998; 138:1009-1014.
42. Williams R, Havoonjian H, Isagholian K, et al. A clinical study of hair removal using the long-pulsed ruby laser. Dermatol Surg 1998; 24:837-842.
43. Lask G, Elman M, Noren P, et al. Hair removal with the Epitouch ruby laser—a multicenter study. Lasers Surg Med 1997; 9(suppl):32.
44. Sommer S, Render C, Sheehan-Dare R. Facial hirsutism treated with the normal-mode ruby laser: results of a 12-month follow-up study. J Am Acad Dermatol 1999; 41:974-979.
45. Campos VB, Dierickx CC, Lin TYD, et al. Long term efficacy of normal-mode 694 nm ruby laser and 800 nm diode laser for hair removal. Lasers Surg Med 1999; 11(suppl):22.
46. Liew SH, Grobbelaar A, Gault D, et al. Hair removal using the ruby laser: clinical efficacy in Fitzpatrick skin types I-V and histological changes in epidermal melanocytes. Br J Dermatol 1999; 140:1105-1109.
47. McDaniel DH, Lord J, Ash K, et al. Laser hair removal: a review and report on the use of the long-pulsed alexandrite laser for hair reduction of the upper lip, leg, back, and bikini region. Dermatol Surg 1999; 25:425-430.
48. Nanni CA, Alster TS. Long-pulsed alexandrite laser-assisted hair removal at 5, 10, and 20 millisecond pulse durations. Lasers Surg Med 1999; 24:332-337.
49. Goldberg DJ, Ahkami R. Evaluation comparing multiple treatments with a 2-msec and 10-msec alexandrite laser for hair removal. Lasers Surg Med 1999; 25:223-228.
50. Boss WK, Usai H, Thompson RC, Fiorillo MA. A comparison of the long-pulse and short-pulse alexandrite laser hair removal systems. Ann Plast Surg 1999; 42:381-384.

51. Nanni C, Brancaccio R, Cooperman M. The subjective and objective tissue effects of long-pulsed alexandrite laser irradiation: comparisons at 5 and 20 millisecond pulse durations. Lasers Surg Med 1999; 11(suppl):24.
52. Dierickx CC, Grossman MC, Farinelli WA, et al. Hair removal by a pulsed, infrared laser system. Lasers Surg Med 1998; 10(suppl):42.
53. Dierickx CC, Grossman MC, Farinelli WA, et al. Comparison between a long pulsed ruby laser and a pulsed, infrared laser system for hair removal. Lasers Surg Med 1998; 10(suppl):42.
54. Grossman M, Dierickx C, Quintana A, et al. Removal of excess body hair with an 800 nm pulsed diode laser. Lasers Surg Med 1998; 10(suppl):42.
55. Gold MH, Bell MW, Foster TD, Street S. Long-term epilation using the EpiLight broad band, intense pulsed light hair removal system. Dermatol Surg 1997; 23:909-913.
56. Weiss RA, Weiss MA, Marwaha S, Harrington A. Hair removal with a non-coherent filtered flashlamp intense pulsed light source. Lasers Surg Med 1999; 24:128-132.
57. Sadick NS, Shea CR, Burchette JL, Prieto VG. High-intensity flashlamp photoepilation: a clinical, histological, and mechanistic study in human skin. Arch Dermatol 1999; 135:668-676.
58. Bencini PL, Luci A, Galimberti M, Ferranti G. Long-term epilation with long-pulsed neodymium:YAG laser. Dermatol Surg 1999; 25:175-178.
59. Goldberg DJ, Samady JA. Evaluation of a long-pulse Q-switched Nd:YAG laser for hair removal. Dermatol Surg 2000; 26:109-113.
60. Grossman M, Wimberly J, Dwyer P, et al. PDT for hirsutism. Lasers Surg Med 1995; 7(suppl):44.
61. McCoy S, Evans A, James C. Histological study of hair follicles treated with a 3-msec pulsed ruby laser. Lasers Surg Med 1999; 24:142-150.
62. Hasan AT, Eaglstein W, Pardo RJ. Solar-induced postinflammatory hyperpigmentation after laser hair removal. Dermatol Surg 1999; 25:113-115.
63. Nanni CA, Alster TS. Laser-assisted hair removal: side effects of Q-switched Nd:YAG, long-pulsed ruby, and alexandrite lasers. J Am Acad Dermatol 1999; 41:165-171.

CHAPTER 14

Liposuction

DARLENE S. JOHNSON
PATRICK J. LILLIS
MICHAEL S. KAMINER

SECTION ONE

History and Scientific Review

BACKGROUND AND HISTORY

Adipose tissue is deposited in human subcutaneous tissue as an energy reservoir and serves to provide the body with temperature and vibratory insulation. It is deposited and reabsorbed as part of normal homeostasis, and its sites of deposition are in large part genetically predetermined. Two general body shapes are known to exist: gynecoid and android (Fig. 14-1). The gynecoid body type is the usual female shape, with fat preferentially deposited peripherally in locations such as the thighs and hips. The male android body type tends to deposit fat centrally in the intraabdominal region. There are certainly exceptions to both, as well as substantial cross-over in fat distribution patterns between men and women. However, a person may be near his or her ideal body weight yet still have disproportionate, localized adipose deposition. It is for such a patient that liposuction is ideal.

Liposuction is the aesthetic removal of undesirable localized collections of subcutaneous adipose tissue.[1] The concept of liposuction was first introduced in Rome in 1976 by Georgio and Arpard Fischer,[2] and suction equipment was further developed by Yves-Gerard Illouz in France.[3] Early liposuction techniques were "dry," relying on general anesthesia for pain control. This early technique was plagued with complications due to extreme fluid shifts, excessive blood losses necessitating transfusions, and an extended recovery time. The American dermatologist Jeffrey Klein introduced the extremely wet, or "tumescent," technique for liposuction in 1987.[4] This technique of infiltrating large volumes of dilute lidocaine and epinephrine obviated the need for general anesthesia, virtually eliminated the need for blood transfusions, and decreased patient recovery time.[4-6]

The evolution of liposuction over the past decade has been driven by the desire to increase safety and allow the procedure to be performed in an outpatient setting. Klein's work in developing the anesthesia system for liposuction has been invaluable to the practicing liposuction surgeon. It is now possible to treat larger surface areas of the body under purely local anesthesia with liposuction. This has dramatically decreased the complication rate for liposuction and improved aesthetic outcomes. Surgeons are able to use extremely small cannulas, some less than half the size of those used with the original dry technique. The use of small cannulas, in a subcutaneous compartment that has been expanded with fluid, gives the surgeon the ideal platform on which to perform his or her work. The tumescent technique allows the procedure to be performed by a wide array of surgeons, and it has obtained an enviable safety record.

Data from the American Society of Dermatologic Surgery (ASDS) tumescent liposuction survey published in 1995 demonstrated the high safety profile for this procedure.[7] Of the 15,336 patients treated, no deaths, blood transfusions, or hospital admissions were reported. Recently the *New England Journal of Medicine* reported adverse outcomes due to lidocaine toxicity, but careful inspection of the data suggests that that is likely to be an erroneous conclusion.[8]

Ultrasonic liposuction, both internal and external, has recently been developed and hailed by some to be superior to the standard tumescent technique. However, experience has shown that although ultrasound can be a useful adjunct to tumescent liposuction, it has not replaced it as the treatment of choice. The high cost of the ultrasound equipment, larger incisions needed for internal ultrasound-assisted liposuction (UAL), and the steep learning curve have put UAL out of the reach of many surgeons. For these reasons it will not be discussed further in this chapter. New machinery and techniques are certain to evolve in time, but tumescent

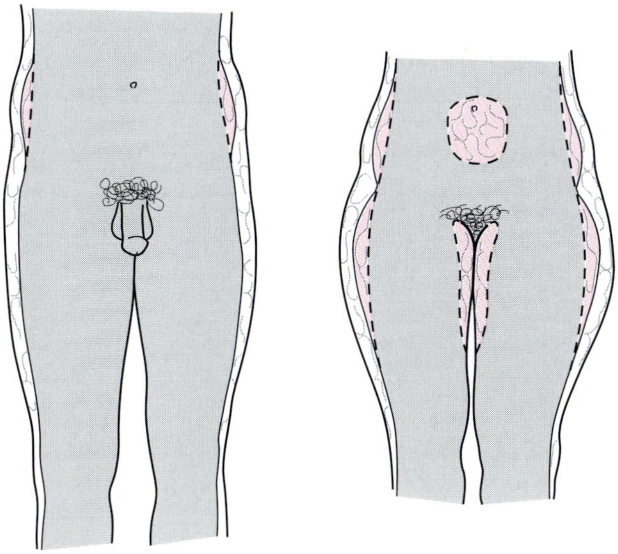

FIG. 14-1
Android *(left)* and gynecoid *(right)* body types. Pink areas denote zones of adipose deposition.

liposuction remains the standard for liposuction surgery as we begin the twenty-first century.

BASIC SCIENCE

Lidocaine toxicity is the most significant factor that limits the amount of anesthesia used in tumescent liposuction. Traditional dosing of lidocaine with epinephrine for dermal or local infusion is 7 mg/kg.[9] Using the tumescent technique, lidocaine doses of 35 mg/kg were shown to be safe and effective.[10] A recent study has shown that dosages up to 55 mg/kg can be used with minimal risk of lidocaine toxicity.[11] That same study also suggests that even higher doses of lidocaine can be used, and some liposuction surgeons around the country have safely used lidocaine in doses of 70 to 80 mg/kg and higher. The very dilute nature of the lidocaine (0.05% to 0.1%) in the tumescent solution, the slow rate of infiltration, the relatively avascular subcutaneous fat compartment, the vasoconstrictive effect of epinephrine, the high lipid solubility of lidocaine and its strong binding affinity to adipose tissue, and the vascular compression due to tissue tumescence all combine to delay systemic uptake of lidocaine.[10,12-14] The peak plasma concentration has been shown to be 8 to 12 hours after infusion, estimated by this formula[11]:

$$\text{Peak plasma lidocaine concentration } (\mu g/ml) = [\text{Dose (mg)}/1000] - 1.25.$$

Lillis initially reported on the safe use of lidocaine doses of 60 to 90 mg/kg,[5] but this was based on plasma lidocaine levels monitored over a 60-minute period. Moy showed in 60 patients that liposuction with a lidocaine dose of 55 mg/kg is safe, with no evidence of lidocaine toxicity over a 24-hour period.[15] The peak plasma lidocaine concentrations obtained from these patients were below 5 μg/ml, under the threshold for when recognizable signs of lidocaine toxicity develop.

Pharmacokinetics relies on not only the concentration but also the rate of delivery. A recent study on the rate of tumescent fluid infiltration evaluated 18 patients receiving 7.4 to 57.7 mg/kg over a period of 5 minutes to 2 hours at rates ranging from 27.1 mg/min to 200 mg/min. Serum lidocaine levels were measured every 15 minutes for the first hour, and at 2 hours. The lidocaine levels for all patients remained below 2 μg/ml.[16] However, the relatively short duration of posttreatment measurements (2 hours) did not completely assess lidocaine levels when they may have been at their peak, up to 12 to 24 hours postoperatively. Clinically, rate of infusion is titrated to patient comfort, which is often directly correlated to degree of sedation.[17] The percentage of lidocaine removed during the liposuction procedure ranged from 1% to 10% of the initial volume infused.[11]

Lidocaine is an amide anesthetic that blocks sodium channels, thus inhibiting the propagation of the neural impulse. It is rapidly and efficiently eliminated by hepatic metabolism via the cytochrome P-450 enzyme CYP3A4. Patients should be screened for concomitant use of medications that are known P-450 CYP3A4 inhibitors, such as erythromycin or ketoconazole.[18] Lidocaine toxicity has been reported in one patient taking sertraline hydrochloride (Zoloft) and flurazepam (Dalmane) who had liposuction performed using 58 mg/kg tumescent lidocaine. At 10 hours, she had clinical symptoms of nausea, vomiting, anxiety, and impaired short-term memory with total blood plasma lidocaine concentration of 6.3 μg/ml.[18] Zoloft and other serotonin re-uptake inhibitors have been shown in vitro to inhibit the activity of cytochrome P-450 3A4 and 2D6.[19] In general, some physicians recommend decreasing the lidocaine dose by 30% to 40% in patients concurrently taking medications that interfere with the P-450 complex.[18] Whether this is actually necessary in clinical practice has not been definitively determined.

The initial clinical manifestations of lidocaine toxicity are perioral numbness or tingling (Table 14-1). As lidocaine levels rise, the patient may develop slurred speech, tinnitus, somnolence, or confusion. At terminally high levels, the patient may have cardiac collapse. Lidocaine suppresses the myocardium at a cellular level, depressing diastolic depolarization and automaticity in the ventricles.[20]

The advent of tumescent liposuction has eliminated the need for intravenous fluid replacement during the procedure, and substantial fluid shifts are not common

Table 14-1 Total Plasma Lidocaine Levels and Corresponding Clinical Signs and Symptoms[20]

Total Plasma Lidocaine Level (μg/ml)	Clinical Signs and Symptoms
<1.5	Idiosyncratic
1.5-4	Mild CNS
4-6	Mild CNS and cardiovascular toxicity
6-8	Major CNS and cardiovascular depression
>8	Seizures, hypotension, respiratory and cardiac depression

BOX 14-1 Most Common Areas of Liposuction for Men and Women[27]

Men
Flanks/love handles (56%)
Abdomen (32%)
Neck/jowls (11%)
Breast (5%)

Women
Abdomen (55%)
Outer thighs (38%)
Hip/waist (10%)
Neck/jowls (3%)

with this technique. Saline is used as the foundation for liposuction anesthesia, and when placed in the subcutaneous space is absorbed slowly into the microvasculature. This form of volume replacement, known as hypodermoclysis, is the mechanism for volume replacement during tumescent liposuction surgery. Since the fluid is absorbed slowly over hours and not minutes (as with intravenous fluids), it allows the patient to mobilize and excrete fluids at a rate controlled by normal homeostatic mechanisms. This allows for long-term hydration of the patient over the immediate postoperative period, yet virtually eliminates the risk of fluid overload. However, the surgeon must use caution when placing subcutaneous fluids during liposuction. It is possible to use such high volumes of local anesthesia (greater than 5 to 6 liters of fluid) that the patient is at risk for volume overload, particularly patients with a history of cardiac or renal disease.

Epinephrine has a threefold importance for tumescent liposuction. It provides excellent hemostasis, slows the rate of lidocaine absorption, and prolongs local analgesia. Unlike lidocaine, there is no described limitation for epinephrine dosing.[21] For treatment of anaphylaxis, the recommended therapeutic dose is 0.01 mg/kg body weight.[22] With the tumescent technique for liposuction, total epinephrine doses as high as 10 mg have been used without adverse effects.[21] Epinephrine toxicity is initially manifested by patient anxiety, agitation, or palpitations. With increased levels, hypertension, tachycardia, or arrhythmias may occur. A study of 20 patients undergoing liposuction, monitored at 3, 12, and 23 hours after tumescent fluid infiltration, demonstrated that the peak serum epinephrine levels occurred at 3 hours. Peak levels were three to five times the upper limit of normal (normal resting values: 0 to 133 pg/ml; patients with pheochromocytoma: 200 to 12,700 pg/ml).[23] The majority had returned to normal at 12 hours. The only reported side effect was anxiety.[21]

CLINICAL STUDIES

Liposuction is one of the most commonly performed aesthetic surgical procedures.[24] In the United States 33% to 40% of adult women and 20% to 24% of adult men are trying to lose weight. Another 28% of each group are trying to maintain their weight.[25] Whereas women cite appearance as more important than fitness, the reverse is true for men.[26] The areas most commonly treated are different for women and men (Box 14-1).

Though cases of megaliposculpture (with the removal of more than 10 L of fat) have been reported,[28] we prefer to perform serial sessions with a range of 2 to 6 L of fat removed on average. Patients must be reminded that liposuction of subcutaneous tissues does not halt deposition of fat. A study of 51 normal weight to mildly obese women studied absolute and relative changes in total body fat and visceral adipose tissue after large-volume (>1000 ml) liposuction. Aspiration of 1.5 ± 0.7 kg of lipid removed 9.2% ± 3.2% of body fat, corresponding to a 12% increase in the ratio of visceral to subcutaneous adipose tissue. The results in 12 men were similar.[29] Increased visceral adipose tissue is a risk factor for metabolic complications of obesity.[30] Compensatory increases in the size of remaining fat deposits have been reported after liposuction.[31] The long-term metabolic changes after liposuction remains an area requiring further study.

DISCUSSION

Indications for liposuction published by the ASDS are cosmetic body contouring, diseases involving the subcutaneous tissue (lipomas, lipodystrophy, axillary hyperhidrosis), and reconstruction.[1] Ideally, liposuction should be used in conjunction with an exercise program and not as a substitution for weight loss by diet control. Many patients pursue liposuction for specific body locations that disturb them. For 87% of female patients, their family history is a good predictor of localized adipose deposition that is resistant to diet and exercise.[27] The physician should take the patient's wishes into consideration, as well as the overall proportions of the patient. Proportion, contour, flow, and symmetry of body lines are essential parts of liposuction planning. Patients with localized irregular contours or localized fat deposits are superb candidates for liposuction and tend to do quite well. The surgeon's role is to identify those body areas that can be contoured with liposuction to create an overall aesthetic and contour improvement. Because of these global considerations, liposuction has been referred to as *liposculpting*. This is one of the most challenging aspects of liposuction surgery.

For some patients, skin laxity, muscle flaccidity, or location of fat pads deeper than the subcutis (i.e., intraabdominal) may not make them good liposuction candidates. One judges skin laxity by the "snap test" (Fig. 14-2). To perform this test, the surgeon pinches 1 to 3 cm of skin, retracts, and releases. Ideally, there should be instant recoil of the skin to its prior location. Slow recoil or excess laxity may be an indicator that the patient will have redundant skin folds or surface irregularities after liposuction. This needs to be explained to the patient, and in some cases a combination of procedures may enable the patient to obtain the anticipated results. For example, abdominoplasty in addition to abdominal liposuction can improve the final contour of the abdomen. However, risk and morbidity are increased by the addition of abdominoplasty to the surgical plan.[32,33] For this reason, recognition of those patients at risk for poor skin retraction is essential. Age is not the sole predictor of skin retraction, and even adults over age 40 can achieve smooth postoperative contours.[34] Locations that are at particular risk for poor skin retraction (in the patient with poor skin tone) are the neck, upper arms, lower abdomen, and inner and outer thighs. We refer to patients with less than optimal skin elasticity as having *soft skin*. This can be recognized as the preoperative appearance of cellulite and dimples on the outer thigh, ridges or folds on the abdomen, hanging neck skin, or wrinkled inner thigh skin. Patients with soft skin must be treated with caution, and they should be counseled as to the expected outcome of surgery. Aggressive suctioning in these patients can produce less than optimal results. However, even patients with good skin tone and elasticity can experience poor skin retraction, most commonly on the upper abdomen, distal anterior thighs, and the anterior axilla.

Tumescent liposuction has evolved to be a very safe, reproducible method for selective fat removal and body contouring. A thorough understanding of the surgical concept, as well as extensive training in the procedure, offer the surgeon a unique opportunity to create aesthetically pleasing contours with fat removal.

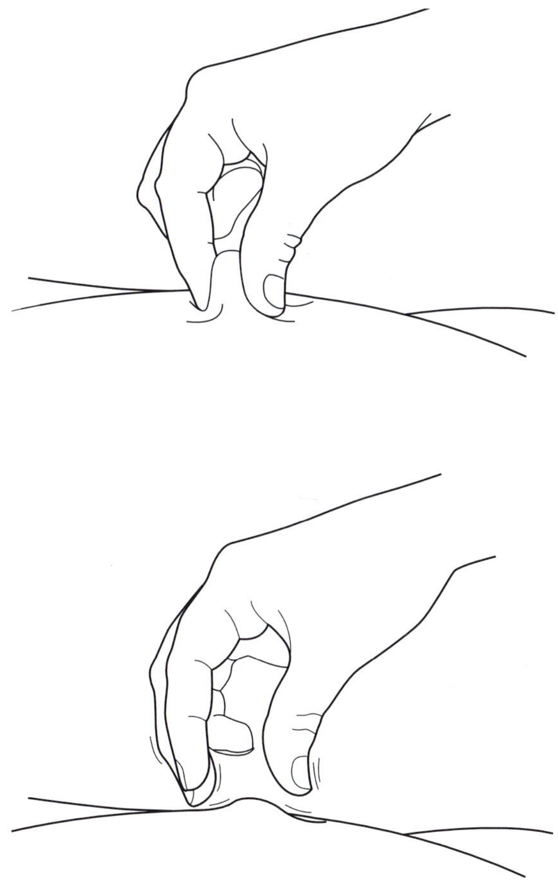

FIG. 14-2
The "snap test" to determine skin laxity. The *top* figure represents the initial pinch of skin, and the surgeon observes recoil as the skin is released (*bottom* figure).

SECTION TWO

Atlas of Surgical Procedures

PREOPERATIVE CLINICAL CONSIDERATIONS

Through written information, informative videotapes, and patient discussions, a physician strives to inform the patient about the procedure of liposuction, including realistic goals, expectations, and possible side effects and complications. Good surgical judgment must be used to determine if the patient has realistic expectations and will participate responsibly with preoperative and postoperative care. As with other cosmetic procedures, it is advisable to be wary of patients who are overanxious or demanding on staff or who the physician thinks will be satisfied only if they obtain a perfect result. All staff, from the front office receptionists to the nursing staff, should be encouraged to inform the physician of any idiosyncrasies they may notice. Patients with suspected eating disorders or body dysmorphism should be referred for appropriate counseling.

As with any procedure, liposuction requires the participation of both patient and physician. The initial patient interview with careful history and physical examination should prepare the patient and answer all of his or her questions. The patient should be given information regarding what medications to avoid for 2 weeks prior to the procedure (Appendix A) and what to expect on the day of the procedure. This helps to alleviate anxiety and minimize confusion.

A thorough medical history is essential to evaluating undue risk of bleeding, infection, emboli, thrombophlebitis, edema, and past surgeries that may complicate the technique.[1] Not only should current medications and medication allergies be recorded but also any history of hepatitis, hepatotoxic chemotherapy, and use of birth control pills or cytochrome P-450 competitors. A complete skin examination should be done, noting adipose distribution, quality of skin tone, and elasticity. All treatment sites should be evaluated for preexisting hernias, varicosities, scars, asymmetry, or other findings. Because of the forces of gravity, evaluation should be done with the patient standing. Some physicians also examine the patient sitting and in the supine position with the hip flexed.

Laboratory studies are done to screen patients for general health, bleeding disorders, and underlying disorders that may affect the metabolism of medications used throughout the procedure. Typical studies include liver function tests, hepatitis profile, electrolytes, complete blood count, prothrombin time, partial thromboplastin time, and pregnancy test for premenopausal women. Other tests may include urinalysis, bleeding time, or infectious disease studies such as for the human immunodeficiency virus.[1]

Preoperative and postoperative care are truly part of the art of medicine and vary with each physician. The results of the 1995 ASDS study of physicians performing liposuction showed 88% started antibiotics 1 day preoperatively, of which more than 80% used a cephalosporin. Oral sedation was used by 53% of physicians, including diazepam (Valium) and lorazepam (Ativan). Preoperative vitamins were recommended by 24% of physicians participating in the study, most commonly vitamins C and K, as well as a multivitamin.[27] To minimize local bacterial flora, some physicians have the patient wash at home with antibacterial soap (Hibiclens, Zeneca Pharmaceuticals, Wilmington, DE) each of the 3 days before the procedure.[35]

At present, there is no required certification to perform liposuction. It is solely dependent on the ethical standards of physicians and medical communities to monitor the procedure. One may read the literature, study instructional materials, and attend practical or hands-on courses, but performing the technique under the guidance of an experienced physician is invaluable. The nuances of the procedure, patient's emotional requirements, managing complications, and the "normal" healing phases must be understood by the physician prior to beginning a liposuction practice. Although the safety record for tumescent liposuction is superb, it remains an invasive surgical procedure. Physicians with good surgical skills and fundamentals can master the basics of the procedure. However, the art of tumescent anesthesia and cannula motion for liposuction are not always intuitive and can be a challenge to even the most skilled surgeon. For these reasons, preceptored experience, such as a hands-on course or a surgical fellowship, are essential to developing solid fundamental skills for liposuction surgery.

PROCEDURAL TECHNIQUES

Before the procedure, laboratory examinations should be reviewed and confirmed, an informed operative consent signed (Appendix B), and last-minute questions answered. The initiation of preoperative antibiotics should be confirmed, as well as the discontinuation of medications that can promote bleeding (Appendix A). The patient's weight should be obtained on the day of surgery and used both as a reference for postoperative visits and to calculate maximum lidocaine dosage for the procedure. If preoperative calculations are performed by nursing staff or assistants, the surgeon should be certain to verify calculations, including the conversion of pounds to kilograms and the calculation of lidocaine dosage.

Although many doctors perform liposuction in office examining rooms, it is advisable to have a larger room (approximately 140 square feet or larger) in which to perform liposuction. It should have good surgical lighting and an adjustable operating room table. Monitoring is not essential for all cases, especially those without sedation and less than 1000 ml of aspirate. Oxygen saturation, blood pressure, and pulse should be monitored intraoperatively for cases exceeding 1000 ml of aspirate or when sedation is used.

A set of preoperative photographs of the area being treated should be taken from at least two angles. Whether these are 35 mm, instant (Polaroid), or digital, they should be stored for future reference. Some physicians have the photographs available during the procedure for reference. Having the photographs available for comparison postoperatively is essential when evaluating possible complications or patient concerns. For this reason it is important to be able to obtain reproducibly good results with consistent distancing, focus, and lighting.

We have begun to use a digital camera system (Canfield, Fairfield, NJ) that has several advantages: convenient and easy photo storage on computer and the ability to instantly view photographic quality preoperatively. The camera is relatively easy to use, but the vagaries of computer usage and backup systems can make this a challenge for some offices.

Marking the areas to be treated is an interactive procedure between the physician and patient. As mentioned above, the patient has a desired outcome in mind, and the physician must weigh this with the overall cosmetic appearance of the patient as well as functional anatomy and treatment "danger zones." While the patient is alert and standing, sitting, and supine the physician should clearly mark the treatment areas. The physician needs to be able to clearly mark areas to be aggressively treated, areas not to be treated, and areas to be "feathered," or lightly treated. One may use different-colored marking pens, or different types of marks with one color, as long as it is clear to the surgeon (Fig. 14-3). We have found that a fine to medium point black Sharpie pen (Sanford, Bellwood, IL) works well, does not come off during the procedure, yet fades during the following few days. Because this marking procedure relies on the patient being cognitively alert, we wait to administer any preoperative sedation until after everything has been confirmed with the patient.

The patient is prepped in a sterile manner with a surgical scrub and paint (Betadine, Purdue Fredrick Co., Norwalk, CT, or Hibiclens, Zeneca Pharmaceuticals, Wilmington, DE) to minimize skin flora and risk of infection. Although cellulitis is rare, it can be a devastating complication. Areas not to be treated are covered with sterile drapes, exposing only the treatment area(s). Some physicians consider liposuction a clean procedure and do not follow full sterile technique guidelines. We prefer to use sterile technique. Many patients become chilled during the procedure, so it is helpful to have a table heating device in place under the patient (Gaymar hydrocollator heating pad, George Tieman & Company, Hauppauge, NY, or the Bear Hugger Warmer, Augustine Medical Inc., Eden Prairie, MN) and maintain careful control of room temperature. Additional options for keeping the patient warm during the procedure are stocking caps to contain body heat and prevent loss through the scalp, as well as warm socks.

The equipment used for tumescent liposuction varies greatly between practitioners depending on style, training, treatment site, patient factors, and desired aggressiveness of liposuction. Common items are an infusion mechanism and cannula for infusion of the tumescent anesthetic solution, suction apparatus, and suction cannulas of specified diameters and tip designs (Box 14-2 and Table 14-2).

There are many ways to deliver the tumescent anesthesia. Peristaltic mechanical pumps such as the Klein pump (Wells Johnson Co., Tucson, AZ) are able to de-

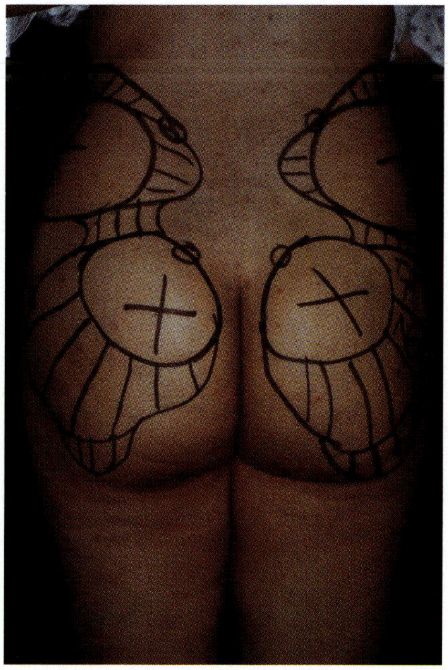

FIG. 14-3
Preoperative markings of the female hips and buttocks. Note lines of flow and markings to guide the surgeon intraoperatively.

BOX 14-2 Cannulas

Aggressive Cannulas: Larger Diameter, Numerous Holes, Holes Placed Toward Tip of Cannula in Direction of Suctioning
Keel Cobra: 3 or 3.7 mm
Capistrano, Mercedes, Pinto, Toledo: 10 or 12 gauge

Intermediate Cannulas: Medium Diameter, Distal Holes Oriented Away from Dermis
Accelerator/Triport: 3 mm
Klein (dual port): 12 gauge
Capistrano: 14 gauge
Keel Cobra, Texas, Dual Port, Fournier: 2.5 mm

Least Aggressive Cannulas: Small Diameter, Distal Holes Oriented Away from Dermis
Capistrano: 16 gauge
Klein (dual port): 14-16 gauge
Spatula: 2-3 mm

Table 14-2 Gauge and Millimeter Equivalents for Liposuction Cannulas

Gauge	Equivalent (mm)
8	4.2
10	3.4
12	2.8
14	2.2

BOX 14-3 Commonly Used Suction Pumps

Aspirator III (Wells Johnson, Tucson, AZ)
Hercules (Wells Johnson, Tucson, AZ)
Reliance (Bernsco, Hauppauge, NY)

liver up to 5 to 6 L of fluid in 15 to 20 minutes. However, a rate of less than 100 ml/min is commonly used (a setting of 2 to 3 on the Klein pump).[6] Roller pumps, spring return syringes, and pressurized infusion bags can also be used. The cannula for infusion of the tumescent anesthetic solution is usually a 6- to 12-inch, 12- to 14-gauge diameter, blunt tipped instrument with a sprinkler-type hole distribution (Fig. 14-4). Spinal needles (18- to 20-gauge) can also be used for infusion of tumescent solution.

Many suction pumps are available for use (Box 14-3). Factors influencing choice include types of compatible tubing, noise made by the machine, reliability, and size. It is interesting to note that suction pumps tend to work more efficiently at sea level than at higher elevations (personal observation, 1999), presumably due to differences in atmospheric pressure. Suction cannulas vary in length, diameter, tip style, and orifice placement. All of these components factor into the aggressiveness of the suction cannula. More aggressive cannulas are wider in diameter and shorter, have an open or pointed tip rather than blunt tip, and have more and larger orifices for aspiration. Nearly all cannulas are designed to be used with the suction holes directed away from the underside of the dermis (Fig. 14-5).

The tumescent technique is a method of delivering large volumes of dilute lidocaine with epinephrine in buffered saline via subcutaneous infiltration to achieve adequate local anesthesia and assist with hemostasis (Fig. 14-6).[4] Table 14-3 lists the standard preparations.

Epinephrine, without the addition of sodium bicarbonate, will make the tumescent solution acidic, which may cause burning with infusion. Also, lidocaine action may be more efficient when it is in solution near its p*K* (p*K* of lidocaine = 7.7).[5] Tumescent solution is also buffered because sodium bicarbonate added to lidocaine in vitro augments the bactericidal activity of lido-

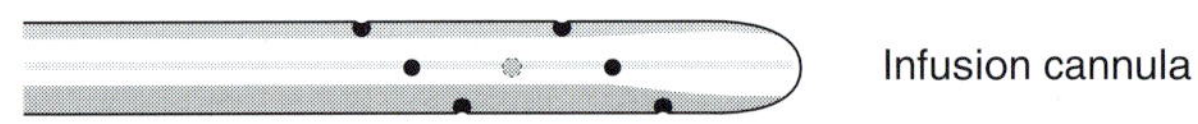

FIG. 14-4
The sprinkler tip tumescent anesthesia infusion cannula.

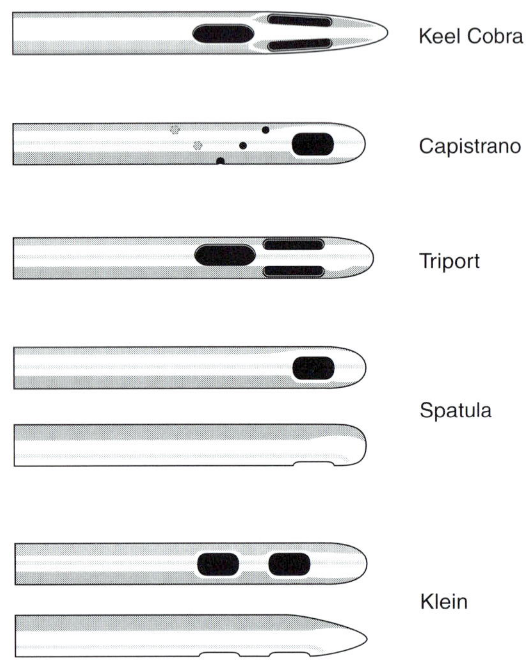

FIG. 14-5
Liposuction cannulas.

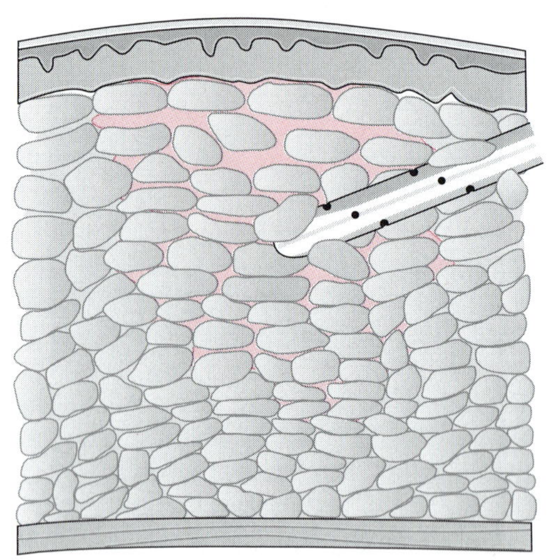

FIG. 14-6
Infusion of subcutaneous tumescent anesthesia. The pink color represents anesthetic fluid hydrodissecting and expanding the adipose compartment.

Table 14-3 Tumescent Anesthetic Solution[6,11]

Constituent	Amount
0.1% Solution	
Normal saline (0.9%)	1 L
Lidocaine 2%	50 ml (final concentration 0.1%)
Epinephrine 1:1000	1 ml (1 mg) (final concentration 1:1,000,000)
Sodium bicarbonate 8.45%	12.5 ml (final solution pH 7.4)
Triamcinolone acetonide	10 mg
0.05% Solution	
Normal saline (0.9%)	1 L
Lidocaine 2%	25 ml (final concentration 0.05%)
Epinephrine 1:1000	1 ml (1 mg) (final concentration 1:1,000,000)
Sodium bicarbonate 8.45%	12.5 ml (final solution pH 7.4)
Triamcinolone acetonide	10 mg

caine.[36] Lidocaine has been shown to be bactericidal for organisms isolated from the skin.[37] Concentrations greater than 0.5% lidocaine provide a dose-dependent inhibition of bacterial growth, gram-negative greater than gram-positive organisms.[38] In dilutions of 0.05%, lidocaine is bacteriostatic for *Staphylococcus aureus*.[39] In in vitro studies using suspensions of bacteria (105 cfu/ml), all gram-positive organisms, including *S. aureus*, had significantly lower colony counts in 0.05% lidocaine.[40] When tumescent anesthesia is used, infection is a rare complication.[41]

The higher concentration of lidocaine (0.1%) is used for more sensitive areas, such as the abdomen, lateral thighs, knees, inner thighs, periumbilical area, neck, flanks, and back.[11,17] Some physicians choose to utilize only the 0.05% lidocaine formula for liposuction to decrease total lidocaine dosage and enable them to treat larger surface areas. However, 0.05% lidocaine is not as efficient at producing anesthesia as the 0.1% concentration. Therefore, an increase in sedation is often required when using 0.05% lidocaine for local liposuction anesthesia. It is a matter of physician preference to determine whether to use the 0.1% solution to treat smaller areas with less sedation, or to use the 0.05% solution with increased sedation. We have recently begun using 0.075% lidocaine anesthesia with excellent results. The 0.075% solution retains much of the anesthetic activity of the 0.1% solution but with 25% less lidocaine, allowing larger areas to be treated in one session. The 1:1,000,000 concentration of epinephrine is more commonly used, but some surgeons have used concentrations as low as 1:2,000,000 epinephrine with good results.

A randomized, double-blind cross-over study demonstrated that warming of local anesthetic solution for tumescent liposuction significantly reduces pain on infusion as perceived by the patient.[42] A randomized, double-blind prospective trial of adult volunteers serving as their own controls showed that warmed, buffered lidocaine was significantly less painful to infuse than either plain lidocaine, buffered lidocaine, or warmed lidocaine.[43]

Tumescent anesthesia fluid is delivered by blunt-tipped small-diameter cannulas (12 to 14 gauge). These are less traumatic than conventional sharp-tipped needles and preserve the neurovascular structures.[44] They also minimize risk for penetrating deeper structures. In skilled hands, 18- to 20-gauge spinal needles can also be used for infusion. Appropriate incision sites should be planned to account for the length of the liposuction cannula to be used, to provide adequate access to all treatment areas, and to facilitate draining of the tumescent fluid during the postoperative period. The surgeon can maximize the use of anatomic landmarks during this phase of the procedure, such as hiding an incision adjacent to the umbilicus.

Using a fine-gauge needle with a small-caliber syringe, each cannula incision site should be anesthetized. Some physicians use buffered 1% lidocaine with epinephrine, but we prefer to use the same solution as that which will be used to provide tumescent anesthesia. An approximately 3 to 4 mm incision with a No. 11 blade serves as a cannula insertion site.[6] Insert the No. 11 blade only partially and at an angle to avoid trauma to deeper tissues. A 1.5 to 2 mm punch biopsy tool is another alternative that may have the advantage of remaining patent longer than traditional incision sites to facilitate drainage. However, we have not found this to be necessary. The blunt-tipped small-diameter infusion cannula is inserted, attached to the peristaltic motorized pump, pressurized infusion bag, or other delivery system. As discussed earlier, the infusion rate may vary and is titrated to the comfort of the patient, most commonly less than 100 ml/min.

The rate of infusion can be increased proportionately to the amount of premedication given.[17] Varying combinations of sedatives and analgesics are given (Box 14-4), but each patient will respond to and metabolize medication at varying rates. Therefore, dosages and choice of medications used should be titrated to each patient individually.

It is best to criss-cross paths of anesthetizing both horizontally and vertically within the depth of the adipose tissue to ensure complete anesthesia. Caution should be used so as not to create excess friction on the incision sites, as this can impair healing. The infusion

BOX 14-4 Commonly Used Sedatives and Analgesics[17]

Diazepam (5-15 mg PO)
Lorazepam (1-2 mg PO)
Triazolam (Halcion: 0.25 mg PO)
Hydroxyzine hydrochloride (Vistaril: 25-50 mg IV or IM)
Midazolam hydrochloride (Versed: 2.5-5 mg IV or IM)
Promethazine hydrochloride (Phenergan: 25 mg IV or IM)
Meperidine hydrochloride (Demerol: 25-50 mg IV or IM)

cannula is moved slowly within the subcutaneous space to thoroughly anesthetize each region. Areas closer to the infusion incision are anesthetized first to allow the cannula to move comfortably to distal regions. The anesthetic fluid also serves to hydrodissect the tissue, creating a plane for the cannula to move in.[6] Trying to change directions, or angling the cannula while in midstroke, should be avoided. A change in cannula direction during its motion can cause tenting or dimpling of the overlying skin. This can be particularly problematic during the suctioning phase and can produce contour irregularities.

The end point for infusion is reached when the tissue becomes firm to hard and indurated (Fig. 14-7). For both infusing tumescent anesthesia fluid and suctioning, one hand moves the cannula and the other serves as a "smart hand" to guide and feel the cannula position. This usually nondominant hand lies on the skin and palpates, constantly assessing the movement of the cannula, depth in the tissue, and degree of tissue induration. The end point for infusion can also be assessed by blanching as a result of vasoconstriction. The amount of tumescent anesthesia fluid infiltrated will depend on the anatomic location (Table 14-4). The surgeon must be cautioned that there is no absolute rule as to how much anesthesia is required to fully treat an area. Factors that can affect volume of infiltration include body weight and the amount of fat in a particular anatomic area; the amounts listed in Table 14-4 represent averages based on our experience. Clearly, certain patients will require more or less local anesthesia depending on individual anatomic variation.

Infusion patterns for men and women are different. Adipose tissue in women tends to lie in the mid to deep subcutaneous space, and therefore anesthetic solution should be directed to these locations. Men tend to have fibrous subdermal fat that requires aggressive suctioning to remove adipose tissue, as well as mid subcutaneous space adipose tissue (Fig. 14-8). For this reason, it is essential to add 0.1% tumescent anesthetic solution to the subdermal fat in sensitive areas for men (breasts, abdomen, love handles), in addition to anesthetizing the mid and deeper subcutaneous compartments.

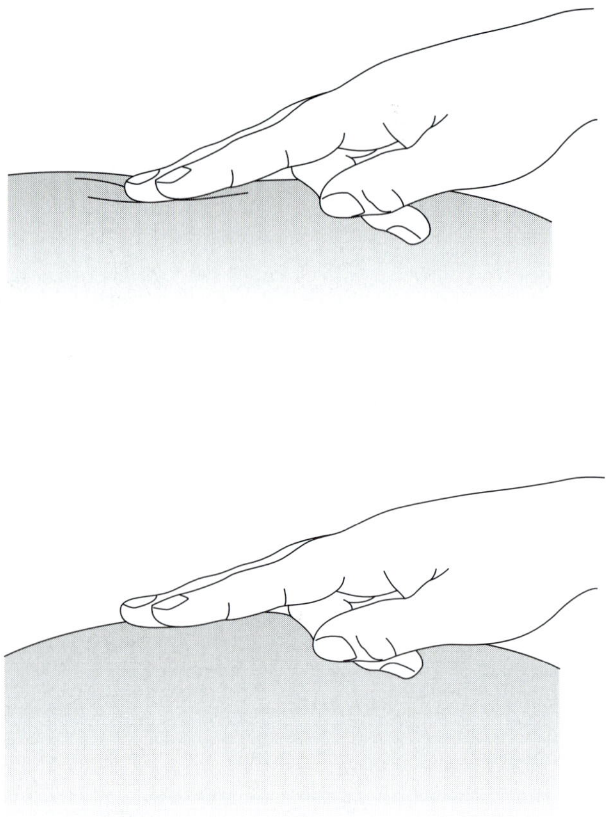

FIG. 14-7
Determining the end point for tumescent anesthesia infiltration. Prior to infusion *(top)* the skin is soft, but when infusion is complete *(bottom)*, the skin is firm and resists downward pressure.

Table 14-4 Approximate Volume of Anesthesia Used According to Body Site

Site	Volume (L)
Neck	0.4
Arms	1.0 per side
Upper abdomen	0.75
Lower abdomen	1.0
Hips	0.75 per side
Love handles	1.0 per side
Flanks	0.75 per side
Outer thighs	1.0 per side
Inner thighs	0.75 per side
Knees	0.5 per side
Calves and ankles	1.0 per side

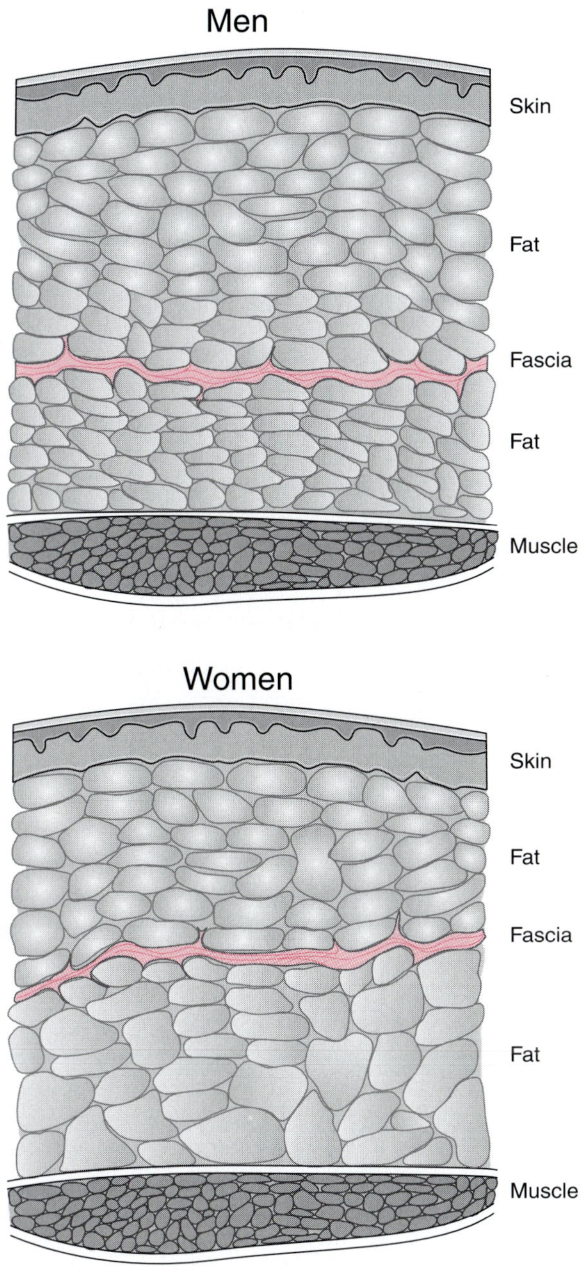

FIG. 14-8
Relative location of fat in men and women (anterior lower abdomen as example). Note relative size/proportion of fat above and below superficial fascia in men and women.

The ideal time delay between tumescent infusion and liposuction varies from patient to patient, and from location to location. Approximately 15 minutes is needed to establish adequate vasoconstriction.[17] A good indicator of the appropriate time delay is the visible blanching that occurs in the tumesced sites.[44] However, a minimum of 30 to 45 minutes is required to establish the profound anesthesia that is essential for performing adequate and careful suctioning. The areas anesthetized should extend beyond the border of the intended liposuction sites to prevent tenderness at the periphery, and to allow for feathering.

BOX 14-5 Liposuction Cosmetic Units

- Neck, submental region, and jowls
- Posterior upper arm
- Posterior axillary line and upper back
- Upper abdomen
- Lower abdomen
- Hip or love handles
- Waistline and mid back
- Outer thigh
- Inner thigh extending to knee
- Anterior thigh
- Posterior thigh
- Calf and ankle
- Breast

The concept of liposculpture is evolving as physicians treat not just one cosmetic unit, but adjacent cosmetic units (Box 14-5), blending the treatment sites to result in a more natural symmetry of proportions. Preoperative markings help the surgeon to delineate areas to be treated, with an improvement in the overall aesthetic appearance as the goal of surgery. However, it is the intraoperative technique that ultimately determines the final result. The surgeon must pinch, feel, inspect, move, and contour the subcutaneous tissue in a manner that will produce an improved skin contour. As liposuction surgeons, we rely on the skin's remarkable ability to contract and drape over the underlying soft tissue. It is imperative to keep the patient's unique physical characteristics and skin type in mind while suctioning. Skin that has poor elasticity will not recontour as well as skin with good tone, and this is part of the art of liposuction/liposculpture. The surgeon factors in all of these issues to determine just how much fat to remove, and from which areas, to produce the final result.

Body position during the procedure must be changed frequently, the physician's as well as the patient's. The physician should use all sides of the operative table to examine and treat the patient, accessing areas from a minimum of two directions, preferably three. We refer to this method of suctioning as *triangulation.* Patient position should also be changed during surgery if the physician needs to access the fat. An advantage of tumescent liposuction surgery is that the patient is awake and therefore able to follow commands. The patient can be asked to change body position during the procedure to make it easier for the surgeon to treat an area of the body. The central premise is that the surgeon must be certain to treat all marked areas in a manner that will yield smooth contours. Asking the patient to change position on the table is one part of the process.

The concept of triangulation is central to obtaining smooth liposuction results (Fig. 14-9). The surgeon should think of each unit area of fat as a compartment that needs to be treated, and linking these areas will produce smooth contours. Each unit area should be accessed and suctioned from three directions (triangulated) in order to avoid producing ridges. When an area is suctioned from one direction it is possible to leave ridges, as small areas of fat between the cannula tunnels remain. Suctioning from two directions helps to reduce this risk, but the third vector dramatically reduces the appearance and feel of residual fat and ridges.

The nondominant smart hand is one of the most important elements of liposuction surgery. This hand is used to guide the cannula, as well as assess cannula position and depth within the fat, bring fat into the can-

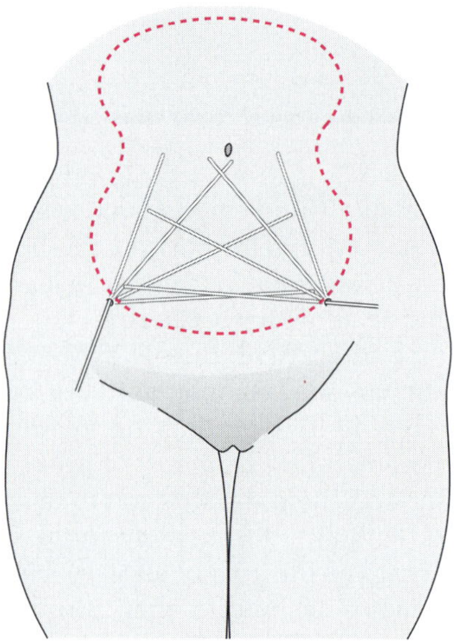

FIG. 14-9
Triangulation of liposuction cannulas.

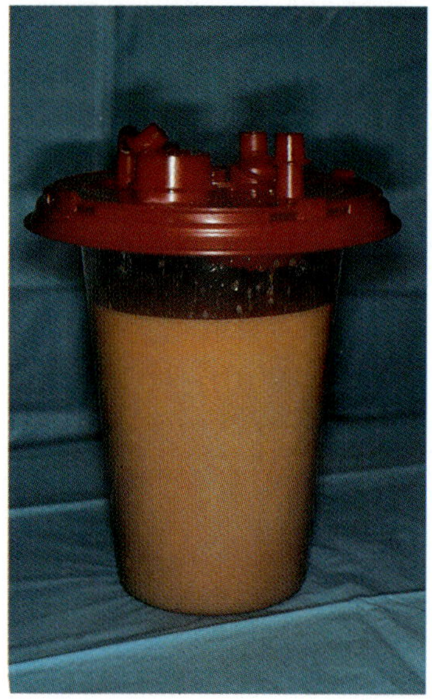

FIG. 14-11
Liposuction aspirate demonstrating nearly 1.5 L of fat without any significant bleeding.

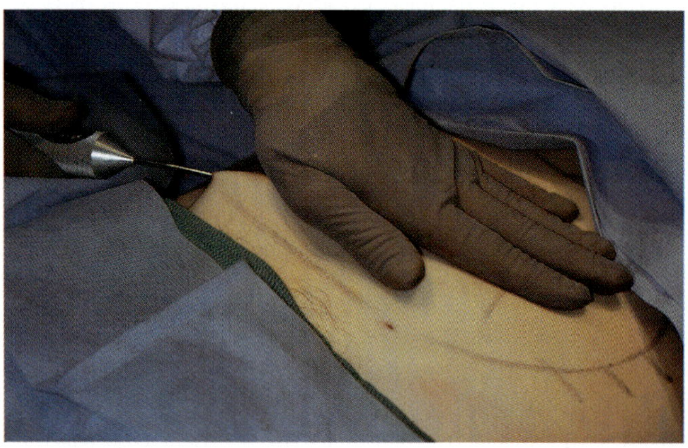

FIG. 14-10
Use of the smart hand. The surgeon uses the nondominant hand (left in this photograph) to palpate the skin and give tactile feedback.

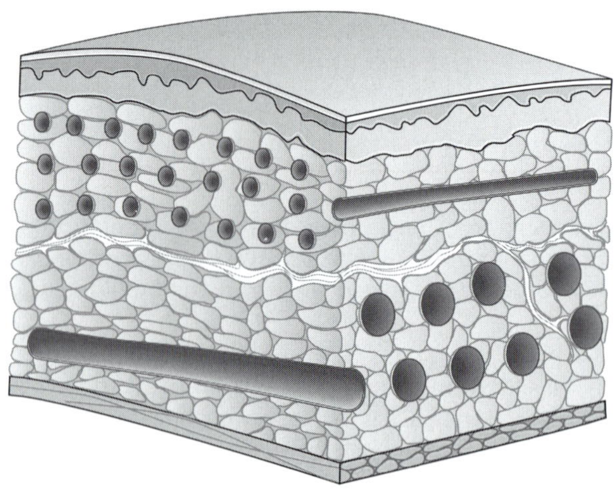

FIG. 14-12
Orientation and placement of liposuction cannula tunnels. Smaller cannula diameters are often used to remove superficial fat after deeper fat is suctioned with larger diameter cannulas.

nula path, stretch or stabilize skin, and in general serve as the sensory input from the patient back to the physician (Fig. 14-10). Visual clues are also extremely helpful for liposuction contouring, but the smart hand is an invaluable link between the surgeon and patient. A surgeon's mastery of the smart hand concept is likely to improve liposuction results significantly.

With the use of tumescent anesthesia, blood loss is minimal. The physician should continuously be monitoring the aspirate for quantity and quality of adipose (Fig. 14-11). If the amount of blood increases in the aspirate at any time during the procedure, active suction of that area should be discontinued. Klein has reported that approximately 12 ml of blood is lost for each 1000 ml of fat that is aspirated using the tumescent technique.[45]

Adequate tumescent anesthesia should make the procedure nearly painless. The use of large cannulas initially takes advantage of the period of maximal anesthesia. Smaller cannulas cause less pain as they are advanced through the adipose tissue and offer more options for fine-tuning and removing the remaining adipose tissue (Fig. 14-12). Changing the angle, direction, diameter of the cannula, altering the patient position, or applying manual traction with the smart hand may allow treatment of tender areas, avoiding the need to use further anesthesia to an area.[6]

The structure and function of each body region necessitates variations in the liposuction technique. Local anatomy, the quality of adipose tissue (soft or fibrous), thickness of the dermis, and skin elasticity all factor into the approach to a liposuction cosmetic unit. The following discussions focus on the unique approach we take for different anatomic regions (Box 14-6).

BOX 14-6 Anatomic Sites and Liposuction Aggressiveness[46]

Aggressive: 80% to 100% Removed
Love handles
Back/flanks
Male breasts
Medial knees
Upper and lower abdomen

Moderate: 50% to 80% Removed

Hips	Inner thighs
Arms	Calves/ankles
Outer thighs	Neck
Buttocks	Jawline

Light: Less than 50% Removed
Mid inner thighs
Jowls
Anterior distal thighs and knees
Posterior knees

Liposuction of the Neck and Jowls

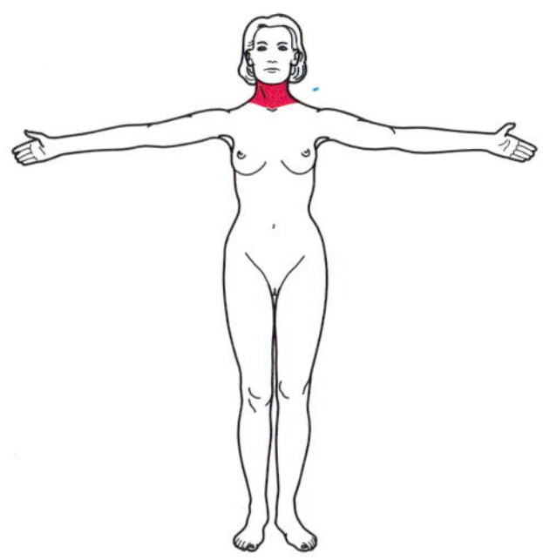

The neck and jowls are difficult but rewarding areas to treat with liposuction. Traditional methods of treatment for the aging neck have primarily included face and neck lifting procedures. However, for selected patients, liposuction can be a definitive treatment. The ideal patient has good skin tone and elasticity, moderate submental fat, mild jowl formation, and a high-set hyoid bone.

There are two basic physical findings of patients who are candidates for neck liposuction: aging and obesity. Patients with neck obesity often have excess adipose tissue in other areas of the body, but many are interested in treatment of the neck to define their facial features for appearance enhancement. These patients often do extremely well with liposuction, in part because many are young (under age 45) with superb skin elasticity (Fig. 14-13). Aging can be challenging to treat with neck liposuction but is perhaps the most common indication for therapy. These patients are often older (over age 40), have mild to moderate jowl formation, fair to good skin tone and elasticity, and mild to moderate submental fat. Lentigenes, poikiloderma, and telangiectasia do not improve with liposuction. However, rhytides will often improve following careful and aggressive suctioning, and neck contours can be greatly improved (Fig. 14-14).

Since liposuction is not a skin-tightening procedure, patients must be carefully evaluated. The patient is asked to clench the teeth, which will tighten the platysma muscle and define fat location. The surgeon pinches the submental skin between thumb and forefinger to assess both quantity and location of fat. Submental fat can be either preplatysmal or postplatysmal. Preplatysmal fat can be suctioned through a small submental incision, but post- (or retro) platysmal fat must be excised directly. Asking the patient to place the tongue up against the hard palate will also help the surgeon to identify fat location. The surgeon should also release the skin as part of a *snap test* to determine skin elasticity. If the skin feels loose and does not recoil quickly, then liposuction alone is unlikely to provide maximal benefit.

The clenched teeth test is also useful to evaluate platysma location and banding. As patients age, some will develop vertical subcutaneous bands that represent nondecussating platysma muscle fibers. When these are identified preoperatively, the surgeon can elect to repair the platysma muscle at the time of lipo-

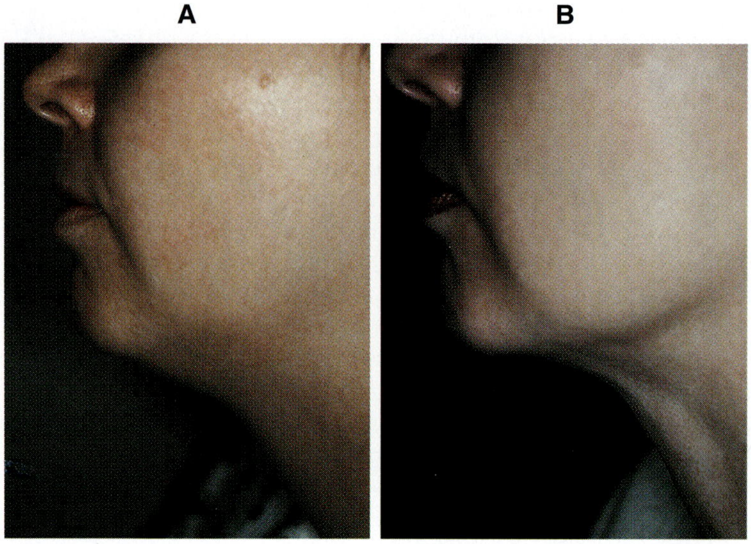

FIG. 14-13
A 28-year-old woman before **(A)** and 6 months after **(B)** neck liposuction.

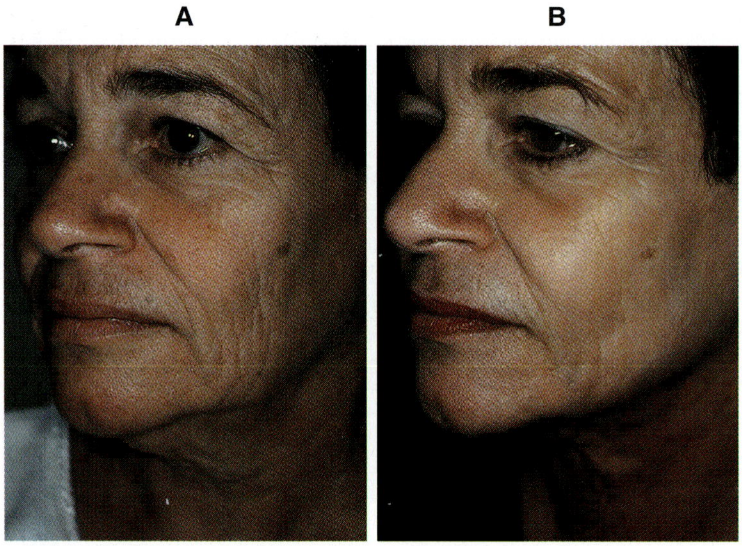

FIG. 14-14
A 52-year-old woman before **(A)** and 6 months after **(B)** neck liposuction.

suction through a submental incision. The surgeon should also evaluate submandibular gland position. Many patients have ptotic submandibular glands that appear as a subcutaneous fullness bilaterally along the inferior portion of the mandibular ramus. These ptotic glands can appear to be jowls, and it is important to identify them preoperatively. Patients are told that submandibular gland position is unlikely to improve with liposuction alone, and that may compromise final results. Platysma repair as well as superficial musculoaponeurotic system (SMAS) plication can improve gland position in some cases, but other surgical procedures are available to definitively correct submandibular gland ptosis. They will not be discussed in this chapter.

The position of the hyoid bone is also an important determinant of postoperative results. The hyoid bone is a central component of neck architecture and musculature, and is an important landmark when evaluating patients preoperatively. Patients with a relatively low hyoid position will tend to have a less well defined cervicomental angle, whereas those with a high-set hyoid are able to obtain greater definition to the cervicomental angle (Fig. 14-15).[47] Although both groups are candidates for neck liposuction, it is helpful to counsel patients preoperatively as to the limits of liposuction if they have a low hyoid position. The authors have found that platysma repair at the time of liposuction can help to improve cervicomental angle formation in patients with both low- and high-set hyoid position (Fig. 14-16).

For patients with poor skin tone or severe jowl and rhytide formation, full or partial face lift procedures can be of significant benefit. We have developed a technique of SMAS plication and periauricular skin excision for use in such patients.

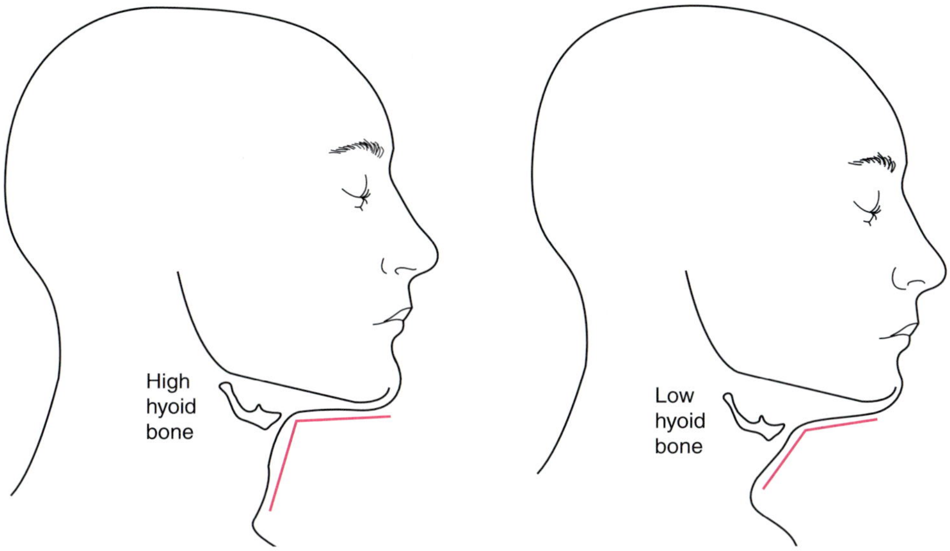

FIG. 14-15
Hyoid bone position. Note the change/improvement in cervicomental angle when the hyoid bone is relatively higher in position.

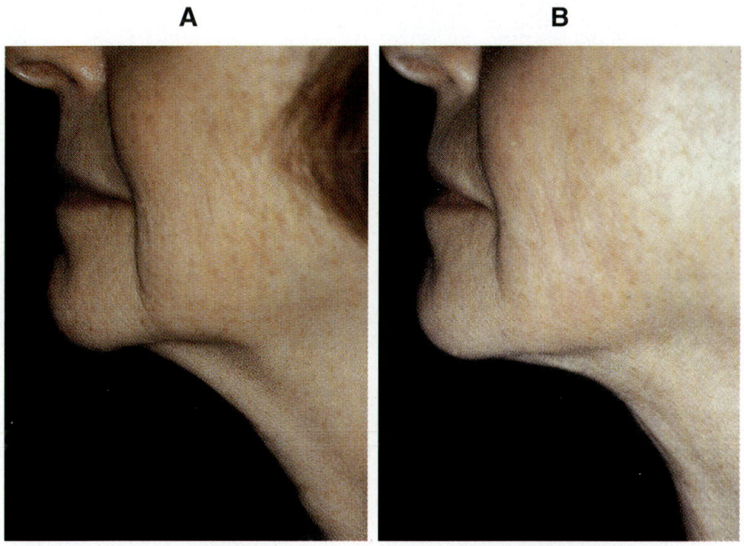

FIG. 14-16
A 62-year-old woman before **(A)** and 6 months after **(B)** neck liposuction with platysma repair.

Liposuction. The neck is marked with the patient in the sitting position (Fig. 14-17). The anterior border of the sternocleidomastoid muscle is defined and outlined, and markings are continued inferiorly across the midline just above the sternal notch. The submental crease is marked, as is the jawline. Care must be taken to identify the jowl bilaterally, as it will extend slightly below the mandibular ramus. The superior extents of the jowl should be marked as well. The extent of submental fat is then identified and marked.

The neck is anesthetized through a 3 to 4 mm submental incision using a short 6-inch sprinkler tip infusion cannula. Anesthesia is performed with 0.1% lidocaine tumescent solution. Care must be taken to anesthetize beyond the skin markings to provide a feather zone and margin for error with cannula motion. The jowls and lateral neck are anesthetized with either the infusion cannula or a 20-gauge spinal needle. This

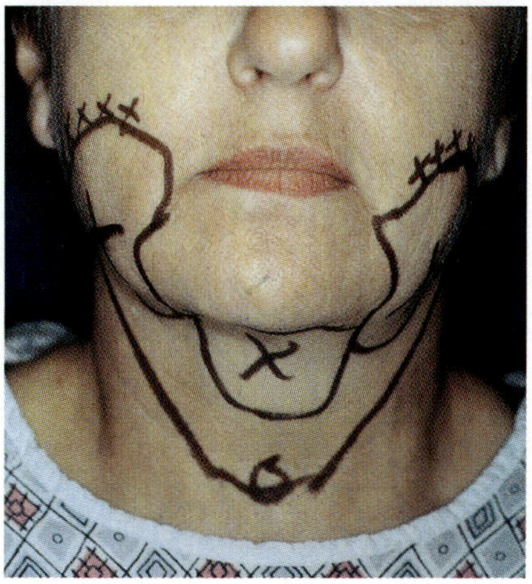

FIG. 14-17
Preoperative markings for neck liposuction.

can be done from a lateral jawline location or an area approximately 1 cm lateral and inferior to the corner of the mouth. Caution must be used when anesthetizing the jowl, since overfilling can theoretically lead to intraoral airway occlusion. Anesthesia is allowed to sit for a minimum of 30 to 45 minutes prior to suctioning.

The patient is asked to hyperextend the neck to provide optimal access. If the patient has difficulty with this maneuver, the headrest of the bed should be dropped to facilitate neck hyperextension. The submental region is suctioned first with either a 12-gauge Klein or 3 mm Accelerator cannula with the holes oriented away from the dermis. The submental region should be machine suctioned thoroughly, including superficial fat (Fig. 14-18). Caution must be used when suctioning in the region of the marginal mandibular branch of the facial nerve. It is most vulnerable to injury below the ramus of the mandible when the neck is hyperextended, as well as along the anterior third of the jawline (Fig. 14-19). Suctioning in a superficial plane in these regions is advised. Suctioning of the neck should not extend beyond the medial border of the sternocleidomastoid muscle to avoid injury to vascular structures. Suctioning of the immediate submental region can be augmented by using a 2 mm spatula-tipped cannula with the suction hole oriented up toward the dermis to remove residual fat.

The jowls and jawline are suctioned as a unit (Fig. 14-20). Initial debulking should be done through a lateral 3 mm incision placed along the jawline. A 2 mm, 3-inch spatula-tipped cannula with 5 ml syringe suction-

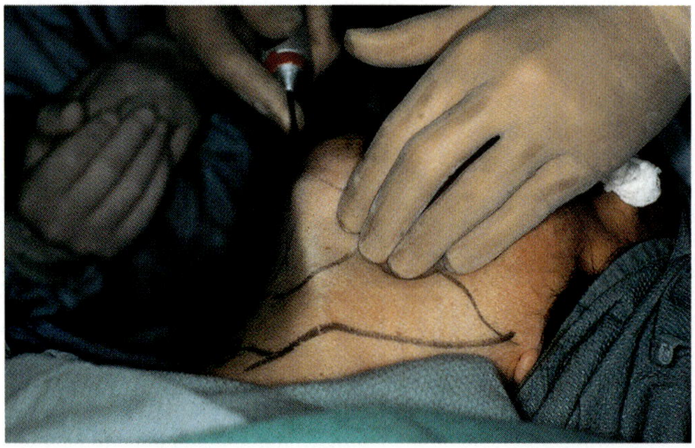

FIG. 14-18
Machine suctioning of submental region. Note surgeon's left hand identifying and protecting the marginal mandibular nerve.

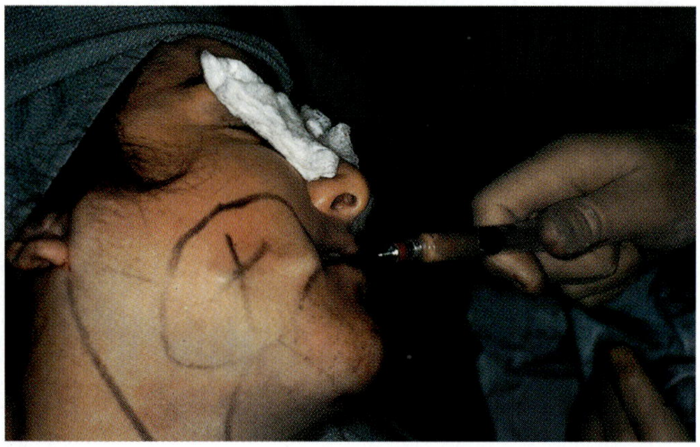

FIG. 14-20
Hand suctioning of the right jowl and jawline.

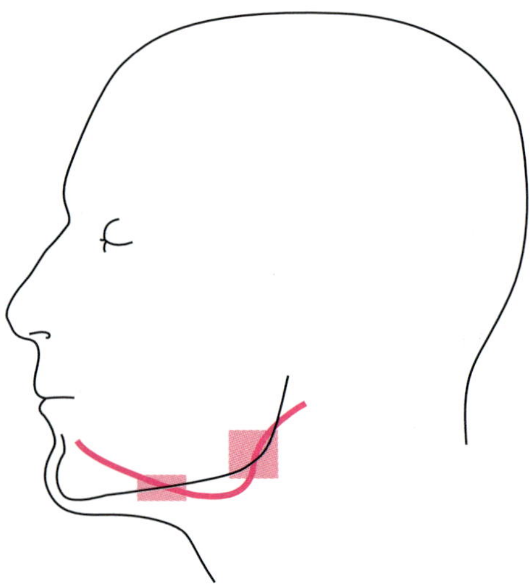

FIG. 14-19
Danger zones (shaded pink boxes) for potential injury to the marginal mandibular branch of the facial nerve (pink line).

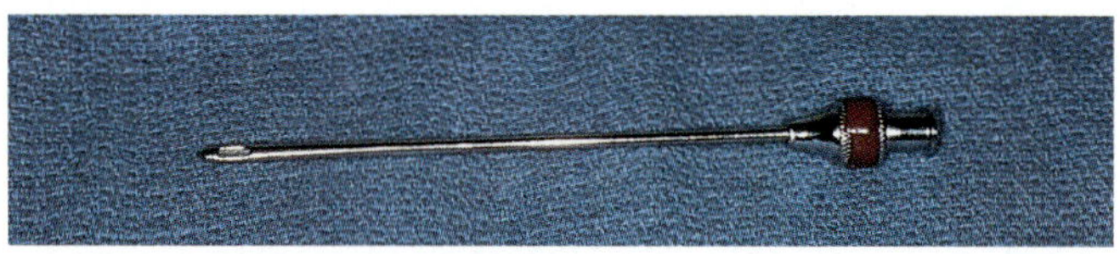

FIG. 14-21
The 2 mm, 3-inch spatula-tipped cannula.

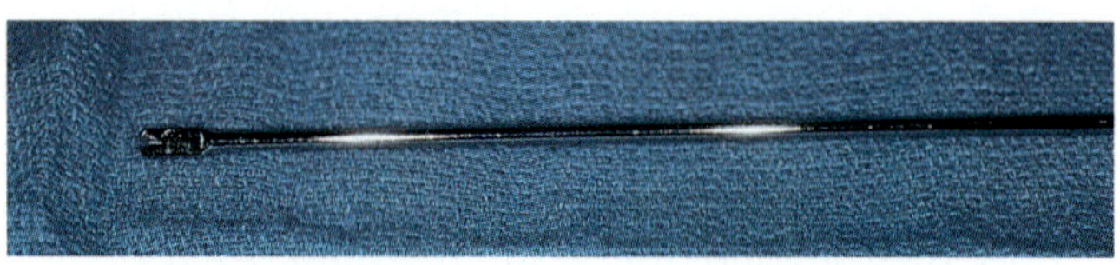

FIG. 14-22
The closed neck dissector. Note V-shaped notch at tip.

ing is used (Fig. 14-21). Caution must be used on the jowl and medial cheek, as overaggressive suctioning of the upper jowl can produce an unnatural dimpled appearance. The cannula should also be used to gently undermine the medial jowl to reduce the appearance of labiomandibular tethering and rhytides. The inferior jowl, jawline, and lateral neck are then aggressively suctioned with the 2 mm spatula-tipped cannula on machine suction. Caution must be used to stay in the superficial fat to avoid nerve injury. The cannula orifice can be oriented both toward and away from the dermis. Particular attention should be paid to the medial fibrous fat that is located just inferior to the ramus of the mandible along the medial jowl. Failure to adequately suction this area can produce an unnatural bulge.

After suctioning has been completed, submental fibrous bands should be released. We have found that this greatly reduces the appearance of puckering of the neck postoperatively. Although skin contraction and puckering tend to improve and resolve over the 6- to 12-month postoperative period, patient satisfaction improves as the healing time is reduced. Submental fibrous bands can be released under direct vision if additional surgery is to be performed (such as platysma repair), or they can be eliminated with a closed neck dissector (Byron, Tucson, AZ) (Fig. 14-22). This instrument has a sharp V-shaped notch at its distal tip that is gently advanced in the superficial fat to catch and cut fibrous bands (Fig. 14-23). Caution should be used to avoid aggressive treatment and increased bleeding. The closed neck dissector should not be used to treat the lateral neck or jawline, as this may increase the risk of permanent marginal mandibular nerve injury (Fig. 14-24). The marginal mandibular nerve function should be assessed before, during, and after the procedure by having the patient grimace to show the lower teeth, pucker, or protrude the lower lip.

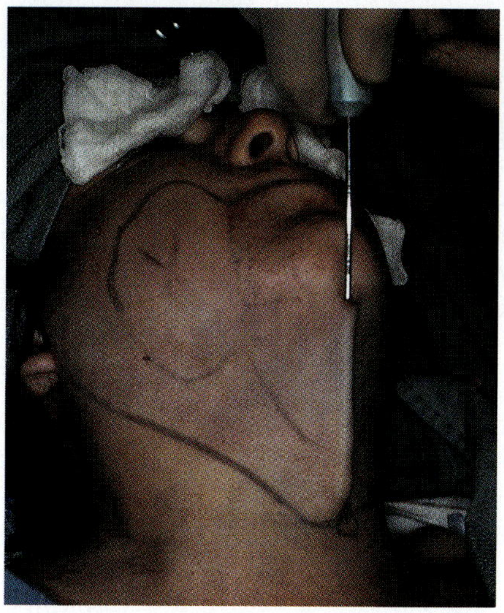

FIG. 14-23
Superficial dissection of fibrous bands of the neck with the closed neck dissector.

Platysma Repair. Repair of the platysma muscle can be performed through a submental incision when platysmal bands are present. Numerous techniques can be utilized to eliminate platysmal bands, but we have found this technique to be quick, reliable, and reproducible.[48,49] An approximately 3 cm elliptical incision is made with a No. 15 blade encompassing the 3 mm stab wound in the submental crease. The skin ellipse is excised, and the submental region visualized. Hemostasis is obtained with electrocautery. A headlamp is useful for this part of the procedure.

The medial borders of the platysmal bands are identified with blunt dissection extending from the submental incision inferior to the level of the thyroid cartilage. If subplatysmal fat is present, it is removed under direct vision with electrosection or sharp dissection (Fig. 14-25). The platysma is then plicated in the mid-

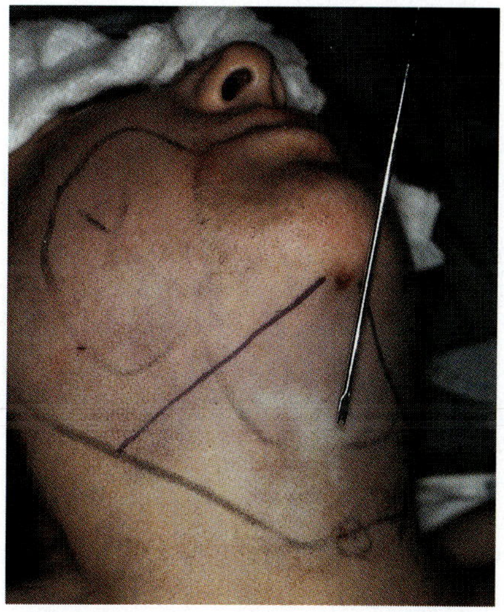

FIG. 14-24
Lateral borders of area to be treated with closed neck dissector. Superior edge of dissection is marked in black at approximately 45-degree angles from the submental incision, extending to sternocleidomastoid bilaterally.

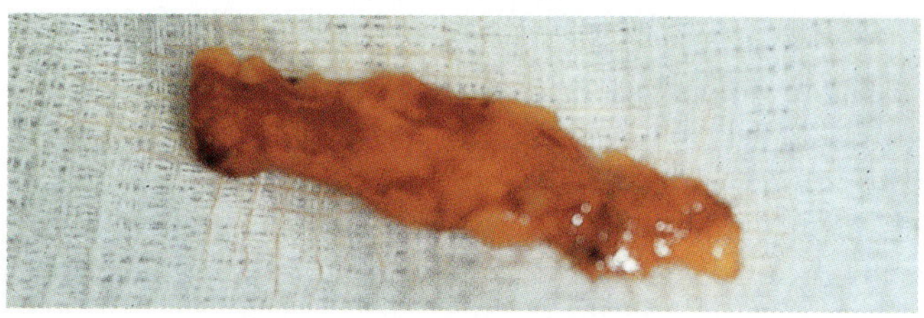

FIG. 14-25
Retroplatysmal fat pad after dissection and excision.

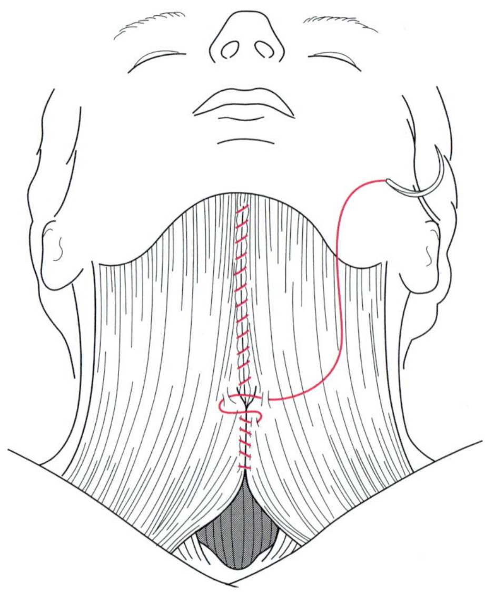

FIG. 14-26
Platysma plication. Note initial running suture (pink) from superior to inferior, with continuation of the running suture in an oversewn plication from inferior to superior. Suture is tied on itself at superior end.

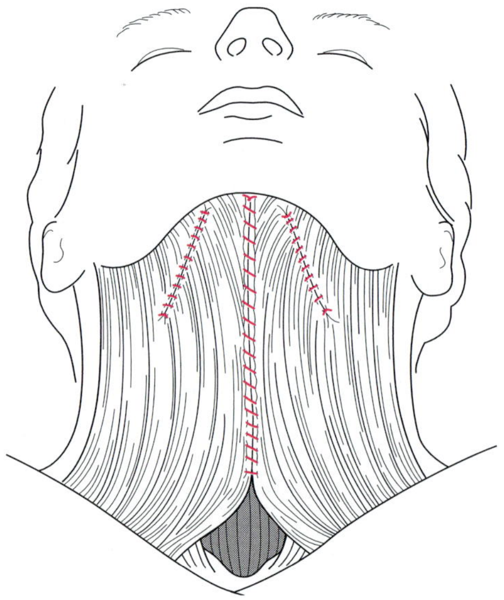

FIG. 14-27
Final appearance of platysma plication. Central two-layer plication produces majority of tightening. Bilateral oblique plication sutures augment platysma tightening as well as help to suspend and elevate submandibular glands.

line using a running 3-0 Mersilene or comparable suture. The plication is performed in a superior to inferior direction, with a buried superior knot. When plication reaches the level of the thyroid cartilage, the repair is then turned in a fold-over maneuver from inferior to superior (Fig. 14-26). The surgeon should be certain to maintain constant tension on the plication suture to ensure adequate platysmal tightening. The fold-over is performed by taking bites outside of the initial plication seam (on either side of the seam) to imbricate the platysma over the initial superior to inferior running suture. The suture is continued superiorly to the initial buried knot and tied to the free strand of that knot. Additional plication sutures can be placed bilaterally in the region of the submandibular glands to both tighten the platysma further and elevate the ptotic submandibular gland (Fig. 14-27). Hemostasis is obtained and confirmed, and the submental wound closed with subcutaneous 5-0 Vicryl (polyglactin 910, Ethicon, Somerville, NJ) and 6-0 Prolene (polypropylene, Ethicon, Somerville, NJ) skin sutures.

SMAS Plication and Skin Excision. Many patients with submental adipose tissue also have prominent jowl formation. A subset of these patients has poor skin elasticity, oftentimes patients over the age of 50 to 60. Patients with prominent jowls and good skin tone can be effectively treated with liposuction alone. However, patients with compromised skin elasticity will often benefit from SMAS plication and skin excision in addition to neck liposuction.[50] These patients often require platysma repair as well, and we prefer to repair the platysma in all patients who have SMAS plication. The net effect of tightening the platysma and SMAS is an overall aesthetic improvement in neck and jawline contours (Fig. 14-28).

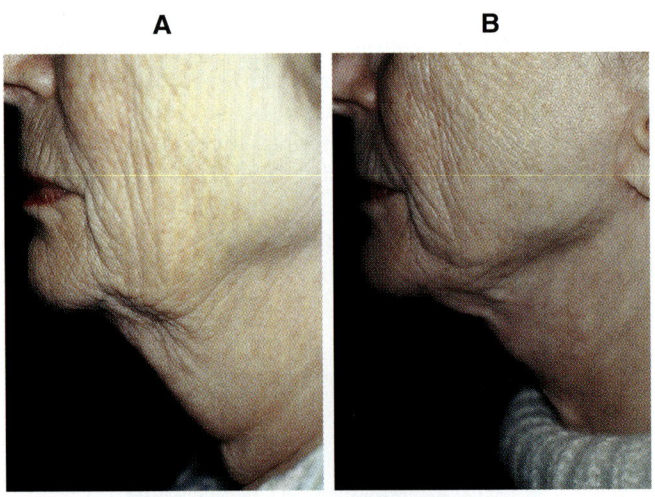

FIG. 14-28
A 72-year-old woman before **(A)** and 4 months after **(B)** neck liposuction, platysma repair, and SMAS plication with skin excision.

Following platysma repair, the preauricular and postauricular regions are anesthetized with 1% lidocaine with 1:100,000 epinephrine. This area is also anesthetized with 0.1% tumescent lidocaine anesthesia at the time of initial anesthesia for neck liposuction. An

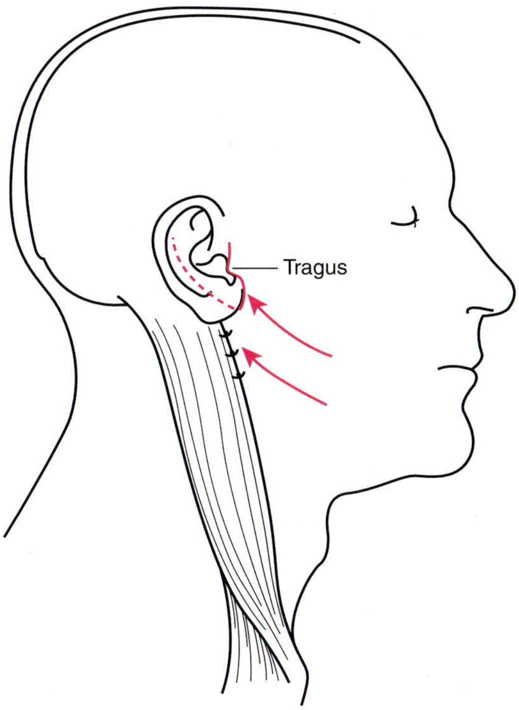

FIG. 14-29
SMAS plication with skin excision. Note extent of incision (pink solid and dotted line). The dotted line represents the retroauricular portion of the incision. Arrows denote direction of skin and SMAS motion.

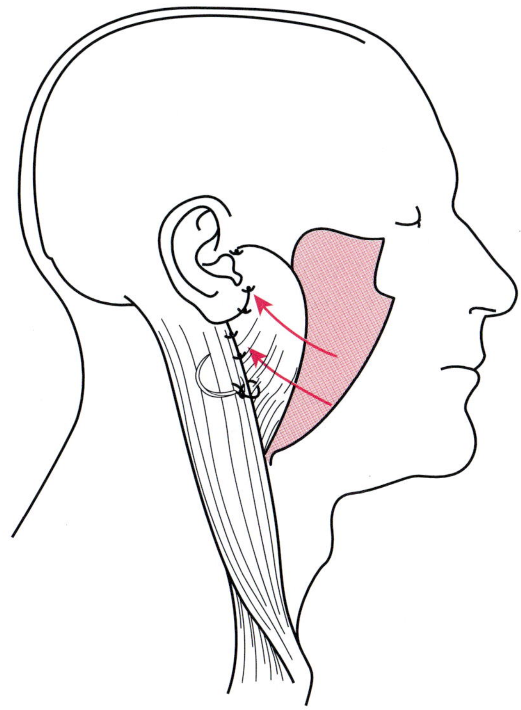

FIG. 14-30
SMAS plication with skin excision (intraoperative diagram). Note position of deep sutures for SMAS plication from tragus extending down along sternocleidomastoid muscle.

incision with a No. 15 blade is made extending from the superior tragus, along the posterior rim of the tragus, anterior and inferior along the front of the earlobe, under the lobe and posteriorly along the postauricular sulcus (Fig. 14-29). The posterior incision extends along approximately 30% to 50% of the postauricular sulcus. A small nick incision is made along the inferior aspect of the earlobe to aid with placement for repair. The superior aspect of the skin incision is made along the posterior aspect of the tragus to minimize postoperative scar appearance.

The cheek and upper neck skin is undermined in the mid subcutaneous plane approximately 3 to 4 cm medial to the incision line. The resultant flap is elevated and hemostasis achieved. The white fibrous surface of the SMAS is identified and plicated along the preauricular sulcus utilizing 8 to 10 3-0 Mersilene (or comparable) sutures with buried knots. Approximately 3 cm of the SMAS is plicated in an anteroposterior direction, with the vectors of plication oriented to maximally contour the jawline. The extent of plication extends inferiorly along the anterior border of the sternocleidomastoid for approximately 3 to 4 cm (Fig. 14-30). This helps to fully tighten the platysma muscle, which in combination with platysma plication produces superb platysma and neck contours.

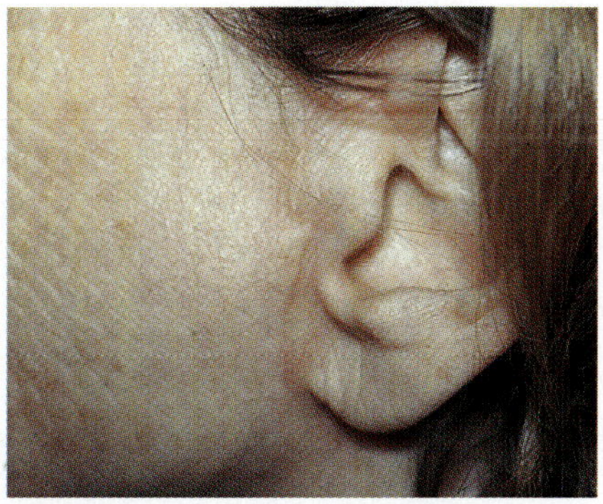

FIG. 14-31
Natural earlobe position with well-healed incision 4 months after SMAS plication with skin excision.

After maximal SMAS plication under moderate tension, the skin is redraped and redundant skin excised. It is important to reposition the earlobe in a natural location without tension (Fig. 14-31). In addition, sutures along the inferior earlobe sulcus should be placed to allow for some skin contraction as the scar matures. Failure to allow for scar contraction can produce an elongated earlobe, often referred to as an *elf ear deformity.* An absorbable suture placed deep in the preauricular sulcus can help to contour the area and recreate the natural crease present in front of the ear.

Skin excision and redraping can be a challenge, since this technique utilizes a short periauricular skin incision of approximately 6 to 7 cm. We have found it useful to reposition the skin of the preauricular region first, with careful attention paid to natural earlobe position. The postauricular skin can be manipulated to account for excess skin and dog ear formation. The wound edges are then closed with subcutaneous 5-0 Vicryl and 6-0 Prolene skin sutures.

Postoperative Compression. A double layer compression garment is placed postoperatively to improve skin contraction and reduce postoperative bleeding. Reston foam or french tape can also be applied under the garments to further improve results. Adequate compression along the jawline for a minimum of 7 to 10 days is essential to obtaining adequate tissue adherence and contraction.

Liposuction of the Arms

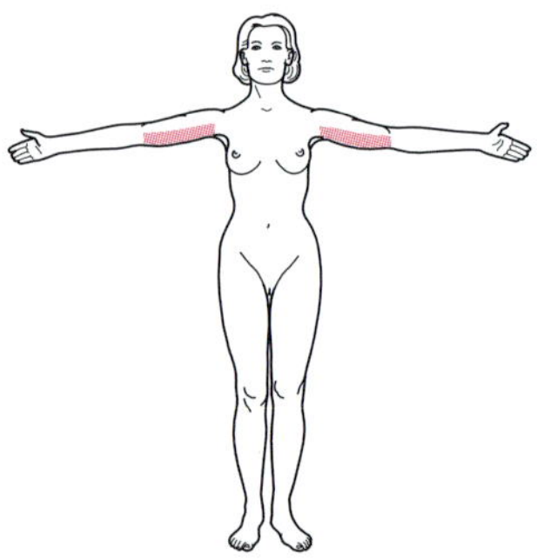

Women with significant lipodystrophy of the proximal arm often have to wear blouses two to three sizes larger than they might otherwise need to have the arms fit. For this reason, even modest improvements result in significant patient satisfaction (Fig. 14-32). In our experience, it is a misconception that liposuction of the upper arms often results in postoperative irregularities with poor skin retraction.[51-53] Liposuction of the arms is performed almost exclusively on women, with the posterior and posterolateral aspects of the arm involved more often than the anterior and medial upper arms. On occasion, a localized fat deposit on the ulnar side of the proximal forearm requires treatment as well. Conservative but thorough fat extraction is obtainable without undue trauma due to the soft quality of the fat in the area. Avoiding trauma to the subdermis with correct cannula choices and minimal use of the smart hand will minimize irregularities.[54] Skin of the upper arm has good potential for significant skin contraction. Therefore, liposuction may be performed primarily for skin tightening even when very little fat is present. Brachioplasty (arm lift) and the resultant scar can produce such an unattractive and uncorrectable result that liposuction, and even a second liposuction session, are often preferable alternatives.

The patient is evaluated in a standing position with arms extended horizontally with the thumb pointing up, or elbows bent, to maximize the laxity of the posterior and posterolateral compartments. As with other sites, skin tone and texture must be evaluated. If skin tone is poor preoperatively, the patient may still achieve significant skin contraction if thorough fat removal is performed, but texture will often not improve. For some patients, concurrent treatment of the upper back and anterior and posterior axillary regions is performed as well.

At least two incision sites are needed for infusion of 0.1% tumescent anesthesia. For infiltration of the posterior and posterolateral arm, incision sites are just proximal to the elbow and at the mid posterior arm. The soft, loose tissue of the upper arms can often be infiltrated more rapidly than other areas. The total amount of tumescent anesthesia may vary greatly, with an expected range of 500 to 1000 ml per arm.

Three incision sites across the mid posterior upper arm are used for aspiration. For large-volume cases

A

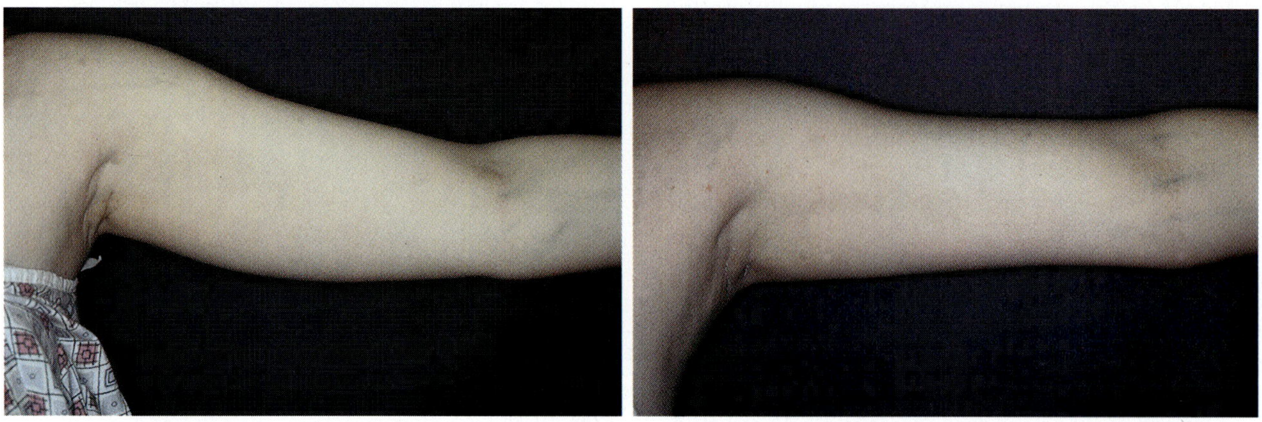

B

FIG. 14-32
A 34-year-old woman before **(A)** and 6 months after **(B)** arm liposuction.

(over 400 ml removed), initial very cautious debulking may be done with the 3.7 mm Keel Cobra cannula (30 cm long). In smaller-volume cases, we find the 3 mm Accelerator or 12-gauge Klein cannula is preferable for debulking. Pinching, lifting, and downward pressure from the smart hand is not necessary in this area and may increase the risk for subdermal fibrosis, adhesions, puckering, and indentations. The 3 mm Accelerator (Eliminator) or 12-gauge Klein cannulas have a relatively nonaggressive tip and with their recessed openings placed away from the dermis are ideal for residual fat removal after debulking. Particular attention must be paid to thoroughly treat the proximal upper arm and fat overlying the medial epicondyle, as incomplete treatment of these areas is the most common cause for patient dissatisfaction. An incision site just distal to the fat overlying the medial epicondyle provides access to that area as well as the more fibrous fat just proximal to the elbow. This may be the only area of the upper arm that may necessitate use of the smart hand to assist with fat aspiration, due to the fibrous nature of this area. For final assessment, the patient is instructed to hold her arms straight up, occasionally exposing residual pockets of fat in the posterolateral compartment.

In the rare case in which the anterior upper arm needs treatment, the 3 mm Accelerator (Eliminator) or 12-gauge Klein cannula is preferred because of the thin dermis in this area. Incision sites in the anterior axilla and just distal to the area of fat to be removed are used. Postoperative pain of the arms is minimal compared with other areas and may be increased with poorly fitting compression garments.

Liposuction of the Trunk

It is useful to consider trunk anatomy and cosmetic contours from two views: anterior and lateral. The lateral view will reveal contour irregularities of the upper and lower abdomen. The anterior view will allow the surgeon to view the upper waist and back, waist, and hips. Patients will often discuss areas of the trunk that bother them, such as the lower abdomen, but it is the responsibility of the surgeon to identify which adjacent regions might benefit from suctioning. Also, the surgeon should consider whether any areas, if they were to gain weight, might look unnatural juxtaposed with the treated area. For these reasons, we have found that this anterior and lateral classification is useful. Patients interested in lower abdominal liposuction are evaluated for possible upper abdominal liposuction. Those interested in treatment of the hips or waist are evaluated to determine whether treatment of the entire lateral waistline unit is indicated.

The abdomen can thus be divided into cosmetic units, many of which are interrelated. The upper and lower abdomen are separate cosmetic units, but often treated together in one session (Fig. 14-33). The hip is another cosmetic unit, and the waist and mid-lower back (below the bra line) is a cosmetic unit as well. The hip and waist and mid-lower back are considered the lateral area of the trunk, and these two cosmetic units are often treated in one session. The upper back (above the bra line) is most often treated in conjunction with the arms and posterior axilla and is not considered part of the abdomen-trunk cosmetic region. The result is a total of four cosmetic units of the abdomen and trunk. In some patients, treatment of all four cosmetic units in one surgical session is indicated. This helps to maximally contour the abdomen-trunk by removing adipose tissue in three dimensions. In addition, postoperative healing and skin contraction along suction vectors provides maximal improvement of the abdominal pannus and waistline (Fig. 14-34).

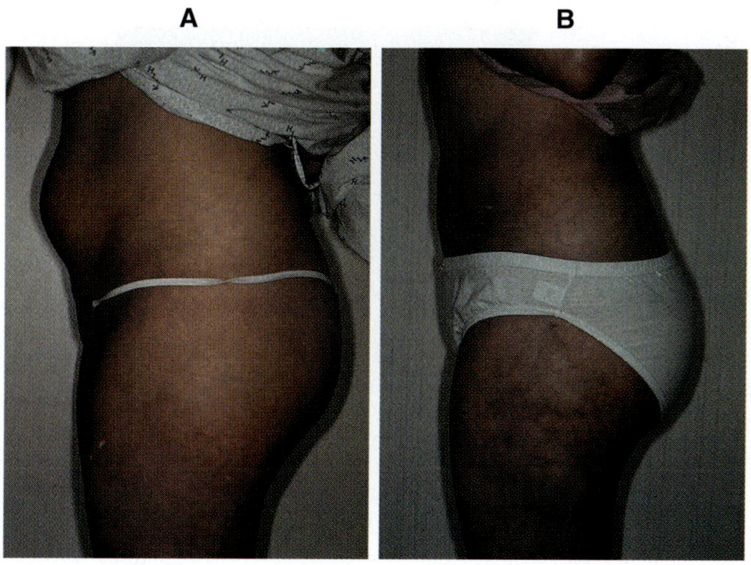

FIG. 14-33
A 35-year-old woman before **(A)** and 6 months after **(B)** upper and lower abdominal liposuction.

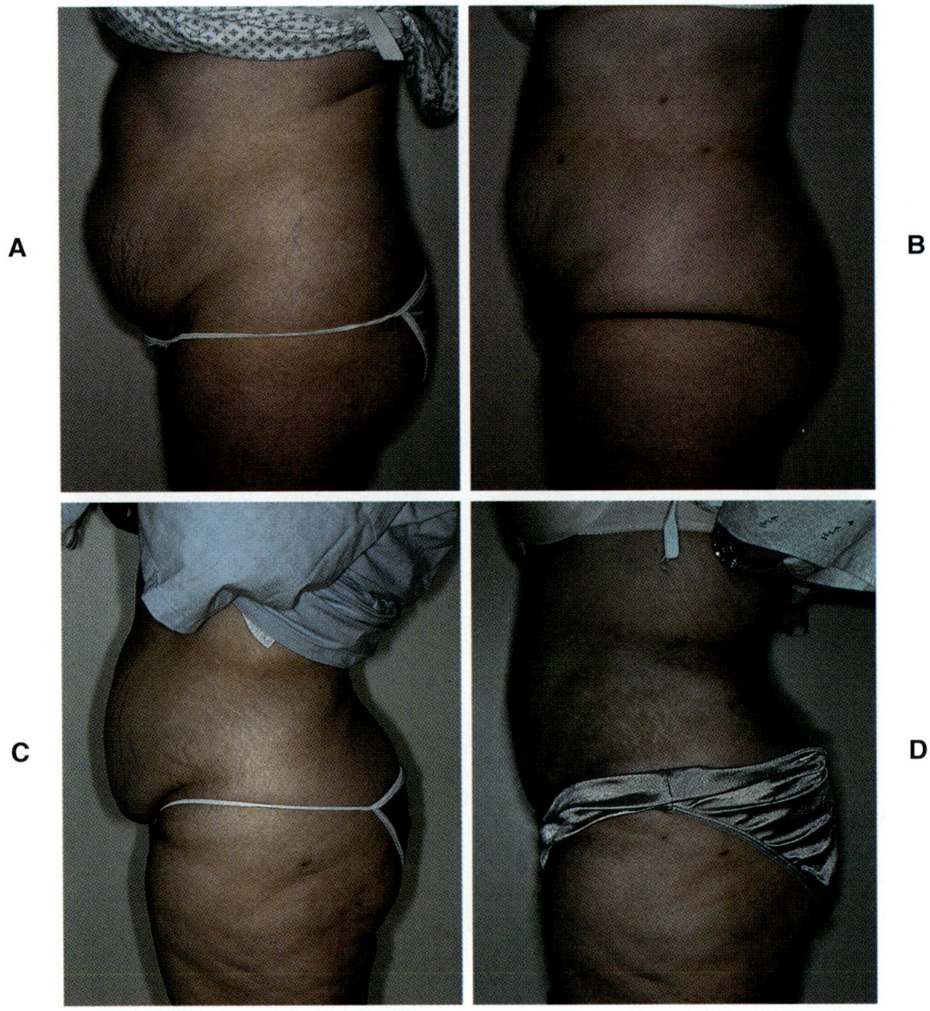

FIG. 14-34
A 43-year-old woman before **(A)** and 6 months after **(B)** upper and lower abdomen, hips, waist, and back liposuction. A 42-year-old woman before **(C)** and 6 months after **(D)** same procedure. Note retraction of pannus in both patients without the need for abdominoplasty.

Upper and Lower Abdomen. Prior to suctioning, the patient must be evaluated for abdominal hernias and scars. Ventral hernias including umbilical, postsurgical, and spigelian (lateral rectus sheath) should be ruled out through clinical examination. Preoperative markings should reflect the extent of suctioning, areas to be suctioned, and localized collections of adipose tissue (Fig. 14-35). The lower abdomen, when suctioned alone, is often clearly demarcated and easily outlined. When the lower and upper abdomen are to be treated together, the extent of

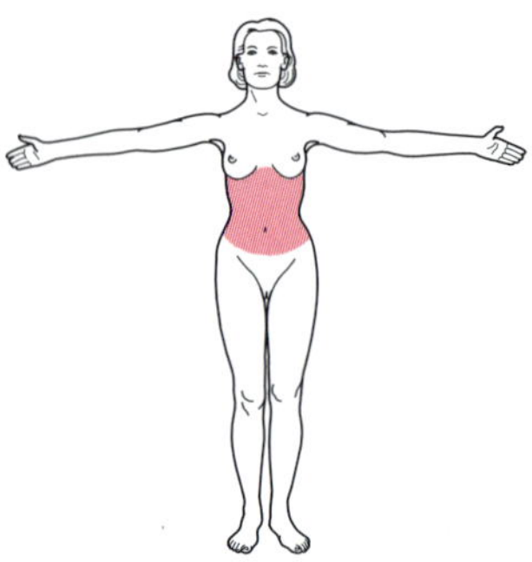

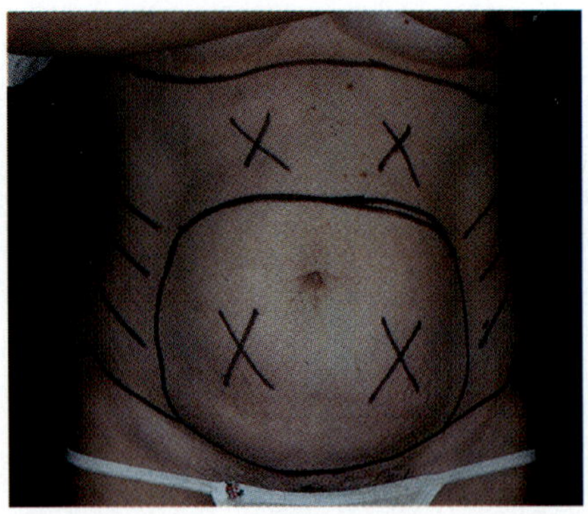

FIG. 14-35
Preoperative markings for abdominal liposuction. Note use of flow lines and markings (large X to denote areas of adipose concentration) to aid surgeon intraoperatively.

A

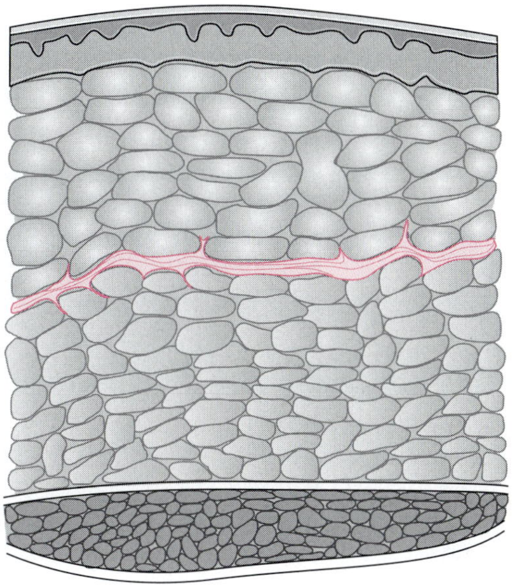

B

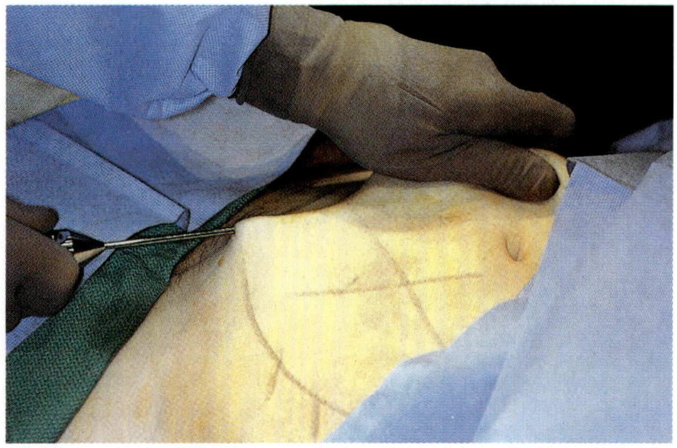

FIG. 14-36
Removal of deep anterior lower abdomen fat. **A,** Location of fat on anterior lower abdomen both above and below superficial fascia. **B,** Smart hand maneuver to elevate skin and expose deep adipose compartment for suctioning.

suctioning extends from under the breasts to the suprapubic region.

Anesthesia is obtained through two incisions placed along the suprapubic region, as well as from mid abdominal sites along the lateral aspect of the area to be treated. Anesthesia is placed in the mid subcutaneous space and allowed to sit for a minimum of 30 minutes prior to suctioning. Tumescent 0.1% lidocaine anesthesia is used for the upper abdomen, especially the areas over the costal margin. When possible, 0.1% lidocaine should be used for the lower abdomen, but this area can be anesthetized with 0.05% lidocaine and suctioned effectively. The cannula will often pass through and under older scars without difficulty, but caution should be used with newer scars.

Suctioning is performed with the 3.7 mm swan neck Keel Cobra cannula for debulking larger patients. The 3 mm Accelerator cannula can be used to debulk smaller patients. Triangulation of areas is essential to produce smooth contours, as 100% fat removal is the goal of therapy. The 12-gauge Klein cannula is used to feather treatment sites and ensure maximal smooth fat removal.

It is essential to thoroughly suction the periumbilical region, as well as the deep fat of the upper and lower abdomen. Many patients will have well-defined adipose collections that lie on the rectus sheath deep to Camper's and Scarpa's fascia, both superior to the umbilicus and inferolateral to the umbilicus. Suctioning of these areas is essential to producing a flat abdomen (Fig. 14-36). It is often necessary to lift the skin with the smart hand and carefully advance the cannula into a deep adipose plane to access this fat. Clearly, caution is needed to prevent subrectus suctioning. We have found it helpful to use short cannula strokes and avoid any cannula motion lateral to the rectus sheath when attempting this deep fat maneuver. Avoiding cannula motion lateral to the rectus reduces the chances of becoming subrectus with cannula position. It is also imperative that cannula position be superficial when it crosses the costal margin to prevent injury in that location.

Postoperative compression can be augmented with ½-inch Reston foam pads (3M, St. Paul, MN) placed for the first few days on the anterior abdomen. These pads are placed on the skin under the liposuction compression garment. They often will aid in skin placement, adherence, and bruising reduction.

Hips. The hips are treated either alone or in combination with the upper back and waistline. Some women will also have the lateral thighs treated in combination with the hips to recontour the lateral silhouette (Fig. 14-37). Correction of the *double-bulge* of the hips and lateral thighs can have a profound impact on body shape. However, many women will benefit from suctioning of the hips alone. These women typi-

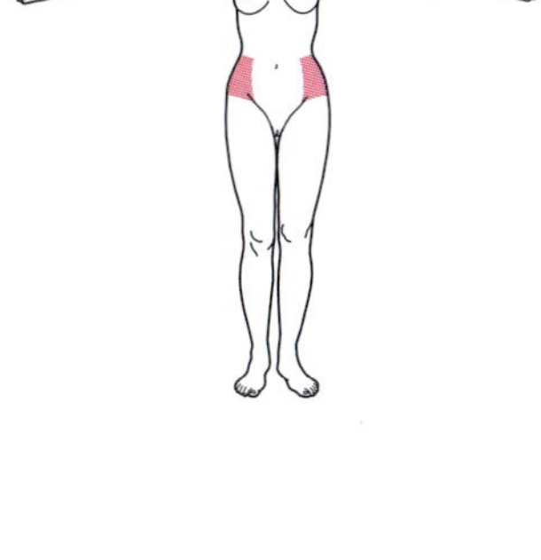

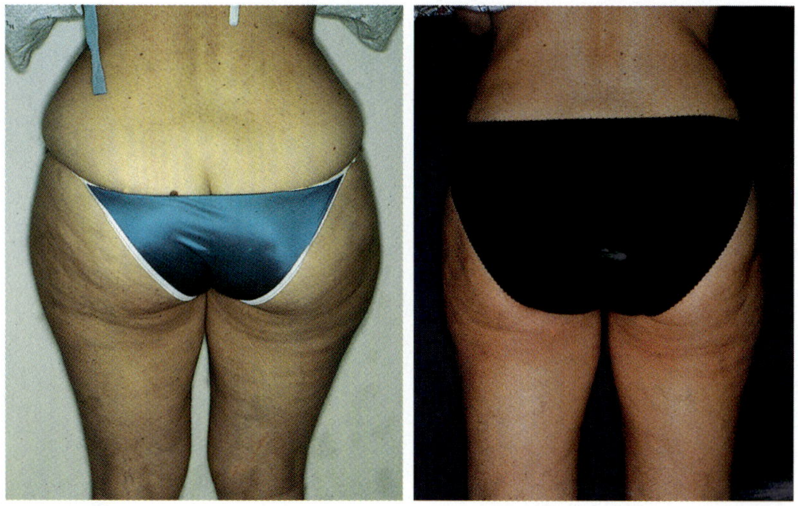

FIG. 14-37
A 41-year-old woman before **(A)** and 6 months after **(B)** hip and outer thigh liposuction.

cally have an athletic build and have isolated hip adipose deposits. Some will have mild outer thigh fullness, but their athletic shape makes treatment of this area less necessary.

The hip is outlined bilaterally with the patient in the standing position. The inferior border of the area to be treated is often easily recognized as a distinct junction between hip and upper lateral thigh. This pseudogroove should not be treated, even when combining hip and lateral thigh liposuction, since this can produce disfiguring depressions. The anterior and posterior hip are also usually distinct, and the surgeon can feel for the boundaries of the hip with the pinch technique. Typically, the amount of fat you can pinch diminishes substantially as you move away from the central area of hip adipose tissue. The superior hip can have an indistinct border, and it is for this reason that hip liposuction is often combined with treatment of the waistline. When you treat the hip alone, it is important to feather suctioning up into the waistline.

Anesthesia is placed with 0.1% or 0.05% tumescent lidocaine and allowed to sit for 30 minutes. The right hip is anesthetized (and suctioned) with the patient lying on the left side, and vice versa for the left hip. Initial debulking can be performed with the 12-gauge Klein or 3 mm Accelerator cannulas. Final blending is done with the 12-gauge Klein cannula. Triangulation is essential, and the goal of therapy is creation of a smooth contour in harmony with the lateral thigh, buttock, and waistline. Sufficient fat is removed to achieve this result and can vary significantly. For most patients, 50% to 80% fat removal from the hip is adequate. Occasionally, near 100% fat removal is needed to obtain the desired contour.

Mid-Lower Back and Waistline. Contouring of the waist can produce beautiful aesthetic results, and a

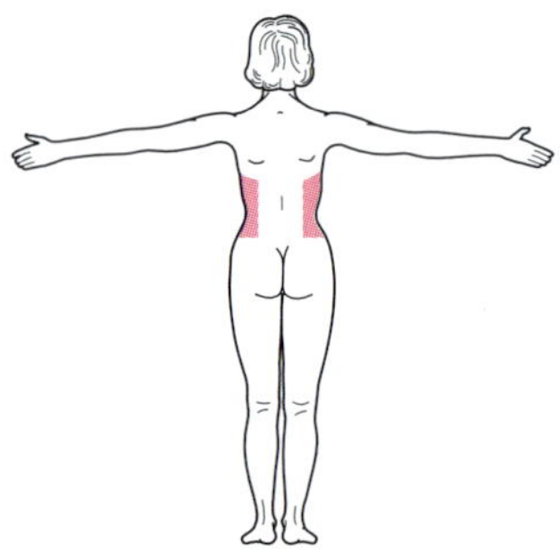

shapely waistline is one of the things appreciated most by patients after their liposuction surgery. To adequately contour the waistline, the surgeon must also treat the back in the vicinity of the bra line. For most patients, suctioning of the hip at the same time is necessary to achieve optimal results. This allows the surgeon to maximally contour the lateral abdomen, blending it into the flank and ultimately the back. Volumetric reduction of fat in three dimensions along the abdomen, flank, waistline, and back is essential for creating substantial improvements in shape and contour.

The patient is marked in the standing position, with vectors of suctioning clearly marked (Fig. 14-38). It is important to suction along intended vectors of skin retraction to promote skin redraping postoperatively. The surgeon can pinch the lower back fat to localize it, and this area is marked. Incisions along the mid waist, posterior mid back, and under the lateral breast are used for anesthesia and suctioning. Additional incisions are placed as needed at the inferior zone of treatment to promote triangulation and facilitate drainage. Anesthesia is obtained with 0.1% lidocaine and allowed to sit for 40 to 45 minutes. It is advisable to allow the tumescent solution in this region to sit for slightly longer than other areas to provide maximal anesthesia. The waistline and mid-lower back can be a particularly sensitive area to treat due to the very fibrous nature of the fat. Some surgeons prefer to use external ultrasound in this area (and other areas with fibrous fat) to make fat removal easier, but we have found this to be cumbersome and unnecessary.[55,56]

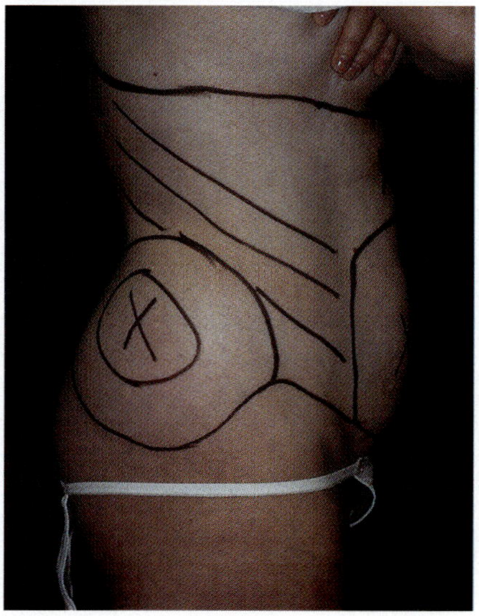

FIG. 14-38
Preoperative markings for liposuction of the back and waistline. Note use of markings to aid surgeon intraoperatively, and suctioning vectors (three black lines on waistline) to contour the waistline and produce retraction of the pannus and skin.

The goal of waistline and upper back suctioning is near 100% fat removal. Initial debulking is performed with either the 3.7 mm Keel Cobra or 3 mm Accelerator cannula. The surgeon must be certain to suction the very deep fat that lies just superficial to the muscular fascia, similar to the technique for the upper and lower abdomen deep fat. The smart hand is sometimes used to lift the skin of the waistline to allow the cannula to access the deeper fat. Final blending and contouring can be done with a 12-gauge Klein cannula, but for many patients the 3 mm Accelerator is adequate for this task. It must be emphasized that triangulation and aggressive suctioning are needed to fully contour the waistline. A few extra minutes of attention to detail in this region can produce dramatic improvements in results.

Liposuction of the Buttock

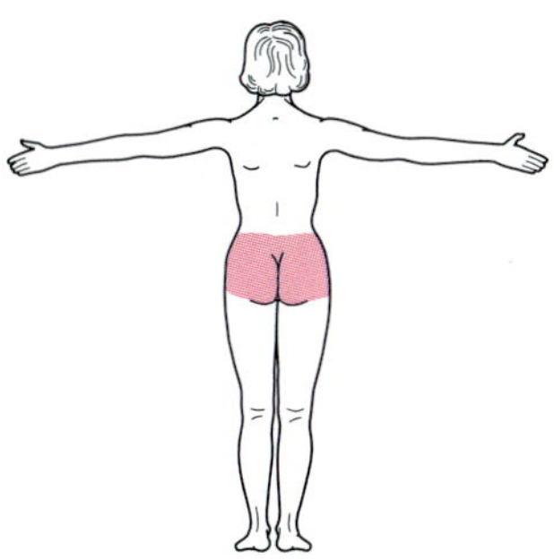

The buttock is a challenging area to suction and is almost exclusively done in women. Many women are interested in reducing the overall size of the buttock but often have difficulty verbalizing exactly what it is that bothers them. The usual concern is size, but the buttock has so many different contours, projecting in both a lateral and posterior direction, that definition of treatment parameters can be difficult. Therefore it is buttock shape, symmetry, and proportion that should guide surgical judgment, and not absolute size. The goal is to treat the buttock so that it fits in harmony with the shape and silhouette of the patient. For these reasons, treatment of the buttock is often combined with treatment of the hips and lateral thighs, considering this to be an extended cosmetic liposuction unit. Preoperative markings are essential and serve as a road map and guide for the surgeon.

Caution must be used to avoid the inferomedial buttock in the vicinity of the sciatic nerve as well as the medial buttock near the gluteal cleft. In addition, suctioning and cannula motion should never cross the inferior gluteal crease where the buttock meets the upper posterior thigh. Suctioning of the inferior buttock–upper thigh crease can disturb the fibrous junction in that region and lead to an unnatural ptosis of the buttock. Blending of the buttock with the lower back, hip, and outer thigh can produce superb contours (Fig. 14-39). Oversuctioning can produce a flattened buttock with irregular contours, which is not desirable.

After appropriate surgical markings have been made, anesthesia is achieved with 0.1% lidocaine tumescent anesthesia bilaterally. The patient is often positioned in the prone position for anesthesia, occasionally rocking gently onto one hip to allow anesthesia of the contralateral buttock. Incision sites should be placed in the lateral infragluteal crease, the upper medial buttock, and the upper lateral buttock to promote triangulation. Anesthesia is placed predominantly in the mid and deep fat of the buttock.

Anesthesia is allowed to sit for a minimum of 30 minutes before suctioning begins. Caution must be used to remain in the mid and deep fat of the buttock, avoiding superficial suctioning. Treatment of the superficial fat can quickly lead to contour irregularities in this technique-sensitive region. The main theme that should guide the surgeon is to retain the contour and convexity of the buttock while decreasing size and improving contours. Mid and deep fat liposuction are essential tools for the physician. Initial gentle debulking can be done with a 3 mm Accelerator cannula in most patients, while larger patients can be treated with the more aggressive 3.0 or 3.7 mm Keel Cobra cannula. Following debulking, the mid fat is contoured with a 12-gauge Klein cannula.

Final results will often depend on the ability of the surgeon to blend the buttock with the hip, lower back, and lateral thigh. The challenge of buttock liposuction is to judge the amount of fat removal correctly and to precisely contour the junction of the buttock with the hip and outer thigh. Actual percentages for fat removal

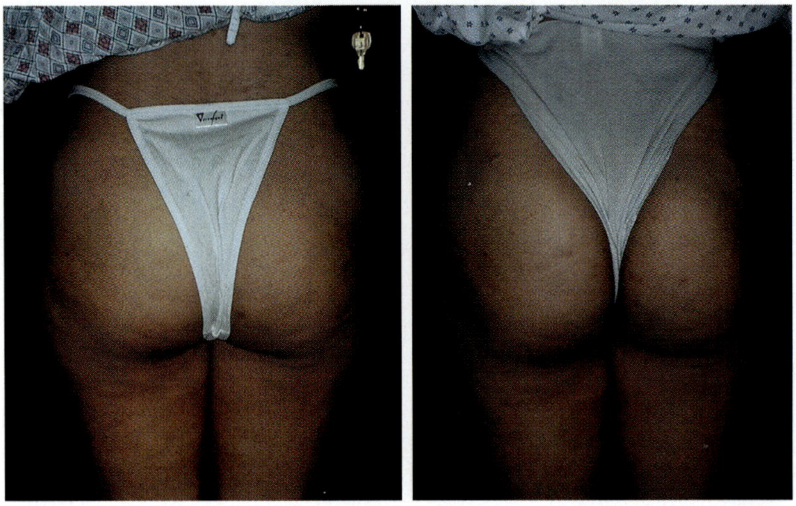

FIG. 14-39
A 32-year-old woman before **(A)** and 6 months after **(B)** liposuction of the buttock.

are less important than the aesthetic result, and this is judged through intraoperative surgical *feel,* both visual and tactile (with the smart hand).

Liposuction of the Legs

Localized adipose deposits of the legs are particularly well suited to liposuction surgery. Although some people (usually women) have diffusely large legs with abundant adipose tissue, many have well-shaped legs with discrete collections of fat. It is for these women that liposuction is ideal. Thorough contouring of these localized fat deposits can dramatically change the shape and flow of leg lines. Clothing fits better, and patients usually feel much more comfortable with their shape in general. As opposed to truncal obesity, many women struggle with the shape of their thighs for years, even when close to their ideal body weight. Genetics plays a significant role in determining leg shape.

Women with generalized leg obesity can be improved with liposuction surgery, but many have underlying bone and muscle anatomy that will not support the appearance of a thin, shapely leg. These women must be counseled preoperatively that although liposuction can alter leg contours and perhaps thin their legs, it is unlikely that they will convert from someone with an obese leg to one with a thin leg. Naturally, there are exceptions to this rule, but we have found this to be true in general. Also, there is a subset of women who have *soft skin.* This term refers to women who have abundant cellulite in the setting of a relatively obese leg. The limiting factor for women with soft skin is that overaggressive suctioning can produce rapid and dramatic skin depressions. Caution, and if anything undertreatment, are the rules for such patients.

It is useful to think of the leg as having discrete cosmetic liposuction units. These include the (1) outer thigh, (2) inner thigh extending down to and including the knee, (3) anterior thigh, (4) posterior thigh, and (5) calves and ankles. With lidocaine toxicity as the limiting factor, the surgeon must factor in anatomy, patient desires, and surgical reality in determining which cosmetic units to treat. The outer thigh, inner thigh, and knee are commonly treated in one session together. Occasionally the outer thigh is treated alone in the absence of other leg obesity, but in many cases the outer thigh and hip are treated together.

Outer Thighs. The goal of therapy is creating a flow of skin that allows the outer leg to blend naturally with the hip, buttock, and trunk (Fig. 14-40). Suctioning of the outer thigh must be approached with caution, as taking too little fat will yield a disappointed patient and taking too much a disfigured patient. The outer thigh is a landmark area, one that is used as a reference point by those casually observing a woman's shape to determine overall body type, thinness, and aesthetic contour. When the outer thigh is large or unnatural in shape, it tends to stand out and be noticeable to the eye. Therefore, improvement in outer thigh contours can have a profound effect on body shape and patient self-image (Fig. 14-41).

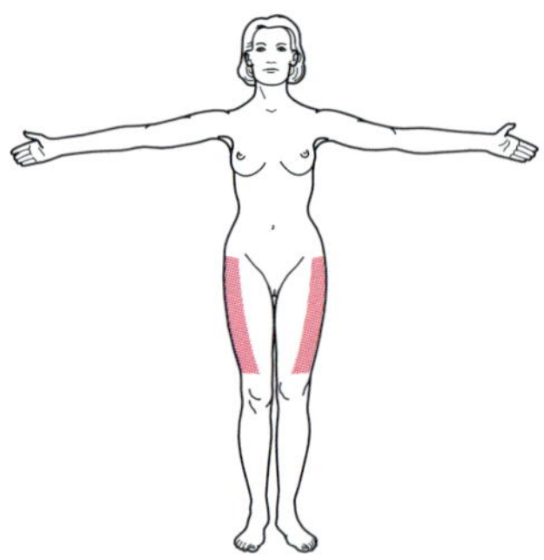

The patient is marked in the standing position (Fig. 14-42). Anesthesia is obtained with 0.05% or 0.1% lidocaine and allowed to sit for 30 minutes. Each leg is anesthetized and treated with the patient lying on the contralateral thigh. Three to four incisions are used, the most common in the lateral aspect of the gluteal crease.

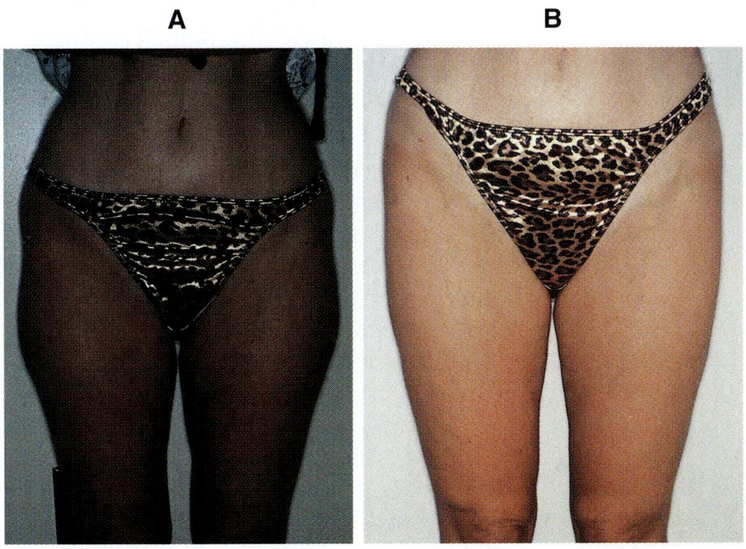

FIG. 14-40
A 40-year-old woman before **(A)** and 6 months after **(B)** liposuction of the outer thighs and hips.

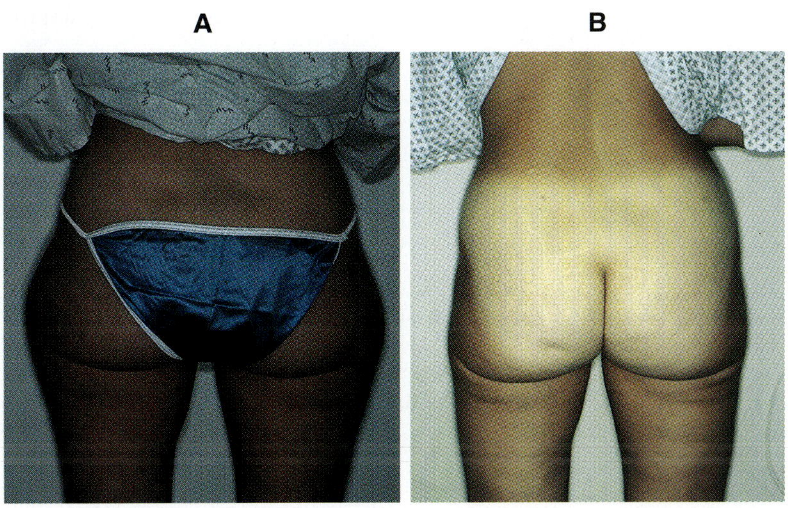

FIG. 14-41
A 38-year-old woman before **(A)** and 6 months after **(B)** liposuction of the outer thighs.

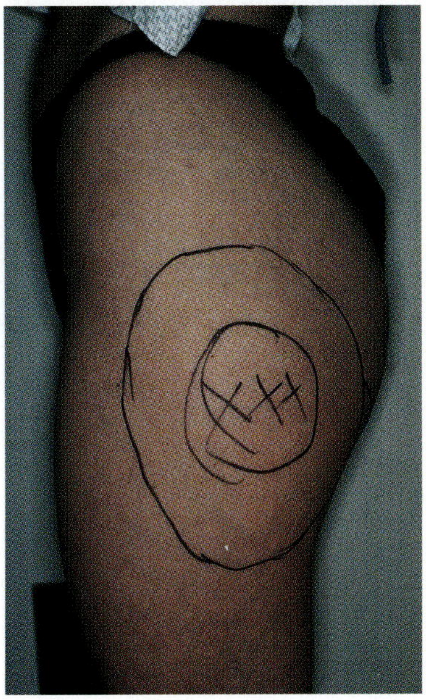

FIG. 14-42
Preoperative markings for liposuction of the outer thigh. Central circle with three X marks is the area with the most adipose tissue, and the outer circle denotes the feather zone.

The other incisions are placed at 2, 8, and 10 o'clock around the typical oval drawn to mark the outer thigh.

Initial debulking is performed with the 3 mm Accelerator cannula in most individuals, but with the 12-gauge Klein in thin women. The 12-gauge Klein is then used to suction more superficially and to perform final blending and triangulation. Although relatively superficial liposuction is performed, it is advisable to leave a narrow zone of intact subdermal fat to retain optimal contours.

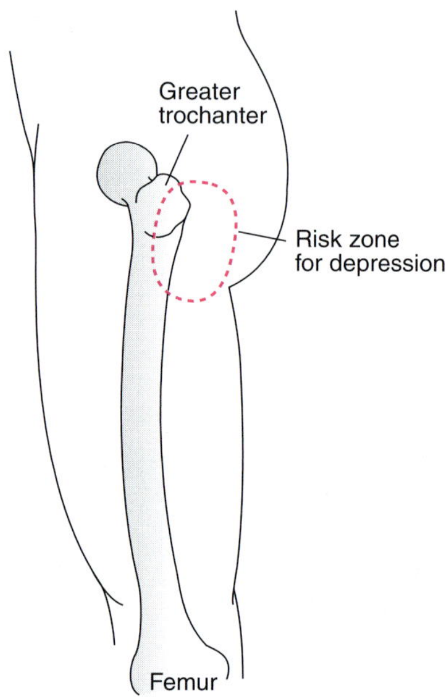

FIG. 14-43
Gasparotti's point. The area posterior to the greater trochanter is a risk zone for liposuction-induced depressions and soft tissue deformities.

Areas to be cautious about include the upper lateral thigh, distal lateral thigh, and Gasparotti's point.[57] The upper lateral and distal lateral thigh are susceptible to oversuctioning and ridging or dimpling, particularly around cannula insertion holes. It is important to move the cannula from one insertion hole to the next with regularity to avoid oversuctioning through one incision and creating a dimple under that incision. Gasparotti's point is just posterior to the greater trochanter, and depressions in this location result from aggressive suctioning of the deep fat (Fig. 14-43). Abduction and internal rotation of the leg are useful to drop the greater trochanter out of the surgical field and thus protect against a Gasparotti point depression. Numerous devices are available, including the triangular wedge pillow, that promote this leg position and aid the surgeon (Well's Johnson, Tucson, AZ). We prefer to have an assistant abduct the leg.

The end point for outer thigh liposuction is subjective. Contour and flow are the most important concerns, and the smart hand pinch technique is invaluable. The surgeon pinches other areas of the leg that appear to be well contoured and determines how many finger-widths (using the index finger) of skin is contained in the pinch (Fig. 14-44). This becomes the set point of the leg and is often 1 to 1.5 finger-widths. The goal of outer thigh suctioning becomes bringing the outer thigh pinch test to match that 1 to 1.5 finger-widths. But the surgeon must use the pinch test in conjunction with visual and other tactile clues to determine the optimal liposculpture end point.

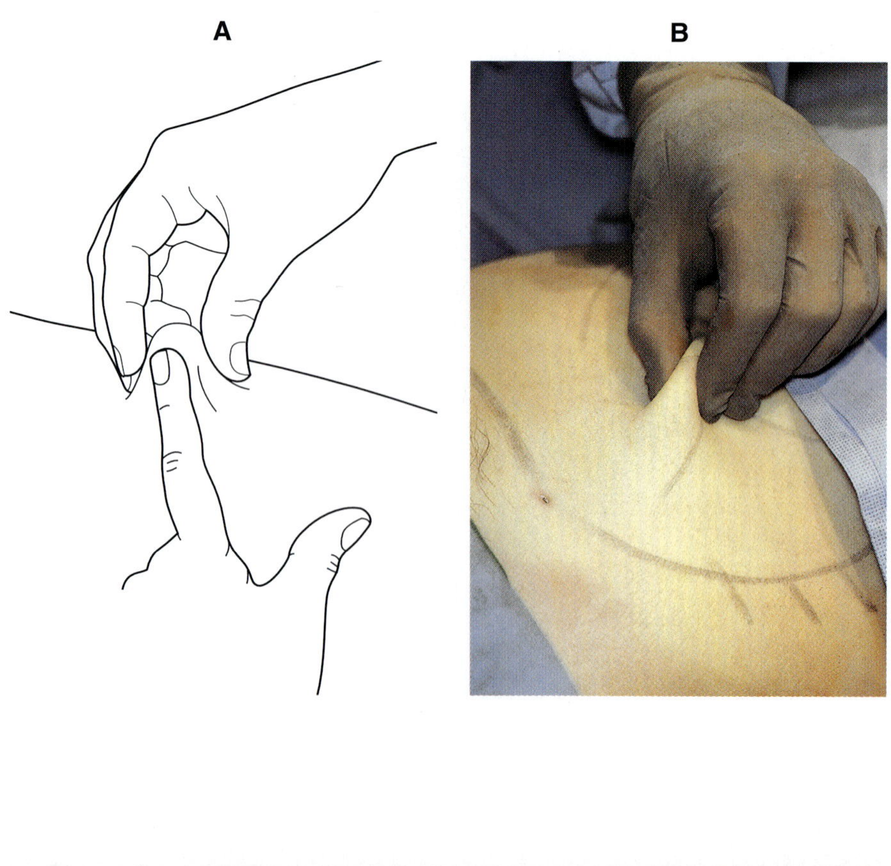

FIG. 14-44
The pinch technique to evaluate liposuction endpoints. **A,** Use of the index finger as a measuring device to determine amount of remaining fat. **B,** Pinch technique showing little remaining subcutaneous fat on the lower abdomen (less than 1 finger).

Inner Thighs and Knees. For many women, the inner thigh region is a difficult place to lose weight and improve contours. Diet and exercise programs can have some limited success, but liposuction is a superb treatment option for this anatomic region (Fig. 14-45). When evaluating the inner thigh and knee, the surgeon must determine both the amount of fat removal to be performed as well as the extent of surface area to treat. Specifically, a decision must be made either to treat the entire inner thigh and knee region as one unit or to treat the upper inner thigh and knee as separate cosmetic units.

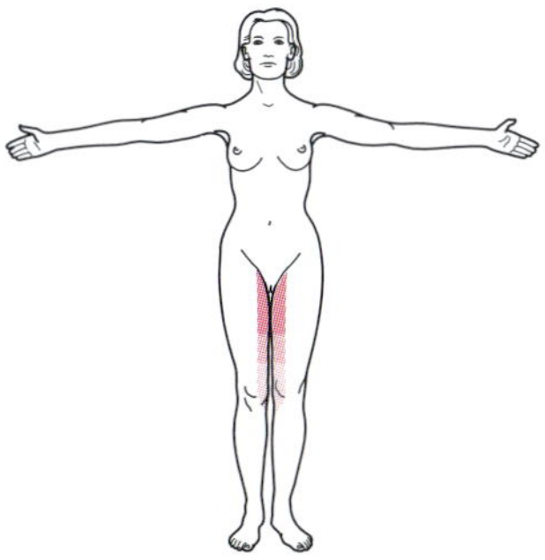

The difficulty with treating the inner thigh or knee as a distinct entity is that the risk of contour irregularities and step-offs increases. Blending of the knee or inner thigh with the mid thigh can be challenging, and the amount of fat that can be removed from these regions is limited if the surgeon must prevent a line of demarcation at the junction with the mid thigh. Suboptimal cosmetic results can be more frequent when the mid thigh is not treated.

For these reasons, the authors have developed a preferred method for treating the entire inner thigh and knee as one cosmetic unit, extending from the inguinal crease down to the superomedial calf. Gentle suctioning of the mid thigh region allows more thorough fat removal from the upper inner thigh and knee, improves blending and feathering into the mid thigh, and increases patient satisfaction by contouring and debulking the entire medial upper leg.

The patient is marked in the standing position with the knee fully extended and the leg advanced forward (a modified lunge position) and externally rotated (Fig. 14-46). The fat pads of the medial knee and upper inner thigh are identified and delineated, as is the inguinal crease. Markings should include the proximal medial calf, as treatment of this area helps to define knee contours and improve the flow of skin lines. The surgeon should be certain to mark and identify the posterior knee and posterior upper thigh fat pockets, as failure to treat these areas will lead to less than optimal postoperative contours. Adequate contouring of these posterior adipose collections is essential, since these fibrous areas will dominate the postoperative appearance if not removed. Also, reduction of these compartments allows the remainder of the inner thigh and knee skin to *fall* into position after suctioning rather than being tented by these posterior fibrous adipose collections. The anterior and posterior borders of the region to be treated should also be marked and are loosely used as feathering guides into the anterior and posterior thigh. Careful feathering is essential to maintain normal thigh contours and flow.

Anesthesia is obtained with 0.1% tumescent lidocaine anesthesia through multiple incision sites. The

A

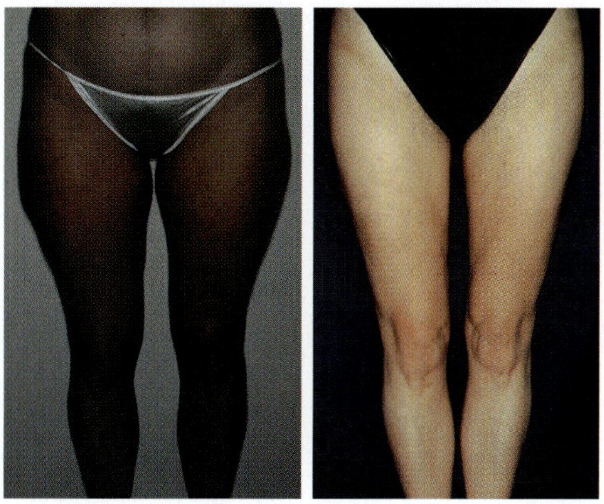

B

FIG. 14-45
A 43-year-old woman before **(A)** and 6 months after **(B)** inner thigh and knee liposuction. Note preoperative distance between inner thighs with feet apart, and increased postoperative space with feet together. Patient has also had outer thigh liposuction.

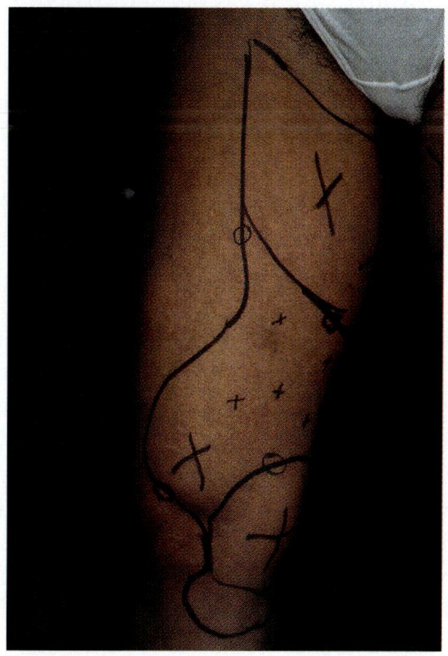

FIG. 14-46
Preoperative markings for inner thigh and knee liposuction. Note the three zones to be treated: upper inner thigh, mid thigh, and knee extending to superior calf.

mid thigh can be anesthetized with 0.05% lidocaine, since it is slightly less sensitive than the remainder of the inner leg. Incision sites below the knee should be avoided because they often do not heal as well as those above the knee. Thorough anesthesia of the fibrous posterior knee and inner thigh regions is helpful for improving patient comfort. Anesthesia should be placed 2 to 3 cm beyond the anterior and posterior markings to allow for feathering. Anesthesia should sit for a minimum of 30 minutes prior to suctioning.

The knee is suctioned first, with the patient in the frog-leg position and slightly rotated onto the side being treated. The degree of convexity of the medial femoral condyle and the tibial plateau may create a pseudolipodystrophy in an area devoid of fat. Palpation upon physical examination will differentiate the depth of the fat pad from the underlying bony prominences. A 12-gauge Klein cannula is used to treat the knee, with near complete fat removal as the goal. The surgeon should feather this treatment area into the proximal calf and the mid thigh. It is useful to perform the feather maneuvers during the intitial phases of suctioning, as this can allow for more thorough and even fat removal from the knee and upper inner thigh. Early feathering tends to improve the surgeon's feel during the procedure, often eliminating the need to "chase" a persistent ridge or depression. Treatment of the posterior fibrous knee fat is performed with the 12-gauge Klein cannula, but in some patients a more aggressive cannula such as the 12- or 14-gauge Capistrano cannula is needed to debulk this area.

The proximal inner thigh is initially gently debulked in the deep fat with the Capistrano cannula. The 12-gauge Capistrano is used for most patients, but thinner patients can be debulked with the 14-gauge. Caution is a must when using the Capistrano cannula in this region. Its benefit is that it can quickly and thoroughly debulk the upper inner thigh, including the very fibrous and resistent posterior inner thigh fat. However, overzealous or superficial use of this cannula can produce persistent ridges and contour irregularities. The surgeon should limit the number of cannula strokes performed from any single incision with the Capistrano cannula, so triangulation is essential with this instrument. The upper thigh is then fine-tuned with the 12-gauge Klein cannula, with blending and feathering into the mid thigh. Fat removal from the upper inner thigh should not be 100%, but more in the 50% to 80% range. This is one area where *flow* and the surgeon's aesthetic sense are essential determinants of the end point of treatment.

The mid thigh is the medial region located between the upper inner thigh and the knee. It should be viewed as a connector, essentially a bridge between the upper and lower inner thigh region. For this reason, treatment of the mid thigh helps the surgeon to blend and contour the inner leg. The overall contour changes of the inner leg come from suctioning of the upper inner thigh and knee, but the mid thigh is the *glue* that holds the cosmetic unit together. Suctioning of the mid thigh should be performed gently in the mid fat with a 12-gauge Klein cannula, taking only what comes very easily. The end point of treatment is when the upper thigh and knee blend smoothly with the mid thigh, as well as when the entire inner thigh blends smoothly with the anterior and posterior thigh. Caution should be exercised in the vicinity of Hunter's canal and the femoral artery, since aggressive suctioning in this area can produce a very unnatural postoperative fullness (lump) in the area. Final blending with the upper inner thigh, posterior upper thigh, and knee is performed during the final stages of mid thigh suctioning. The rule of thumb is that it is better to remove too little rather than too much fat from the mid thigh.

It is useful for the surgeon to think of the inner leg as an entire cosmetic unit during the final stages of suctioning. Taking a literal step back to view the flow and contours of this region can help the surgeon see areas that require further treatment and blending.

Postoperative compression of the upper inner thigh is especially important, and the surgeon should be certain to choose garments that provide adequate support in this area. Some garments have a cutout in the groin area to facilitate toilet use, but this opening can hinder compression of the upper thigh and should be eliminated as soon as possible postoperatively.

Anterior and Posterior Thighs. The authors infrequently treat the anterior and posterior thighs. The anterior thigh is occasionally treated as an extension of the knee, and in most cases involves gentle suctioning of the distal anterior thigh from two incisions placed in the medial and lateral suprapatellar regions. The so-called *banana roll* of the upper posterior thigh is occasionally suctioned very gently. Overtreatment of this area can produce a very unnatural ridging. Gentle mid to superficial suctioning of the fat can improve contours and encourage skin tightening with a good safety margin. The 12-gauge Klein cannula is used for both regions.

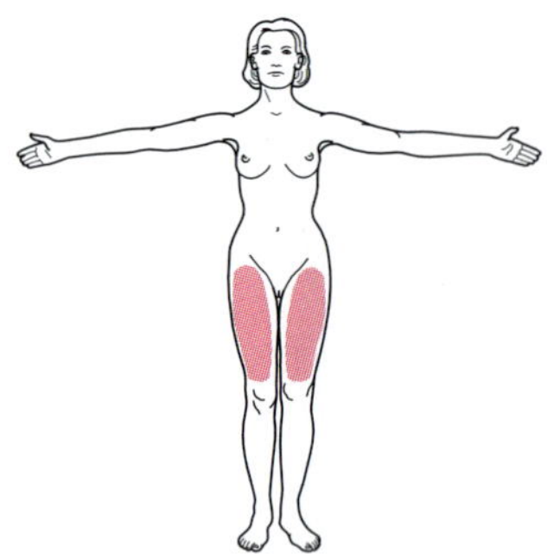

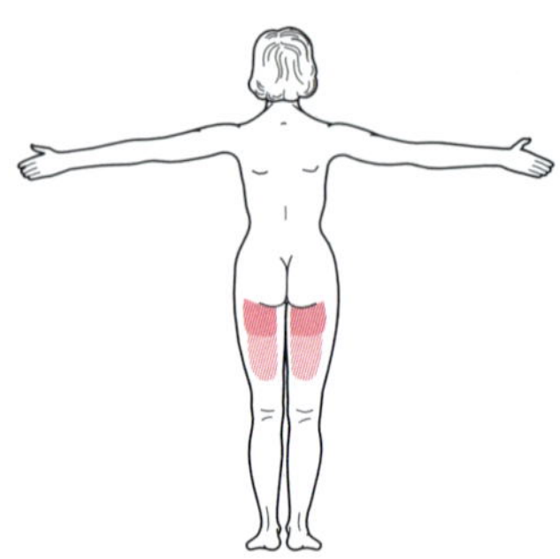

Calves and Ankles. Lipodystrophy of the calves and ankles is often not dependent on body weight and is usually present from early adolescence. Fatty deposits of the calves and ankles often make patients look much heavier than they really are, but fortunately liposuction can help in this area. With the use of tumescent anesthesia, smaller cannulas, and good postoperative compression, excessive bruising, persistent swelling, and irregularities occur infrequently.[58] The challenge of calf and ankle liposuction is treating a small convex surface so that at the end of the procedure the patient has an even smaller, natural appearing, shapely convex lower leg. Patients with a history of deep venous thrombosis (DVT), hypercoagulable state, angina, past myocardial infarction, or large varicose veins are not candidates for liposuction of the calves and ankles.

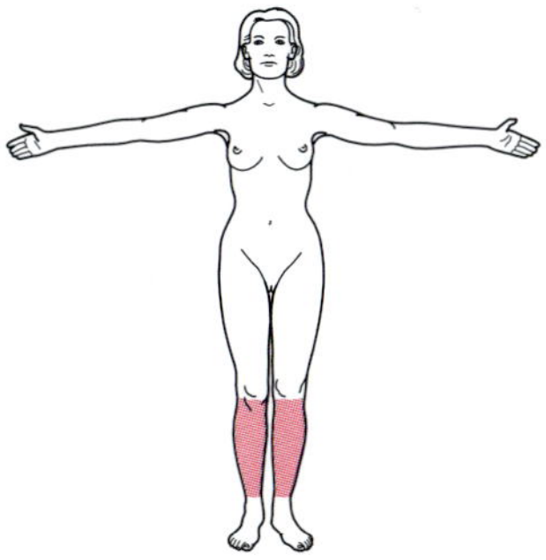

The patient is marked in the standing position. It is often useful to have the patient stand on a stool or low bench. The anterior leg in the pretibial area is rarely treated due to the almost universal absence of fat in this region. Tumescent anesthesia is obtained with 0.1% lidocaine and allowed to sit for 30 to 45 minutes.

Suctioning is performed with small cannulas, usually a 12-gauge Klein or 3 mm spatula cannula. Incisions are kept to a minimum (usually four to eight per leg), since lower leg incisions often do not heal as well as those placed in other areas. Areas to focus on include the lateral and medial upper calf, as contouring of this area will often substantially improve leg shape. Further debulking of the posterior calf can reduce circumference and provide additional contour improvements. Moderate liposuction around the ankle region can refine distal lower extremity contours.

The goal of calf and ankle liposuction is gentle but thorough fat removal. The surgeon must use caution so as to avoid injury to the underside of the dermis, which can produce unnatural ridging and become quite noticeable in this region. Therefore it is advisable to treat the calf and ankle as one cosmetic unit, leaving a small amount of subdermal fat while enhancing contours through targeted suctioning of the areas discussed above.

Postoperative compression garments and leg elevation are essential following calf and ankle liposuction. Patients are encouraged to ambulate and perform leg exercises to prevent DVT. Despite the best efforts of both patient and surgeon, postoperative lower leg edema is to be expected and often will persist for many months. Evaluation for DVT should be performed regularly during the first 2 postoperative weeks, and necessary studies should be performed when indicated. Postsurgical swelling resolves slowly, and patient counseling can be invaluable during this time.

Liposuction for Men

The male breast and love handles are areas commonly treated with liposuction. In some male patients, the upper and lower abdomen will benefit from suctioning as well. The guiding principle in men is that fat is much more fibrous than in women and therefore often requires more aggressive suctioning to remove. In addition, male fat tends to *hang* off the underside of the dermis in a more superficial location than female fat does. Men also have mid and deep adipose tissue, but this superficial fat is often quite difficult to access without substantial subdermal tissue trauma.

The advantage of treating men is that their skin/dermis is often quite thick and resilient, responding quite well to aggressive treatment. The one exception is neck skin, which does not retract and redrape as well as in women. The surgeon is often able to suction with the goal of 100% fat removal in men without producing unnatural ridges or surface irregularities. Naturally, extreme care must be exercised to produce optimal skin contour and flow, but skin and fat in men can, for the most part, be treated more aggressively than in women.

Male Breast. The male breast responds well to liposuction. A careful history screening for breast cancer in the patient and close relatives is essential. Some, but not all, physicians also advocate mammograms preoperatively. Screening for fibrous subareolar glandular tissue is also helpful, as patients with extensive glandular tissue will often benefit from sharp excision under direct visualization. Marking is performed with the patient in the standing position. Asking the patient to contract/flex the pectoral muscles often helps to delineate the extent of the area to be treated. The superomedial breast area often requires minimal suctioning, with the most fat removed from the lateral and infrareolar and subareolar breast regions. Some men will also benefit from suctioning axillary and upper back adipose connections to the breast area.

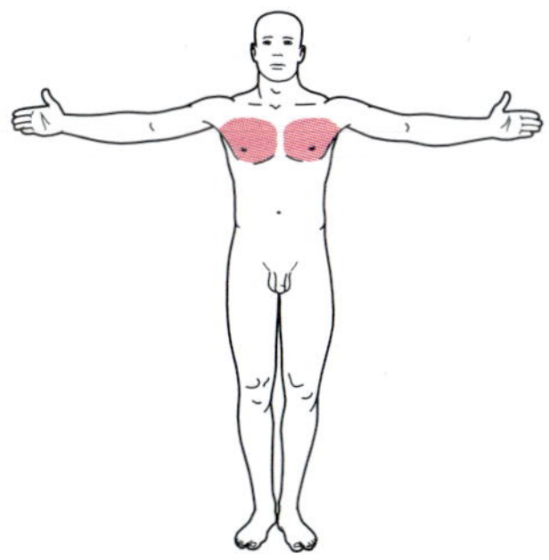

Of interest, liposuction for the female breast is an emerging procedure with some very attractive features. Breast reduction with liposuction eliminates the unsightly scars associated with traditional breast reduction surgery, has a much more rapid recovery period, and can produce superb contours. The most appropriate women candidates are those with good skin tone, an anteriorly oriented nipple complex and absence of nipple ptosis, and relatively fatty breast tissue with the absence of a prominent glandular component.

Anesthesia is obtained with 0.1% tumescent lidocaine anesthesia and allowed to sit for 30 to 45 minutes. Incisions should be placed in concealed areas, such as the inframammary crease and axillary folds. Initial suctioning is performed with the 3 mm Accelerator cannula from multiple incision sites and with careful triangulation. Thorough suctioning under the areola is important for enhanced contours, and more aggressive or sharper cannulas are sometimes required (e.g., Pinto cannula). In our experience, injury to the nipple complex is rare with liposuction alone. Final contouring is performed with the 12-gauge Klein cannula. If glandular tissue persists under the nipple after healing is complete, it can be removed under direct visualization during a follow-up procedure, utilizing a 1- to 2-inch curvilinear infraareolar incision. However, the need for surgical excision of residual glandular tissue following liposuction is uncommon. Direct excision of glandular tissue at the time of liposuction surgery is avoided because it can induce necrosis of the nipple complex due to aggressive suctioning and subdermal trauma to that area.

The optimal amount of breast fat to be removed is sometimes difficult to determine. In younger patients, more aggressive treatment is often beneficial, as the skin will redrape well. Older patients tend to have less skin elasticity, and in these patients thorough, smooth fat removal is indicated to produce optimal skin retraction. Some patients will benefit from selective suctioning and liposculpting to enhance the definition of chest contours and further define underlying pectoral muscles. The male breast can also have a pseudocapsule, creating a diffuse mound of tissue that tends to move as the cannula approaches it. Stabilization of this mound with the smart hand is essential.

Postoperative compression is important. It is obtained with either a standard male breast liposuction garment or conventional 9- to 12-inch abdominal binders.

Love Handles and Abdomen. Fat removal from the abdomen and love handles should be thorough for men. Most male patients desire and benefit from near 100% fat removal in these areas. However, adipose tissue in these areas is quite fibrous, and aggressive suctioning is indicated. Careful treatment of the superficial fat compartment is often essential in these regions, as failure to remove this tissue can lead to persistent fullness.

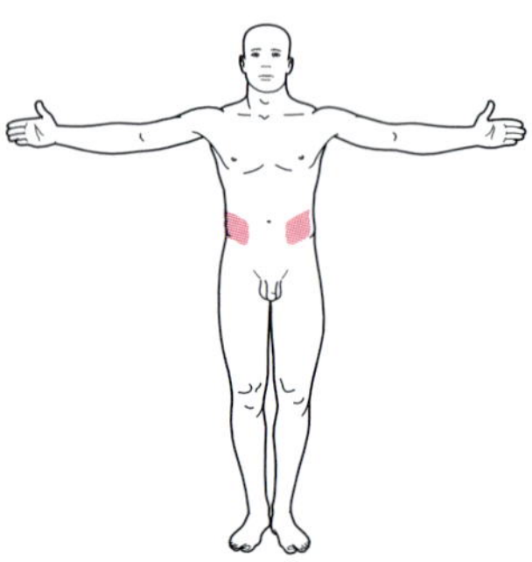

The areas to be treated are marked in the standing position. The love handles can be treated alone or combined with treatment of the upper and lower abdomen. Evaluation for hernias is essential preoperatively (see section on liposuction of the female abdomen). Many men have intraabdominal fat that causes a protuberant abdomen. It is essential to identify this during the initial consultation and educate patients about the location of their adipose tissue. Fat that is deep to the rectus muscle cannot be treated with liposuction. Patients who have fat superficial and deep to the rectus will often be disappointed with their results if they are not counseled preoperatively as to the limitations of treatment. The ideal patient has little to no intraabdominal fat and well-defined adipose collections superficial to the rectus and oblique muscles.

Anesthesia is obtained with 0.1% tumescent lidocaine anesthesia. Allowing the anesthetic to sit for an additional 15 to 20 minutes (45 to 50 total) is helpful in these sensitive areas. Multiple incision sites are used, hiding them in the suprapubic, periumbilical, and hair-bearing regions when possible. Initial suctioning can be performed with the 3.0 or 3.7 mm Keel Cobra cannula in larger individuals, as well as 10- to 12-gauge Capistrano cannulas. Caution must be used to prevent ridging when using these aggressive instruments despite the fact that men tend to have resilient skin. Further suctioning is performed with the 3 mm Accelerator cannula, and superficial fat is removed with either the Accelerator or 12-gauge Klein cannula.

The abdomen is treated with the patient in the flat supine position. Caution should be used when crossing the costal margins. Each love handle is best treated with the patient lying on his contralateral side. Very aggressive suctioning of the deep fat in the love handles is essential for contouring. Many men have firm, fibrous fat in the posterior love handle/lower back region, and this can be a challenge to maximally debulk. Use of aggressive cannulas such as the 10- to 12-gauge Capistrano can be useful.

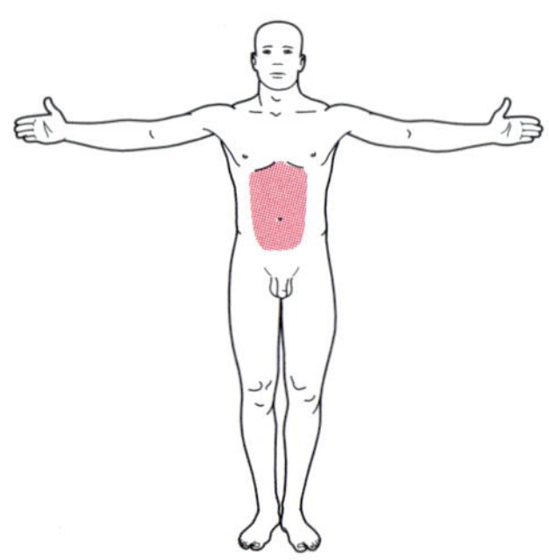

Postoperative compression is obtained with 9- or 12-inch elastic abdominal binders. Male patients are encouraged to wear these garments as much as possible to compress and contour the treated areas.

POSTOPERATIVE CLINICAL CONSIDERATIONS

Patients may be greatly distressed by the quantity of drainage during the postoperative period unless they have been adequately prepared by the medical team. Placement and changing schedules for the various pads and support garments may be easily confused by the sedated patient and should be provided in writing. Any instructions regarding medications (antibiotics and analgesics), and continued avoidance of certain products, should also be provided in writing.

The management style for the postoperative liposuction patient is again unique to each physician. Most patients' postoperative pain is well controlled with acetominophen, requiring acetominophen with codeine or other narcotics only the first few days, if at all.

Support garments applied by the medical team in the operating room will facilitate drainage of the tumescent fluid, provide significant pain control, improve final outcomes and contours, and reduce the risk of seroma formation. These garments should compress all surgical areas; multiple garments may be needed. A compression level between 17 and 21 mm Hg is desired.[59] They should allow the patient to comfortably eat, breath, and use the bathroom. Many companies offer appropriate garments, and even over-the-counter athletic support braces may be sufficient, provided all treatment sites are covered and firm compression is obtained. Adequate circulation and perfusion must be ensured before the patient is discharged. These garments should not be removed by the patient for the first 24 hours. The patient is instructed to return to the office on the first postoperative day, where the medical team assists with removing the garments for the first time. This is best done with the patient supine, and he or she should be closely monitored for hypotension as the pressure garment is removed. Wounds are cleaned, and either the original or a new garment is applied with appropriate bandaging.

Incision sites are not sutured postoperatively and therefore tend to drain copious amounts of fluid. Absorbent pads are applied over incision sites under the support garment. Additional pads may be placed over the garment to facilitate changing by the patient. These may be changed as frequently as necessary to absorb discharge. Some patients have found that sleeping the first two nights on a plastic mattress cover facilitates cleanup. Superabsorbent pads are becoming increasingly available and may provide some advantages over conventional dressings at the incision sites.

The patient is asked to wear the compression garment for 23 to 24 hours a day for the first 7 postoperative days, removing it to shower when needed. After the first week, the patient is instructed to wear the compression garments for 8 to 10 hours a day for the following 3 to 4 weeks. Compression is particularly important for the neck, upper arms, upper inner thighs, and abdomen.

If preoperative antibiotics were initiated, they are usually continued for 7 to 10 days postoperatively. Patients are instructed not to shower for the first 24 to 48 hours to decrease the risk of infection. For the same reason, they should not bathe in a tub until all incision sites have healed. They should be informed of the signs of possible infection, such as fever, chills, increased pain, or redness, and told to notify the physician immediately if there is concern.

Since the lidocaine plasma peak level may actually occur after the patient has left the office, it is imperative that the patient also be aware of the signs of lidocaine toxicity: difficulty speaking, ringing in the ears, tremors or tingling around the mouth, confusion. We prefer to have patients in the company of another person for 12 to 24 hours after surgery so they are not left unattended.

The patients are asked to not drink alcohol for 3 days after surgery, to refrain from smoking for as long as possible, and to avoid strenuous activity for 1 week. They are encouraged to drink fluids and have a soft diet for the first 24 hours, after which they may resume their regular diet.

Edema, ecchymosis, dysesthesias, fatigue, and soreness are common complaints that improve with time. Using a 1.5 to 2 mm punch biopsy for incision sites may decrease edema and ecchymosis by preventing premature closure of incision sites and facilitating drainage.[60] Wearing the compression garments will also improve these symptoms. For this reason, some patients will choose to wear their garments for many weeks after the procedure.

Development of a hematoma, seroma (Fig. 14-47), infection, or drug reaction are indications to see the pa-

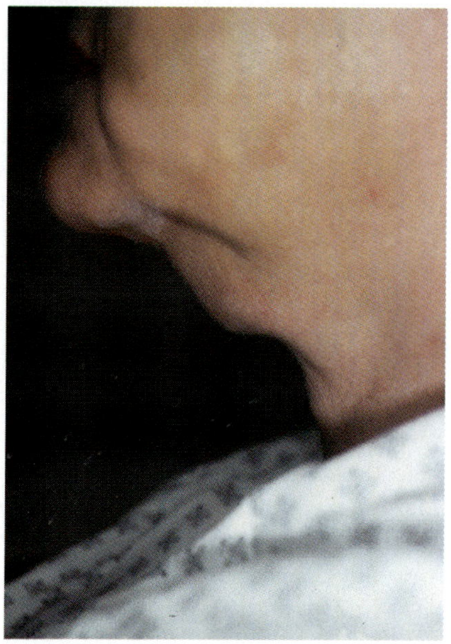

FIG. 14-47
Seroma on postoperative day 3 following neck liposuction.

tient immediately. Early intervention is key. Hematomas may require drainage or even surgical exploration. Seromas require aspiration, often serially over several days. The physician must again confirm that the patient is being compliant with compression garment use, as poor compliance is often a cause of hematoma or seroma formation. Drug reactions may be confused with cellulitis, neither of which should go untreated in the liposuction patient. Antibiotics should be promptly changed if a drug reaction is suspected. Incision site cultures, as wells as urine and blood cultures, should be obtained if systemic infection is suspected. Hospital admission should be considered depending on the clinical scenario.

Some degree of entry site scars should be expected by the patient and followed clinically for improvements over a year. A double-blind study evaluating the healing of cannula incisions with and without sutures demonstrated that the sutured sites healed more slowly and left more visible scars.[61] Therefore, it is recommended that incision sites not be sutured at the conclusion of the procedure. In patients with light skin, incision sites initially turn red by 1 to 2 weeks and fade completely by 3 to 6 months, leaving a small porcelain white scar 2 to 4 mm in length. Patients with olive or dark skin should be told to expect some degree of postinflammatory hyperpigmentation, with resolution over 6 to 12 months.

Persistent edema and dysesthesias (usually hypesthesia) can be troubling to the patient. Lower leg edema is common, particularly following calf liposuction. Leg elevation and properly fitting compression garments are essential. Acute onset edema in the immediate postoperative period necessitates an evaluation for deep venous thrombosis (DVT). Although DVT is uncommon in the postoperative period following tumescent liposuction, women on oral contraceptives and those with a family history of DVT may be particularly at risk. Edema of the distal arm is occasionally seen after arm liposuction and is often due to garment constriction at the forearm. A change in garments will usually correct this, along with elevation of the affected limb.

Reported cases of congestive heart failure, fat emboli, pulmonary edema, and cardiovascular collapse associated with liposuction have been presented as complications of tumescent liposuction.[62-64] However, closer examination of these cases reveals that the patients were placed under general anesthesia with intravenous fluids. By definition, true tumescent technique is a method of delivering local anesthesia, without concomitant intravenous sedation or fluids. It is advised that physicians interpret the literature with this distinction and definition in mind.[65]

After the initial dressing change on postoperative day 1, patients are seen again 1 week postoperatively to assess healing and effectiveness of garments. Modifications can be made to the postoperative plan as indicated, and patients are routinely seen 1 month postoperatively and then again at 3 to 6 months.

What the patient may notice most is any degree of asymmetry, contour imperfections, or dimpling. Preoperative photographs are essential for comparison during the postoperative period. Most patients are not symmetric prior to the procedure, and this can be pointed out to the patient preoperatively. Minor irregularities may improve as the edema improves. More noticeable contour imperfections may be best served with a "touch-up," or additional liposuction to a limited area. Dimpling of the skin can be caused by damage to the reticular dermis, overaggressive suctioning of the deep fat, or poor skin tone.

Patients are encouraged to wait a minimum of 3 months before assessing surgical outcomes. This allows for postoperative edema to resolve and skin contraction to begin. Some patients, especially younger patients with taut skin, will begin to see their results on postoperative day 1. Others will see their results evolve over weeks to months. Touch-up procedures are performed in approximately 10% of patients, and surgeons differ in their approach to touch-ups. Some prefer to intervene early in the postoperative course, while others prefer to wait until the final result has settled. While it is essential to tailor decision making on touch-ups to patient desires, it is often advisable to wait as long as possible before performing touch-ups. This is because skin retraction and redraping in the postoperative period will often improve contours for months after surgery, and an area that appears to need a touch-up 1 month after surgery may look superb at the 6-month mark without any intervention.

In the event that surface irregularities do persist postoperatively, the surgeon has several options. A central premise to liposuction surgery is that it is always easier to remove additional fat than it is to replace fat. Therefore, part of the treatment of postoperative contour irregularities comes during the initial surgical session in the form of conservative fat removal in some areas. This is particularly important in challenging areas such as the inner and outer thighs and upper arms, or any area where less than 100% fat removal is the goal. Since liposuction is a contouring procedure, the goal of treatment is not always to remove 100% of the fat, but rather to leave just enough fat to produce an aesthetically pleasing contour. If the surgeon undertreats slightly, then it is possible to go back for a touch-up procedure and remove additional fat to enhance results. If the surgeon overtreats, then there is a need to either replace fat with fat transplantation, or elevate the skin and improve contours with alternate methods. Clearly, the method of removing more fat is preferrable if a touch-up is to be performed. This point cannot be emphasized enough. Although all surgeons strive to produce superb results each time a procedure is performed, it is the cautious surgeon who plans for worst case scenario.

When replacement of fat is needed, fat transplantation is a good option. Fat can be harvested from other areas of the body and moved to the area to be treated via this relatively simple technique. The authors utilize a 12-gauge Klein cannula to harvest and implant the fat from a 10 cc syringe. It is important to realize that fat will be less likely to maintain permanence in areas of high mobility, such as the outer thighs. Also, some fat is likely to be absorbed during the healing phase, so it is advisable to harvest more fat than is needed and freeze some in the event a fat transplantation touch-up is indicated.

An alternative or complementary solution to fat transplantation is subdermal undermining. This is done with the 12-gauge Klein cannula and can be performed alone or in combination with fat transplantation. The cannula is inserted in a pistonlike motion similar to liposuction and is directed to bound-down or fibrous areas that are in need of elevation. By releasing the tissue in these areas, it is possible to elevate and improve its contours. The body's natural response to injury will cause an inflammatory response that ultimately produces a fibrous reaction, which develops into a form of soft tissue augmentation.

SUMMARY

Liposuction is a challenging surgical procedure that can produce superb aesthetic results when performed properly. Careful suctioning, use of the smart hand, triangulation, and fluid management are all important parts of the liposuction procedure. Final outcomes depend on both the skill of the surgeon and the healing response of the patient. However, it is the responsibility of the surgeon to have thorough knowledge and training in the procedure to minimize the possibility that surgical technique is the contributing factor to less-than-optimal results. It is the blend of physician skill and artistry that ultimately determines outcomes, and the surgeon can create beautiful contours by managing the interplay of skin healing dynamics, cannula motion and position, thoroughness of fat removal, and body shape.

REFERENCES

1. American Society for Dermatologic Surgery. Guiding principles for liposuction. Dermatol Surg 1997; 23:1127-1129.
2. Rischer A, Fischer G. First surgical treatment for molding body's cellulite with three 5 mm incisions. Bull Int Acad Cosmet Surg 1976; 3:35.
3. Illouz RG. Body contouring by lipolysis: a 5-year experience with over 3000 cases. Plast Reconstr Surg 1983; 72:591.
4. Klein JA. Tumescent technique for liposuction surgery. Am J Cosmet Surg 1987; 4:263.
5. Lillis PJ. Liposuction surgery under local anesthesia: limited blood loss and minimal lidocaine absorption. J Dermatol Surg Oncol 1988; 14:1145-1148.
6. Narins RS, Coleman WP. Minimizing pain for liposuction anesthesia. Dermatol Surg 1997; 23: 1137-1140.
7. Hanke CW, Bernstein G, Bullock S. Safety of tumescent liposuction in 15,336 patients. Dermatol Surg 1995; 21:459-462.
8. Rigel DS, Wheeland RG. Deaths related to liposuction. N Engl J Med 1999; 341:1001-1002.
9. Coleman WP III. Liposuction and anesthesia. J Dermatol Surg Oncol 1987; 13:1295.
10. Klein JA. Tumescent technique for regional anesthesia permits lidocaine doses of 35 mg/kg for liposuction. J Dermatol Surg Oncol 1990; 16:248-263.
11. Ostad A, Kageyama N, Moy R. Tumescent anesthesia with a lidocaine dose of 55 mg/kg is safe for liposuction. Dermatol Surg 1996; 22:921-927.
12. deJong RH. Local Anesthetics. St. Louis: Mosby–Year Book, 1994.
13. Covino BG. Clinical pharmacology of local anesthetic agents. In: Cousins MJ, Bridenbough PO, eds. Neural Blockade. Philadelphia: Lippincott, 1988.
14. Tucker GT, Boas RA. Pharmacokinetic aspects of intravenous regional anesthesia. Anesthesiology 1971; 34:538-542.
15. Moy R. Tumescent Liposuction Council Bulletin. Dermatol Surg 1997; 23:214.
16. Butterwick KJ, Goldman MP, Sriprachya-Anunt S. Lidocaine levels during the first two hours of infiltration of dilute anesthetic solution for tumescent liposuction: rapid versus slow delivery. Dermatol Surg 1999; 25:681-685.
17. Hanke CW, Coleman WP III, Lillis PJ, et al. Infusion rates and levels of premedication in tumescent liposuction. Dermatol Surg 1997; 23:1131-1134.
18. Klein JA, Kassarjdian N. Lidocaine toxicity with tumescent liposuction: a case report of probable drug interactions. Dermatol Surg 1997; 23:1169-1174.
19. Nemeroff CB, DeVane LC, Pollock BG. Newer antidepressants and the cytochrome P450 system. Am J Psychiatry 1996; 153:311-320.
20. Grazer FM. Complications of the tumescent formula for liposuction. Plast Reconstr Surg 1997; 11:1893-1896.
21. Burk RW, Guzman-Stein G, Vasconez LO. Lidocaine and epinephrine levels in tumescent technique liposuction. Plast Reconstr Surg 1996; 97:1379-1384.
22. Sifton DW, ed. Physician's Desk Reference. 54th ed. Napa, CA: Epipen Dey, 2000:958.
23. Bouloux P, Perett D, Besser GM. Methodological considerations in the determination of plasma catecholamines by high-performance liquid chromatography with electrochemical detection. Ann Clin Biochem 1985; 22:194.
24. Lewis CM. Lipoplasty in males. Clin Plast Surg 1989; 16:335-339.
25. Serdula MK, Collins ME, Williamson DF, et al. Weight control practices of US adolescents and adults. Ann Intern Med 1993; 119(7 pt2):667-671.
26. Technology Assessment Conference Panel. Methods for voluntary weight loss and control: Technology Assessment Conference Statement. Ann Intern Med 1992; 116:942-949.
27. Hanke CW, Bullock S, Bernstein G. Current status of tumescent liposuction in the United States. Dermatol Surg 1996; 22:595-598.
28. Fournier PF. Therapeutic megalipoextraction or megaliposculpture. Obes Surg 1996; 6:167.
29. Matarasso A, Kim RW, Kral JG. The impact of liposuction on body fat. Plast Reconstr Surg 1999; 102:1686-1689.

30. Terry RB, Stefanick ML, Haskell WL, Wood PD. Contributions of regional adipose tissue depots to plasma lipoprotein concentrations in overweight men and women: possible protective effects of thigh fat. Metabolism 1991; 40:733.
31. Scarborough DA, Bisaccia E. The occurrence of breast enlargement in females following liposuction. Am J Cosmet Surg 1991; 8:97.
32. de Souza Pinto EB, de Almeida AE, Knudsen AF, et al. A new methodology in abdominoplasty and suction-assisted lipectomy. Aesthetic Plast Surg 1991; 15:111-121.
33. Matarasso A. Evaluation and classification in abdominal contour surgery. In: Abdominoplasty, Vasconez LL, ed. Oper Tech Plast Surg 1996; 3:7.
34. Bank DE, Perez MI. Skin retraction after liposuction in patients over the age of 40. Dermatol Surg 1999; 25:673-676.
35. Matarasso A, Matarasso SL. When does your liposuction patient require an abdominoplasty? Dermatol Surg 1997; 23:1151-1160.
36. Thompson KD, Welykyj S, Massa MC. Antibacterial activity of lidocaine in combination with a bicarbonate buffer. J Dermatol Surg Oncol 1993; 19:216.
37. Miller MA, Shell WB. Antimicrobial properties of lidocaine on bacteria isolated from dermal lesions. Arch Dermatol 1985; 121: 1157.
38. Parr AM, Zoutman DE, Davidson JSD. Antimicrobial activity of lidocaine against bacteria associated with nosocomial wound infection. Ann Plast Surg 1999; 43:239-245.
39. Kiak GA, Koontz FF, Chavez AJ. Lidocaine inhibits growth of *Staphylococcus aureus* in propofol. Anesthesiology 1992; 77:A407.
40. Gajraj RJ, Hodson MJ, Gillespie JA, et al. Antibacterial activity of lidocaine in mixtures with Diprivan. Br J Anesth 1998; 81:444.
41. Klein JA. Antibacterial effects of tumescent lidocaine. Plast Reconstr Surg 1996; 104:1934-1936.
42. Kaplan B, Moy RL. Comparison of room temperature and warmed local anesthetic solution for tumescent liposuction: a randomized double-blind study. Dermatol Surg 1996; 22:707-709.
43. Colaric KB, Overton ST, Moore K. Pain reduction in lidocaine administration through buffering and warming. Am J Emerg Med 1998; 16:353-356.
44. Hunstad JP. Addressing difficult areas in body contouring with emphasis on combined tumescent and syringe techniques. Clin Plast Surg 1996; 23:57-80.
45. Klein JA. Tumescent technique for local anesthesia improves safety in large volume liposuction. Plast Reconstr Surg 1993; 92: 1085-1098.
46. Lillis PJ. Liposuction: how aggressive should it be? Dermatol Surg 1996; 22;973-976.
47. Moreno A, Bell WH, Zhi-Hao Y. Esthetic contour analysis of the submental cervical region. J Oral Maxillofac Surg 1994; 52:704-713.
48. Kamer FM, Lefkoff LA. Submental surgery: a graduated approach to the aging neck. Arch Otolaryngol Head Neck Surg 1991; 117:40-46.
49. Feldman JJ. Corset platysmaplasty. Clin Plast Surg 1992; 19:369-382.
50. Alt TH. Facelift surgery. In: Elson ML, ed. Evaluation and Treatment of the Aging Face. New York: Springer-Verlag, 1995:110-168.
51. Grazer FM. Atlas of Suction Assisted Lipectomy. New York: Churchill Livingstone, 1992:140.
52. Illouz YG, de Villers YT. Body Sculpturing by Lipoplasty. Edinburgh: Churchill Livingstone, 1989:281.
53. Pitman GH. Liposuction and Aesthetic Surgery. St. Louis: Quality Medical Publishing, 1993:176.
54. Lillis PJ. Liposuction of the arms, calves and ankles. Dermatol Surg 1997; 23:1161-1168.
55. Cook WR Jr, Cook KK. Manual of Tumescent Liposculpture and Laser Cosmetic Surgery. Philadelphia: Lippincott Williams & Wilkins, 1999.
56. Cook WR Jr. Utilizing external ultrasonic energy to improve the results of tumescent liposculpture. Dermatol Surg 1997; 23:1207-1211.
57. Troilius C. Ten year evolution of liposuction. Aesthetic Plast Surg 1996; 20:201-206.
58. Lillis PJ. Liposuction of the knees, calves and ankles. Dermatol Surg 1999; 17:865-879.
59. Illouz YG. History and current concepts of lipoplasty. Clin Plast Surg 1996; 23:721-730.
60. Klein JA. Post-tumescent liposuction care: open drainage and bimodal compression. Dermatol Clin 1999; 17:881-889.
61. Naris RS, Coleman WP. Liposuction technical tips. Dermatol Surg 1996; 22:973-978.
62. Gilliland MD, Coates N. Tumescent liposuction complicated by pulmonary edema. Plast Reconstr Surg 1999; 99:215-219.
63. Dillerud E. Abdominoplasty combined with suction lipoplasty: a study of complications, revisions and risk factors in 487 cases. Ann Plast Surg 1990; 25:333-338.
64. Ross RN, Johnson GW. Fat embolism after liposuction. Chest 1988; 93:1294-1295.
65. Klein JK. Intravenous fluid and bupivacaine are contraindicated in tumescent liposuction. Plast Reconstr Surg 1998; 102:2516-2517.

APPENDIX A

Medications That May Affect Bleeding

Patient is to avoid use of these agents for 2 weeks prior to liposuction:

Accutane-Alert MD
Advil
Alka-Seltzer tablets
Alka-Seltzer Plus cold medicine
Anacin capsules/tablets
Anacin Maximum Strength capsules/tablets
Anarox
Ansaid
A.P.C. tablets
A.P.C. with codeine, Tabloid (branded tablet)
Arthritis Pain Formula by the makers of Anacin tablets
Ascodeen-30
Ascriptin
Aspergum
Aspirin
Aspirin suppositories
Bayer aspirin
Bayer Children's Chewable aspirin
Bayer Children's cold tablets
Bayer timed-release aspirin
BC Powder
Bufferin
Bufferin Feldene
Butalbital
Celebrex
Cheracol capsules
Clinoril
COPE
Coricidin D decongestant tablets
Darvon
Darvon with aspirin
Darvon-N with aspirin
Disalcid
Dristan decongestant capsules/tablets
Duragesic
Ecotrin
Empirin
Empirin with codeine
Equagesic
Excedrin

Feldene
Fiorinal with codeine
4-Way cold tablets
Goody's Headache Powders
Ibuprofen
Indocin
Lodine
Midol
Momentum Muscular Backache Formula
Motrin
Naprosyn
Norgesic/Norgesic Forte
Norwich aspirin
Panalgesic/Percodan/Percodan Demi tablets
Quiet World analgesic/sleeping aid
Robaxisal tablets
Salsalate
Sine-Aid
St. Joseph Adult Chewable aspirin tablets
Sulindac
Supac
Synalgos-DC capsules
Tolectin
Triaminic
Trilisate
Verin
Vioxx
Viro-Med tablets
Vitamin E
Voltaren

Please notify your doctor of all of the prescription and over-the-counter medications you are taking. If you are uncertain whether you may take a medication within 2 weeks of your liposuction procedure, please contact your physician's office.

APPENDIX B

Liposuction Consent Form

Patient Name: ____________________ Date: __________
Procedure: ____________________
Diagnosis: ____________________

Dr. ______________ and/or his/her staff has explained the nature of my condition, the nature of the procedure, its alternative treatments, and the risks/benefits to be reasonably expected compared with alternative approaches. This document is a written confirmation of this discussion.

By placing my initials next to the following items, I clearly understand and accept the following.

____ 1. The goal of liposuction surgery, as in any other cosmetic procedure, is improvement, not perfection.

____ 2. The final results may not be apparent for 6 to 12 months postoperatively.

____ 3. In order to achieve the best possible result, a "touch-up" procedure may be required. There will be a charge for any "touch-up" operation performed.

____ 4. Areas of "cottage cheese" texture, i.e., "cellulite," are unlikely to improve with the procedure.

____ 5. Liposuction surgery is a contouring procedure and not performed for purposes of weight reduction or skin reduction.

____ 6. Strict adherence to the preoperative and postoperative regimen (i.e., wearing garments for 4 weeks and following instructions) is necessary in order to achieve the best possible results.

____ 7. I have not taken any aspirin or aspirin-containing products, or nonsteroidal anti-inflammatory drugs (i.e., Advil/Motrin or Vitamin E) for 10 days prior to my surgery.

____ 8. The surgical fee covers the operation itself and subsequent postoperative office visits. There is no guarantee that the expected or anticipated results will be achieved.

____ 9. I authorize the taking of photographs or films during the procedure and their use for teaching and research purposes.

Although complications following liposuction are infrequent, by placing my initials next to the following, I understand that they may occur:

____ 1. Skin irregularities, lumpiness, hardness, and dimpling may appear postoperatively. Most of these problems disappear with time and massage, but localized irregularities may persist permanently. If loose skin is present in the treated area, it may or may not shrink back to conform to your new contour.

____ 2. Possible livedo pattern (mottled red and brown coloring) may occur following the procedure.

____ 3. Infection is rare, but should it occur, treatment with antibiotics and/or surgical drainage may be required.

____ 4. Numbness or increased sensitivity of the skin over the treated areas may persist for months. It is possible that localized areas of numbness or increased sensitivity could be permanent.

____ 5. Objectionable scarring is rare because of the small size of incisions used in liposuction surgery, but scar formation is possible.

____ 6. Dizziness may occur during the first week following liposuction surgery, particularly upon rising from a lying or sitting position. If this occurs, extreme caution must be exercised while walking. Do not attempt to drive a car if dizziness is present.

____ 7. Surgical bleeding is very rare, and theoretically could require hospitalization. It is possible that blood clots may form under the skin and require subsequent surgical drainage.

____ 8. Although rare, injury to the facial nerve (for neck liposuction only) may occur.

____ 9. You have arranged for someone to bring you to the office and drive you home. We have cancelled surgeries in the past if the patient didn't have a ride.

_____ 10. You have arranged for someone to stay with you for 24 hours after surgery.

_____ 11. In addition to these possible complications, I am aware of the general risks inherent in all surgical procedures and anesthetic administration.

_____ 12. I am aware that unexpected risks or complications may occur and that no guarantee or promises have been made to me concerning the results of any procedure or treatment.

My signature certifies that I have read and discussed the previous material thoroughly with my physician and/or his staff; and that I understand the goals, limitations, and possible complications of liposuction surgery and I wish to proceed with the operation.

______________________________ ____________

Patient Signature Date

I have explained the above statements to the patient and answered all questions.

______________________________ ____________

Clinical Staff Signature Date

______________________________ ____________

Physician Signature Date

CHAPTER 15

Hair Transplantation

WALTER P. UNGER

SECTION ONE

History and Scientific Review

BACKGROUND AND HISTORY

Hair transplantation was first reported in 1822 in a doctoral thesis published by J. Dieffenbach.[1] At the suggestion of his mentor Carl Unger, he used goose quills as trephines to move around small pieces of skin in order to investigate and successfully prove the concept of autotransplantation of hair, feather, and skin in animals and fowl. For approximately a century after Dieffenbach's early work, sporadic published reports of hair transplantation surfaced in the medical literature from Germany, England, France, and Japan. The majority of these reports described successful transposition of relatively large grafts or pedicle flaps.[2] The two notable exceptions were a German article on eyelash transplantation of single hairs in the early 1900s, and Okuda's 1939 article on punch grafting of hair for human alopecia in the *Japanese Journal of Dermatology*.[3]

Although this early work paved the road for the concept of hair transplantation, the idea for hair restoration surgery *for male pattern baldness* (MPB) belongs to the American dermatologist Dr. Norman Orentreich. Orentreich discovered and defined the phenomenon of "donor dominance" in MPB, and as is often the case, came upon it by accident. He was doing a study on vitiligo, transferring autologous punch skin grafts to investigate the pathogenesis of the disease. Dr. Orentreich noted that a punch graft from hair bearing vitiliginous skin, when placed into a non–hair bearing area, grew hair at the new site. In 1952, the first patient with frontal MPB was treated with 10 round 4 mm grafts harvested from his occipital area. Orentreich's classic 1959 paper[4] reporting the successful transfer of hair to areas of MPB in this and other patients opened the floodgates to a new field of cosmetic surgery.

The "fathers" of modern hair restoration surgery emerged as a result of their relationships with Dr. Orentreich. They include Drs. Hiram Sturm, Jim Burks, Blu Stough, Jean Arouete, Sam Ayres III, Robert Fosnaugh, Jay Pinski, Patrick Rabineau, Robert Auerbach, Robert Berger, and Hillard Pearlstein. A second and larger group of hair transplant surgeons came during the later 1960s and early 1970s. Prominent among them were O'Tar Norwood, Leonard Lewis, Sorrel Resnick, Walter Unger, Rolf Nordstrom, Robert Limmer, Martin Unger, Manny Marritt, Tom Alt, Patrick Frechet, Pierre Pouteaux, Ted Tromovitch and Sam Stegman.[5] To a large extent it is they who refined, taught widely, and popularized the technique of hair transplanting as we currently practice it.

The Hamilton-Norwood classification for MPB established the standard description of degrees of genetically based alopecia in men, while Ludwig's classification did the same for females. Concomitantly, refinements over the past 10 to 15 years in donor area harvesting and in transplanting techniques including minigrafting, micrografting, and follicular unit hair transplanting have revolutionized the approach to patients with MPB. An ever-expanding number of surgeons are now able to consistently create remarkably natural-looking results through the use of these techniques. One of the advantages of now having so many skilled physicians performing hair restoration surgery is the enormous potential for further innovations and refinements. What follows is one experienced physician's view of the currently optimal approach to hair restoration surgery, and the reasoning behind it. The statement "many roads lead to Rome" has, however, rarely been as true as it is for hair restoration surgery. Many different approaches can result in excellent results and the reader is urged to remember that this chapter deals with only one such road.

EVALUATION OF THE HAIR TRANSPLANT PATIENT

MPB is a progressive disorder that in men usually begins in the frontotemporal triangles. Frontal area hair loss progresses medially while in the temporal area it moves posteriorly so that the alopecic frontotemporal triangle gradually becomes larger. Either at the same time, before, or after the frontotemporal thinning, a similar process may begin in the vertex area. With the passage of time the latter also enlarges until it finally may reach the hair loss progressing from the frontal area. Figure 15-1 demonstrates different stages and types of hair loss as described by Norwood. Tables 15-1 and 15-2 indicate the frequency of the various degrees of MPB at different ages as tabulated by Norwood and the author. Planning for hair transplanting should therefore take into consideration present as well as future areas of involvement. The superior border of the "permanent" fringe hair nearly always will run inferi-

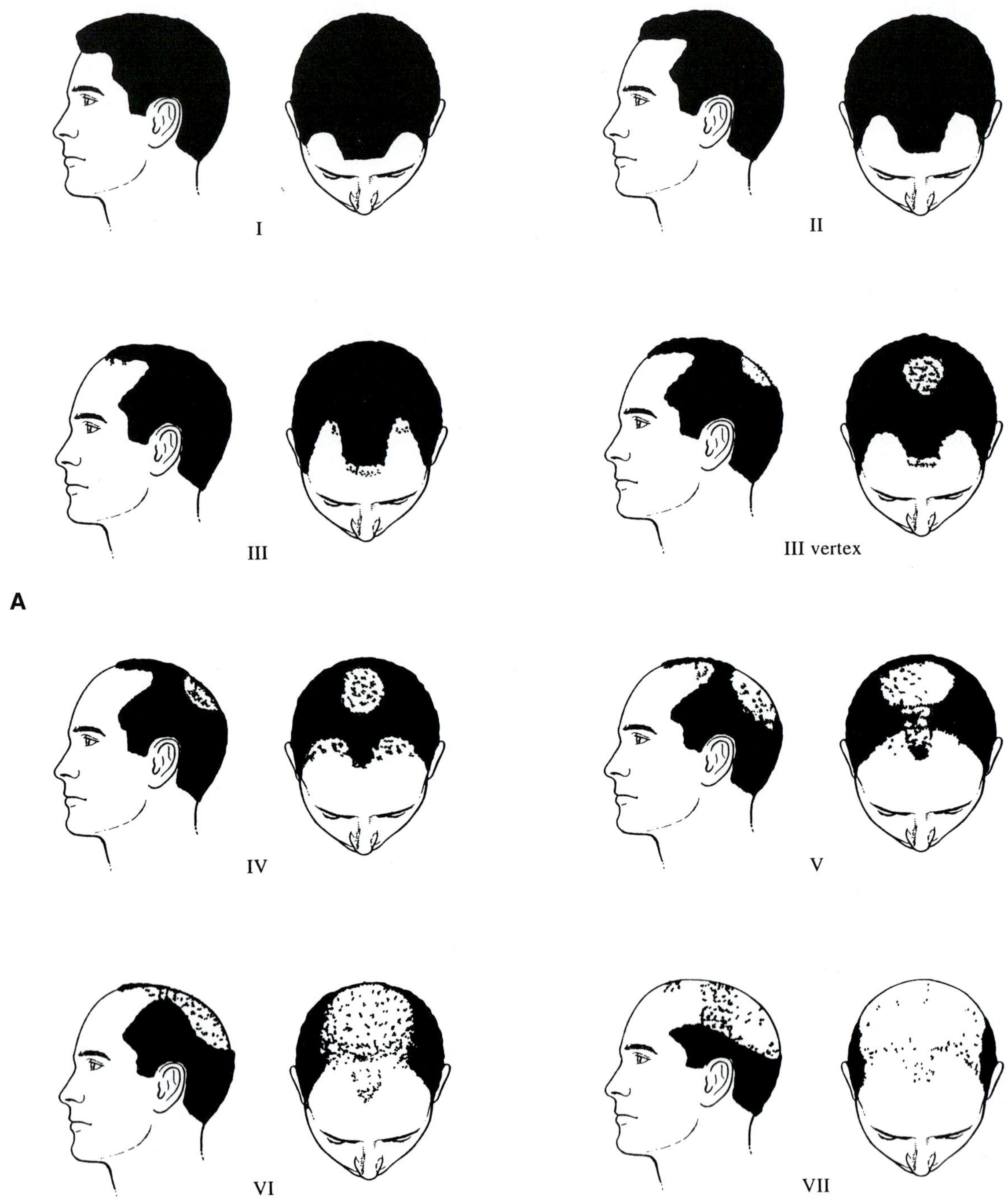

FIG. 15-1
A, Norwood classification of male pattern baldness (MPB). (From Norwood OT, Shiell R, eds. Hair Transplant Surgery. Springfield, IL: Charles C. Thomas, 1984.) *Continued*

orly as one moves posteriorly from the frontal hairline (Fig. 15-2). Your approach therefore ideally should include grafting into areas that are still hair bearing but that can reasonably be expected to lose hair in the future (Fig. 15-3). This will make an almost constant and frustrating "chasing" of an enlarging alopecic area less likely.[6] On the other hand, the "price" for this approach is that a smaller proportion of the currently more clearly thinning areas can be transplanted, unless one employs more grafts. Patients will initially be more impressed with the treatment of a larger proportion of the more obvious areas of thinning (short-term planning), but in the long run the disadvantages of such an objective will become evident. Lack of long-term planning is

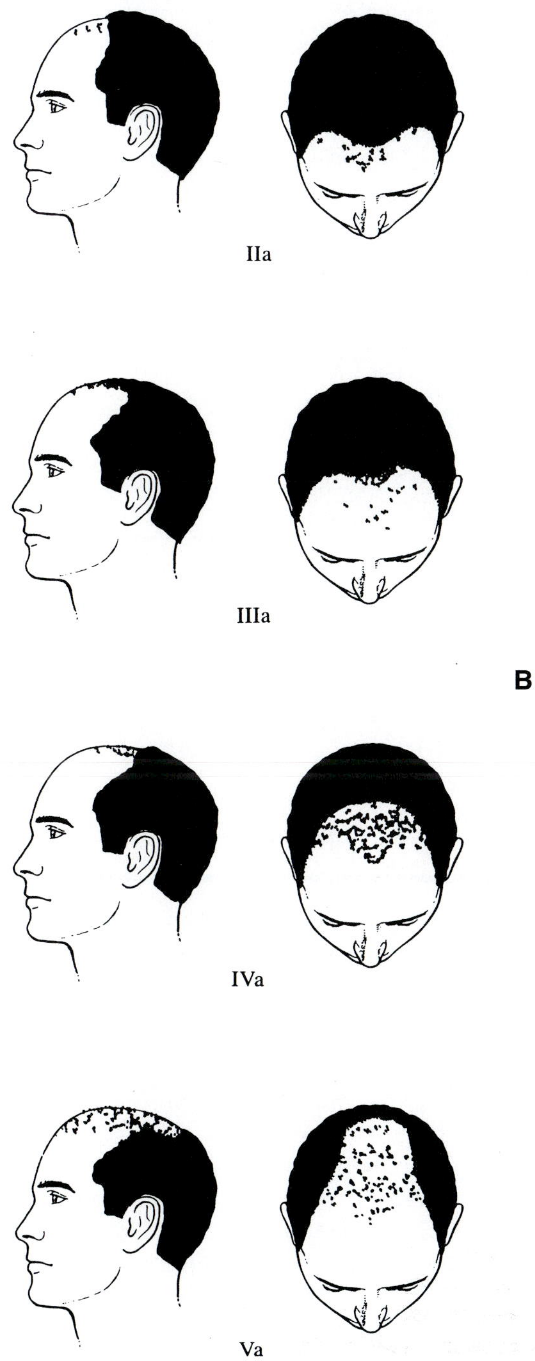

FIG. 15-1, cont'd
B, Norwood classification of type A variant MPB.

Table 15-1 Norwood Survey of Incidence of Different Types of Male Pattern Baldness at Different Ages

	Age (Years)						
	18-29	30-39	40-49	50-59	60-69	70-79	≥80
Type I	110 (60%)	60 (36%)	55 (33%)	45 (28%)	29 (19%)	18 (17%)	12 (16%)
Type II	52 (28%)	43 (26%)	38 (22%)	32 (20%)	24 (16%)	20 (19%)	11 (14%)
Type III	14 (6%)	30 (18%) (3V)*	37 (20%) (15V)*	34 (23%) (15V)*	22 (15%) (10V)*	16 (16%) (7V)*	12 (16%) (8V)*
Type IV	4 (3%)	16 (10%)	15 (10%)	21 (9%)	17 (12%)	13 (13%)	9 (12%)
Type V	3 (2%)	10 (6%)	13 (8%)	15 (10%)	22 (15%)	13 (13%)	9 (12%)
Type VI	2 (1%)	4 (3%)	7 (4%)	10 (7%)	19 (13%)	11 (11%)	10 (13%)
Type VII	0	2 (1%)	5 (3%)	4 (3%)	16 (10%)	11 (11%)	14 (17%)
Total	185 (100%)	165 (100%)	165 (100%)	156 (100%)	149 (100%)	102 (100%)	77 (100%)

*Numbers in parentheses under type III represent type III vertex persons.

From Norwood OT, Shiell R, eds. Hair Transplant Surgery. Springfield, IL: Charles C. Thomas, 1984.

Table 15-2 Unger Survey of Incidence of Different Types of Male Pattern Baldness at Different Ages

	Age (Years)			
Type	65-69	70-74	75-79	80+
I	2 (3.6%)	5 (6.2%)	4 (5.5%)	2 (1.7%)
II	9 (16.4%)	7 (8.6%)	7 (9.6%)	12 (10.1%)
III	4 (7.3%)	15 (18.5%)	18 (24.7%)	11 (9.2%)
IV	10 (18.2%)	16 (19.8%)	8 (11.0%)	10 (8.4%)
V	6 (10.9%)	7 (8.6%)	10 (13.7%)	16 (13.4%)
VI	13 (23.6%)	19 (23.5%)	16 (21.9%)	37 (31.1%)
VII	11 (20.0%)	12 (14.8%)	10 (13.7%)	31 (26.1%)
Total	55 (100%)	81 (100%)	73 (100%)	119 (100%)

Note:

- In age group 65-69, if one excludes types I and II, 33 of the remaining 44 (75%) have types III to VI (83.3% Norwood).
- In age group 70-74, if one excludes types I and II, 57 of the remaining 69 (82.6%) have types III to VI (82.8% Norwood).
- In age group 75-79, if one excludes types I and II, 52 of the remaining 62 (83.9%) have types III to VI.
- In age group 80+, if one excludes types I and II, 74 of the remaining 105 (70.5%) have types III to VI (74.0% Norwood).

From Unger W, ed. Hair Transplantation. 3rd ed. New York: Marcel Dekker, 1995.

the commonest reason why the author sees patients for "correction" of transplanting done elsewhere.

Perfect prognostication of the degree of alopecia that any given patient will develop is impossible, so a reserve of what is expected to be permanent hair-bearing donor area should also be maintained. In addition, the lateral borders of the transplanted areas should always be constructed with small grafts and micrografts (Fig. 15-4), so should one misjudge the ultimate limits of MPB, the patient will be left with a larger than usual isolated frontal forelock (IFF) which will look "natural" standing on its own[7] (Fig. 15-5). Alternatively, because one can never be 100% certain as to who will evolve into a type VI or VII MPB, some surgeons intentionally attempt to produce only an IFF on all or virtually all patients.[8] In my opinion, however, Tables 15-1 and 15-2 show that this is an overly conservative objective and leaves many patients with less of the area of alopecia treated than could reasonably be hoped for. The construction of a "prospective" IFF as described above seems to be a reasonable compromise position. Each patient should be assessed individually, based on the

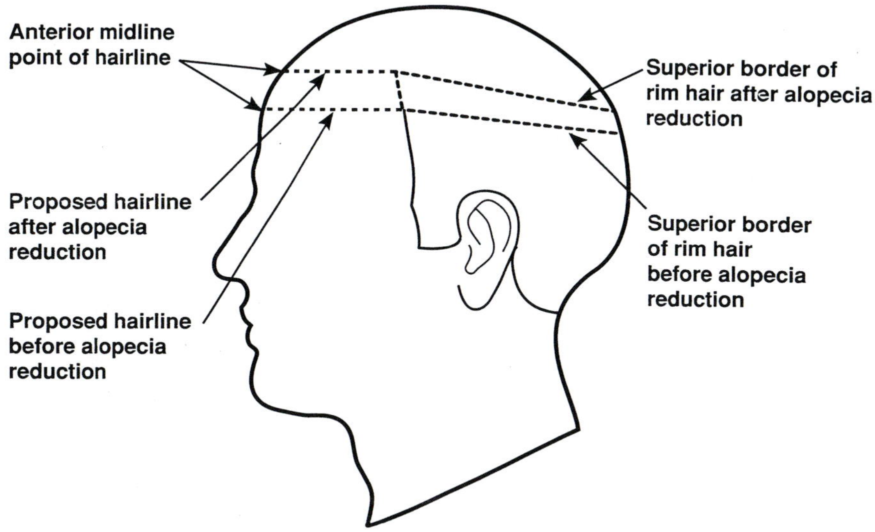

FIG. 15-2
The superior border of the "permanent" fringe hair nearly always will run inferiorly as one moves posteriorly from the frontal hairline. After an alopecia reduction, this border will move superiorly, allowing the anterior midline point of the hairline to be placed more superiorly without affecting the aesthetically appropriate more or less horizontal orientation of the hairline. (From Unger W, ed. Hair Transplantation. 3rd ed. New York: Marcel Dekker, 1995.)

A 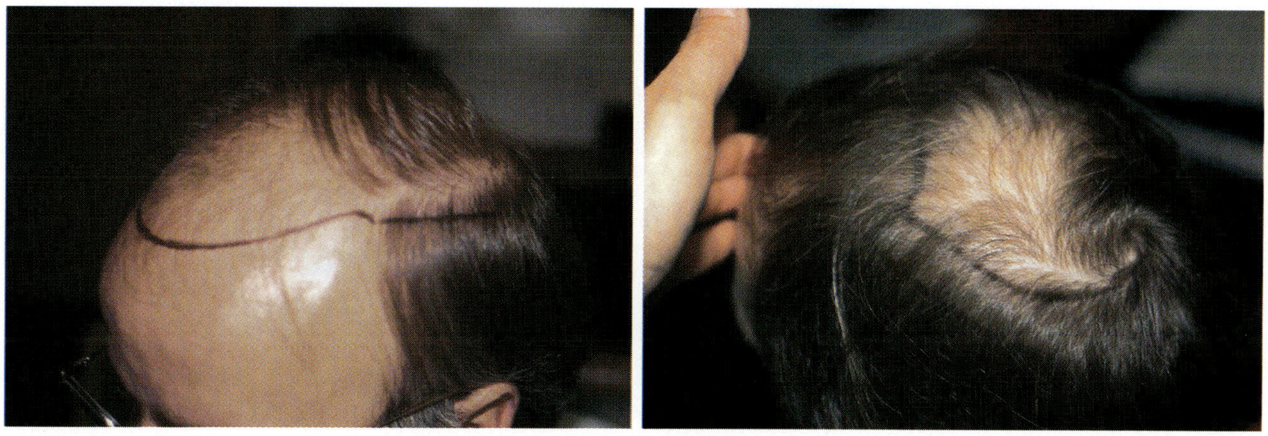 B

FIG. 15-3
A, Transplanting should ideally be carried out through areas of still-existing hair that is expected to be lost eventually. Grafting will be carried out in this patient through the area of existing hair down to the black line that denotes the expected ultimate location of the superior border of the temporoparietal hair. Note also the slight bell shape of the proposed hairline. **B,** Two black grease pencil lines can be seen laterally in the vertex area. The superior one denotes the presently obvious thinning areas; the inferior one is the point to which hair can be expected to be lost in the future. Transplanting should include this presently hair-bearing area. Approximately 50% of the grafts consumed in the treatment of the vertex area are commonly used in such still hair-bearing areas of the vertex.

physical findings on examination, his age, and family history as to the likelihood that he will develop any given degree of MPB. A suitable long-term treatment plan can then be established.

Androgenetic alopecia in females usually occurs in a different form than that described for males, although there are some females who thin in a similar fashion.[9] The classification for androgenetic alopecia in females that is most commonly used is Ludwig's classification, shown in Figure 15-6. Maintenance of at least some hair in the hairline zone while thinning occurs more posteriorly and small round alopecic areas that are scattered throughout the diffuse thinning are hallmarks of MPB in nearly all females. In addition to thinning over the top of the scalp, a significant minority of women also develop thinning in the potential donor areas. This minority of women are not good candidates for hair transplantation. However, a substantial majority of women can be improved with current hair transplanting techniques[10] (Fig. 15-7). Once again the age of the patient, physical examination, and family history should be considered carefully.

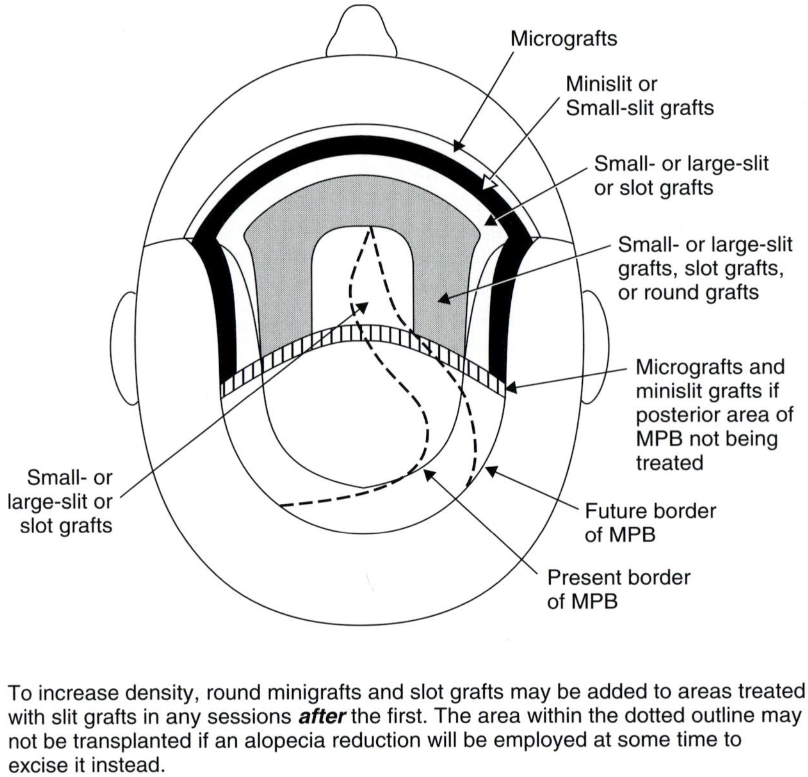

FIG. 15-4
The type of grafts that are used in various zones of the anterior third to half of an area of male pattern baldness (MPB). Note that the lateral and posterior borders of the transplanted areas are constructed with small grafts and micrografts, so should one misjudge the ultimate extent of MPB, the patient will be left with a larger than usual isolated frontal forelock.

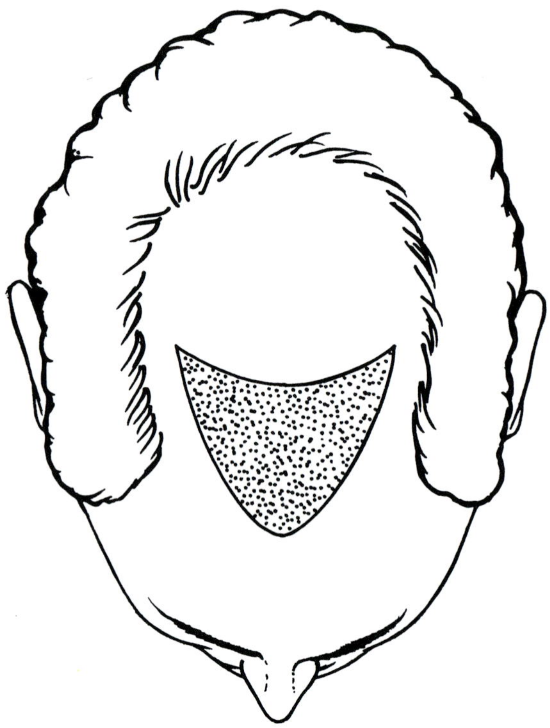

FIG. 15-5
The shape of a typical isolated frontal forelock.

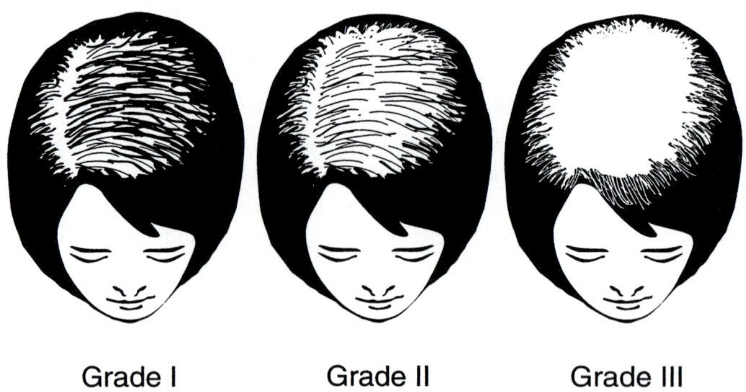

FIG. 15-6
Ludwig's classification of androgenetic alopecia in females. (From Montagna W, Parakkal PF. The Structure and Function of Skin. 3rd ed. New York: Academic Press, 1974.)

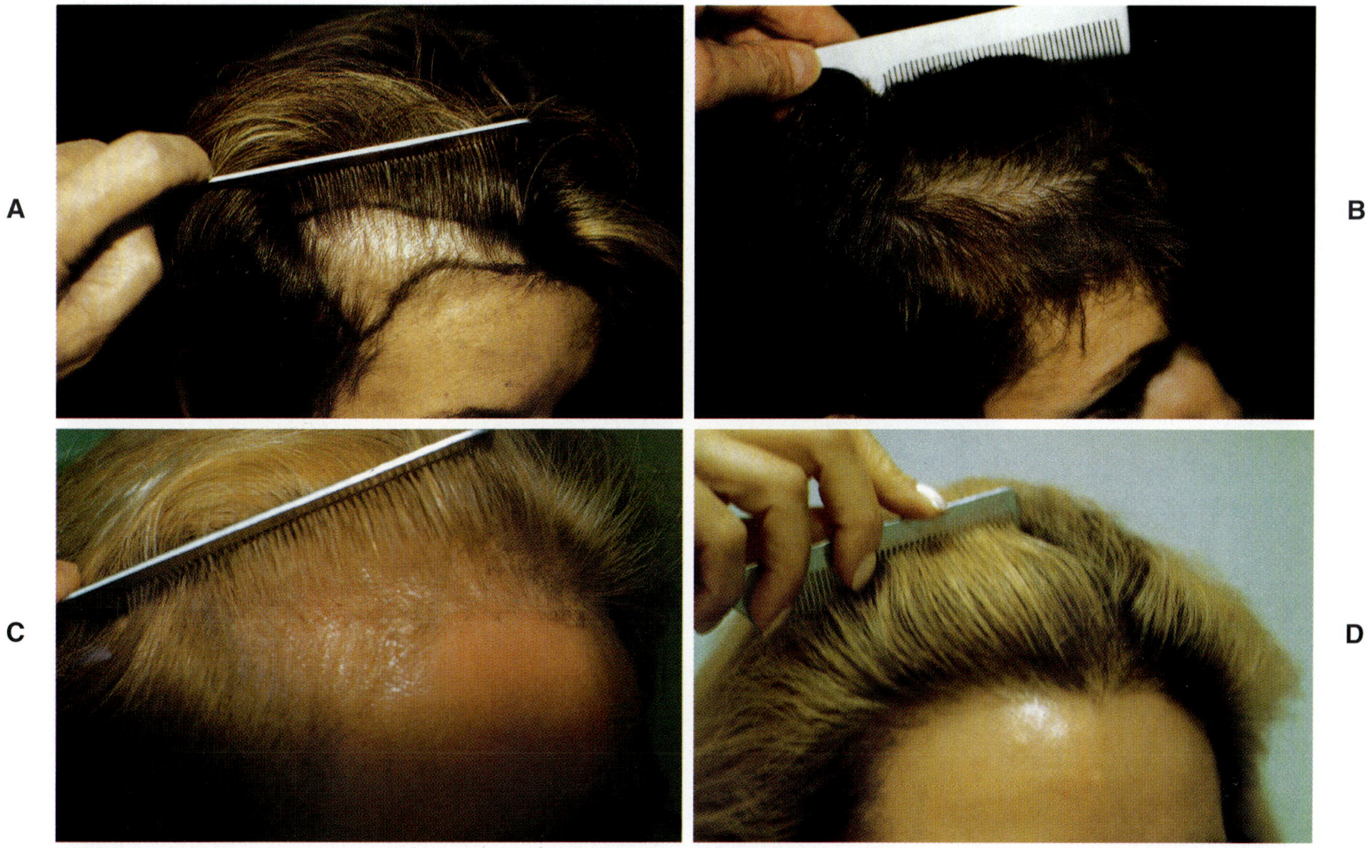

FIG. 15-7
A, A woman with marked thinning in the frontotemporal triangle. **B,** Four and one-half months after a single transplant session consisting of 200 micrografts and 268 minislit grafts. **C,** A woman before her first hair transplant with marked thinning of both the frontotemporal triangles and the frontal hairline zone. **D,** Nine months after the first hair transplant session. This remarkable result is unusually good because of advantageous hair characteristics including dense donor areas, blond coloring, and fine texture. Most women will of course not have results as dramatic as that shown.

It follows from the preceding that the beginning and end of the hairline that is chosen for male patients should ideally be the *eventual* or ultimate anterior/superior most temporal points. The midline point of the hairline should then be located so that when the hairline is viewed laterally, it will run more or less horizontally. You can move this midline point more superiorly, thereby decreasing the length of the area of MPB to be treated, by creating and accentuating a "bell" shape to the hairline (see Fig. 15-3*A*), or by raising the anterior/superior most temporal points with alopecia reductions (AR) (see Fig. 15-2).[11] Using either of these options will allow for a higher midline hairline point without affecting its cosmetically advantageous horizontal orientation. In addition, the anterior most point of the hairline zone should ideally lie within the transition area within which the vertical aspect of the forehead becomes more horizontal. A natural hairline zone also has the following characteristics[12]:

- An irregular anterior border
- Irregular hair density
- Fine hair most anteriorly, coarser hair as one moves more posteriorly
- Often single, fine-textured "sentinel" hairs scattered irregularly anterior to the bulk of the hairline zone (Fig. 15-8).

AR will be discussed more fully later in this chapter, but a few comments on its role in planning are warranted here:

1. Whenever the goal is maximum coverage, use AR or plan to use AR in the future by not placing grafts in areas that you plan to excise later (Figs. 15-4 and 15-9).
2. Do not leave a scar in an area that you do not intend to transplant later.
3. Unless you are using scalp extension, followed by a three-flap "slot correction" (discussed later), do not try to excise all the alopecic area. This will re-

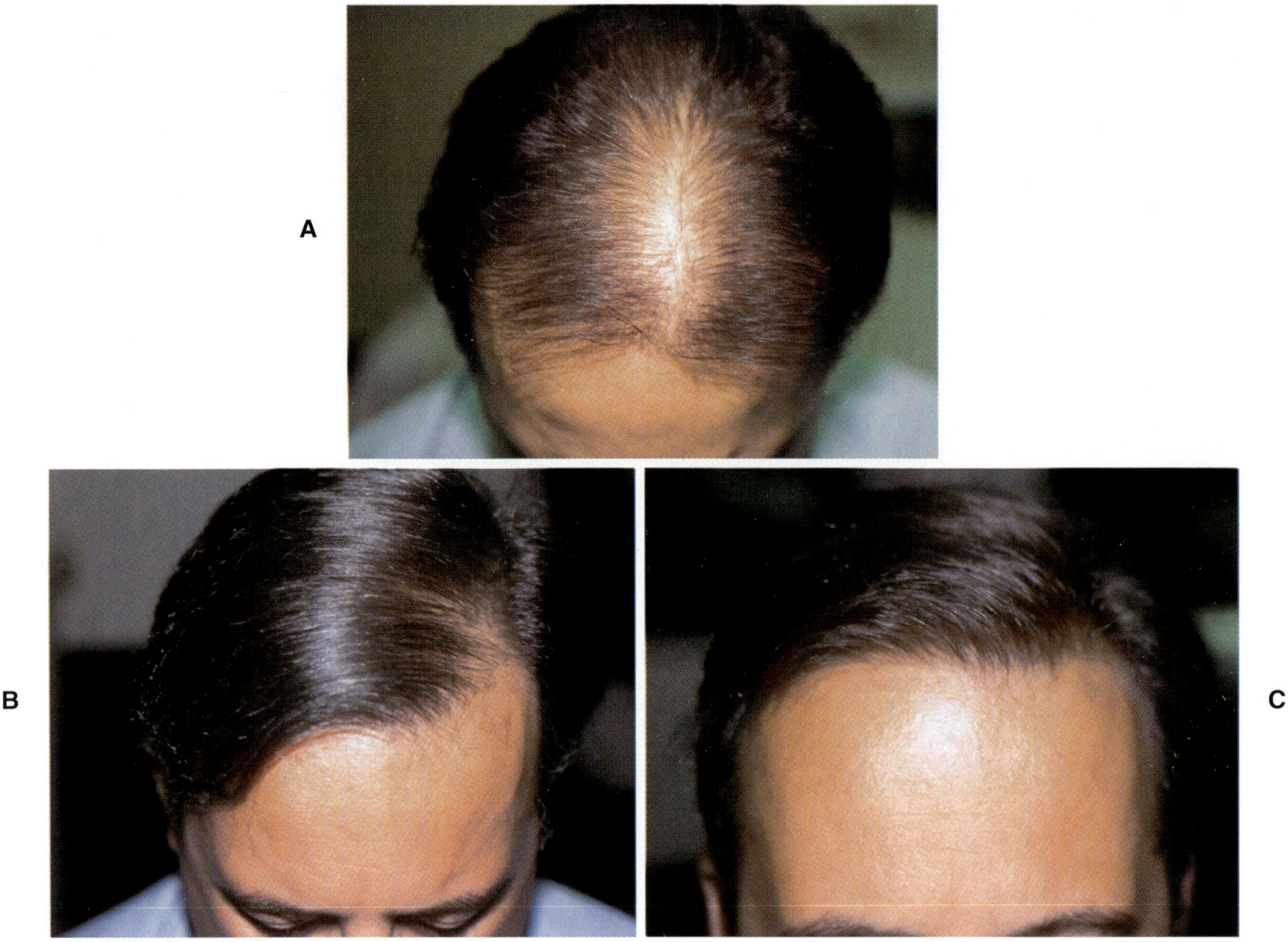

FIG. 15-8
A, A man before hair transplantation. **B,** Nine months after his third transplant session consisting of micrografts, minislit, and small-slit grafts. **C,** Photograph taken at the same time as that shown in **B.** Note that the hairline zone has been constructed with (1) an irregular anterior border, (2) irregular hair density, (3) fine hair most anteriorly with coarser hair as one moves more posteriorly, and (4) single fine-textured "sentinel" hairs scattered irregularly anterior to the bulk of the hairline zone.

sult in an abnormal hair direction at the midline, which has been referred to as the "parting of the Red Sea" effect. If, for example, one eliminates all but a 5 to 6 cm wide area of alopecia, this remaining area can be transplanted with grafts that produce a natural-looking gradual change of hair direction from left to right or right to left.

4. The wider the area of alopecia you eventually remove, the sparser the hair in the stretched "permanent" fringe will become. Fringe hair will also gradually become sparser with age, and this should be factored into your objectives for AR. Despite arguments to the contrary, if the patient has normal healing (as revealed, for example, by prior hair transplanting), this is the only negative consequence of AR that is not completely avoidable. It warrants serious consideration. Two or three modified major AR[13] (or the equivalent) rarely if ever have a significantly negative impact on rim hair density. Anything more aggressive warrants more caution.
5. In the vast majority of patients, if surgical technique is good, there is minimal "stretchback" or loss of some of the gain obtained. Nordstrom reported on 13 patients in whom there was a 30% to 52% stretchback,[14] but he has admitted to closing under considerable tension to maximize the results, and his patients included persons with prior AR. Unger's study on 56 patients, whose excisions were closed with minimal tension, re-

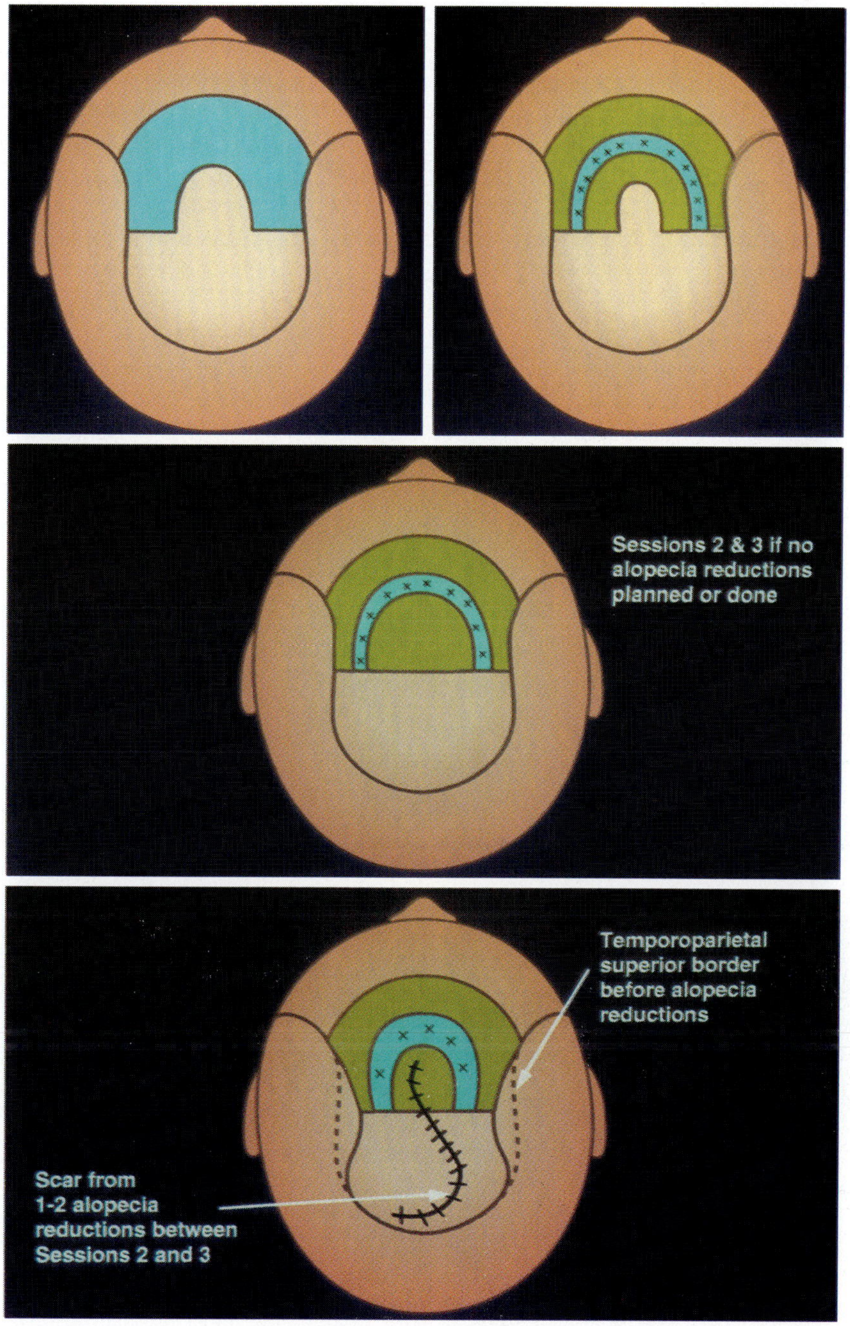

FIG. 15-9
Various patterns of transplanting used during each session. **A,** Session 1. **B,** Session 2: Option A—alopecia reductions planned. **C,** Sessions 2 and 3: Option B—no alopecia reductions planned. **D,** Session 3: Option A—with reductions. (From Unger W, ed. Hair Transplantation. 3rd ed. New York: Marcel Dekker, 1995.)

ported *no* stretchback in 55% and less than 3 mm stretchback in another 43% of the patients treated.[15] Hitzig reported on 40 AR patients, 50% of whom had no stretchback and another 25% of whom had less than 10% stretchback.[16] For some reason Nordstrom's study of 13 patients has inappropriately received far more attention in the literature than these substantially larger ones. More recently, the use of nonabsorbable galeal "anchoring sutures" has further minimized this potential sequela of AR.[17]

6. AR is a useful tool for the treatment of MPB that has extended beyond its originally estimated borders. It is generally unwise to expend a limited

supply of remaining donor tissue to treat unanticipated new areas of alopecia if those areas can be excised instead.

Table 15-3 defines the various types of grafts used in hair transplanting. All grafts are obtained by excising strips of tissue from the donor area and dividing them with varying degrees of magnification into whatever numbers and types are required.

I use micrografts with minislit and *small* slit or minigrafts for all women with androgenetic alopecia (see Fig. 15-7) and whenever the ultimate hair density objective is less than maximum. Obviously the younger the patient, the less certain you can be of the eventual size of the area of MPB (and donor area). Thus you would be wiser to aim for less density by using micrografts with minislit and *small* slit or minigrafts to conserve as much donor tissue as possible while still pro-

Table 15-3 Graft Terminology

	Number of Hairs	Type of Recipient Site	Number of Follicular Units	Tissue Removed
Micrograft (always a single follicular unit)	1-3	Puncture hole	1	No
Minislit graft	2-3	Beaver mini-ES, Sharpoint, or Minde knife	2	No
Minigraft "small"	3-4	Hole or slot	2-3	Yes
Minigraft "large"	5-6	Hole or slot	2-4	Yes
Slit graft "small"	3-4	Blade slit	2-3	No
Slit graft "large"	5-6	Blade slit	2-4	No
Standard graft	8-30	3+ mm hole	6-22	Yes

A

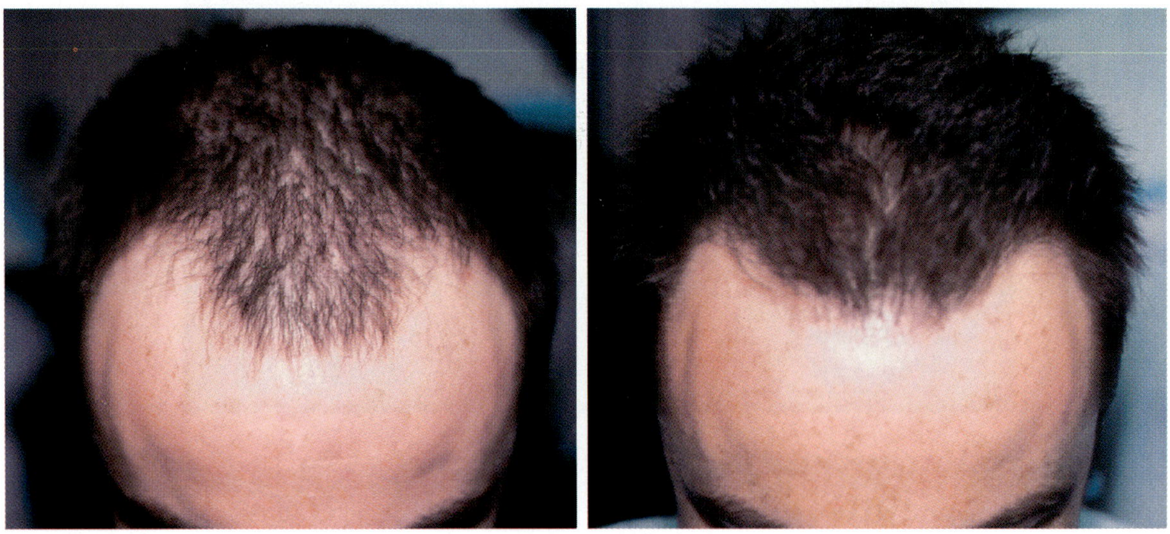

B

FIG. 15-10
A, Before treatment. This patient was in his late 20s and wanted full coverage of the area of male pattern baldness (MPB) as it developed. Because it was impossible to tell how large the eventual size of the area of MPB would be, I chose to aim for less density by using micrografts and minislit, slit, and minigrafts to conserve as much donor tissue as possible while still producing natural-looking coverage in the recipient area. **B,** One year after his first hair transplant session. He had returned for a second treatment but even at this stage had a very natural looking, though light, coverage. *Continued*

ducing natural-looking coverage in the recipient area (Fig. 15-10*A* and *B*). I also virtually always use them in the hairline zone and the posterior half of larger areas of MPB (Fig. 15-10*C*-*E*).

If you choose to use micro-minigrafting, it is worthwhile to make note of the following points:

- For Caucasians, unless the donor hair is white, salt-and-pepper colored, blond, or light brown and the contrast between hair and scalp color is minimal, you should usually limit yourself to using micrografts, minislit and *small*-slit grafts, and *small* round minigrafts.
- For Asians with high caliber hair you usually should use micrografts with minislit, *small*-slit, and *small* round minigrafts.
- For African Americans or for those with naturally curly hair you can use micrografts and small- or large-slit or minigrafts for all sessions.

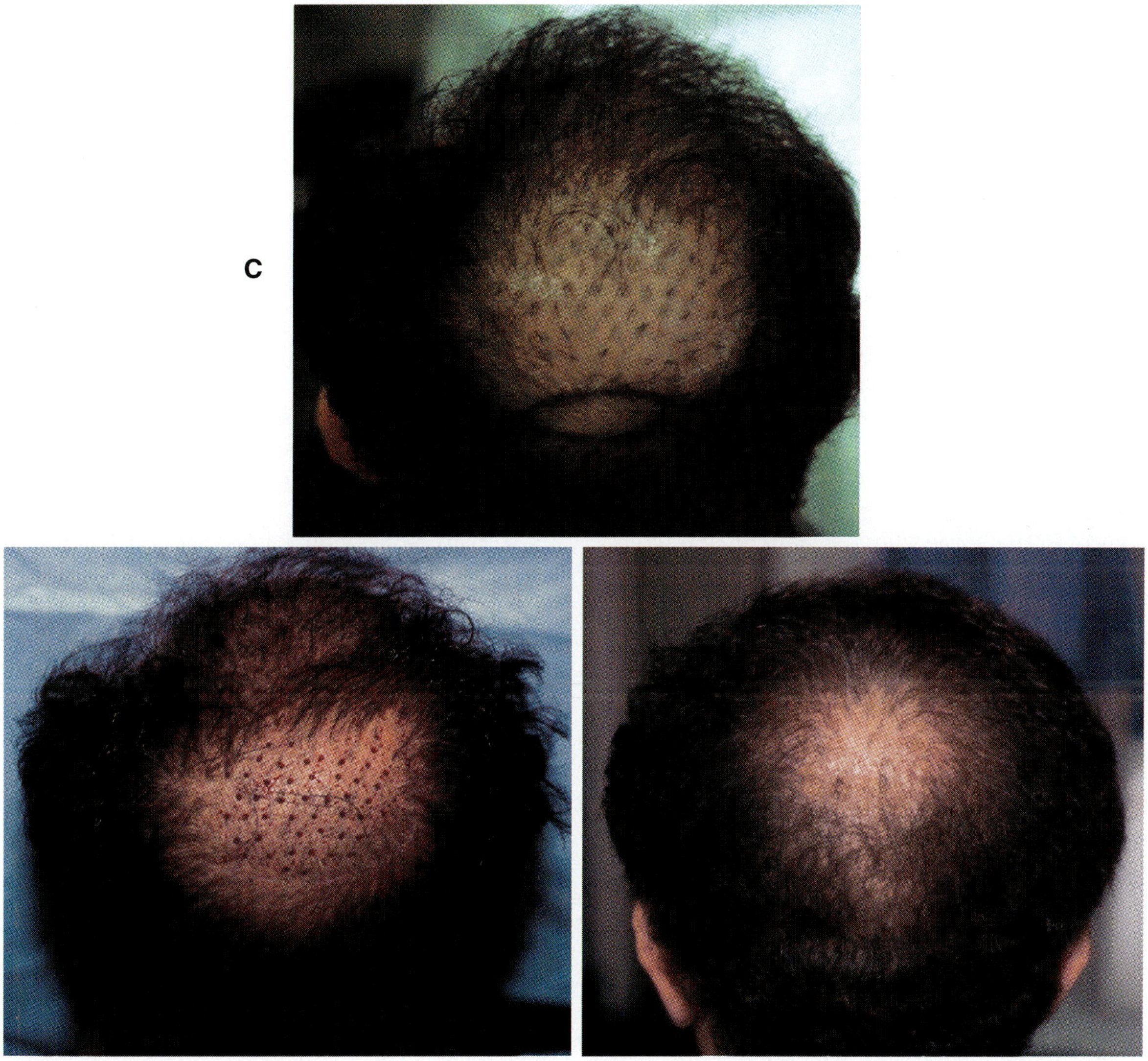

C

D

E

FIG. 15-10, cont'd
C, This patient had his original transplanting carried out elsewhere. The vertex area was treated with standard-size round grafts and had a very pluggy appearance. **D,** A portion of most of the standard grafts was punched out and the tissue obtained was divided into slit grafts, minigrafts, and micrografts. Additional donor tissue was employed to treat the entire developing area of MPB with micrografts, minislit, slit, and minigrafts at the same time. **E,** The same patient shown 1 year after his first repair. A very even light and natural-looking coverage has been accomplished. The hair has been parted for critical evaluation. I use only micrografts, minislit, slit, and minigrafts in the posterior half of larger areas of MPB in most patients to produce a natural-looking coverage while consuming the minimal amount of donor tissue.

- The finer the hair texture or the less contrast between the hair and skin color, the more acceptable *large* slit or minigrafts become.

Micrografts or follicular units (FUs) should be used not only in the hairline zone and the center of the whorl of the vertex *but should also be scattered between minislit and slit or minigrafts during each session,* to produce a more even and natural-looking coverage of hair per session (Fig. 15-11). Note: *This scattering of micrografts between minislit and slit or minigrafts is especially important as part of the first session if the area is alopecic* and in the areas adjacent to the hairline zone, the center of the whorl of the vertex, and the lateral aspects of the recipient area. I also recommend the use of 500 to 1500 micrografts as a component of the last session in any area to provide a background of evenly distributed hair for previously transplanted slit or minigrafts. The more skin contrasts with hair color and the coarser the hair, the more useful these "finishing micrografts" become.

In general, when you are using minislit and slit or minigrafts in male patients, you will find it advantageous to use micrografts and slit grafts instead of round minigrafts for the initial session (see below). After the first session has grown in it is often useful to scatter some round minigrafts between the grafts transplanted in all previous sessions, thus producing more density but minimizing any noticeable temporary plugginess (see Fig. 15-11). You should be prepared to use all types of grafts, depending on patient characteristics and objectives. In women with androgenetic alopecia, micrografts and minislit and small-slit grafts are also the types predominantly used, but some small, totally hairless, round areas are frequently scattered within areas of diffuse thinning; these can be punched out with appropriately sized trephines and filled with round grafts during all sessions.

In general, minislit and small-slit grafts are superior to small round minigrafts in producing even coverage with minimal plugginess. If you are working in an area that still contains some of its original hair—for example, in early MPB in men and in diffusely thinning areas in women—you will also find that micrografts and small-slit grafts will produce a greater increase in hair density than small round minigrafts will (Figs. 15-7, 15-8, and 15-10). This is because making round recipient sites of any size removes some of the original hair, so the net gain in hair is the *difference* between what is removed and what is added. On the other hand, needle holes for micrografts and scalpel incisions for minislit and slit grafts can be made between existing hairs without causing permanent injury to them. Thus the net increase in hair density will be equal to *all* the transplanted hair. However, *in alopecic recipient sites,* round grafts produce greater hair density in the short run as well as the long run, when compared with micrografts and minislit and slit grafts. This is because alopecic skin is being excised at the same time the hair is being added.

Male patients with early MPB

- Will usually prefer the greater initial hair density produced by micrografts and minislit and slit grafts
- Can have small round minigrafts added between previously transplanted minislit and slit grafts when more of the original hair has been lost, thus partially compensating for the long-term density disadvantage of what would otherwise have been produced by exclusive microslit grafting

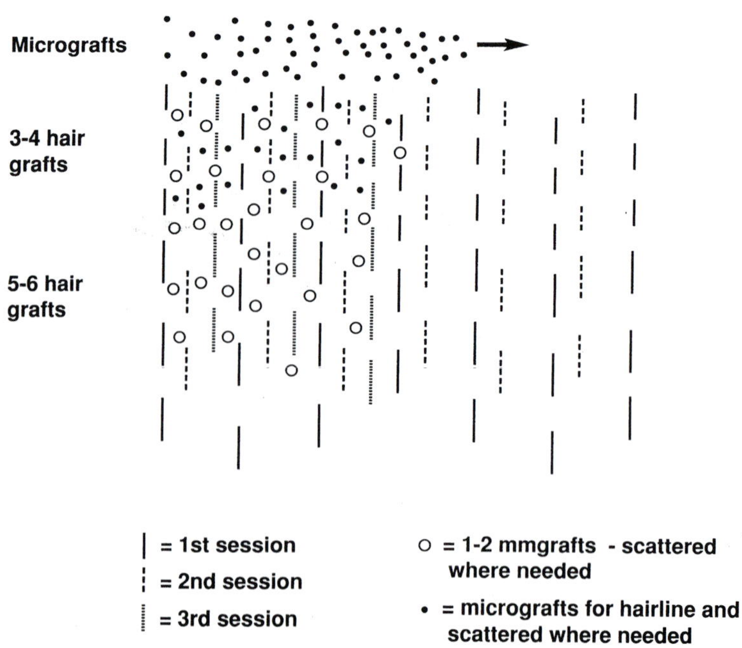

FIG. 15-11
Placement of grafts in each session. Note the "organized disorganization," with even dispersion of recipient sites during each surgery but in an irregular pattern anteroposteriorly. Micrografts should not only be used in the hairline zone and in the center of the whorl of the vertex but also should be scattered between minislit, slit grafts, and minigrafts during each session to produce a more even coverage of hair per session.

After the first session has grown in, it is often useful to scatter some slot grafts or round minigrafts between the grafts transplanted in all previous sessions, thus producing more density but minimizing any noticeable temporary plugginess. (From Unger W, ed. Hair Transplantation. 3rd ed. New York: Marcel Dekker, 1995.)

- May not object to somewhat less hair density when they are older and have lost all of their original hair
- Just *may*—with the passage of time—still have enough donor hair available to do additional sessions that will produce hair density equal to or greater than that achieved with round grafts, although at the cost of more sessions and the use of more donor tissue

Sessions of exclusive micrografts should be used if the objective is to produce the most even and natural distribution of hair in order to complete treatment in two or, less frequently, one session. However, exclusive micrograft sessions are the least efficient way of producing substantial hair density. "Megasessions" of over 1500 and sometimes thousands of follicular units in a single sitting and "dense packing" have been suggested as a means of accomplishing respectively more coverage as well as more hair density per session. Remarkably natural results with hair density that should be satisfactory for most patients can in fact be consistently produced by experts using this technique in two sessions, and if hair characteristics are advantageous (see below), occasionally in a single session. Unfortunately, sessions of 8 to 12 hours or longer are necessary and may be medically unwise for some persons. There are also serious questions as to whether hair survival is as good as it is with standard-size sessions and lower densities of FU/cm^2.

In an effort to overcome the problem of lower densities with exclusive follicular unit hair transplanting (FUHT), proponents of this approach have steadily increased the number of follicular units planted per square centimeter. In areas where greater hair density is the goal, in addition to employing more FU/cm^2 (for example, 40 to 45 FU/cm^2), FUs with 2 to 3 or more hairs are transplanted into each recipient site. However, even if only 2.3 hairs went into each site (FUs contain an average of 2.3 hairs), there should be a hair density of at least 92/cm^2 after a single session of 40 FU/cm^2 (that is, 40 × 2.3). Yet Marritt—in an article that was strongly supportive of FUHT—reported that an average density of only 78 hairs was achieved in 16 patients after *two* sessions carried out in the office of a widely acclaimed expert in the technique.[18] These numbers suggest substantial death rates when FUHT is combined with dense packing. This suspicion has been reinforced by two papers delivered at the 1999 annual meeting of the International Society of Hair Restoration Surgery, one by Michael Beehner[19] and the other by John Cole.[20] They revealed only 65% to 77% regrowth (at 7 to 10 months) of FU hair in small test sites treated by other FUHT experts—despite the fact that those sites were surrounded, not by thousands of additional recipient sites (as would be the case clinically), but by *intact* skin. Finally, FUHT proponents have pointed out in earlier studies that in small test areas (also surrounded by intact skin), if one plants 100 hairs, one can expect 113[21] to 133[22] hairs to eventually grow. This makes the more recent studies' 65% to 77% growth rates, *based on original hair counts,* generous estimates of true apparent survival rates.

Accurate hair counting and other circumstances in such studies are extraordinarily difficult, and the results should not be taken as "gospel." Yet it appears that if one increases the density of FU/cm^2 enough to produce cosmetically acceptable hair densities in only one session, decreased hair growth is more likely. As a result, therefore, I prefer to use densities of no more than 25 FU/cm^2 and to limit use of exclusive FUHT to areas where maximum naturalness is worth any potentially lethal damage to some follicles—the hairline and the center of the whorl of the vertex are the most obvious examples of such areas. As noted above, even two sessions of FUs transplanted 20 FU/cm^2 could yield a very respectable 92 hairs/cm^2 if there was 100% hair survival.

Effect of Choice of Donor Area

Regardless of the type of grafts used, specific donor area hair characteristics are advantageous:

1. The finer the hair texture, the more natural looking low-density coverage will appear.
2. Conversely, an increase in hair caliber will have a surprisingly large positive effect on total hair volume and apparent "fullness." Cole has noted that a mere 0.01 mm increase in hair diameter produces a 36% increase in hair volume.[23]
3. In general, the less contrast between the hair and skin color, the denser the hair coverage will appear. Thus for Caucasians, for example, white, salt-and-pepper, blond, red, light brown, dark brown, and black coloring produce apparent hair density with decreasing effectiveness. Despite the foregoing, if one is using exclusive FUHT, many Caucasians with dark-colored, fine-textured hair can have results that are equal to or even better than that seen with lighter coloring. The reason is unclear to me but may be related to better visualization of dark follicles and consequently less injury to them during preparation.
4. The more wave or curl to the hair, the greater the apparent hair density and naturalness.
5. "Frizzy" hair produces greater apparent hair density and naturalness.

Medical Treatments for Male Pattern Baldness

Numerous medical treatments for MPB have been tried, and at least three are quite helpful in slowing down the rate of hair loss or in fact growing some hair: 1 mg finasteride orally per day,[24] 2% to 5% minoxidil applied twice a day to the scalp,[25] and 0.025% estradiol applied once every 1 to 2 days.[26] Finasteride is recommended only for men and has been shown to produce a decreased rate of hair loss in 88% of patients and some hair growth in approximately 66% of patients if used for 6 months or longer. The initial studies demonstrating this effect were carried out in the vertex area. Results frontally were not scientifically evaluated but were noted by most of the investigators as being substantially less than in the vertex area. Finasteride interferes with the conversion of testosterone to dihydrotestosterone by competing with 5 α-reductase, an enzyme necessary for the conversion process. Side effects include decreased sex drive in 1.8% of patients, erectile dysfunction in 1.3% of patients, and decreased semen volume in 0.8% of patients. These side effects occurred almost as commonly in the placebo group and disappeared in nearly 60% of patients who continued taking the drug. They also disappeared in 100% of patients who discontinued the drug. Unfortunately, long-term side effects are not known at this time but it seems reasonable for patients who are not ready for surgical intervention to use finasteride as a *temporary* "stopgap" measure for 1 to several years, or until such a time as circumstances are suitable for surgical treatment, especially if the area of involvement is the vertex.

Minoxidil was the first preparation approved by the U.S. Food and Drug Administration for the medical treatment of androgenetic alopecia. It is applied topically twice daily and has produced some hair in up to 35% of patients. As with finasteride it is far more effective in the vertex area than frontally. There are essentially no systemic side effects from this medication, although the occasional patient will note palpitations or light-headedness due to a decrease in blood pressure. Both men and women can use it.

A topical solution of 0.025% estradiol is effective in slowing down hair loss.[26] Most women can tolerate applications one or two times daily, although breakthrough bleeding, breast tenderness, and morning nausea occasionally occur. Existing fibroids are a contraindication to its use, and although estradiol does not increase the incidence of breast cancer, it accelerates the growth of such tumors, so monthly breast palpation is mandatory. In most men, applications once every second or third day will also be very effective in slowing down the rate of hair loss. If men use the estradiol more than once every 2 or 3 days, gynecomastia is a common side effect. No new hair growth occurs in men or women.

All of these medications must be continued indefinitely or any benefits disappear quite quickly. Several drug companies are working on other medications for the medical control or reversal of androgenetic alopecia, but currently, in my opinion, the three mentioned are the most useful.

SECTION TWO
Atlas of Surgical Procedures

PREOPERATIVE PREPARATION AND ANESTHESIA

We ask patients to abstain from any medications that could result in excessive bleeding. Alcohol should be avoided for 1 week preoperatively and vitamin E and acetylsalicylic acid preparations for 3 weeks preoperatively. Any medications that are being taken should also be noted, in case they should not be combined with the drugs used during surgery. Monoamine oxidase inhibitors, for example, have been reported as causing fatal reactions when combined with some local anesthetics. We also screen patients for HIV and hepatitis B and C. If anyone in the medical team accidentally gets punctured, a rapid and appropriate response can be decided on without having to wait or ask for patient testing. Prophylactic treatment for accidental HIV contact, for example, is most effective when started within hours of the incident.

The hair is washed the night before and the morning of surgery. Any shampoo may be used. Perioperative antibiotics (usually cefadroxil) have been used for many years, and in view of an infection rate of less than a fraction of a percent, I am reluctant to discontinue it. Other elective cosmetic procedures for which the Centers for Disease Control and Prevention in the United States did not recommend perioperative prophylactic antibiotics have recently been shown to have significantly reduced rates of infection if they are in fact used.[27] Such studies have as yet not been done for hair transplanting, but I prefer to "never argue with success" until they are conducted.

Diazepam (Valium) 20 mg is given orally 30 minutes before surgery to minimize anxiety but more importantly to decrease the possibility of anesthetic toxicity.[28] In addition, 2 ml of methylprednisolone acetate 40 mg/ml (Depomedrol) is administered intramuscularly just prior to beginning surgery in order to minimize postoperative edema. Prednisone 60 to 80 mg each morning for 3 days may also be added for patients particularly concerned about postoperative edema.

A tumescent anesthetic solution is used for the donor area. It is prepared by adding 19 ml of 2% lidocaine with 1:100,000 epinephrine and 1 ml of 1:1,000 epinephrine to a 100 ml IV bag of saline. In addition we use a buffered pH neutral solution of 1% lidocaine with 1:100,000 epinephrine to produce a field block prior to injecting the tumescent solution into the donor area.[28] The donor area should be quite turgid at the completion of infiltration. Occasionally it is necessary to reinforce "hot spots" with 2% or 3% lidocaine with 1:100,000 epinephrine in some patients, but large amounts of tumescent solution always result in minimal bleeding and provide excellent anesthesia for most individuals.

Once the donor area has been harvested and sutured, three injections of 2% lidocaine with 1:100,000 epinephrine are made along the hairline with a 30-gauge needle—one in the midline and one in the middle of the proposed left and right hairline. At intervals of approximately 2 minutes, the wheals raised with these initial injections are slowly enlarged by putting the needle through the anesthetized spot and infiltrating a small distance to the left and then right of each wheal until a complete field block of the recipient area has been accomplished. If this is done slowly enough, the patient feels only the initial three injections. Occasionally 3% or 4% lidocaine with 1:50,000 epinephrine is used for the field block in patients who are particularly difficult to anesthetize. Then 15 to 30 minutes after completion of the recipient area field block, as much as 15 ml of epinephrine 1:50,000 is infiltrated *superficially* in small amounts and in many spots throughout the recipient area to minimize bleeding during surgery.

Occasionally we use premixed and self-administered nitrous oxide 50% and oxygen 50%. Propofol, injected intravenously by an anesthetist, can also be employed in individuals who are apprehensive about "needles." In the latter case, both field blocks are made in 10 to 15 minutes while the patient is unconscious.

A field block of bupivacaine (Marcaine) 0.5% can be used in the donor area before the patient leaves the office to prolong anesthesia at that site. Ketorolac tromethamine (Toradol) 30 to 60 mg is usually administered intramuscularly at the end of the procedure. It eliminates virtually all pain in most patients for 4 to 6 hours postoperatively. It should not be used in patients with a history of asthma or gastrointestinal ulcers. A single dose of Toradol has never been reported as causing acute glomerulonephritis—one of its most serious potential complications.

PROCEDURAL TECHNIQUES

The Donor Area

The importance of improvements in donor area harvesting in approximately the last 10 years cannot be overstated. They have revolutionized what can be accomplished with hair transplanting. Conceptually one excises an appropriately sized donor area as an ellipse or uses a multibladed handle to excise contiguous narrow strips. The ellipse or strips of tissue are removed, the donor site sutured—most often in a single layer—and the tissue is then subdivided into the desired number and types of grafts. The author employs two donor zones in most patients; one inferiorly on the left or right side of the occipital area and the other on the contralateral area more superiorly, extending from the midline of the occipital area into the parietal and posterior temporal areas (Fig. 15-12).[29] Using two donor zones allows the author to obtain hair of different textures and colors to use in the recipient area. It also enables one to take narrower strips than if a single ellipse were excised, and to therefore more easily close the wounds with less tension in order to achieve better scars, especially if galeal sutures are not used.

The schematic drawings shown in Figure 15-12 demonstrate typical excision widths during each of six sessions, with *A* representing the first and *F* the sixth session. Many variations of this pattern, however, are possible. For example, if the density of the hair in the donor area is lower than average one can use the superior zone *A* combined with the superior zone *B* rather than with the inferior zone *A*, creating a longer total donor zone that goes from ear to ear more superiorly. Alternately, if the density is lower than average, wider strips or an additional strip can be excised in one or both donor areas. Any of these approaches will increase the numbers of hairs available for transplanting. In addition, of course, each of the areas marked *A, B, C, D, E,* and *F* may instead be harvested as ellipses without using multibladed knives.

Although the first session is usually taken from the left inferior and right superior donor areas and the second from the right inferior and left superior donor areas, the result after these two sessions should be one long scar extending from ear to ear superiorly, and one more inferior scar line extending from the left to right postauricular area. All subsequent sessions are taken immediately adjacent to the previously produced scar tissue, and the scar is excised as part of the new harvest. Thus no matter how many times donor areas are excised, only two narrow scars are present at any given time. Whenever one is not comfortable about the long-term height of the donor area—for example, in a patient with a family history of type VI or VII MPB—a single donor zone is utilized. This zone will run midway between the superior and inferior border of the donor area and results in one rather than two scars. As can be seen in Figure 15-12 a total of 48.5 mm of donor tissue is typically required for six sessions of micrograft or minigraft strip harvesting, and a total of 57 mm is typically required when the harvesting is intended to produce a combination of standard round grafts and micrografts or minigrafts.

The "permanent" donor area containing hair densities of 8 or more hairs per 4 mm circle is on average 69 mm wide in at least 80% of patients past the age of 65 years,[29] so a substantial "margin of error" is still present if even 57 mm are harvested. In addition, donor sites with fewer than 8 hairs per 4 mm circle can in fact be utilized if necessary. Figure 15-13 is a schematic of the potential "permanent" donor zone. Note that it is widest in the parietal areas, so elliptical excisions should ideally *not* have their widest aspects in the midline of the occipital area, as is common. It is also important to recognize that the quoted measurements were made in nontumesced potential donor areas.

A

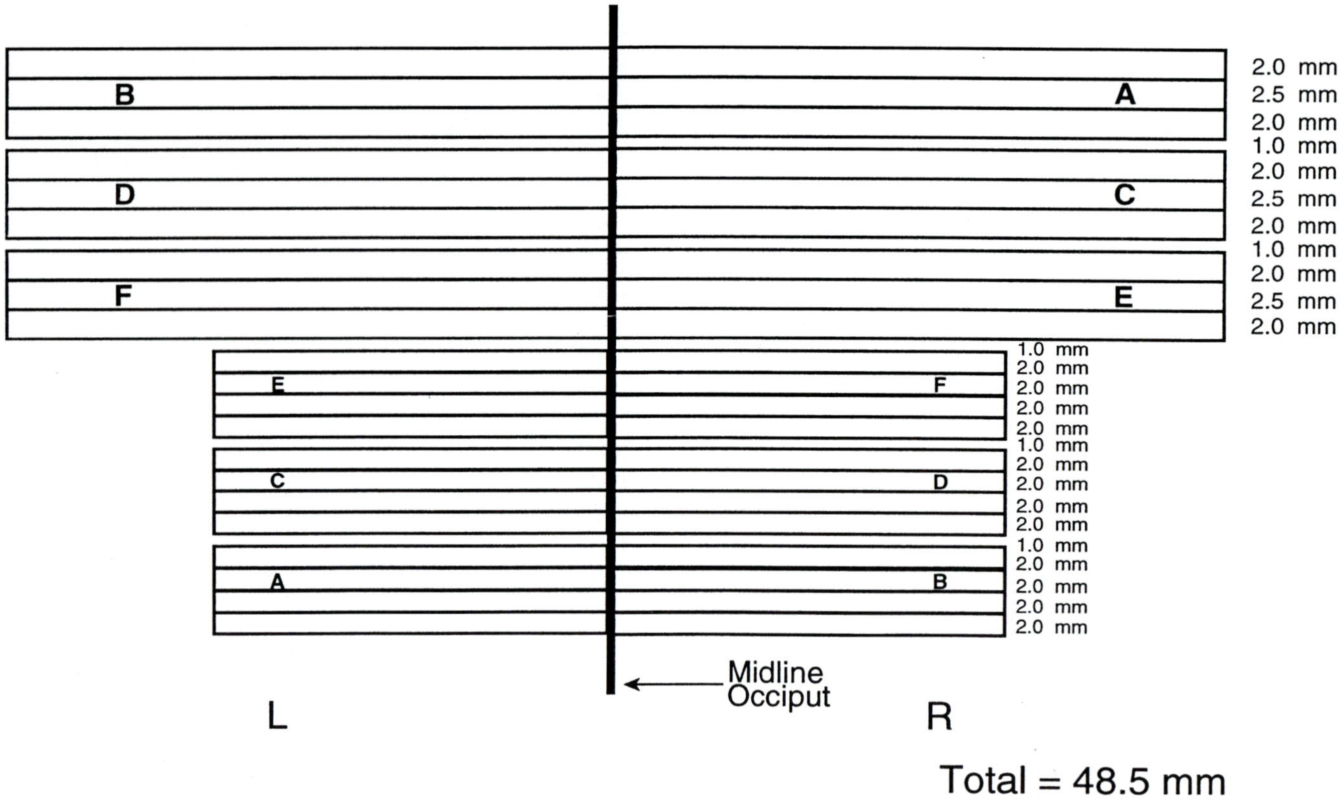

FIG. 15-12
A, An example of "strip harvesting" using six donor zones (*A, B, C, D, E,* and *F* for sessions 1, 2, 3, 4, 5, and 6). The width of the strips is shown on the right side of the drawing. A 1 mm space has been left between donor sites from different sessions and represents scar lines. A total of 48.5 mm of donor tissue would be used for six sessions, each of which would yield approximately 350 to 400 micrografts and 450 to 500 or more minigrafts per session. For each session we usually use an inferior donor zone (for example, inferior *A*) to be used at the hairline or the center of the whorl of the vertex, as well as a superior and contralateral donor zone (for example, superior zone *A*) to obtain coarser, denser hair to be used more posteriorly or peripherally in the vertex area. (From Unger W, ed. Hair Transplantation. 3rd ed. New York: Marcel Dekker, 1995.) *Continued*

When strips are harvested from tumesced tissue, the donor area has been stretched by the tumescent fluid, so, for example, an ostensibly 2.5 mm wide strip actually represents removal of less than 2.5 mm of nontumesced tissue. Thus in practice, although six sessions of micrografts or minigrafts might consume 48.5 mm of tumesced tissue, less than 48.5 mm of the nontumesced potential donor area will have actually been harvested.

Once the strips are carefully removed from the donor sites, any larger bleeding vessels are cauterized with a Hyfrecator set at unipolar delivery and 80 to 90. The wound is usually closed with a running single-layer suture technique using 2-0 Supramid (nylon) on a CL-30 reverse cutting needle, and loops are normally placed 4 to 6 mm apart (Fig. 15-14). If there is any tension on closure, one can either undermine the superior flap or use galeal sutures or interrupted sutures. The length and width of the donor strips, closing tension (rated from 1 to 10), and the numbers and types of grafts obtained are also noted on the operative record as a guide for what amount of donor tissue should be excised in future sessions.

Graft Preparation and Insertion. If a multibladed knife has been used, the strips of tissue are removed from the donor area, carefully separated from each other, and laid out on a moistened tongue depressor or back-lighting box or placed under stereoscopic microscopes (see following discussion). If an ellipse is excised it is first carefully divided into narrow slices using super sharp razor blades much as one would slice

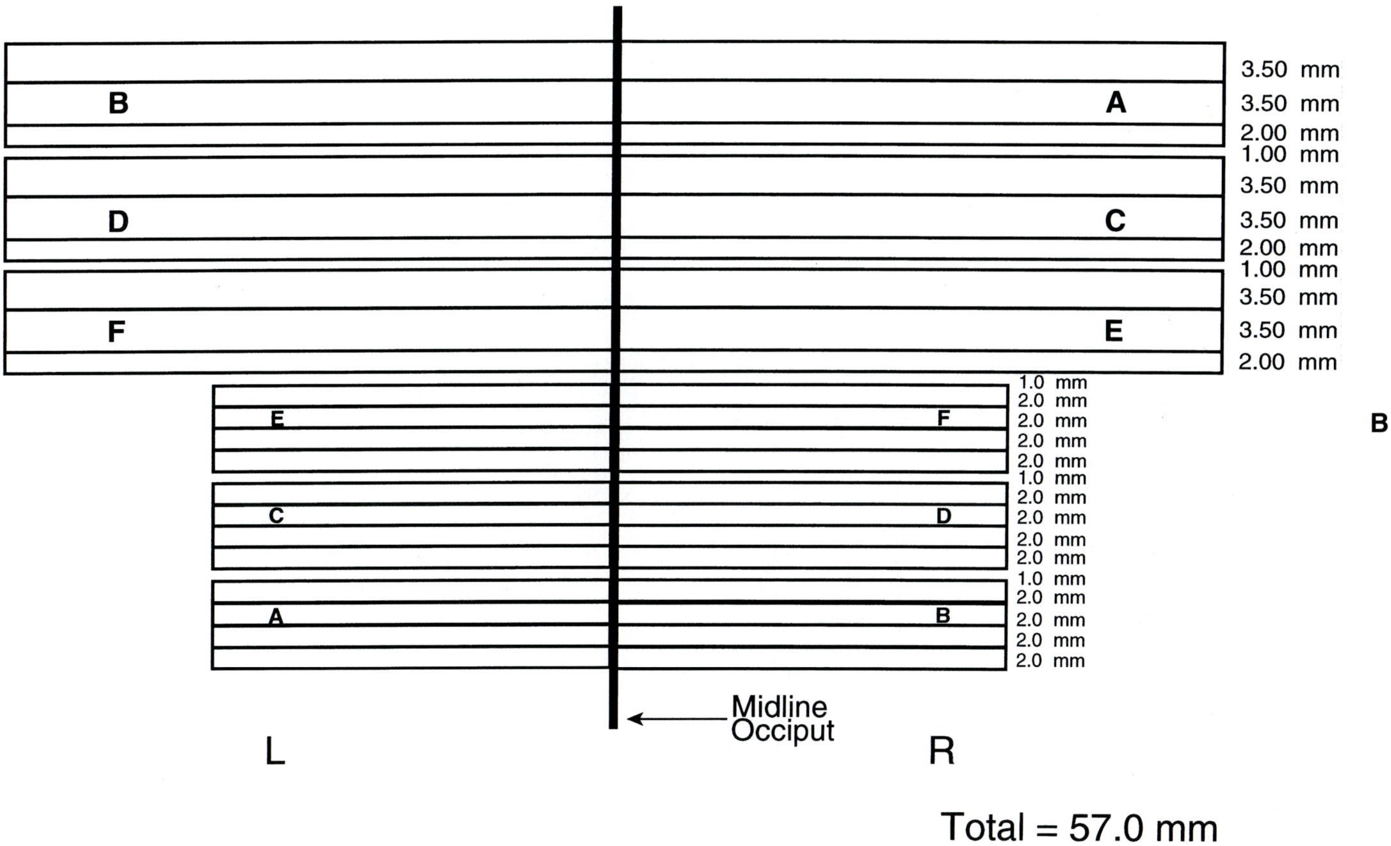

FIG. 15-12, cont'd

B, Typical widths of strips excised for standard round grafts, minigrafts, and micrografts. A total of 57 mm of donor tissue is required to yield six sessions of grafts consisting of approximately 300 to 350 minigrafts, 350 to 400 micrografts, and 50 to 60 standard round grafts per session. Any scar tissue from previous harvests is re-excised during each subsequent harvesting session so that at most only two continuous scars should be left in the donor zone regardless of the number of sessions carried out. The widths of the strips shown in both **A** and **B** may be increased slightly if donor area hair density is lower than average, or decreased slightly if it is higher than average. In areas where fine hair texture is not cosmetically critical or if a larger than usual amount of donor tissue is required, two superior donor zones could be used instead of one inferior and one superior—for example, superior *A* can be combined with superior *B.*

a loaf of bread. These slices are 1 FU wide and are nearly always prepared with ×8 to ×10 magnification so as to ensure this limited width while minimizing FU injury. The donor tissue should be orientated so that a clear view of hair follicles is possible. Then a small jeweler's forceps and the razor blades are used to carefully section the tissue into pieces containing the desired numbers of FUs or hairs. A small amount of subcutaneous tissue should be left below the level of the deepest hair bulbs. Grafts ideally should be grasped by this subcutaneous "tag" when they are being inserted into recipient sites. The rest of the subcutaneous tissue should be sectioned off the grafts as part of the "cleaning" process. Removal of the epidermal portion of each graft is optional. The strip must be kept constantly moist, and after separating the grafts from the strip you should immediately place them into a Petri dish with a 4 × 4 gauze that has been at least half filled with saline or Ringer's injection.

Hair most often emerges from the scalp in small groupings of 2 or 3 hairs and less commonly as single or 4 or 5 closely associated hairs. The follicles of these hairs may sometimes combine as they approach the surface of the skin so as to produce more than one hair emerging from what appears to be a single orifice. More often, however, the hairs exit the surface of the skin as quite closely placed bunches of individual hairs separated from other similar groups by somewhat larger alopecic spaces. Histologically these FUs or groups of follicles are also bound together in a loose

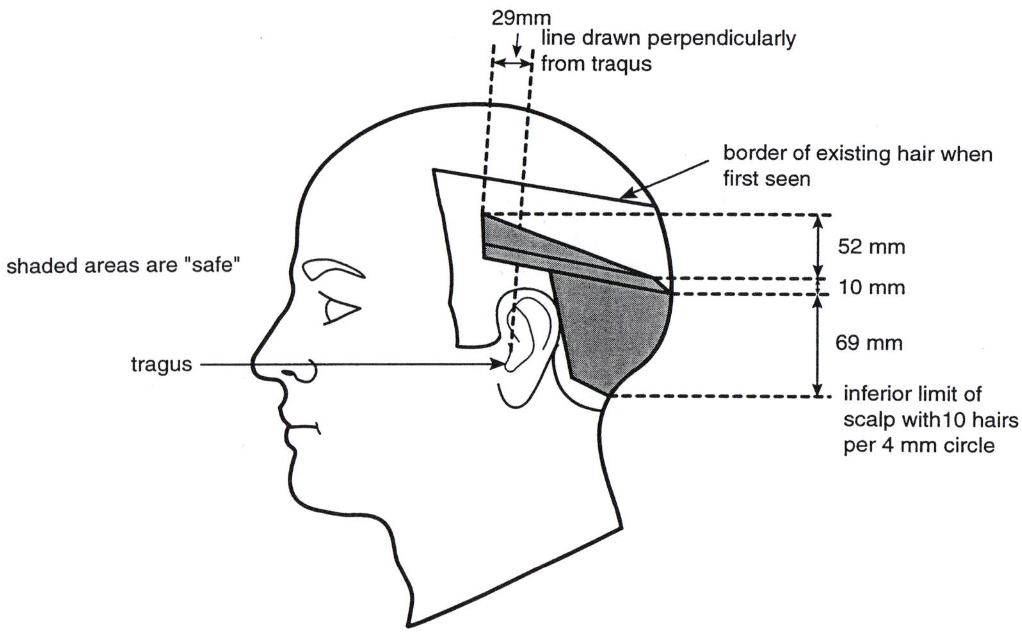

FIG. 15-13
The potential "permanent" donor zone as determined by an examination of hair density in the donor area in 328 randomly chosen men aged 65 years or older. Note that it is 69 mm high in the midline of the occipital area and that hair with fewer than 8 hairs per 4 mm circle is present superior, inferior, and anterior to the shaded "safe" donor area. (From Unger W, ed. Hair Transplantation. 3rd ed. New York: Marcel Dekker, 1995.)

A

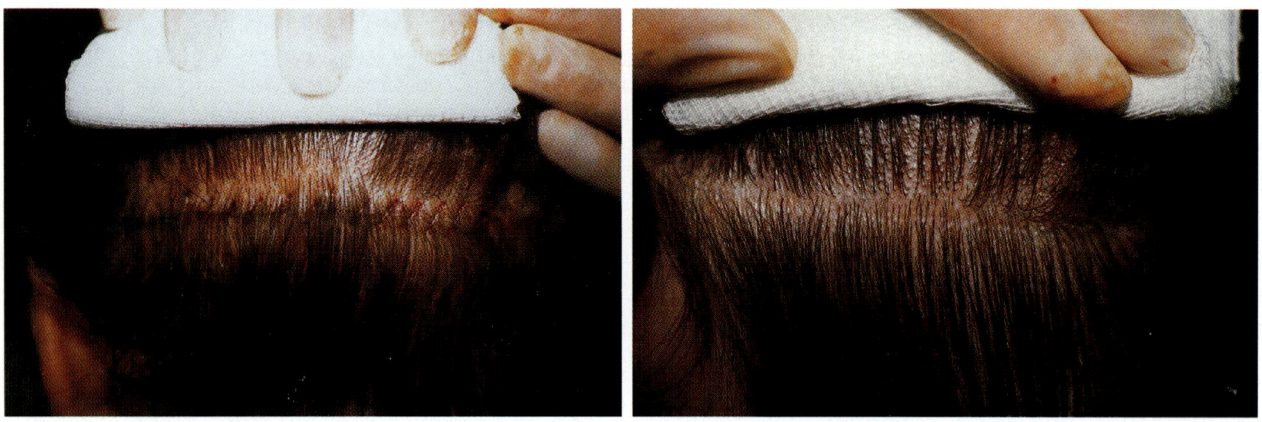

B

FIG. 15-14
A, A donor area immediately after harvesting and suturing. The wound is usually closed with a running single layer suture technique using 2-0 Supramid on a CL-30 needle. **B,** The same donor area 6 months after surgery. Only a narrow, difficult-to-find scar line remains.

adventitial tissue consisting of fine collagen and elastic fibrils as well as nerves and a vascular plexus.[30] If one is attempting to obtain only single FUs, most of the alopecic skin between the FUs is carefully trimmed away from them. Limmer has stated that approximately 50% of a donor strip can be discarded during this process. If slit grafts are being employed, the possibility of "compression" of hair into dense unsightly lines is eliminated by making them only 1 FU wide and 2 to 3 FUs long. Donor strips that are 2.5 to 3 mm wide can often be easily divided into such slit grafts by slicing them into sections that are approximately 0.6 mm wide (Frechet P. Personal communication, 2000). Slot grafts are most often 2 FUs wide, and because tissue is being removed in recipient sites, compression is not a problem. Grafts that are intended for 1.3 to 2 mm holes are prepared from 2 mm wide strips and those that will be inserted into 3 to 3.5 mm holes are generally obtained from 3.5 to 3.75 mm wide donor strips.

Most technicians will prepare grafts with the least damage to follicles by using various degrees of magnification. How much magnification is necessary to produce excellent grafts will vary with the hand-eye coordination of the technician and his or her visual acuity. Norwood, after visiting Jim Arnold's office, commented that "a highly skilled technician can cut follicles or do follicular transplantation without the binocular microscope,"[31] so obviously some experienced technicians can also produce excellent minigrafts without the use of significant magnification. In my office most technicians wear ×1 to ×4 magnification loupes. In addition, four technicians utilize Mantis or ×10 stereoscopic microscopes for the preparation of FUs.

The less one injures follicles during graft preparation the better. However, minimal injury of the follicular architecture seems to have little effect on its survival. The unanswered question is how much FU injury is necessary to actually produce a lethal effect on the follicles. With the exception of dehydration, it appears that a great deal of abuse must be administered to the follicle to actually kill a hair.[32] Even intentional mutilation of follicles will often not deter growth. Kim has demonstrated 80% regrowth of hair when the upper third of the follicle has been totally removed intentionally. (If the lower third is removed, hair survival drops to 60%.) Limmer has shown lower rates of hair survival, and Mayer has demonstrated that when follicles are divided into upper third and lower two thirds and all of the fragments are transplanted, that one will achieve a total of 133 hairs from every 100 hairs transplanted (though these hairs often have a finer texture).[33] Regardless of the variable percentage rates of survival, it is clear that substantial damage can be done to follicles without death of the hair. Minor injuries during graft preparation are not nearly as important as one might surmise, and they appear to be far less important than, for example, excessive handling or dehydration of FUs during "dense packing."

I have discussed in other publications the likelihood that some unseen telogen follicles can be mistakenly discarded as part of the "garbage" between FUs when microscopic dissection of donor tissue is used to remove everything but the visible anagen hairs or FUs.[34] As noted earlier, studies that have shown 33% more hairs growing than were originally counted, when "chubby" rather than "skinny" FUs were transplanted, lend credence to this fear.[19] It would seem wise when producing FUs to leave a cushion of tissue around each FU rather than to make them as "skinny" as possible, in order to insert them into the smallest and most densely packed holes.

The prepared grafts should be gently eased into the recipient sites using small serrated forceps or jeweler's forceps. To avoid damage to the hair matrices the grafts should never be grasped at the proximal end of the follicle. Steady pressure is applied to control any bleeding in the area and to assure that the grafts are flush with the surrounding skin. It is important to be careful to avoid "burying" your grafts beneath the level of the skin. It is far better to leave a graft protruding *slightly* above the level of the surrounding skin than below it, as inclusion cysts or "delling" may result from the latter. Trying to mimic the angle and direction with which the recipient site was made as one inserts the various grafts also minimizes trauma to them. A new suction "pen" has just become available that may eliminate the need for forceps and thereby decrease follicle trauma during insertion. I had not had the opportunity to try it before writing this chapter.

While in most offices all the recipient sites are made before any grafts are inserted, the insertion of a graft immediately after the preparation of the recipient site—either by a needle or scalpel—is generally less traumatic to that graft. The smaller the grafts and the more densely they are being packed, the more important this "stick and place" technique can be expected to be. Thus if one is employing FUHT with dense packing, the "stick and place" method of transplanting would seem advantageous for minimizing trauma to the grafts. But unless the surgeon is a partner to this process, making each site followed immediately by insertion of the graft, the density of grafts as well as the angle and direction are left entirely in the hands of technicians. Most operators are not willing to delegate these decisions to technicians who are less experienced than the physicians and may also be less artistic or careful. A compromise I sometimes use is (1) less than "dense" packing and (2) the creation of FU sites myself that are then dilated by the technicians with a small-bore solid and blunt "needle" just before insertion of the grafts if such dilation is necessary to produce easy introduction of the grafts into the sites. Experienced

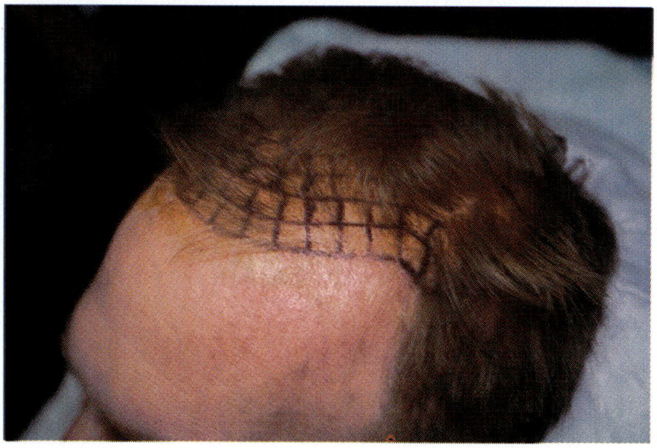

FIG. 15-15
Sandoval has devised a simple solution to the problem of graft density designation for his technicians who use the "stick and place" technique. He divides the recipient area (posterior to the hairline zone, which he does himself) into 1 cm squares and indicates to the technicians how many FUs he wants, evenly spaced, in each square.

technicians are also allowed to create additional needle holes between those made by me, following the same angle and direction of my sites if they feel additional FUs can be inserted without undue trauma to the grafts.

Sandoval has devised an ingenious yet simple solution to the problem of graft density designation for his technicians using the "stick and place" technique. He divides the recipient area (posterior to the hairline zone, which he does himself) into 1 cm squares and indicates to the technicians how many FUs he wants, evenly spaced, in each square (Fig. 15-15).

It cannot be overemphasized that grafts must be kept moist during the entire procedure. Dehydration has been shown to be more lethal to follicular cells than pressure injury. It is also useful to segregate grafts into groups that contain, for example, fine hair, coarse hair, gray hair, and so on, and then further segregate them according to the number of hairs that they contain. By doing this in advance, the ideal graft for any particular recipient site is immediately available to the technician during implantation.

The Recipient Area

I conceptually divide the potential recipient area into three zones: the anterior third, middle third, and posterior third. The anterior third begins at the hairline and ends at a line drawn perpendicularly from the tragus. The posterior third begins at a point that Beehner has called the "transition point," where the more or less flat part of the top of the skull starts becoming more vertical as it drops into the "crown" area. If hair is transplanted as far posteriorly as the "transition point," the person will look like he has full coverage when viewed frontally and almost full coverage when viewed laterally, despite the presence of a bald "crown." There are few patients in whom total coverage should be attempted if he or she is unwilling to undergo AR. However, the older the patient and the better his hereditary factors, the less dogmatic this statement should be. Lower hair density objectives also will increase the proportion of the area of MPB that can be transplanted with a limited number of grafts.

The recipient area can be treated in one of three different general ways: (1) exclusive FUHT, (2) a combination of FU, slit grafts, slot grafts, and minigrafts, and (3) a combination of FU, slit grafts, slot grafts, minigrafts, and round grafts of various sizes. These will be discussed separately.

Follicular Unit Hair Transplanting

The goal of FUHT is to divide all the donor tissue into FUs, discarding what is viewed as excess alopecic tissue between them. The FUs are then inserted into holes made by various sized needles or small blades, thus attempting to recreate what occurs in nature. Orthodox proponents of FUHT go further and state that all donor tissue should be excised only as an ellipse, that multibladed knives are contraindicated, and that grafts should be produced only under stereoscopic magnification in order to minimize damage to the FUs.[35] As has been noted earlier, one of the great advantages of FUHT in fact is that a single session can stand completely on its own and look extraordinarily natural (Fig. 15-16). An additional important attribute of FUHT is that if the MPB extends beyond the initial estimate, the then isolated transplanted area will be transformed into a more natural looking IFF than if larger grafts had been used. This is a less compelling reason for FUHT, as very natural looking IFF and "prospective" IFF can be produced with a combination of FU, slit grafts, and minigrafts of various kinds. Nevertheless, both of these characteristics of FUHT leave the patient and physician with a minimum amount of concern about the unknown future and are compelling reasons for its use. Finally, FUHT enthusiasts have believed that this technique allows them to produce essentially 100% hair survival. Unfortunately, if FUHT is combined with "dense packing," the hair survival rate appears to be substantially less than 100%.

Typically FUs containing a single hair are used most anteriorly, two to three rows deep, and at a density of 20 to 40 FU/cm^2. (I use approximately 20 to 25 FU/cm^2.) FUs containing 2 hairs are transplanted posterior to these and at initially similar densities. As one moves progressively more posteriorly, the FU density decreases and FUs with more than 2 hairs are utilized, except that many FUHT proponents create a midline

A

B

C

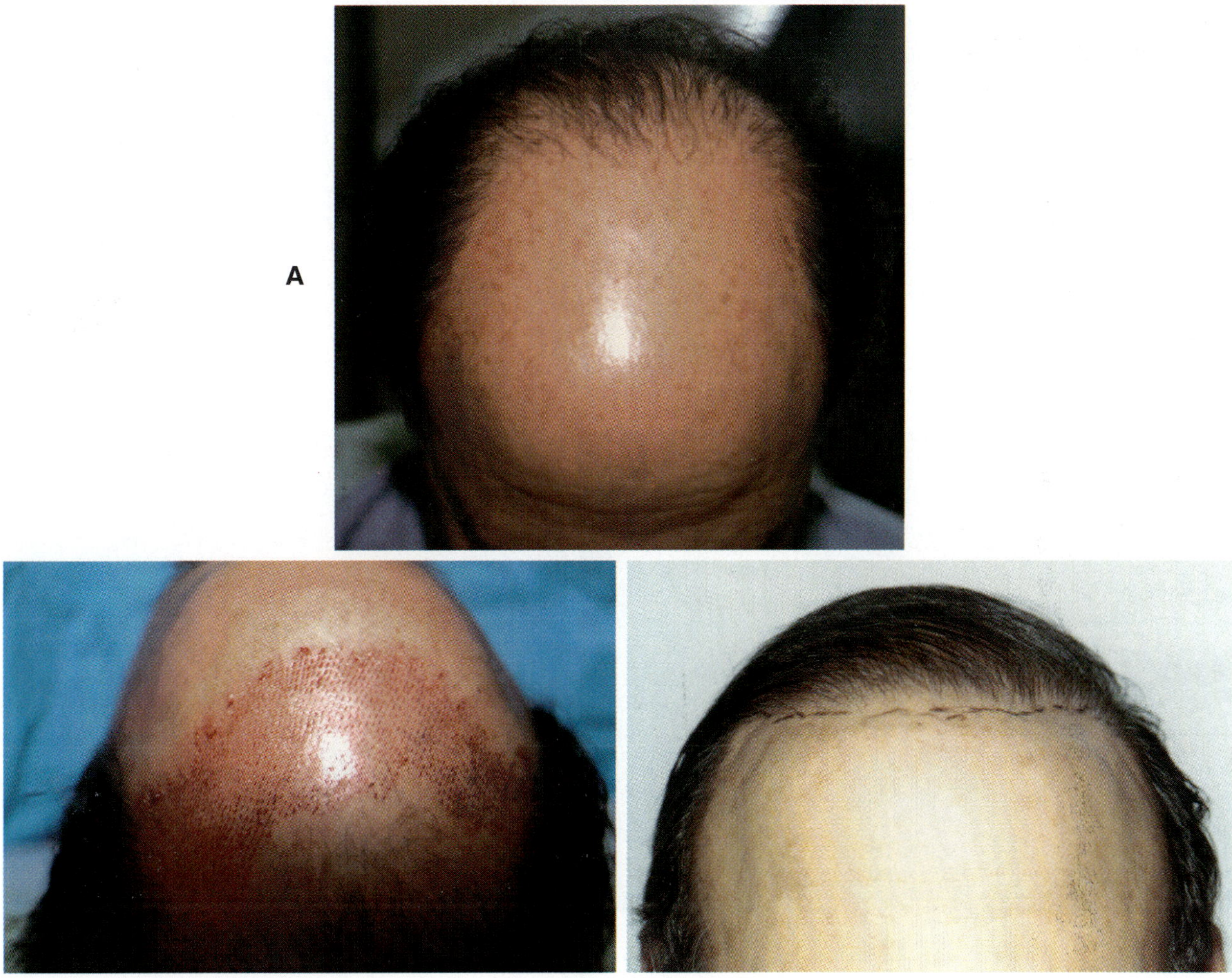

FIG. 15-16

A, A patient before FUHT. "Pluggy" round grafts had been used in the vertex area years before by another surgeon, and the patient refused anything but exclusive micrografts. **B,** Intraoperative photograph showing recipient sites for 1600 follicular units. **C,** Five months after 1600 micrografts were transplanted to frontal area. Black crayon mark denotes suggested advancement of hairline.

roundish zone, just posterior to the hairline zone, that is treated with densely packed FUs containing 3 or more hairs.

There are significant practical disadvantages to FUHT, the most important of which is that large numbers of good to excellent technicians are required and quality control of such a group becomes increasingly problematic as the sessions get larger and the dense packing increases. Nevertheless, if enough hairs are transplanted and packed closely enough together, even the death of as many as 35% of them may still leave one with a very good looking result—hence the popularity of this approach. The author however finds such potentially high levels of hair loss unacceptable given the limited donor area resources that most patients have. It is for this reason that I have generally limited exclusive FUHT to the hairline zone or reserved it for particularly anxious patients. Elsewhere, as indicated earlier in this chapter, I use a combination of other grafts with FUs scattered between them. In addition, when FUs are used, no attempt is made to complete the area in one session, as this requires "dense packing" and potentially entails more follicular death. Although some hairlines will look very good after one or two sessions, most often hairline zones are transplanted three times to produce ideal results (Figs. 15-8*B* and *C*, 15-17, and 15-18).

FUHT Combined with Minislit, Slit Grafts, Slot Grafts, and Minigrafts

When a combination of FU, slit grafts, slot grafts, and minigrafts is used, the hairline zone is constructed with

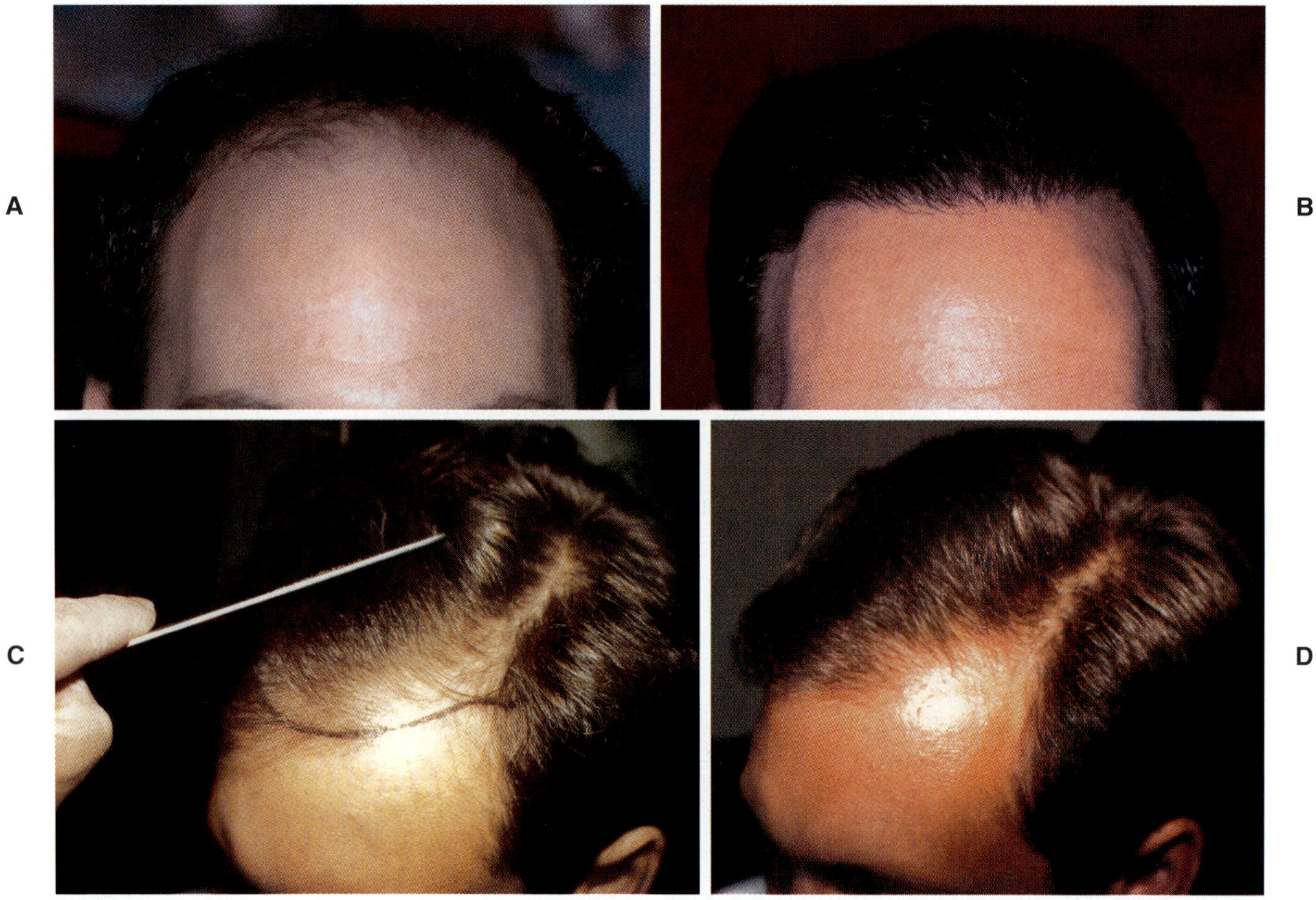

FIG. 15-17
A, A man before his first hair transplant. **B,** Seven months after his second hair transplant consisting of micrografts, slit grafts, and minigrafts. Although some hairlines will look good after two sessions as shown above, most often hairline zones are transplanted three times to produce ideal results. **C,** A man before hair transplanting. **D,** The same patient 9 months after his first transplant session consisting of micrografts and minislit grafts. This result was satisfactory for the time being because the hair was both fine textured and relatively light colored.

FUs that are five to six sites deep in a manner similar to that described above for FUHT. These are then followed by one to two rows of minislit grafts and then one to two rows of small-slit grafts posterior to the latter (Fig. 15-18). *Additional micrografts are scattered between the minislit grafts and small-slit grafts* (see Fig. 15-11). The first two rows of slit sites are prepared with a Beaver ES miniblade or a 1.3 to 1.8 Minde knife, the small-slit-graft recipient sites usually are prepared with a No. 15 blade, and the FU recipient sites are prepared with a Nokor needle or a 16- to 18-gauge needle. One or two hair micrografts usually fit easily into 18-gauge holes, while 3 or more hair micrografts are usually less traumatized during insertion into the holes made by a Nokor or 16-gauge needle. After 4 to 6 or more months have elapsed, a similar session of minislit and small-slit grafts as well as micrografts should be placed between those transplanted during the first session. In addition, small round minigrafts or slot grafts can be scattered here and there between the small-slit grafts if you seek to produce greater density posterior to the hairline zone and if hair characteristics are suitable—the finer the hair texture, the more curl, and the less color contrast between skin and hair, the better. At this point the hair growing from the first session will help to camouflage any slight plugginess the round minigrafts or slot grafts might otherwise have produced.

If the hair within any of the previously transplanted grafts is accidentally too coarse or dense, a small round punch or slot punch can be used to excise that graft

A B C

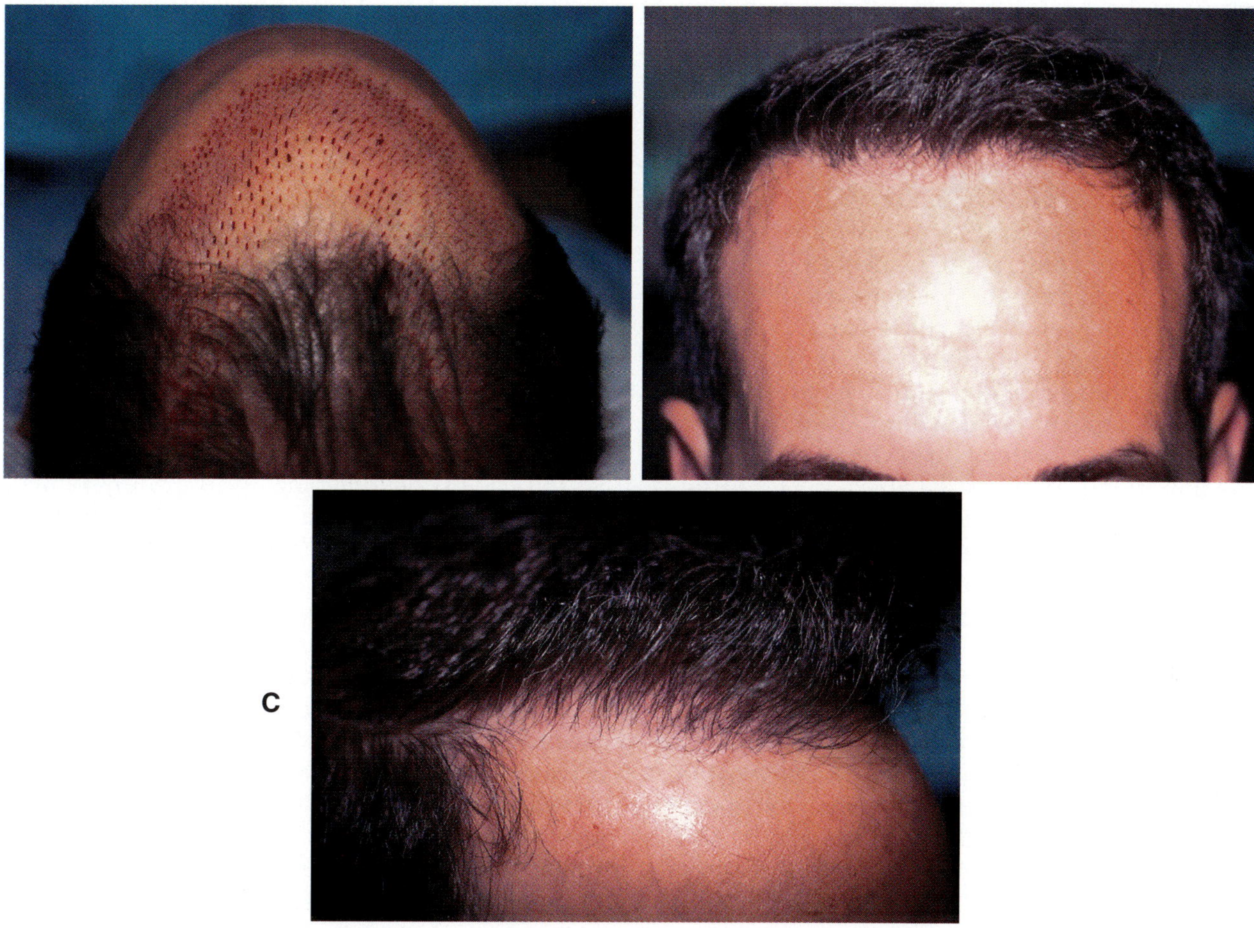

FIG. 15-18
A, When a combination of micrografts or follicular units (FUs), slit grafts, and minigrafts is used, the hairline zone is constructed with FUs that are five to six sites deep. These are followed by one to two rows of minislit grafts and then one to two rows of small-slit grafts posterior to the latter as shown above. In addition, in the patient shown in the photograph, five rows of slot grafts (3 mm long) were used to produce more density more posteriorly. **B,** Six months after the second session. **C,** Close-up photograph of the hairline taken at the same time as **B.** Note that the micrografted zone has an irregular anterior border with triangular or rounded areas of grafts protruding here and there.

(which is then transplanted into a more suitable site), and it is replaced with one containing finer or less dense hair. Four to six or more months later, a third session, similar to the second, is usually done to complete the hairline zone and the area posterior to it. You may use intervals as short as 6 weeks between sessions if your patient is completely alopecic when treatment begins, though as described above, the longer intervals will allow you to adjust what you do in subsequent sessions according to what you see growing from previous ones. You can also employ intervals of longer than 6 months between sessions, especially if there is a reasonable amount of hair still present in the recipient area. The author most often prefers to do sessions in the same area 5 to 6 months apart, thus allowing the patient to see more hair from previous treatment(s) and creating a more gradual transition from sparser hair to thicker hair. Longer intervals also result in more postoperative camouflage from longer transplanted hairs.

It is important to note that although you are ultimately trying to produce a random and therefore natural-looking distribution of hair, an "organized disorganization" creates a more natural-looking short-term as well as long-term appearance. The micrografted zone should have a very irregular anterior border with triangular or rounded areas of grafts protruding anteriorly here and there (see Figs. 15-8*B* and *C*, 15-17*D*, and 15-18*B*). Minislit and slit grafts should be placed approximately 3 mm apart from each other as well as 1 mm anterior or posterior to their lateral neighbors.

This produces the most even distribution of hair while not creating a straight line (see Fig. 15-11). During the second session you should place the grafts approximately midway between those of the first session, again "juggling" them slightly anterior or posterior to their neighbors. During the third session use a similar approach. Thus an even distribution of hair over the entire surface can be created by each session, without some grafts being closer to the neighboring graft on the left side than on the right side, for example. Inconsistent density, one of the characteristics of natural hairlines, is produced only wherever it is wanted. At the same time, the juggling of grafts slightly anterior or posterior to adjacent grafts will produce a random natural-looking distribution of hair. Two other parameters are important: (1) follow the direction of the original hair in that area and (2) mimic the angle at which any persisting or previously transplanted hair exits the scalp.

In summary, the cutting of the slit sites should satisfy four parameters: (1) they should be 3 mm apart laterally, (2) they should be 1 mm anterior or posterior to their neighbor, (3) they should follow the direction of the existing hair in that area, and (4) the angle at which they exit the scalp should mimic that of the existing hair in that area. Micrografts, slot grafts, and round minigrafts (if you are using the latter) should be scattered *randomly* between the carefully spaced slit grafts and should follow their direction and angle. I routinely spend between 45 and 70 minutes preparing recipient sites—depending on the type and number of grafts and the amount of hair present in the recipient area. I was surprised to be told recently by a surgeon who prefers to remain anonymous that only 10 to 20 minutes is spent on this task in many offices.

Conceptually, I divide the frontal one-third of the recipient area into two zones: (1) the hairline zone, which is approximately 2.5 cm wide and has been discussed above, and (2) the main body of the recipient area. In approximately 85% to 90% of my patients the same types and distributions of grafts will be used for the *entire* recipient area including the "main body" of the recipient area. Large-slit grafts and slot grafts may also be used in the more posterior midline aspect of the recipient area in second and later sessions—especially if hair texture is fine or there is minimal contrast between hair and skin color. Thus in a sizable majority of patients, approximately 400 to 550 micrografts and 350 to 400 minislit, slit, or slot grafts and round minigrafts will be employed during each session—although the third session may be composed of a far higher proportion of micrografts. In female patients nearly all grafts will be minislit, slit grafts, and micrografts. As indicated earlier, round minigrafts are employed only in small more or less round areas that are completely alopecic.

The vertex area of MPB should similarly be treated only with slit grafts, micrografts, and the occasional small round minigraft. Micrografts are used to prepare the center of the whorl of the vertex, minislit grafts are used for two to three rows peripheral to the micrografted area, and minislit or small-slit grafts are used for the rest of the vertex area—minislit grafts if hair characteristics are not good, and small-slit grafts if they are good (Fig. 15-19). In second and later sessions, small- and large-slit grafts may be used, as well as the occasional slot graft and 1 to 2 mm round graft.

"Mixed" Micrograft, Slit Graft, Minigraft, and Round Graft Sessions

As implied by the foregoing, in 10% to 15% of male patients, posterior to the hairline zone you may want to switch to an organized pattern of round grafts if your objective is greater hair density.[36,37] In such cases, each session will usually require 400 or more micrografts, 250 to 350 minislit and slit grafts, and either 100 to 120 slot grafts or 100 to 120 2 mm grafts or 50 to 60 standard grafts—or a combination of them. The 2 mm round grafts should be used instead of standard grafts when the recipient area is alopecic or nearly alopecic or when the hair is particularly dense or coarse or dark. They should be spaced much the same way described for standard grafts below (Figs. 15-20 to 15-22). Generally, double the number of slot grafts or round minigrafts will be required when they are used instead of standard grafts in any given area.

Space does not permit a detailed description of the technique used to produce solid filling of the round grafted zones. A full description is available in the third edition of my text (1995)[37] and more recent publications.[36,38] It is, however, important to stress that whenever such grafts are utilized the intention should be solid filling of that zone in four sessions. If this is done, no plugginess will be noted even when all the original hair is lost and the hair is wet and parted or wind blown. Despite this recommendation, only a minority of patients actually request the fourth session in the area treated with round grafts, because hair density is sufficiently great that a single sweep of fingers through the transplanted area is nearly always adequate to overcome any otherwise noticeable plugginess. Less than solid filling of a round grafted area is far less cosmetically problematic when round grafts are being used posterior to a zone treated with micrografts, minislit, and slit grafts than it was in the past when round grafts were being used to create a hairline.

To minimize the interruption of blood supply to the grafts in the central portion of the frontal third of the recipient area, I usually do not transplant grafts in a solid hemispheric pattern during any individual session. A

U-shaped pattern followed by an untreated area followed more posteriorly by another U-shaped pattern, or a U-shaped pattern plus an island in the midline is used instead (see Fig. 15-9). When one leaves an untransplanted zone in the midline of the U, one also leaves open the possibility of an AR excising that area instead of transplanting it later. Quite often the decision whether to use AR or not is made only after the first one or two sessions have been completed. At that point the patient is well aware of any disadvantages associated with hair transplanting and can see the results. He is in a better position to realistically decide whether he wants to attempt to treat the entire area of alopecia, or only the anterior one third or two thirds of the area of alopecia. Thus a decision with regard to transplanting the peninsula between the arms of the U is often delayed until growth of the first or second session has been observed, despite the fact that AR has been discussed and photographs of the effects of AR have been shown during the first consultation. Because of heavy negative advertising and commentary in the media and in medical journals, many patients are unwilling to con-

A B

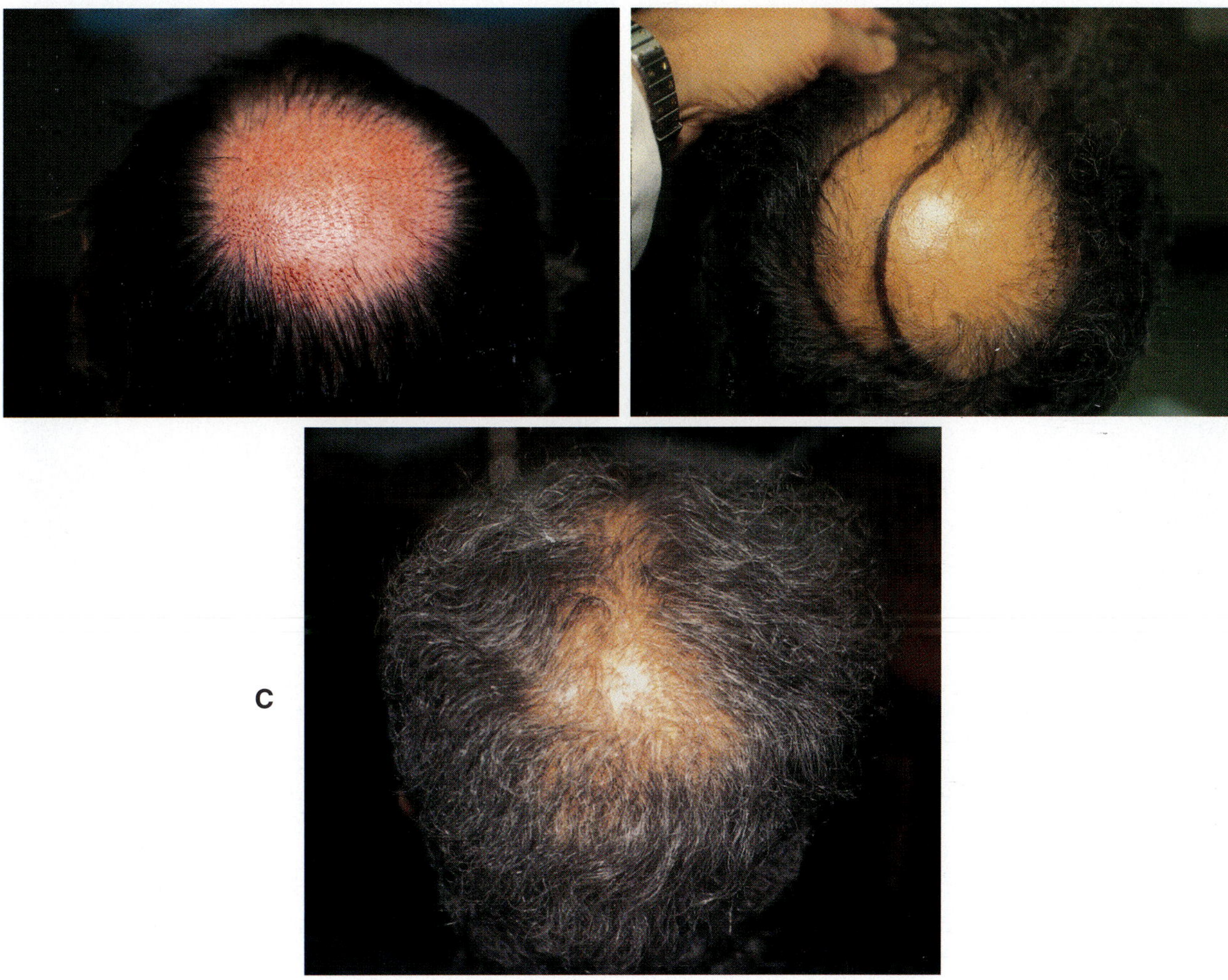

C

FIG. 15-19

A, Vertex area with recipient sites made. Note that micrografts are used between the minislit and slit grafts and to prepare the center of the whorl of the vertex—located in this patient on the left side just short of half way anterior to the posterior border of the vertex. Minislit grafts are used for two to three rows peripheral to the micrografted area, and small-slit grafts have been used in the rest of the vertex area. If hair characteristics had not been good, minislit grafts would have been used throughout the remainder of the vertex area instead of small-slit grafts. In the second session somewhat larger grafts and the occasional slot graft or small round graft may be used to increase hair density. **B,** The vertex area of a patient with a proposed alopecia reduction (AR) outlined on the left side. **C,** After a single AR and two transplant sessions, with the hair parted for critical evaluation.

A B C D

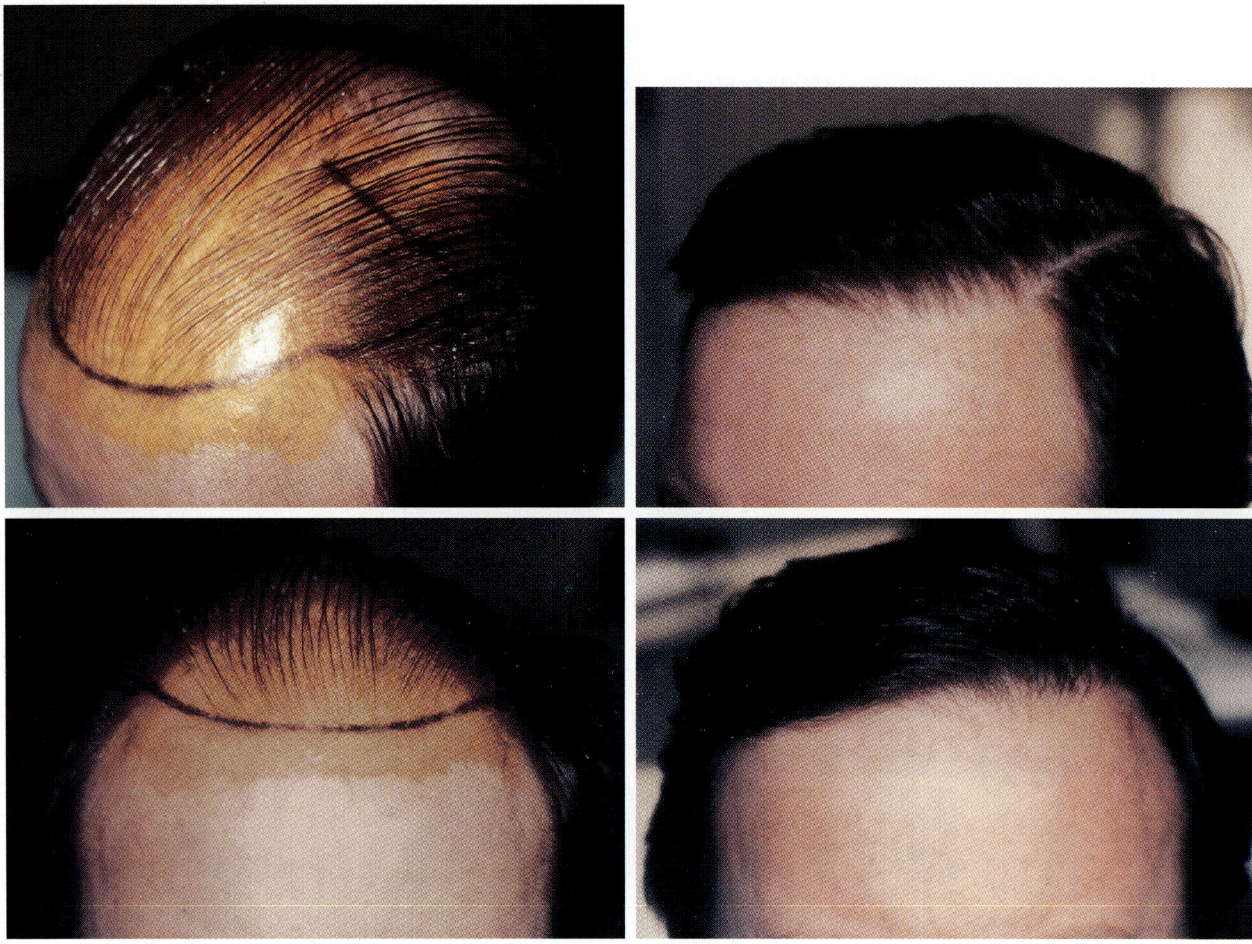

FIG. 15-20
A, Before treatment. We opted to use a mixture of micrografts, slit grafts, and 2 mm round grafts in this patient in his early 40s who wanted high-density results. **B,** The same patient shown 1 year after his third frontal hair transplant. **C,** A front view before treatment. **D,** One year after his third frontal transplant. (Two transplant sessions had also been carried out in the posterior half of the area of male pattern baldness.)

sider the option of AR until a trusting relationship has been established between the physician and patient.

If the patient decides that he is not going to attempt to transplant the entire area of alopecia, then the option of treating the middle third of the recipient area is discussed. Usually only two sessions are required at that site, although the patient may opt for one or three. As has been noted earlier, in general, one should not attempt to transplant the entire ultimate area of MPB unless the patient is willing to undergo AR at some point during the course of treatment. Exceptions to this general rule are older patients whose extent and pattern of hair loss is more certain than in younger individuals, those who are seeking relatively less dense coverage of larger areas, and those with exceptionally good prognoses based on family history and physical examination. Even in the latter group, acceptance of perhaps less dense coverage should be anticipated as a *possible* necessity.

For the majority of patients in whom AR will not be used, limiting transplanting to the anterior two thirds of the area of MPB is a more reasonable and cosmetically very acceptable goal—especially if only micrografts, slit grafts, and minigrafts are utilized. The posterior border of the middle third of the area of MPB should be curved so as to leave a normal, oval, or round shape to the remaining vertex area and should be completed with micrografts and minislit grafts in a posterior "hairline zone" fashion.

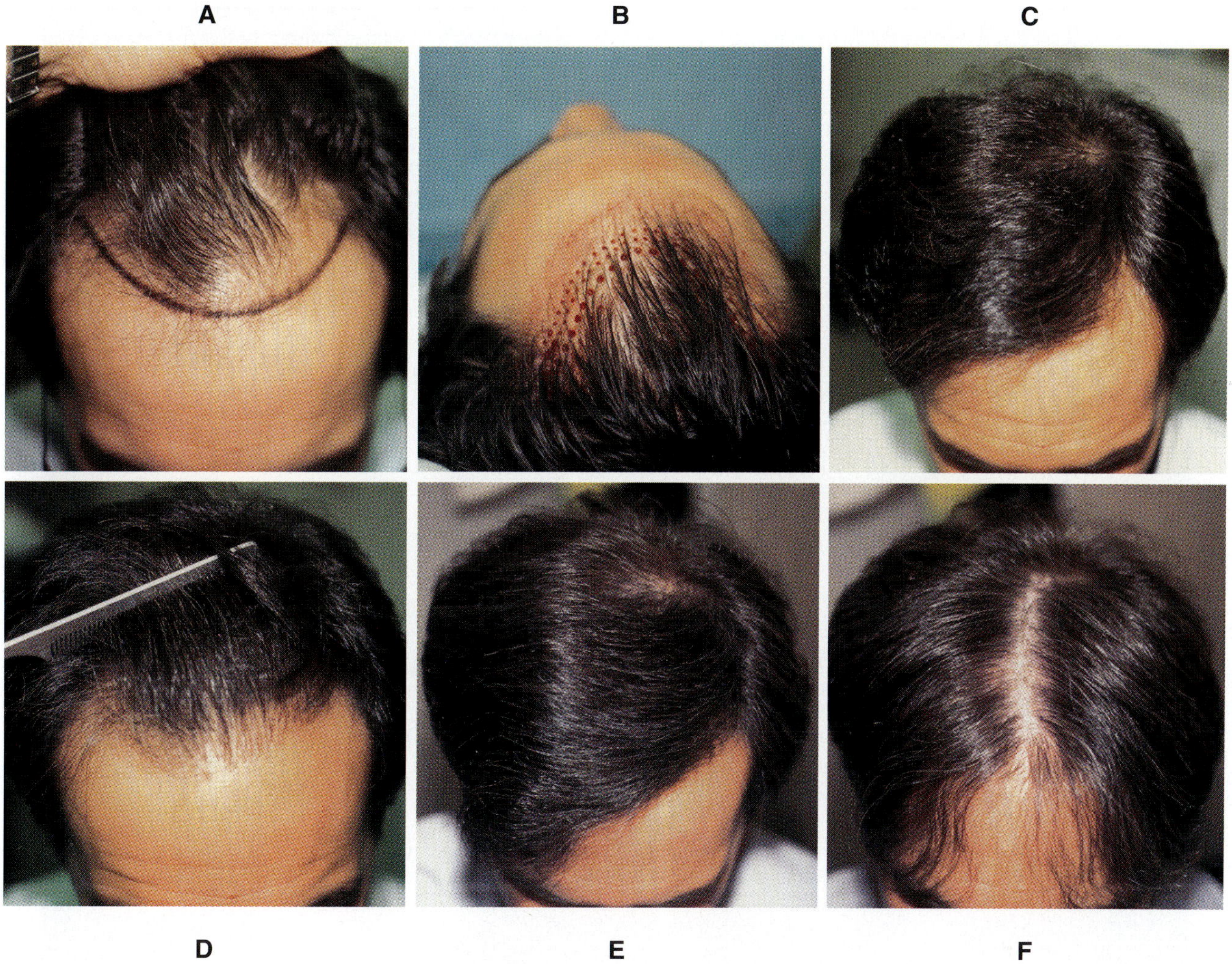

FIG. 15-21
A, Before treatment. **B,** Intraoperative photograph of patient's first session in 1991; 60 micrografts, 162 slit grafts, 100 2 mm grafts, and 22 standard grafts were employed. **C,** One year after the first treatment. **D,** One year after the first treatment with his hair combed straight back for critical evaluation. Note the absence of obvious plugginess despite black hair, pale skin, and a single session. **E,** One year after his third transplant with the hair combed as it was normally worn. **F,** One year after the third transplant with the hair parted for critical evaluation.

Tissue turgor is as important in the recipient area as it is in the donor area if you are to minimize injury to hair adjacent to the recipient sites being prepared during any given session. Just as in the donor area, significant amounts of saline may be necessary for this purpose. *A secondary advantage of maximum tissue infiltration in micrografted areas is that once the fluid dissipates the grafts will move closer together and more density will be produced.* Last, good control of bleeding in the recipient area is likewise an important component of good hair transplanting. The more bleeding present during the actual surgery, the more the grafts have to be handled and the greater the potential damage to follicles within them.

Ultrapulse carbon dioxide lasers can be used to make recipient sites for slit grafts or round grafts. Carbon dioxide lasers allow you to produce recipient sites with less bleeding and probably less edema and postoperative pain. The use of a laser to produce round holes, however, will not result in superior cosmetic results but eliminates the need to remove tissue from the hole and therefore speeds up the process. The chance that some of the tissue may be left behind to cause epidermal cysts is also eliminated. When slits are made with a laser, tissue is ablated. Thus the density and absence of compression as seen with round grafting are combined with the cosmetically superior linear shape of a slit graft. Remarkably natural-looking results are possible with only

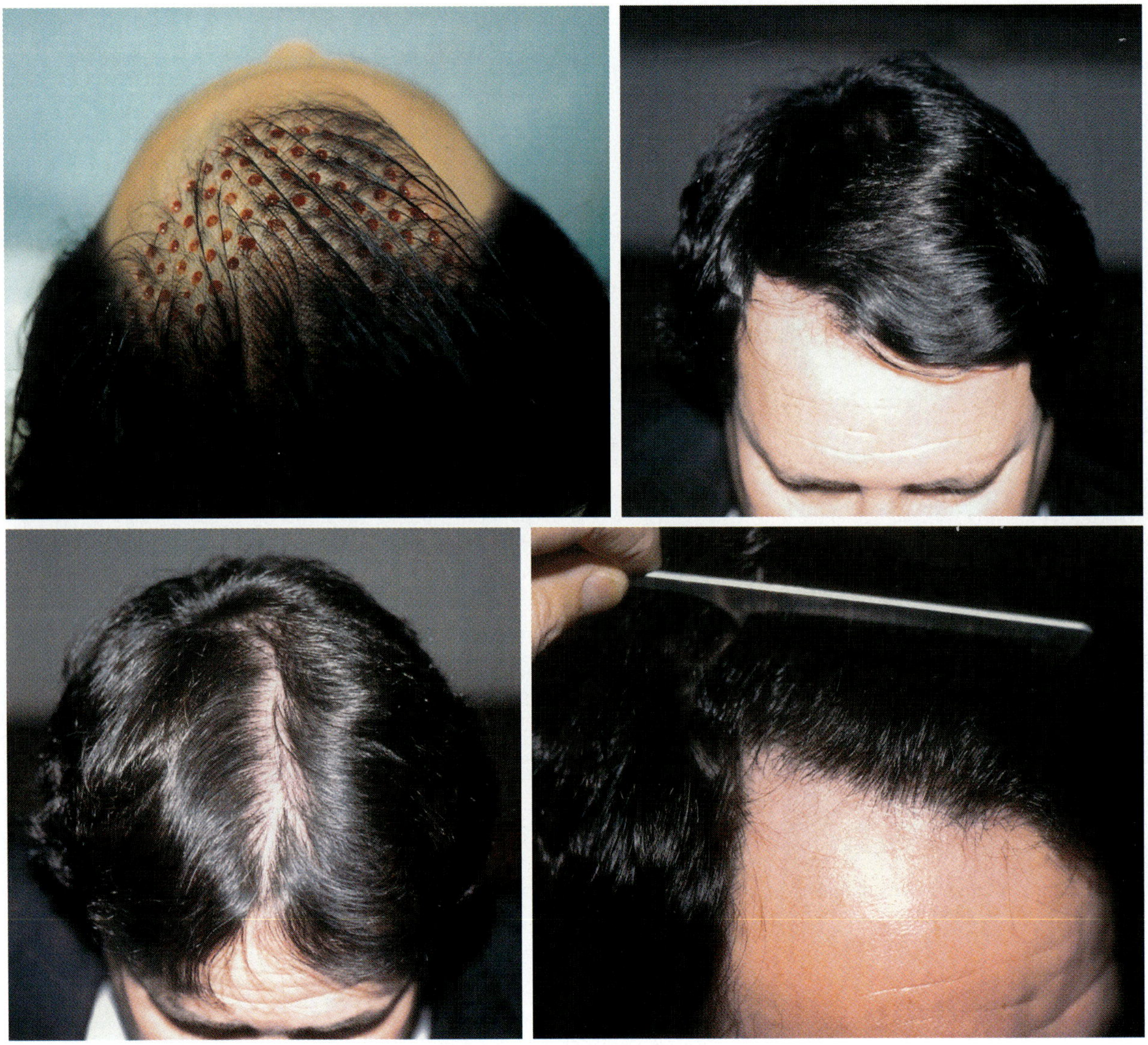

A B C D

FIG. 15-22

A, Before photograph of a patient who wanted maximum hair density. This patient began his transplanting in 1987 and was initially treated with only micrografts and standard grafts. **B,** Seven months after the last of four and a half sessions to the frontal half of his male pattern baldness (MPB). **C,** Seven months after the last of four and a half sessions to the frontal half of his MPB with his hair parted for critical evaluation. **D,** Close-up of the patient's transplanted hairline taken at the same time as **C.** The remarkable density shown in these photographs was produced because of the preponderance of standard grafts that were utilized.

one session, surpassing the naturalness of conventional slit grafting or round grafting while achieving the density of the latter (Fig. 15-23). On the other hand, there is usually some additional early crusting over the grafts and a delay of 2 to 6 weeks before hair growth begins, as compared to when a laser is not employed. Unfortunately, hair survival rates of grafts placed into laser sites are not consistently good.[39] A new slot punch creates recipient sites and therefore results similar to those of laser slits.[40] Because of both of the above, I discontinued laser transplanting after 5 years of experimentation. New erbium lasers for hair transplanting will probably result in more consistently good hair yields. However, these lasers currently produce only round sites and therefore cannot offer superior cosmetic results.

Alopecia Reduction (AR)

AR is defined as the excision of an area of alopecia or prospective alopecia. The size of the area that can be ex-

A B C D
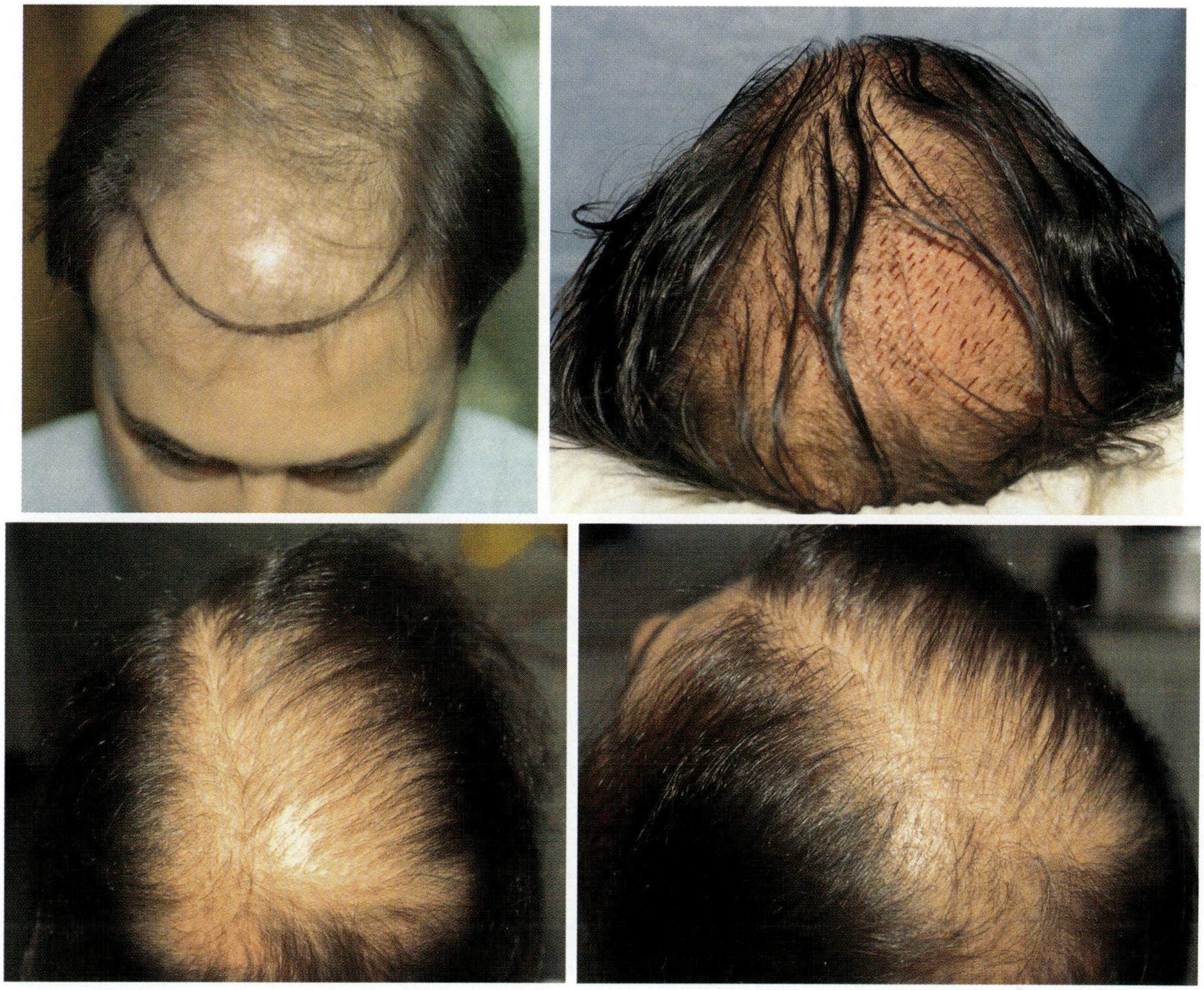

FIG. 15-23

A, Before hair transplanting. **B,** The same patient shown in the middle of a session in which 111 laser recipient sites had been made on the right side of his mid scalp and a comparable number of conventional slit grafts on the left side of his mid scalp. (Hair anterior to these sites had been transplanted in previous sessions.) Note that the laser sites are more "slot"-like than "slit"-like. **C,** Seven months later the hair is shown growing in both conventionally and laser treated sites. The right side, which had been prepared with an UltraPulse laser (Lumenis, Santa Clara, CA), shows a more even, slightly denser looking, and more natural looking growth of hair than the left side that had been conventionally prepared. **D,** A different view taken at the same time as **C** showing the denser, more even coverage on the laser-treated side and the somewhat "stringy" lighter coverage on the conventionally treated side. Unfortunately, such results were not consistently seen with laser transplanting.

cised varies with (1) the degree of natural scalp laxity and (2) the extent of surgical undermining or (3) the amount of prior stretching of the hair-bearing rim or "biological creep" created by scalp expansion or extension prior to AR. The larger the area that can be removed, the smaller the remaining area of alopecia will be, with the result that fewer grafts will be required to transplant it.[41] In general I recommend that AR be employed any time the objective of the patient is complete coverage of frontal, midthird, and vertex alopecia. The more AR that is done, the more likely it becomes that one will not run out of available donor tissue before the entire area of alopecia is treated.

In some persons another important function of AR is to raise the superior border of the hair-bearing temporal and parietal areas. If the patient intends to use "a part," for aesthetic reason it should begin at a line drawn vertically from the lateral canthus of the eye or at some point medial to this. If the anterior superior most point of the temporal hair is inferior to where the part line should aesthetically begin, the part will therefore pass through transplanted areas. This is less optimal than having a part pass through nature's higher-density perfectly even distribution of hair that would occur if the temporal and parietal areas could be raised to the appropriate location.

There has been a great deal of debate in the medical community as to whether a significant amount of the gain obtained with an AR is subsequently lost as the scalp laxity returns postoperatively. I cannot state strongly enough that although some stretchback is a component of every AR, the ultimate benefits obtained will always far outweigh the stretchback that may occur postoperatively *if the AR has been carried out properly,* and stretchback can be virtually nonexistent if "anchoring sutures" are utilized.

A variety of AR patterns have been described, but the most common patterns employed are the ellipse, inverted Y, and more recently, a flattened S shape.[41] The inverted Y pattern should be used if one anticipates insufficient donor tissue to transplant the entire bald area even after AR. This design prevents the production of scar in the areas that cannot later be covered with transplanted hair. Usually AR is carried out after the first two transplants have been completed. But occasionally AR will be done before any transplanting is started. This will occur most often in the following situations:

- There is a great deal of scalp laxity, making it likely that the shape of the hairline will be significantly altered by the AR.
- The area of alopecia is particularly large and therefore requires several ARs to raise the superior border of the temporoparietal hair to an appropriate level.
- The crown is the recipient area and the patient is relatively young and might need the grafts saved by the AR for other areas of future alopecia (Fig. 15-24).
- One is correcting poorly planned transplanting in which new areas of alopecia have developed without sufficient donor grafts having been left to treat them.
- One is treating large areas of cicatricial alopecia.

Technique. AR is usually carried out on an outpatient basis under sterile conditions. The patient is given 15 to 20 mg of oral diazepam 30 minutes prior to surgery. The pattern to be excised is drawn out using a marker such as a Micropoint Super Marker and the outline is then infiltrated with 2% lidocaine with 1:100,000 epinephrine. The same solution is used to produce a circle of anesthesia around the circumference of the head inferior to the expected extent of undermining.

If the pattern is an ellipse or a variant of an ellipse, an incision is made down to and through the galea along one side of its entire length, usually in a staged fashion, stopping to control bleeding with cautery where required. Care is taken to angle the blade so as not to injure any adjacent follicles, and if previously transplanted grafts are nearby, a 2 mm margin of safety is utilized.

Mayo scissors are used to undermine between the periosteum and galea aponeurotica, which is then completed to at least 10 cm or more on either side by blunt figure dissection. There is usually little bleeding encountered during this stage of the surgery except in the vertex area, where two or more perforators are frequently transected and must be ligated or cauterized.

The amount of redundant scalp tissue is estimated by overlapping the tissues, followed by perpendicular in-

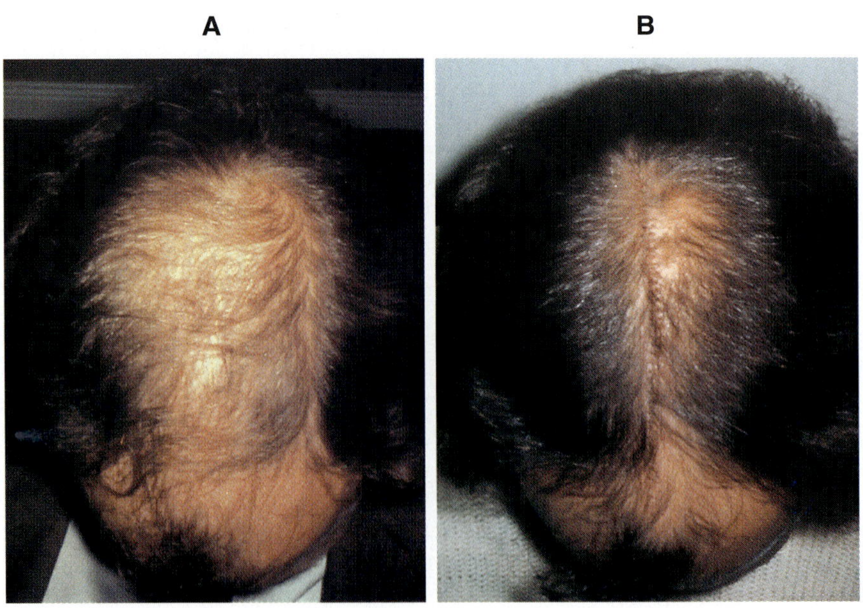

FIG. 15-24
A, Patient before alopecia reduction (AR). This person had an extraordinarily lax scalp. **B,** The same patient immediately after a single AR. Note that virtually the entire bald area has been removed. In this person, AR was carried out before any transplanting because it was anticipated that any hairline that had been transplanted prior to AR would be significantly altered by the AR because of his marked scalp laxity. More commonly AR is carried out after the first or second transplant session to the frontal third to half of the area of MPB. (Courtesy Martin Unger, MD, Toronto, Ontario.)

cisions made through the top flap stopping at the points where the flaps meet. The perpendicular points are then joined by a linear incision and the excess tissue is thereby removed. If the AR is done in the shape of an inverted Y—a far more common pattern than the ellipse—each "arm" of the Y is treated as a separate ellipse.

ARs are closed in two layers using interrupted 2-0 Dexon or Vicryl sutures for the galea and running 4-0 chromic catgut sutures for the skin.

Many names have been used for what I refer to as "major reductions." These include bilateral occipital parietal flaps and bilateral temporal flaps.[42] Major reductions are distinguished from the standard AR described above by more extensive undermining involving the severing of temporal, postauricular, and occipital arteries and nerves bilaterally as part of the undermining process. Although the efficacy of these procedures in excising substantial areas of alopecia is beyond question, the morbidity and relative safety of carrying them out has caused a great deal of discussion among physicians and has limited their use. When carried out by experienced and skillful surgeons, however, surgical complications are uncommon.

In AR preceded by soft tissue expansion, specially designed balloonlike tissue expanders are inserted as a separate procedure, usually 6 weeks to 3 months prior to a planned AR.[43] They are then gradually inflated with injections of saline every 1 to 2 weeks. At the end of approximately 6 weeks to 3 months the expanders are removed and the AR is carried out at the same time (Fig. 15-25). The use of such expanders has enabled physicians to excise as much as 10 to 12 cm of alopecia with one AR. Unfortunately, the cosmetic disability caused by the gradually inflated expanders has almost completely limited tissue expansion prior to AR to individuals with cicatricial alopecia. Unger has described a variation of tissue expansion prior to AR that he has termed a "PATE" reduction.[44] The acronym PATE stands for *p*rolonged *a*cute *t*issue *e*xpansion. In this procedure the surgery is similar to that described for a standard AR except that a tissue expander is inserted under the galea, the wound is closed, and while the scalp is still anesthetized the expander is repeatedly filled with saline to a preselected pressure over a period of 1 to 2 hours. This produces "mechanical creep" and enough tissue laxity, once the expanders have been removed, to allow for the excision of nearly double the amount of tissue that could formerly be excised with a standard AR.

Despite the obvious advantages of AR, a large number of patients and physicians refuse to consider AR as a component of treatment because of unsatisfactory prior experience or the overwhelming amount of information in the medical literature that is negative. As fully trained surgeons and plastic surgeons begin hair restoration surgery, the popularity of this procedure is likely to increase, because the benefits for someone who wants maximum coverage is undeniable.

Scalp Extension

In 1993 Frechet described a procedure in which a Silastic sheet or "extender" with metal hooks at either end was stretched to double its original width and hooked into the underside of the galea beneath the left and right side "permanent" rim hair. This process was carried out as a component of an otherwise conventional elliptical AR. Over a period of approximately 30 days the Silastic sheet tried to revert to its original size, bringing both sides of fringe hair closer to each other in the process. During a second AR, after 30 days, he was able to remove twice the amount of alopecic skin usual in a conventional AR; another "extender" was often inserted to improve the results of a third AR that was carried out 30 days later. He called this technique "scalp extension" and typically was able to excise as much as

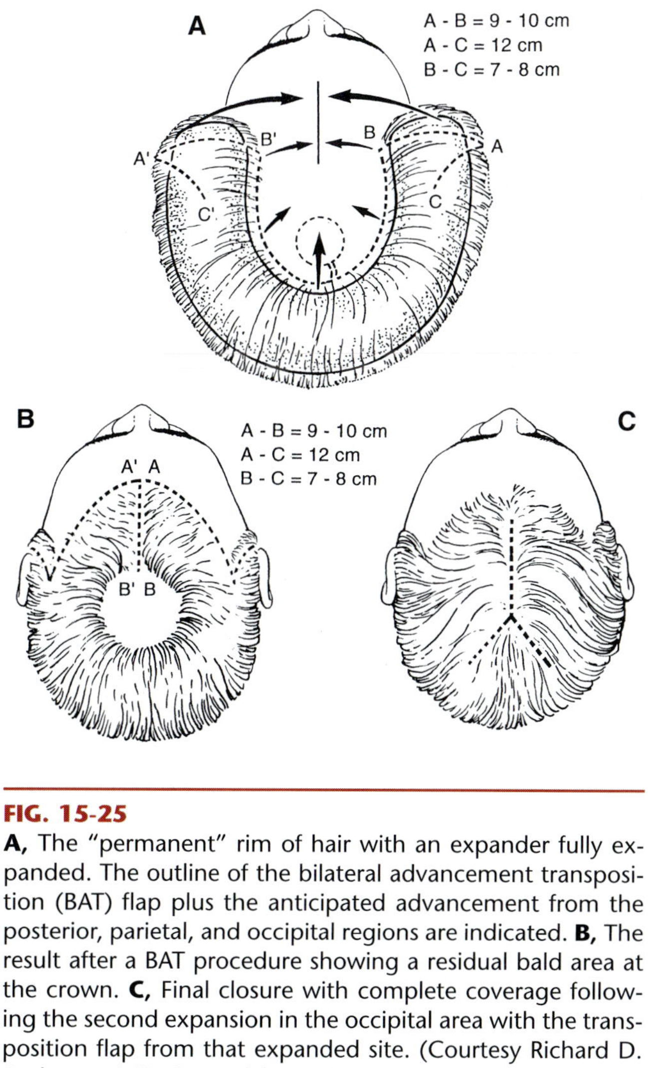

FIG. 15-25
A, The "permanent" rim of hair with an expander fully expanded. The outline of the bilateral advancement transposition (BAT) flap plus the anticipated advancement from the posterior, parietal, and occipital regions are indicated. **B,** The result after a BAT procedure showing a residual bald area at the crown. **C,** Final closure with complete coverage following the second expansion in the occipital area with the transposition flap from that expanded site. (Courtesy Richard D. Anderson, MD, Scottsdale, AZ.)

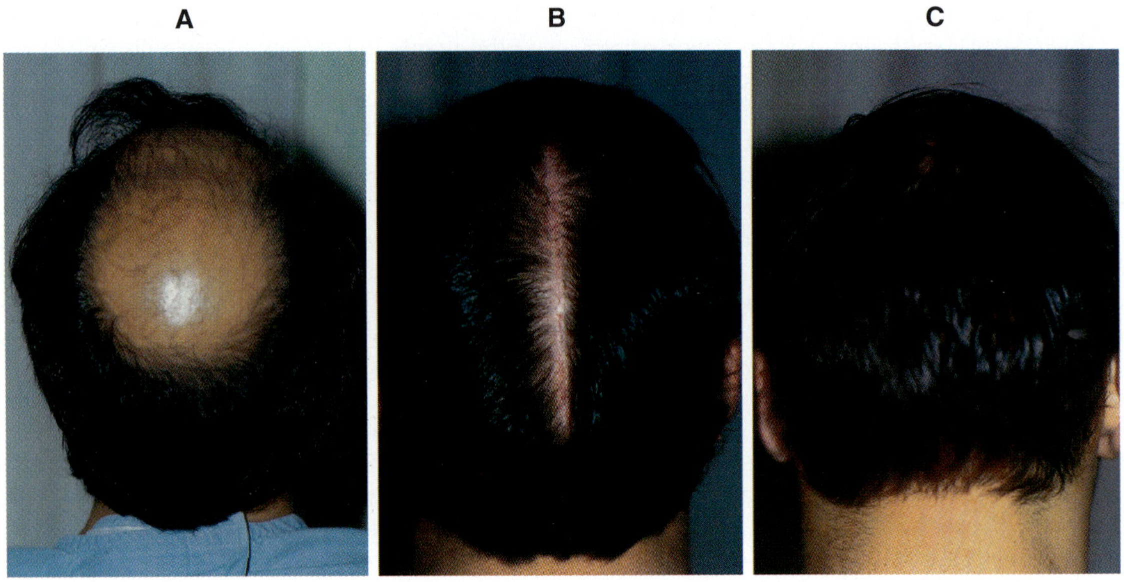

FIG. 15-26
A, Patient before scalp extension. **B,** Sixty days later, after three alopecia reductions and two scalp extensions. All of the alopecic area has been excised, intentionally creating the "slot" defect seen above. **C,** The same patient after a Frechet three-flap corrective procedure. Frechet now carries out this procedure as part of the final reduction, thus eliminating the need for another surgery. (Courtesy Patrick Frechet, MD, Paris, France.)

12 cm of alopecic skin in 60 days.[45] The object of scalp extension is the removal of "all" alopecic skin. The resulting abnormal hair direction is corrected by another type of surgery he described and called a "three-flap corrective procedure."[46]

Space does not allow a full description of the procedures here, but results are impressive (Fig. 15-26), and a more complete account of the techniques are easily found in the noted references.[45,46] I recently suggested that Frechet shorten his excision to stop just posterior to the middle of the vertex and limit his objectives to eliminating all but an approximately 5 cm wide area of alopecia. This would allow for a rapid major reduction in the area of alopecia while avoiding a slot defect that would require the technically demanding three-flap procedure that has deterred many from employing scalp extension.

Practical Approaches to the Vertex

Hair restoration surgery in the vertex area is, in my opinion, considerably more demanding than frontal hair transplanting. Hair direction and angling are far more difficult to mimic if there is existing hair or to create in a natural pattern if there is very little or none present. The whorl-like direction of hair allows for none of the usual benefits of overlapping hair that is seen frontally and in the middle third of the scalp. I utilize only FUs in the center of the whorl, where even the slightest plugginess or compression would be noted. The recipient area at that site is infiltrated with either saline or 1:50,000 epinephrine to produce maximum turgor and vasoconstriction so that the needle holes, once the infiltration has dissipated, will move closer together and produce greater hair density at that site. Excellent control of bleeding is particularly important in order to minimize trauma to the FUs during their insertion. Peripheral to the center of the whorl of the vertex, minislit grafts are used followed by small-slit grafts more peripheral to them (see Fig. 15-19). FUs are extensively used between all slit sites whether produced for minislits, small slits, or large slits. Unless hair characteristics are advantageous, few slot grafts or round grafts are used. Unless the patient is past middle age or has a particularly advantageous family history and physical findings, I do not transplant the posterior third of an area of alopecia unless the patient agrees to some type of AR as a component of the treatment plan. In addition, all patients are advised that because of natural hair direction there is little opportunity for overlapping of hair in the crown region and that therefore they should be prepared to accept the appearance of a somewhat lower density at that site. Fortunately, the vast majority of patients are satisfied with the appearance after one or two sessions of a combination of micrografting combined with slit grafting and minigrafting in the vertex area (see Fig. 15-19).

REFERENCES

1. Dieffenbach JF. Nonnulla de regeneratione et transplantatione. Disseration inauguralis, 1822.
2. Davis JS. Scalping accidents. Bull Johns Hopkins Hosp 1911; 16:257.
3. Okuda S. Klinische und experimentelle Untersuchungen über die Transplantation von lebenden Haaren [in Japanese]. Jpn J Dermatol 1939; 40:537.
4. Orentreich N. Autografts in alopecias and other selected dermatological conditions. Ann NY Acad Sci 1959; 83:463.
5. Unger W. The history of hair transplantation. Dermatol Surg 2000; 26:181-189.
6. Unger W. Hair transplantation and alopecia reduction. In: Freedberg IM, et al, eds. Fitzpatrick's Dermatology in General Medicine. 5th ed. New York: McGraw-Hill, 1999:2972-2980.
7. Beehner M. The frontal forelock: conception in hair transplantation. Am J Cosmet Surg 1997:125-132.
8. Marritt E, Dzubow L. A redefinition of male pattern baldness and its treatment implications. Dermatol Surg 1995; 21:123.
9. Dawber R, Van Neste D, eds. Androgenetic Alopecia in Hair and Scalp Disorders. London: Martin Dunitz, 1998:96-106.
10. Cotterill P. Application and approach to hair transplantation in females. Am J Cosmet Surg 1997:137-141.
11. Unger W, Knudsen R. General principles of recipient site organization and planning. In: Unger W, ed. Hair Transplantation. 3rd ed. New York: Marcel Dekker, 1995:105-158.
12. Rose P. It's not just a line: the subtleties of the hairline area. Sixth annual meeting of the International Society of Hair Restoration Surgery; September 16-20, 1998; Washington, DC.
13. Unger MG. The modified major scalp reduction. J Dermatol Surg Oncol 1988; 14:80.
14. Nordstrom R. "Stretch-back" in scalp reductions for male pattern baldness. Plast Reconstr Surg 1984; 3:422.
15. Unger MG. Alopecia reduction and stretchback. Clin Dermatol 1992; 10:345.
16. Hitzig GC, Sadick NS. A new technique for curvilinear scalp reduction. J Dermatol Surg Oncol 1989; 15:1108.
17. Seery GE. Anchor scalp reduction. Dermatol Surg 1996; 22:1009-1013.
18. Marritt E. The death of the density debate. Dermatol Surg 1999; 25:654-660.
19. Beehner M. Hair survival of FU grafts at World Hair Society Spring Live Workshop. Seventh annual meeting of the International Society of Hair Restoration Surgery; October 23, 1999; San Francisco.
20. Cole J. Graft dissection: loupes versus dissecting microscopes. Seventh annual meeting of the International Society of Hair Restoration Surgery; October 23, 1999; San Francisco.
21. Norwood O. Limmerization. Hair Transpl Forum Int 1996; 6:12.
22. Beehner M. A comparison of hair growth between follicular-unit grafts trimmed "skinny" vs. "chubby." Hair Transpl Forum Int 1999; 9:16.
23. Cole J. Mathematics of follicular hair transplantation. Sixth annual meeting of the International Society of Hair Restoration Surgery; September 16-20, 1998; Washington, DC.
24. Kaufman KD. Clinical studies on effects of oral Finasteride. In: Van Neste D, Randall VA, eds. Hair Research for the Next Millennium. Amsterdam: Elsevier Science, 1996:363-365.
25. Olsen EA, Weiner MS, Amara IA, DeLong ER. Five-year follow-up of men with androgenetic alopecia treated with topical minoxidil. J Am Acad Dermatol 1990; 22:643-646.
26. Orfanos CE, Vogels L. Lokaltherepie der Alopecia Androgenetica mit 17a Ostradiol. Dermatologica 1980; 161:124-132.
27. Manuskiatti W, Fitzpatrick RE, Goldman MP, Krejci-Papa N. Prophylactic antibiotics in patients undergoing laser resurfacing of the skin. J Am Acad Dermatol 1999; 40:77-84.
28. Unger W. Anesthesia. In: Unger W, ed. Hair Transplantation. 3rd ed. New York: Marcel Dekker, 1995:165-181.
29. Unger W. The donor site. In: Unger W, ed. Hair Transplantation. 3rd ed. New York: Marcel Dekker, 1995:183-187.
30. Headington JT. Transverse microscopic anatomy of the human scalp. Arch Dermatol 1984; 120:449-456.
31. Norwood O. Kudos. Hair Transpl Forum Int 1997; 7:9-11.
32. Gandelman M, Abrahamson PA. Light and electron microscopic analysis of controlled crushing injury of micrografts. Abstract from 1997 annual meeting of the ISHRS. Dermatol Surg 1998; 24: 789.
33. Mayer MA. Follicular regeneration. Sixth annual meeting of the International Society of Hair Restoration Surgery; September 17, 1998; Washington, DC.
34. Unger W. The telogen war: the "condemned" replies. Hair Transpl Forum Int 1999; 9:22-24.
35. Bernstein R, Rassman W. The logic of follicular unit transplantation. Dermatol Clin 1999; 17:277-296.
36. Unger W. Different grafts for different purposes. Am J Cosmet Surg 1997; 14:177-183.
37. Unger W. The recipient area. In: Unger W, ed. Hair Transplantation. 3rd ed. New York: Marcel Dekker, 1995:215-321.
38. Unger W. Treatment for baldness. In: Aston S, Beasley R, Thorne C, eds. Grabb and Smith's Plastic Surgery. 5th ed. Philadelphia: Lippincott-Raven, 1977:569-585.
39. Unger W. Laser hair transplanting. Am J Cosmet Surg 1997; 14: 143-148.
40. Hitzig G. Linear (slot) grafting: my 3-year retrospective. Hair Transpl Forum Int 1998; 8:22-23.
41. Unger M. Scalp reduction. In: Unger W, ed. Hair Transplantation. 3rd ed. New York: Marcel Dekker, 1995:509-569.
42. Brandy DA. New various approaches for the treatment of extensive baldness. Am J Cosmet Surg 1990; 7:129-139.
43. Anderson R. New expanded scalp flap techniques for elimination of male pattern baldness. In: Unger W, ed. Hair Transplantation. 3rd ed. New York: Marcel Dekker, 1995:673-691.
44. Unger M. Prolonged acute tissue expansion (PATE). Am J Cosmet Surg 1995; 12:231-240.
45. Frechet P. Scalp extension. In: Unger W, ed. Hair Transplantation. 3rd ed. New York: Marcel Dekker, 1995:662-642.
46. Frechet P. Occipito-frontal transposition flap combined with scalp extension for extensive baldness. Int J Cosmet Surg 1998; 6:50-56.

CHAPTER 16

Soft Tissue Augmentation

MADELINE KRAUSS
ARNOLD WILLIAM KLEIN

SECTION ONE

History and Scientific Review

BACKGROUND AND HISTORY

Patients frequently come to dermatologists, and physicians of other specialties, in search of cosmetic improvement. Magazine articles, television news stories, and advertisements fuel patients' interest and have made aesthetic procedures more socially acceptable than previously. Many practitioners are becoming trained in cosmetic surgery and are offering these services as part of their office practice. Courses in cosmetic surgery techniques are becoming extremely popular at medical meetings. Soft tissue augmentation has become increasingly important as more individuals seek aesthetic improvement without major surgery or significant recuperation time.

Much of the reinterest in filling agents stems from success with Botox (Allergan, Irvine, CA) in rejuvenating the upper face. The dichotomy between a youthful-appearing upper face and an older-looking lower face is aesthetically unappealing, however. Soft tissue augmentation in combination with Botox provides physicians with the ability to treat the entire face.

The rebellion against the two-dimensional look of the overpulled face is also fueling renewed interest in filler substances. The youthful face has a much fuller look, not a tight, flat appearance. Many patients prefer to obtain this more natural effect with augmentation, rather than subject themselves to a major surgical procedure possibly resulting in an unnatural result. Additionally, affordable outpatient surgery has replaced much of the expensive hospital-based surgery. Less-invasive techniques provide a catalogue of therapeutic options for the multitudes.

In keeping with the public's quest to appear more youthful, the desire for lip enhancement is here to stay. Perioral rejuvenation is the Number 1 indication for injectable fillers. Soft tissue augmentation allows us to achieve this goal without the risk of significant scarring, further stimulating interest in this area.

As a result of the foregoing developments, we have seen a renaissance of interest in tissue augmentation. Today, physicians have a much larger armamentarium of techniques and implant materials with which to improve facial contours, ameliorate wrinkles, and stall the telltale signs of the aging face. Although the perfect material has continued to elude us, more and more viable options have become available. We must heed the lessons of the past, however, when choosing what should and should not be implanted in our patients. Only with time and experience will we be able to determine which of these substances deserve a position of importance in our aesthetic armamentarium.

The history of modern soft tissue augmentation begins in the late 1800s. Injectable fat is the oldest material used for tissue augmentation.[1,2] In the early part of the twentieth century, free fat grafts were used for tissue augmentation until the technique was displaced by the use of pedicle flaps and the subsequent use of paraffin and silicone as filling agents.[3-5]

The use of injectable paraffin became popular during the early 1900s. The high incidence of undesirable foreign body granuloma formation caused paraffin to be abandoned prior to 1920[6,7]except in the Orient, where its use persisted into the 1960s.[8] Despite initial failures, the need for a successful material for soft tissue augmentation motivated investigation of autologous, allogenic, xenogenic, and synthetic substances for this purpose.

Synthetic materials have been heavily investigated because they are not resorbed, can be manufactured to fill particular surgical needs, reduce operating time of harvesting and donor site morbidity, and are available in adequate supply. The history of silicone implantation began in the 1940s with attempts to augment the breasts in Latin America and the Orient.[9] Adulterated forms abounded, most often administered by nonphysicians, including combinations with olive oil and paraffin to induce fibrous encapsulation. An investigational new drug application was granted in 1965 to Dow Corning for medical grade, sterile, purified silicone. In the hands of qualified medical personnel, particularly those involved in the trials, microinjections of small volumes of medical grade silicone induced a self-limited fibroblastic response with collagen deposition. The technique was very useful in eradication of depressed scars, rhytides, hemifacial atrophy,[10] and even for cushioning between bony prominences and corns.[11]

A number of issues involving silicone breast implants, as well as injections, received great attention. These included anecdotal reports of human adjuvant connective tissue disease,[12,13] and proven migration of silicone to synovium, skin, and alveolar macrophages.[14] Even medical grade silicone has resulted in chronic inflammatory reactions[15] and swelling requiring persistent systemic steroids.[16] Nonmedical grade silicone has been reported to cause severe fibrotic reactions,[17] ulceration,[18,19] granulomatous hepatitis, and even death,[20] although silicone has never been shown to be carcinogenic.[10] Because of myriad concerns, the Food and Drug Administration revoked its authorization for investigational cosmetic use of silicone for injection. Solid silicone rubber implants have a great deal less surface area and less tendency for shedding of small particles than do breast implants or microinjections, and they are still in frequent use today.

Difficult lessons have been learned from other synthetic materials. Proplast (Dupont, Wilmington, DE) is a combination of porous graphite combined with Teflon (polytetrafluoroethylene or PTFE), widely used in the 1980s. Temporomandibular joint implants were created from Proplast, but these were unable to withstand the tremendous physical stresses placed on them over time. Erosion and small-particle shedding caused macrophages to ingest Proplast particles between 20 and 60 μm and then die with release of intracellular enzymes, leading to chronic inflammation and eventually absorption of surrounding bone.[21] Severe sequelae resulted for some patients with these implants, and all eventually required surgical removal.

The image and reputation of synthetic materials in soft tissue augmentation was bolstered by successful reports of the use of expanded polytetrafluoroethylene (ePTFE) or Gore-Tex (W. L. Gore, Flagstaff, AZ) for aesthetic enhancement. Three decades of historical data have proven its safety in humans for other indications. It is commonly used today in soft tissue augmentation, enhancement of bony prominences, and in general and vascular surgery.

The most important development in soft tissue augmentation in the twentieth century has been the introduction of an easy-to-use xenograft. Injectable bovine collagen has been in use in the United States since 1977.[22] In July 1981, Zyderm Collagen Implant (McGhan, Santa Barbara, CA) received FDA approval. This was the first time an FDA-approved injectable device was available for soft tissue augmentation. This approval renewed interest in the entire field of filling substances.

In the years since approval of the first form of injectable collagen, information regarding new products, techniques, and indications has continued to be promulgated at an ever-increasing pace. This process will continue as newer techniques and filler substances become available and existing materials are reevaluated.

BASIC SCIENCE

One of the visible consequences of time, smoking, sun exposure, and gravity is a loss of dermal collagen in the skin, with resulting wrinkle formation. Patients often seek cosmetic procedures to eradicate the signs of aging that appear on the part of the body most seen by others: the face. Age-related changes of the lips and mouth include atrophy of both the upper and lower lips, actinic changes of the mucosal surface and vermilion border, and atrophy at the corners of the mouth with resulting downturn. Subtle improvements in the lips and their surrounding tissue can produce astounding results by rebuilding the perioral structure and producing a more youthful, rested look. Another early sign of aging is the development of nasolabial lines and folds. Filler substances to reduce or eradicate these furrows produce excellent results unattainable even by cervicofacial rhytidectomy.

Wrinkles come in various shapes and sizes, and treatment needs to be specifically tailored to the anatomy of the individual region.[23] Failure to determine the precise cause and depth of a wrinkle will put the physician at a distinct disadvantage before treatment is ever begun. Fine, superficial rhytides respond best to therapy at the intradermal level. Deeper, more substantial wrinkles typically have a subcutaneous component, with or without a muscular element, and are best approached from the subcutaneous space. Oftentimes a wrinkle will have both a superficial and deep component, as in the nasolabial fold, and both of these components need to be addressed to obtain optimal results.

Rhytides in the upper one third of the face are largely dynamic in nature. They are the result of muscle movement, as opposed to sun damage and chronological aging alone. Therefore glabellar furrows, forehead creases, and crow's feet are best treated by botulinum toxin (Botox) injections as first-line therapy. It is impossible to properly discuss rhytide therapy without Botox as a central component. An understanding of the anatomy of wrinkles will help the physician to determine whether botulinum toxin alone will do the job. Combining Botox therapy with resurfacing or filler substances can dramatically improve efficacy.

Once the physician has evaluated a patient's facial anatomy and goals, the choice of procedure will follow. If soft tissue augmentation is the best means of attaining aesthetic improvement, alone or in conjunction with other procedures, the selection of an appropriate implant must ensue. This choice requires a thorough understanding of the materials available and their specific risks and benefits. No available material is best for all patients, or all indications.

The ideal filler substance must have both a high "use" potential, producing pleasing cosmetic results with a minimum of untoward reactions, and a low "abuse" potential, such that widespread and possibly incorrect or indiscriminate use should not result in significant morbidity.[24] The material should be natural looking, nonpalpable, and able to provide adequate correction without migration. The agent must provide proven and predictable results through reproducible implantation techniques. There should be minimal risk and recuperation time from the procedure itself, no significant donor morbidity, and no risk of infectious agents harbored within the implant. The ideal filler must be noncarcinogenic, nonimmunogenic, and unable to cause a chronic inflammatory reaction. In addition, it should be cost-effective with adequate quantities available and have a conveniently long shelf life. If not autologous, the substance, agent, or device should be FDA approved.

The duration of correction with any filling substance depends on multiple factors. The material implanted, procedural technique, amount utilized, type of defect, and mechanical stresses at the insertion site all influence persistence of correction. The ideal filler should be biodegradable but long lasting enough to avoid frequent touch-up procedures despite the listed variables. If permanent, the material should be retrievable in the event of overcorrection, misplacement, or migration.

Autografts are obtained from a patient for use in the same patient. The advantage of autogenous grafts is their excellent safety profile. There is decreased risk of nosocomial infection and no possibility of rejection. However, there is often significant donor site morbidity, limited quantity, and frequent resorption of autografts utilized for soft tissue augmentation. Fat is a good alternative for the patient with deep furrows or hollows who desires minimum recuperation time, does not mind the need for multiple procedures, and understands that there may not be permanent improvement. Autologous dermis or Autologen are options when excess skin is available from concurrent procedures such as rhytidectomy and abdominoplasty.

Allografts are derived from another individual of the same species. This category of implant has received new attention with materials obtained from banked dermis and fascia. These extensively treated materials now can adequately ensure against transfer of pathogens and also prevent the rejection previously seen with nonprocessed tissue. AlloDerm, Cymetra, and Fascian have renewed interest in this category of solid and injectable fillers.

Xenografts are derived from other species and have the risk of allergic reaction by the human recipient. Bovine collagen is the most prevalent example of this type of implant. In the future, recombinant human collagen may replace the bovine, as it would carry no risk of allergic reaction, will not require skin tests, and cannot harbor animal pathogens such as the feared spongiform encephalitis. Hyaluronic acid is identical across species but its derivatives may be produced from animal sources or via fermentation.

The search for the perfect material to eradicate rhytides, smooth scars, and fill traumatic defects continues. Many options are adequate for a given task, satisfy patients, and offer excellent safety profiles. New products appear, sometimes with great fanfare, and often fail to fulfill the promise of a better alternative to what we use now. For this reason, an in-depth understanding of implant materials is necessary for any physician performing soft-tissue augmentation procedures.

CLINICAL STUDIES AND REVIEW OF MATERIALS

The list of filling substances has increased in length and breadth from about five substances a decade ago to an encyclopedia of agents available today. To choose among the plethora of available fillers, the physician must first determine the defect. This will define the substance. A very deep nasolabial furrow may be best treated with autologous fat, but a more superficial nasolabial crease will require Zyderm I or II, possibly layered over Zyplast collagen. A physician's comfort level with a particular augmentation tool must also be taken into account. Author Klein's experience has focused on the use of bovine collagen, particularly in conjunction with Botox. Where others might not use collagen for a particular defect, a physician with a high level of mastery may achieve optimum augmentation with this agent. Prior to the procedure, physicians must counsel patients as to the risks and benefits of the filler substance to be implanted or injected. Skin testing, recuperation time, treatment expectations, and alternatives must be fully reviewed.

Box 16-1 is a list of agents available worldwide, although new products are continually emerging. In the United States, Zyderm and Zyplast collagen are the most popular substances used for soft tissue augmentation. Other materials in use include autologous fat, AlloDerm, Autologen, Dermalogen, Fascian, Gore-Tex, and SoftForm. In Europe and Canada, hyaluronic acid

BOX 16-1 Filling Agent

AcHyal (hyaluronic acid)
AlloDerm (acellular dermal allograft)
Artecoll (PMMA and collagen)
Arteplast (PMMA)
Autologen (autologous collagen)
Biocell Ultravital (silicium)
Bioplastique (silicone rubber)
Cymetra (micronized AlloDerm)
Dermal Grafting (autologous dermis)
Dermalive (hyaluronic acid and acrylic)
Dermalogen (human collagen matrix)
Endoplast-50 (elastin peptides, collagen)
Fascian (freeze-dried human fascia lata)
Fat (autologous)
Fibrel (porcine gelatin)
Gore-Tex (ePTFE)
Human Placental Collagen
Hylaform Gel (hyaluronic acid)
Hylan Rofilan Gel (hyaluronic acid)
Isolagen (autologous fibroblasts)
Koken Atelocollagen (bovine collagen)
Meta Crill (PMMA)
New-fill (polylactic acid)
Perlane (hyaluronic acid)
Permacol (porcine collagen sheets)
Plasmagel (autologous plasma)
PMS-350 (silicone)
Profill (synthetic copolymer)
Recombinant Human Collagen
Resoplast (bovine collagen)
Restylane (hyaluronic acid)
  Restylane-fine
Reviderm-intra (dextran beads)
Silicone (illegal in United States)
  Adatosil-5000
  Silikon-1000
SoftForm (ePTFE)
Zyderm and Zyplast Collagen (bovine collagen)

derivatives such as Restylane and Hylaform gel are ubiquitous, but not yet FDA approved for sale in the United States.

AcHyal (not FDA approved)

AcHyal is a 1% solution of the sodium salt of hyaluronic acid. It is provided in 2.5 cc prefilled syringes with 30-gauge needles. It can be stored at room temperature and has a shelf life of 3 years. Indications are wrinkles, scars, and lip and contour deformities. Adverse reactions are listed as reddening, inflammation, or bruising, which generally dissipate in 2 to 3 days. There is no experience with the material in the United States. It is manufactured by Tedec Meiji Farma, S.A. Ctra. M-300, KM 30,500 28802, Alcalá de Henares, Madrid, Spain.

AlloDerm (FDA approved for reconstruction)

AlloDerm acellular dermal allograft is a solid material for soft tissue augmentation derived from screened cadavers. Tissue is obtained from American Association of Tissue Banks regulated sources, then treated with a series of detergents to destroy cellular components and their associated targets of rejection, the major histocompatibility antigens. Additional viral deactivation steps are employed. The resulting material is then freeze dried by a technique that spares the protein matrix of the dermis, including intact collagen, elastin, lamina densa, and glycosaminoglycans. The resulting acellular dermal graft comes in sheets up to 1 mm thick and of varying sizes, and may be kept refrigerated for 2 years.

AlloDerm was first used in conjunction with very thin split-thickness skin grafts in third-degree burn patients. Excellent functional and cosmetic results were realized from decreased wound contracture. Harvesting thinner skin grafts limited hypertrophic scarring, pain, and infection in the donor site.[25,26]

After rewarding experiences with AlloDerm in burn patients, interest quickly turned to its use in reconstructive and cosmetic procedures. The dermal allograft is easy to cut and can be stacked, rolled, and folded into an appropriate shape for many indications. Once implanted, it is quickly revascularized, does not have the tendency for extrusion as do firmer synthetic materials such as Gore-Tex (ePTFE), and is not rejected. In 1996, Jones et al reported successful results of AlloDerm use in revision rhinoplasty, lip augmentation, glabellar contouring, and scar revision.[27] At follow-up from 2 to 12 months, 1 of 25 patients experienced graft resorption in the lower lip. Minimal postoperative discomfort was noted. Three suture site infections were associated with attempts to anchor the implant to the cutaneous entry and exit sites, and all cleared with oral antibiotics and trimming of the implant, without requiring implant removal. In another series, Achauer et al treated 11 children and adults with scarring or soft tissue defects.[28] Mean follow-up was 13 months with no graft mobilization, absorption, rejection, or extrusion seen. The author emphasized the distinct advantage of avoiding donor site surgery in the pediatric population.

Lip augmentation has always been a challenging area in aesthetic surgery. Mucosal advancements and excisional lip lifts may increase vermilion show, but at the risk of visible scarring and significant recuperation time. The mobility and vascularity of the lips is thought to decrease the longevity of bovine collagen and autologous fat injected into the perioral region. Patients are keenly aware of the palpability of any foreign material in this area as well, leading to dissatisfaction in some individuals with synthetic Gore-Tex implants. Tobin and Karas followed 12 patients with AlloDerm lip augmentation from 3 to 12 months after implantation.[29] All patients were pleased with the results of surgery. Induration resolved by 3 months. The authors suggested that 20% shrinkage in the graft was to be expected over 4 to 6 weeks with subsequent stabilization of correction.

Castor et al attempted to quantify vermilion show in patients undergoing AlloDerm implantation submucosally in conjunction with intramuscular fat transplantation, compared with fat transplantation alone.[30] They used digital imaging to demonstrate a 61% increase in vermilion show with combination treatment at 3-month follow-up compared with only 13% in fat transplantation alone. Resorption was not seen beyond 1 month in the combination group. Larger, long-term studies on the use of AlloDerm in soft tissue augmentation have not yet been published.

Advantages of the material include its lack of allergenicity, immunogenicity, and foreign body reaction. There are no reports of extrusion, migration, or cyst formation. Although some resorption may occur, and patients must be warned of this, the great majority of patients appear to have stable results that may prove permanent. The integration of the implant into host tissue allows the surgeon to repeat the procedure in the future for more augmentation without having to manipulate around, or remove, synthetic implants. The material also has a long shelf life, allowing a physician to keep it on hand to use as needed. Contraindications to AlloDerm include an infected or avascular recipient site, allergy to gentamicin used in storing the material, and collagen vascular disease.

AlloDerm's uses are increasing as more specialties are exposed to its advantages over autologous and synthetic tissue. Periodontists now may employ AlloDerm for reexpansion of keratinized gingival tissue, avoiding the need for painful tissue harvesting from the palate.[31] Acellular dermal matrix is helpful in septal perforation repair and reconstruction, facilitating the procedure by eliminating the need for autologous temporalis fascia or mastoid periosteum.[32] Animal studies have shown promise in utilizing AlloDerm for neonatal diaphragmatic hernia repair[33] and as a dural replacement instead of autologous pericranium.[34]

AlloDerm can be an important tool in developing an in vitro skin substitute in conjunction with cultured keratinocytes. Potential clinical use includes wound management, closure of surgical defects, and treatment of genetic bullous diseases such as epidermolysis bullosa simplex (EBS).[35,36] Further work will be directed to see if stem cells harvested from patients with EBS or similar disorders can be genetically manipulated with a wild type keratin gene, grown in specific conditions on AlloDerm, and grafted back to the patient. If these stem cells have a growth advantage over cells with defective keratin genes, the potential for effective treatment of these debilitating genetic disorders may be in sight. Oral keratinocytes have been successfully cultured on acellular dermis as an ex vivo mucosa equivalent.[37]

AlloDerm is manufactured by LifeCell Corporation, The Woodlands, TX, and has a corporate office at 1 Millennium Way, Branchburg, NJ 08876-3876. Tel 800-367-5737. Website: www.lifecell.com

Artecoll and Arteplast (not FDA approved)

Resoplast is monomolecular bovine collagen. Arteplast is a vehicle containing polymethylmethacrylate (PMMA) microspheres, also known as Plexiglas or Lucite beads. Artecoll is a combination of the two. PMMA is used extensively in medicine for bone cement, dentures, and artificial eye lenses. Polymerized PMMA is formed into smooth-surfaced spheres 30 to 40 μm in diameter and then suspended in the vehicle. The collagen serves as a bridge for the deposition of the beads and is eventually degraded with permanent deposition of PMMA. Company literature claims that the microspheres will be encapsulated within 2 to 4 months after injection and that these nonbiodegradable particles are too large and smooth to be phagocytized and thus cannot migrate.

Gottfried Lemperle, the developer of Artecoll, and colleagues published results of a prospective study in 118 patients.[38] Overall, 90% of patients who answered a survey were satisfied with the result of treatment, with 64% reporting striking and lasting improvement (follow-up approximately 2 years). Another 10% reported no improvement or adverse side effects. Swelling, redness, and moderate pain were common over the first few days. Longer-lasting redness occurred when the injection was too superficial. Itching in an unspecified number of patients subsided within weeks or months. Some patients with lip augmentation reported pain in the cold and lip tightness. Two patients required surgical removal of hypertrophic scars after dorsal lip augmentation. Other studies[39,40] have disputed Lemperle's results, and some authors claim that particles of this size can be phagocytized, with the subsequent death of the engulfing macrophage and release of enzymes leading to a chronic inflammatory response. Lemperle states that this is less likely given the smooth surface of PMMA microspheres.

There have also been problems reported with the collagen vehicle used for this product.[39] The collagen was found to have nonhelical molecules subject to rapid degradation in vitro. Other impurities from the manufacturing process were also found in the vehicle.

Artecoll is injected deeply with a 27-gauge needle at the junction between dermis and subcutaneous fat and can be molded with finger-tip pressure. According to the manufacturer, it is indicated for deeper wrinkles and furrows, deep glabellar furrows, nasolabial lines, perioral lines, radial lip lines, lip and philtrum augmentation, scar revision, and other dermal, subdermal, and osseous defects. Patients must be skin tested for allergy to bovine collagen prior to use. It is contraindicated in patients who form keloids, who have atrophic skin diseases, and who have very thin, flaccid skin because of the risk of permanent superficial irregularities. Nodularity in the lip may be palpable indefinitely after augmentation.

The product is manufactured and distributed by Rofil Medical International B.V., Stationstaat 1B, 4815 NC Breda, The Netherlands. Tel 31-76-531-5670, Fax 31-76-531-5660. In the United States, Rofil Medical USA, Inc., 7500 Hudson Blvd., Suite # 130, Oakdale, MN 55128.

Autologen

Autologen is true autologous collagen. It is a sterile suspension of intact collagen fibers prepared from a patient's own tissue. Harvested skin is forwarded to the manufacturer for processing into a suspended autologous fibrillar material. The prefilled syringes contain a solution of approximately 3.5% collagen, the maximum concentration easily extruded through a 30-gauge needle. Three square inches of skin produces 1 ml of Autologen within these parameters. Individual concentrations can be formulated at the physician's request.

Autologen may be used for fine lines, wrinkles, depressions, and lip augmentation. In the past, the material was very difficult to extrude, easily leading to hand fatigue in the physician. The present formulation is much more injectable than previously and does give persistent, predictable correction when placed in the proper position in the dermis. The material cannot be placed quite as superficially as Zyderm I, but if it is placed deeply like Zyplast, it is ineffective. Autologen has been used in 1100 individuals. The manufacturer states there is a greater longevity of correction than with bovine collagen because its autologous composition retards degradation. Controlled studies are not available.

To produce Autologen, skin is harvested from the patient (preferably from a procedure such as rhytidectomy or abdominoplasty), stored in a freezer for up to 2 weeks, and shipped to Collagenesis (address below). Storage is $250 per year. When needed, the material is ordered. The resultant syringes can be refrigerated at 2° to 8°C for up to 6 months. The current cost is $1095 for processing each batch. A 27- or 30-gauge needle is used to inject, although author Klein uses only a 30-gauge needle with eutectic mixture of local anesthetic. Manufactured by Collagenesis, Inc., 500 Cummings Center, Beverly, MA 01915. Tel 800-411-9440. Website: www.collagenesis.com

Biocell Ultravital (not FDA approved)

Also known as Biopolymere III, this product was developed in Switzerland and contains Silicium (a derivative of silicon). According to the manufacturer, there is no need for allergy tests prior to treatment and results may be permanent. It is commonly used in South America. It is distributed by Biocell Laboratoires, CH 593 Vaduz, Lichtenstein.

Bioplastique (not FDA approved)

Bioplastique is a suspension of textured solid vulcanized methylsiloxane rubber particles from 100 to 400 μm in size suspended in a carrier vehicle of biocompatible plasdone hydrogel. It is an investigational material for soft tissue augmentation with a controlled foreign body response. The large size of the particles reportedly reduces migration. Several reports of granulomas in the lips requiring excision have been reported.[41] Therefore, it was suggested that the material may be better suited for augmenting areas with bone contact such as the chin and dorsum of the nose. Because of the controversy and resultant bad press surrounding silicone gel implants, it is unlikely to be FDA approved. It is used in Europe and Australia, particularly for injection into the bladder neck for female stress incontinence.[42] Bioplastique is manufactured by Uroplasty, Inc., Minneapolis, MN. Website: www.uroplasty.com

Cymetra (FDA status identical to AlloDerm)

Cymetra is micronized AlloDerm produced by a cryofracturing process. The material is rehydrated with 1 ml of lidocaine. According to the manufacturer, no allergy prescreening or testing is required. It is implanted with a 26-gauge needle into the subcutaneous space, then gently massaged. Preliminary clinical studies on 200 patients to date demonstrated no allergic or immunologic reactions. Adverse reactions include bruising, redness, swelling, and wrinkling of skin. A 50% overcorrection is recommended for lip augmentation.[43] Cymetra is significantly more expensive than Zyplast collagen. More data will be necessary to determine whether it is longer lasting, thus compensating for its higher price. LifeCell Corporation, The Woodlands, TX, and its corporate office at 1 Millennium Way, Branchburg, NJ 08876-3876. Tel 800-367-5737. Website: www.lifecell.com

Dermal Grafting

This is a unique process championed by Dr. James Swinehart.[44] Dermal grafts are particularly convenient for autologous augmentation when excess skin is available, such as in rhytidectomy or abdominoplasty. Alternatively, dermis can be harvested inconspicuously from the retroauricular area, lower abdomen, and groin crease. The epidermis and subcutaneous fat are removed via scalpel or carbon dioxide laser.[45] Risks include epidermal inclusion cysts or fistula formation, graft resorption, and hematomas requiring drainage.[46,47] Hinderer and Escalona described a technique for smaller defects, whereby the harvested dermis is divided into the smallest possible pieces, then placed into a syringe with a large-bore needle. The material is then injected into a space created by a trocar.[48]

Dermalive (not FDA approved)

Dermalive is composed of hyaluronic acid and acrylic hydrogel fragments. It is nonanimal in origin. The particle sizes are 45 to 65 μm. Skin tests are reportedly unnecessary. It is produced by Dermatech, 28 Rue de Caumartin, 75009 Paris, France.

Dermalogen

Dermalogen is human tissue collagen matrix derived from the dermal layer of cadaveric skin specimens. Collagen fibrils are suspended in a neutral pH buffer. Other matrix proteins such as elastin are also found within the injectable substance. Dermalogen is sterilized and undergoes viral inactivation procedures and a prion inactivation step. HIV and hepatitis tests are performed. The source of the donor skin is certified by the American Association of Tissue Banks (AATB). Nearly 2 million AATB certified tissue and organ transplants have been done without any cases of retroviral disease transmission. Despite the human origins of the collagen and proteins, some physicians perform skin tests because of reported cases of sensitization, perhaps to a preservative or treatment agent used in the manufacturing process. The incidence of erythema and positive skin tests have decreased over time as the manufacturing process has been fine-tuned. The manufacturer no longer recommends performing skin tests. The material is produced in a nominal 3.5% concentration with no local anesthetic added (although the true concentration is about 5%). A newer 2.8% concentration form of Dermalogen is on the horizon and may ameliorate the difficulty in injecting this substance. Placement somewhere between the level of injection of Zyderm and Zyplast yields the best results. A topical anesthetic is recommended prior to use.

Patients have been followed for up to 6 months after injection with Dermalogen with some increase of longevity over bovine collagen reported. At 12 months, results were equal. Dermalogen's great advantage, however, lies in its use for patients who are allergic to bovine collagen. It is distributed by Collagenesis, Inc., 500 Cummings Center, Beverly, MA 01915. Tel 800-411-9440. Website: www.collagenesis.com

Endoplast-50 (not FDA approved)

This is a new product of solubilized elastin peptides with bovine collagen for intradermal injection. Two skin tests are performed at 15-day intervals prior to treatment. Test syringes are available. The material is provided in 0.5 or 1 cc syringes for use with a 30-gauge needle. A serial puncture technique is utilized in the reticular dermis and the area is then massaged. After treatment, inflammation is expected for 24 to 48 hours. The material is purported to influence proliferation of fibroblasts to produce collagen, similar to Fibrel, with duration of correction said to be 8 to 12 months. Distributed by Laboratories Filorga, 79 Rue de Miromesnil, 75008 Paris, France.

Fascian

Freeze-dried cadaver fascia lata has been used since 1960 for a variety of surgical procedures in orthopedics, and later in ophthalmology for correcting ptosis.[49] Its use in dermatology was popularized by Burres in 1996 when he described a recollagenation procedure for acne scars.[50] Irradiated, freeze-dried fascia lata from screened human cadavers is cut to an appropriate size and then inserted into a recipient pocket. Ten percent of patients required retreatment at 6 weeks follow-up. The number of patients treated was not specified. No allergic reactions were reported and seromas were seen rarely.

The same author later reported on the use of fascia lata for lip enhancement.[51] Mucosal stab incisions were used to pass 4 to 6 mm squares or rectangles of diced fascia into the submucosal tissue. Some transient graft lumpiness and postoperative paresthesia occurred. An unknown number of patients were treated, with enhancement obvious in "most" patients for 6 to 12 months after treatment. An unspecified percentage of patients also acknowledged continued enhancement years later, though photographs of such patients were not included in the publication.

An injectable form of freeze-dried, irradiated fascia is now available as Fascian. This product comes in particulate sizes from 0.25 to 2 mm. A 50 to 80 mg pellet of the material is packaged in a sterile 3 cc syringe to be hydrated with saline or lidocaine, agitated for 20 minutes, and injected with a 14- to 22-gauge needle depending on particle size. Because of the large needle required, recipient sites must be anesthetized prior to injection. Clogged tips require withdrawal of the syringe and aspiration of more saline, or a change of needle. A recipient site may be prepared by subcision,[52] though this is not mandatory. No allergy testing is required, and the material can be stored at room temperature for 3 to 4 years.

Burres treated 81 patients with injectable particulate fascia lata over a 9-month period. Fifty-nine were examined at 3 to 4 months, with 11 additional patients followed up by phone only. No patients experienced hypersensitivity reactions or infections. Firmness was present for 1 to 2 months but was not visible. Although results were not objectively quantified, Dr. Burres stated that subjects were very satisfied and that in almost all cases, graft persistence was evident at 3 to 4 months follow-up. Though the safety profile of preserved fascia is excellent, longer-term data from a variety of sources will be necessary to more fully evaluate the role that Fascian will have in our armamentarium of soft tissue augmentation materials. Manufactured and distributed by Fascia Biosystems, LLC, 465 North Roxbury, Suite 1012, Beverly Hills, CA 90210. Tel 888-3FASCIA. Website: www.fascian.com

Autologous Fat Transplantation

The popularity of tumescent liposuction has brought renewed interest in fat transplantation for soft tissue augmentation. Fat allows a patient to benefit from autologous tissue without risk of allergy, rejection, or possible transmission of viral or retroviral infection. Resorption of transplanted material remains the greatest concern. Differences in harvest sites, methods, preparation of material, technique and location of implantation, and means of evaluation have made measurements of longevity difficult.

Exposure to lidocaine and epinephrine is not harmful to the donor adipose tissue.[53] Syringe-suctioning of fat appears to add no more trauma to the fat cells than does excision en bloc[54] and may allow better revascularization. Bacteria in harvested samples at room temperature were first measurable at 8 hours, and saline was necessary to maintain viability of the adipocytes over the same period of time.[55]

Implanting thin strands of adipocytes increases the likelihood of survival. In an important study by Carpaneda, collections of surviving adipocytes were of a maximum 1 to 2 mm in thickness histologically and adjacent to zones of necrosis and inflammation when fat was grafted into patients prior to abdominoplasty.[56] Location of transplanted fat may also play a role in survival. Guerrerosantos found subfascial and intramuscular fat grafts work better for patients with combined liposuction and lipoinjection for contour improvement in the gluteal and lateral femoral areas.[57] Illouz felt only 40% of patients achieved stable correction of liposuction defects after one or more fat injections.[55] Patients with idiopathic subcutaneous fat atrophy have been reported to do well after fat transplant intramuscularly as well as subcutaneously, but may initially require substantial overcorrection.[58,59] Sydney Coleman has reported on his experience in over 1000 cases of fat transplantation to accentuate malar and mental prominences, jawlines, atrophic areas, and traumatic defects. Many of his patients have been followed longer than 8 years with persistent improvement subjectively suggesting permanence, though results may be subtle.[60]

Fulton et al suggests that fat transplants stabilize after 60 days and remain as long as 10 years. They achieve longer-lasting results in augmentation of the chin, cheekbones, and buccal fat pads, with more transient results in the lips and nasolabial folds, perhaps due to mobility in these areas.[61] Pinski and Coleman reported long-lasting results in furrows, scars, and dorsal hands when using outer thigh fat harvested with the tumescent technique.[62] In the future, growth factors added to harvested fat may increase survival of transplanted adipocytes.[63]

Mechanically processed fat injected intradermally can improve finer defects via fibrosis causing deposition of new collagen,[64] a procedure coined *lipocytic dermal augmentation.* The tissue reaction leading to augmentation may be identical to the mechanism of silicone, subcision procedures,[52] and lanolin and paraffin injections of the past.[65] As described by William Coleman, harvested material is processed to break the adipocytes and to separate the ruptured cell walls from the other material. The resultant material can then be injected using a 23- or 25-gauge needle. A major advantage of lipocytic dermal augmentation is its ability to be layered over microlipoinjection. This two-level approach may allow more complete correction than does the use of a dermal or subcutaneous filler alone.

Although fat transplantation is generally a safe, straightforward procedure, serious side effects have been reported. Ocular embolism has occurred alone[66] and in conjunction with hemiplegia after injection into the glabellar area.[67] Parotitis,[60] persistent edema, lipoma, calcification,[68] bacterial infection,[61] and overcorrection later requiring liposuction[58] have also been reported. Retrograde filling of a defect without force, the use of a blunt instrument for injection, and avoiding injections into traumatized tissue (e.g., after rhytidectomy) or into high-risk areas such as the glabella may minimize the chance of intravascular injection and trauma to underlying structures.

Fat transplantation for breast augmentation can create microcalcifications on mammography that are indistinguishable from radiologic changes seen with carcinomas.[69] Inflammatory masses, pseudocysts, and sinuses may also result. Therefore autologous fat is not an appropriate material for breast augmentation.

Fibrel

Bailey and Ingraham first used "fibrin foam" as a surgical hemostatic agent in 1944. In 1957 Spangler reported the efficacy of fibrin foam in treating depressed scars in 23 patients. Subsequently, he reported good to excellent results in treating 7000 patients with this substance.[70] The composition and fabrication of Fibrel, the modern descendant of fibrin foam, was further delineated by Gottlieb.[71] Autologous plasma, gelatin, and aminocaproic acid were utilized in combination to stimulate collagen synthesis and to elevate depressed scars.

Fibrel works by creating a clot that becomes colonized with fibroblasts. The patient's plasma serves as a supplemental source of clotting factors, the gelatin provides the framework on which a clot forms, and aminocaproic acid is added to prevent its lysis. The process is believed to then stimulate fibroblasts near the site to synthesize collagen, with resultant replacement of the clot formed by the implantation of Fibrel. Unlike bovine collagen, where the material remains as a relatively inert implant, Fibrel is believed to induce a local wound healing response that ultimately leads to new host collagen formation. It is to be expected that a certain degree of swelling and inflammation will occur during this process. Additionally, the use of Fibrel can be uncomfortable, and local anesthesia prior to its application is frequently utilized by those experienced in its use. Fibrel was manufactured by the Mentor Corporation, Goleta, CA, and is no longer available.

Gore-Tex

Gore-Tex, or expanded polytetrafluoroethylene (ePTFE) (W. L. Gore and Associates, Flagstaff, AZ), is a soft, pliable, synthetic material of nodes and interconnecting fibrils manufactured by the extrusion of Teflon (Dupont, Wilmington, DE). The material can be reinforced with fluorinated ethylene propylene to create a more rigid implant appropriate for malar and mental augmentation. The original material is produced in sheets, patches, sutures, and tubes for a multitude of indications.

Gore-Tex has an excellent safety profile as proven in over 3 million patients and 3 decades of historical data in cardiac, vascular, and general surgery. It is inert, exhibits minimal capsule formation, elicits no allergic reaction, and may be steam or gas sterilized. Pores of 22 to 30 μm allow passage of air, despite the hydrophobic properties that have won it acclaim in foul weather gear. These pores also allow a small amount of fine tissue incorporation, minimizing postsurgical shifting. The lack of extensive incorporation into surrounding tissues is helpful when the implant needs to be removed, as in cases of infection.

In 1991, ePTFE was reported to be a useful material for correction of the nasolabial folds and other rhytides.[72] Both the sheet and suture forms of the material were implanted. In 100 patients treated, one infection required treatment with antibiotics without removal of the ePTFE. Over a 5- to 9-year follow-up, three patients maintained 50% to 90% improvement.[73] In another series of 400 patients followed for 5 years, seven patients required removal of Gore-Tex because of infection.[74] Both ePTFE sutures[75] and strips[76] have been used to augment the vermilion border and philtrum. One of 11 patients required removal of ePTFE strips because of infection. In another series of 21 patients with lip augmentation, one seroma required treatment.[77] No infections, extrusion, inflammation, capsule formation, or loss of sensation resulted.

Individual cases of disfiguring scarring after ePTFE placement in the lips have been reported in the literature[78] as well as case reports of extrusion and cellulitis in the glabella. Multiple complications have been reported in using ePTFE on the dorsum of the nose and other superficial locations.[79]

The constant motion of the oral region makes lip and nasolabial fold augmentation with ePTFE particularly challenging. Although results are permanent, extrusion may occur if the ends of the implant are not properly buried, or if the patient does not follow postoperative instructions to minimize movement in the area. Failure to keep the ePTFE subcutaneous and not intradermal can also cause surface irregularities. Perioperative and postoperative antibiotics in conjunction with sterile technique is imperative in preventing infection, which may require removal of all material placed. In addition, patients must be cautioned that although the aesthetic results may be excellent, the implant will likely be palpable indefinitely. Manufactured by W. L. Gore and Associates, P.O. Box 2300, Flagstaff, AZ 86003-3200. Tel 888-914-4673. Website: www.gore.com

Human Placental Collagen (not FDA approved)

Gamma-irradiated amnion collagen from human placentae has been suggested as an injectable soft tissue augmentation material and tested in animal studies.[80] Human placentae are readily available and contain abundant collagen. Author Klein conducted studies for the Collagen Corporation (recently purchased by McGhan Medical) on human placental collagen obtained from France. The substance worked extraordinarily well. Because of concerns about public perception of infection risk and acceptability, the product will likely never come to market.

Hylaform Gel (not FDA approved)

Hyaluronic acid derivatives are exciting new materials for soft tissue augmentation with great future potential. Hyaluronic acid is a mammalian polysaccharide found naturally in the dermis. Its ability to bond water assists in hydration and provides skin turgor. Unlike collagen, it is identical across all species and is produced by many types of cells.

Hylan gels are composed of cross-linked hyaluronan polymer molecules with very high molecular weights. Hyaluronic acid itself is broken down quickly within the dermis, then eliminated by the lymphatics and eventually the liver. Hylan gels have longer dwell times in tissues but are eventually broken down into their original molecules and eliminated in the same fashion.[81]

Piacquadio[82] reported the use of cross-linked hyaluronic acid (Hylan B gel) in 150 patients enrolled in a multicenter clinical study initiated in 1991. Patients with distensible scars or wrinkles received an initial treatment and a touch-up at weeks 2 to 4. At week 12, 84% showed moderate (33% or greater) improvement and 80% of patients reported moderate or higher satisfaction. Adverse reactions, including persistent erythema and ecchymosis, were rare. Using a guinea pig model, Hylan gel was seen histologically in 87% of sites at week 26, whereas bovine collagen was present in only 25%.[83]

Hylaform gel, also known as Hylan B gel (Genzyme Biosurgery, formerly Biomatrix, Inc., Ridgefield, NJ) is processed from the cock's combs of domestic fowl. In clinical trials in wrinkles and scars, 80% reported moderate or greater satisfaction at 12 weeks. Hylaform is used for facial augmentation throughout most of the world (Canada, England, Europe, Australia). It is especially popular for volume augmentation of the lips. However, it is not available for this purpose in the United States. It is available in a more concentrated form as Synvisc in America for use in osteoarthritis of the knee. Clinical trials for Hylagel-Nuro in lumbar surgery have been approved by the FDA. This variation of Hylaform gel purportedly minimizes scarring and adhesions in a number of important surgical applications.

Adverse reactions have been less than 2% and include persistent redness, ecchymosis, and acne. While the major problem reported by the company has been the occurrence of a certain degree of redness, others have verbally reported significant reactions resembling hypersensitivity, though the product is touted to be nonimmunogenic. Because of these anecdotal nonpublished reports, some practitioners have opted to continue skin testing. Hylaform gel is manufactured by Genzyme Biosurgery of Cambridge, MA (Tel 617-252-7500. Website: www.genzymebiosurgery.com). It is distributed in Europe by Collagen International, Inc., Avenue Gratta-Paille 2CP430, CH-1000 Lausanne 30 Grey, Switzerland.

Hylan Rofilan Gel (not FDA approved)

This gel is composed of hyaluronic acid cross-linked with a natural acid instead of a chemical compound. The product is manufactured and distributed by Rofil Medical International B.V., Stationstaat 1B, 4815 NC Breda, The Netherlands.

Isolagen (not FDA approved)

Isolagen Technologies cultures autologous fibroblasts in a similar manner to that used to propagate cells for burns, cartilage repair, and marrow transplants. It is suggested for fine lines, depressions, and lip augmentation. A 3 mm punch biopsy of skin is taken from the postauricular area, although some use the back of the neck, and author Klein obtains it from the buttock. It is shipped in an iced thermos; a test dose is returned in 6 weeks, and treatments are begun at 8 weeks. A multilevel injection into the superficial dermis, mid dermis, and dermal-subcutaneous junction is necessary for most wrinkles and scars. Topical anesthetic and icing the area assist in preventing pain associated with these injections. Generally two to three treatments are required, although four treatments are suggested for lip enhancement. The cost to the physician is $500 per treatment.

The concept behind this novel agent is the placement of fibroblasts at the site of soft tissue deficit in order to eventually create collagen and other matrix proteins where needed. The advantages are the abundant supply of fibroblasts available by culturing, the absence of lumpiness after injection, and its ability to be used in concert with Zyderm (but not Zyplast). Isolagen cannot be used in patients over 70 years old or those with autoimmune disorders, systemic disease, or malignancies.

The company states that Isolagen has persisted for 5 years in a human wrist and for 22 months therapeutically in patients. It has also been reported by Dr. William Boss, its inventor, that there was no resorption and results were apparent 3 to 10 months after the injection. He saw continual, gradual improvement over 16 to 18 months, and all patients acknowledged results, with a 92% satisfaction with no overgrowth, lumps, or allergy. Other investigators, including author Klein, have not been able to duplicate these results. West and Alster reported improvement in only 2 of 12 patients.[84]

Production of Isolagen has been halted, as the presence of growth factors added to the cells may require classification of Isolagen as a medical device. It will likely be necessary to obtain FDA approval for this product, which is no longer considered simply autologous tissue. It is manufactured and distributed by Isolagen Technologies, Inc., 22 Madison Ave., Paramus, NJ 07652. Tel 201-291-0147.

Koken Atelocollagen (not FDA approved)

Koken Atelocollagen implant is a 2% monomolecular solution of bovine collagen from Japan. It is supplied in cartridges to be injected with a dental syringe through a 30-gauge needle. The indications, contraindications, testing, and injection techniques are the same as those for Zyderm collagen implant. Unlike Zyderm, Koken Atelocollagen does not contain lidocaine. It does not contain fibrils of collagen as does Zyderm. It is manufactured by the Koken Co., Ltd., 3-14-3 Mejiro, Toshima-KM, Tokyo 171, Japan.

Meta Crill (not FDA approved)

Meta Crill is composed of microspheres of methacrylate in a colloidal suspension without protein. It is similar to Arteplast, the precursor to Artecoll. It is distributed by Nutricel, Rua Sampaio Viana, 299-Rio Comprido, Rio de Janeiro/RJ, Cep: 20,261-030, Brazil. Website: www.metacrill.com.br/us/usaber.htm

New-fill (not FDA approved)

New-fill is a polylactic acid not of animal origin. It is provided as freeze-dried material and can be stored at room temperature. After reconstitution with water, it is 4.45% polylactic acid. The material is biocompatible, biodegradable, and immunologically inert. It is injected into the superficial dermis or subdermally using a 26-gauge needle. Indications include nasolabial folds, lips, lipodystrophy of cheeks, acne scars, wrinkles, hands, and liposuction contour deformities. It is manufactured by Biotech Industry S.A., Siège social, 38 Ave du X Septembre, L2550 Luxembourg, and is available from Imadis, 50C Av du Roule, 92200 Neuilly s/S, France.

Perlane (not FDA approved)

Perlane is a more robust form of Restylane for use with a 27-gauge needle. It is placed at the subcutaneous-dermal border. It is manufactured and distributed by Q-Med AB, Seminariegatan 21, S-752 28 Uppsala, Sweden. Tel 011-46-18-474-90-00. Website: www.q-med.com

Permacol (not FDA approved)

Permacol is a permanent, cross-linked solid porcine collagen implant presently available only in sheets for surgical insertion. It allows ingrowth of host tissue cells and blood vessels. In Europe it is a CE Mark Class III and is thus approved for implantation. No U.S. studies exist on this porcine product. It is available in 5 × 5 cm and 5 × 10 cm sheets in two thicknesses, 1.5 mm and 0.75 mm. It may become available in an injectable form in the future. The extremely attractive cost is a major advantage, currently about \$6 (US)/cm^2. The product is manufactured and distributed by Tissue Science Laboratories, Ltd., Greyholme House, 49 Victoria Rd., Aldershot, Hants GUII ISJ, United Kingdom.

Plasmagel

Plasmagel is an autologous, blood-derived augmenting material. Ascorbic acid and lidocaine are added to blood plasma. The material is heated to form a gel and injected. It is applicable for wrinkles, contour defects, acne scars, and lip augmentation.[85]

PMS-350 (not FDA approved)

PMS-350 achieved CE certification in Europe after 15 years. It is silicone with a viscosity of 350 centistokes. It is indicated for glabellar lines, nasolabial folds, perioral lines, lip augmentation, atrophic disorders, and scars. It is distributed by Vikomed in Germany.

Profill (not FDA approved)

Provided as a translucent gel, Profill is a block copolymer of polyoxyethylene and polyoxypropylene with mineral salts, amino acids, and vitamins. The material contains no animal proteins. It is provided as a liquid that can be refrigerated until used. After injection the liquid turns into a gel and can then be molded. No skin test is required. It is provided in 1 ml syringes and injected with a 30-gauge needle with a serial puncture technique. Several hours of erythema are expected after treatment. Correction reportedly lasts 6 to 9 months. Profill is frequently used in concert with Endoplast-50. It is manufactured and distributed by Laboratories Filorga, 79 Rue de Miromesnil, 75008 Paris, France.

Recombinant Human Collagen

Research efforts are under way to create a recombinant human collagen. This type of collagen would eliminate the risk of donor viral or prion contamination, eradicate the need for proteolytic cleavage of animal collagen with its attendant degradation, and have no potential for allergy. One area of research involves human collagen produced within the cow and subsequently separated from the cow's milk. Cohesion Technologies (Palo Alto, CA) has recently reported the ability to produce human collagen in the laboratory without an animal carrier. No clinical studies have been reported.

Resoplast (not FDA approved)

Resoplast is bovine monomolecular collagen in solution. Concentrations of 3.5% and 6.5% are available. Indications and techniques of implantation are similar to Zyderm collagen. A skin test is provided. It is distributed by Rofil Medical International B.V., 4811 D H Breda, The Netherlands.

Restylane (not FDA approved)

The hyaluronic acid derivative Restylane has been available for soft tissue augmentation in Europe for over 4 years. Restylane is stabilized, partially cross-linked hyaluronic acid created via bacterial fermentation from streptococcal bacteria and, thus, does not require an animal source. It is biocompatible and biodegradable. It is indicated for rhytides, depressions, and lip augmentation. Restylane has a higher concentration of hyaluronic acid than Hylaform gel (20 mg/ml of stabilized hyaluronic acid). Despite its higher concentration, the material itself has a lower molecular weight, so comparisons with Hylaform gel are difficult.

One clinical study involved 113 European patients receiving injections of Restylane to 285 facial wrinkles.[86] Physicians rated the degree of correction to be 82% at 3 months and 66% at 1 year, with similar patient opinion. Side effects were minimal, including erythema when injected too superficially and technique-related unevenness. There were no reported allergic reactions.

Another study consisted of 158 patients treated in 273 facial sites. Thirteen of 78 patients (17%) experienced intermittent swelling of the lips after augmentation in that area.[87] Patient and physician satisfaction was reported as 60% at 52 weeks. Studies were performed with the first generation of this product. Improvements initiated in the second generation of this product have reportedly reduced the swelling problems previously encountered. Recent anecdotal unpublished reports of patients with extrusion of the material from facial sites after large-volume injection are also of concern but are not fully substantiated.

Restylane is indicated for rhytides, depressions, and lip augmentation. It is provided in 0.7 cc preloaded syringes containing 20 mg/ml of stabilized hyaluronic acid. A linear threading or serial puncture technique may be utilized with a 30-gauge needle. No overcorrection is necessary. Restylane may be placed into the potential space at the vermilion border of the lip and then into the mucosa itself, creating excellent volume lip enhancement. Restylane-fine is a new, less viscous form of Restylane for use with a 32-gauge needle. It is manufactured and distributed by Q-Med AB, Seminariegatan 21, S-752 28 Uppsala, Sweden. Tel 011-46-18-474-90-00. Website: www.q-med.com

Reviderm-intra (not FDA approved)

Reviderm-intra contains 40 to 60 μm dextran beads of the Sephadex type in hylan gel. It is of nonanimal origin. The material is nonimmunogenic, biocompatible, and biodegradable. Company literature reports that an initial macrophage response is seen at 30 days accompanied by fibroblast proliferation and new collagen formation. Intradermal injection is performed with a 30-gauge needle. A topical anesthetic can be used. No overcorrection is necessary. The material can be molded after injection to disperse the beads. In a clinical study, 274 patients showed the material to be resistant to resorption and migration.[88] The product is manufactured and distributed by Rofil Medical International B.V., Stationstaat 1B, 4815 NC Breda, The Netherlands.

Silicone (not FDA approved)

Silicones are synthetic compounds and do not occur naturally. The liquid silicones used for medical purposes are long polymers of dimethylsiloxanes. Siloxane is an acronym used to describe compounds containing repeating units of silicon, oxygen, and methane. During the 1940s there was a large German, Swiss, and Japanese experience with injectable silicone.

There have been two major American protocols involving the use of highly refined liquid silicone. In 1965, Dow-Corning conducted a trial involving seven investigators and 1334 patients. This trial was halted by the FDA in 1967 due to concerns about product quality, use methodology, and inadequate animal toxicity data. A second trial was conducted by Dow-Corning in 1978 involving 27 investigators and 144 patients.

Silicone has a high use potential, providing pleasing aesthetic results in many patients, but unfortunately, it also has a high abuse potential. Numerous disastrous complications have resulted from the use of adulterated or impure silicones. Foreign body type siliconoma can occur up to 11 years after implantation, even with the highly refined, medical grade Dow-Corning MDX4-4011 and microdroplet technique.[89] Other adverse reactions reported are movement or drift of the implant, "peau d'orange" of overlying skin, visible or palpable beading, discoloration, site reactions in 12% to 14% of patients, and immunologic reactions.

Dr. Norman Orentreich claims that silicone injections are permanent,[90] although other investigators have reported a loss of material from the injection site. He also maintains that it is applicable for all facial sites. Others report that it is contraindicated in lips and eyelids. Techniques also vary from injector to injector. Some prefer fanning, some serial puncture with microdroplets, some tattooing or superficial placement, and some threading.

Despite injectable silicone's long history of use in the United States, the FDA declared its use for soft tissue augmentation illegal. Nevertheless, two forms of silicone—Adatosil-5000 (Escalon Medical, Wayne, PA) and Silikon-1000 (Richard-James, Peabody, MA)—were recently approved as ophthalmic devices. When injected into the eye, these highly viscous agents provide prolonged retinal tamponade in selected cases of complicated retinal detachment (see January 13, 1999, transcript of the FDA Ophthalmic Device Panel). The numbers in the product names refer to the viscosity in centistokes (cs). Water has a viscosity of 100 cs. Mineral oil has a viscosity of 350 cs.

Despite legal implications, some physicians are injecting this high-viscosity material into the skin of the face. Adatosil-5000 requires a 26-gauge needle with an assist device to inject. Dr. David Duffy reports that postinjection dispersion is difficult (personal communication). Caution must be exercised when injecting into the lip and glabella. Before considering these materials for use, a physician should contact his or her malpractice carrier in case the procedure is not covered. Some states have laws with significant penalties to dissuade practitioners from attempting use of these agents.

SoftForm

The success of e-PTFE (Gore-Tex) in soft tissue augmentation led to attempts at improving its ease of use and risk profile. Maas et al noted a significant reduction in extrusion and inflammation when tubular implants were utilized as opposed to strips and rolled sheets of ePTFE in a porcine model.[91] Fibroblastic ingrowth filled and anchored the implant at 6 months after the procedure but still allowed removal when necessary by dividing the fibrous tissue at the poles of the hollow structure. These studies led to development of the SoftForm facial implant.

SoftForm is preloaded on a protected trocar to facilitate implantation without contaminating, stretching, or dragging the tubular ePTFE with or without pretunneling. Promising anecdotal reports of good results, particularly in the perioral region, have been published,[92] but long-term studies are not yet available. SoftForm is distributed by McGhan Medical Corporation, 700 Ward Drive, Santa Barbara, CA 93111. Tel 800-MCGHAN 1 (624-4261), 805-683-6761, Fax 805-967-5839. Website: www.mcghan.com

Zyderm and Zyplast Collagen

Injectable bovine collagen has come to be regarded as the "gold standard" of injectable fillers. The normal human dermis is composed largely of collagen proteins. A team of investigators at Stanford University in the early 1970s began work on the development of a clinically useful collagen implant material.[93] This led eventually to the development of Zyderm I Collagen Implant (ZC I) and eventually Zyderm II (ZC II) and Zyplast (ZP) Collagen Implant. Since that time an estimated 1,900,000 individuals worldwide have received injectable collagen implants.

Zyderm and Zyplast are sterile, purified fibrillar suspensions of bovine dermal collagen. The products are suspended in phosphate-buffered physiologic saline containing 0.3% lidocaine. It should be noted that these substances are all taken from the skin of a closed American herd of cattle, negating the possibility of contamination with the bovine spongiform encephalopathy virus or prion.[94]

ZC I, the original material produced, is 3.5% by weight bovine collagen, whereas ZC II, introduced in 1983, is 6.5%. In ZP, bovine dermal collagen is lightly cross-linked by the addition of glutaraldehyde, resulting in a more robust implant that is essentially an injectable latticework of bovine collagen.[95] As a result of this cross-linkage, ZP is more resistant to proteolytic degradation, less immunogenic, and more applicable for deeper contour defects.[96]

The products are provided in preloaded syringes that are stored at low temperature (4°C) so that the dispersed fibrils remain fluid and small. This allows passage of the products through small-gauge needles. Once implanted, the human body temperature causes the products to undergo consolidation into a more solid gel.

Proper patient screening and skin testing are of the utmost importance in the application of bovine collagen therapy. Persons who have lidocaine sensitivity, a history of an anaphylactoid event, or previous sensitivity to bovine collagen are excluded from testing and treatment. The safety and contraindications of the various injectable collagen formulations have been described elsewhere.[96]

Potential allergenicity to injectable collagen is reliably determined by skin testing. Approximately 0.1 ml of Zyderm is administered in a tuberculin manner in the volar forearm. The site is evaluated at 48 to 72 hours and again at 4 weeks. A positive skin test is defined as swelling, induration, tenderness, or erythema that persists or occurs 6 hours or longer after test implantation. This is a definite contraindication to treatment. A positive skin test response will be seen in 3% to 3.5% of individuals. Seventy percent of these reactions will become manifest in 48 to 72 hours, indicating a preexisting allergy to bovine collagen.[97,98] Most authorities now recommend a second test as an additional precaution.[99-101] It is administered 2 to 4 weeks after the initial test. The volume utilized for the second test is the same as that used for the first test. Since the majority of treatment-associated hypersensitivity reactions occur shortly after the first treatment, double testing greatly reduces the frequency of this most undesirable sequela. Additionally, treatment-associated hypersensitivity reactions that occur after two negative skin tests tend to be milder. Single retesting of individuals who have not been treated for more than 1 year or who were successfully tested or treated elsewhere is strongly recommended. After retesting, a minimum of 2 weeks is recommended for test site evaluation before commencing treatment.

Adverse treatment responses to injectable collagen can be divided into non-hypersensitive and hypersensitive reactions. Nonhypersensitive reactions include bruising, reactivation of herpetic eruptions, and bacterial infection. Additionally, local necrosis due to vascular interruption at the treatment site has been noted with ZP and rarely ZC I/ZC II.[102] Fifty-six percent of these locally necrotic events occur in the glabellar area while using Zyplast; thus physicians are cautioned against using ZP at this site. Local necrosis may also occur in scarred, less vascular areas. If, upon injection, a physician notes severe blanching of the area and pain, he or she should immediately stop injecting because compression of, or injection into, local vessels may have occurred. The value of massage, warm compresses, or nitroglycerin gel in this situation is, as yet, unsubstantiated.

Two reports of partial vision loss after Zyderm Collagen therapy have been noted.[103,104] These are probably the result of an occlusive event involving the retinal artery. These serious consequences of a cosmetic procedure underscore the need to inject bovine collagen only in the dermis and not subcutaneously.

Treatment-associated hypersensitivity reactions to bovine collagen implants consist of redness and swelling at the treatment site. Rarely, mild systemic symptoms can accompany these reactions. Hypersensitive reactions are almost uniformly associated with anti-Zyderm antibodies.[105,106] These antibodies do not cross-react with human collagen.[107] Cyst-abscess formation is a rare but severe hypersensitivity response lasting as long as 2 years.[105] This type of reaction is usually associated with ZP and rarely ZC I/ZC II. Eighty-six percent of these individuals have associated anti-bovine antibodies. An expert panel convened by the FDA has found no supporting evidence that bovine collagen may induce connective tissue disease in the human host.

For all causes, 70% require touch-up treatments at intervals of 3 to 12 months, whereas 30% may have some persistent improvement up to 18 months.[96] Correction with all forms of bovine collagen is temporary and requires periodic maintenance. Acne scars appear to retain correction the longest.

Variation in longevity is influenced by continued mechanical stress at the treatment site, lesion location, and, possibly, the patient's individual response to collagen implants. Histologic studies with both ZC I and ZP have shown excellent human biocompatibility with minimal inflammation at sites of implantation. Although histologic studies of ZP, as opposed to ZC I/ZC II, have revealed some deposition of host collagen, there is no convincing evidence that this deposition contributes to longevity of correction.[108] Indeed, correction with all forms of bovine collagen appears to be lost as the material is displaced from its site of implantation in the dermis into the subcutaneous space.[109] Developing an injectable collagen technique is an evolutionary process for the treating physician. In author Klein's experience with roughly 70,000 patients, correction now requires fewer visits and less material.

Zyplast and Zyderm collagen is now available through McGhan Medical after that company purchased Collagen Aesthetics. McGhan Medical, 700 Ward Dr., Santa Barbara, CA 93111-2936. Tel 800-624-4261. Website: www.mcghan.com

DISCUSSION

Efforts to develop the perfect soft tissue augmentation material continue. New products and techniques are constantly appearing and evolving. An accelerated rate of new product introduction is likely the result of an understanding by the cosmetically oriented physician that the three-dimensional aspect of the face must be preserved for the best aesthetic result. We, as physicians and guides for our patients, must resist jumping on the bandwagon of every new fad or implant material.

There are many substances available for soft tissue augmentation. Although one must be familiar with all of the techniques, materials, and options, we feel that it is best to become proficient in two or three different methods so that you can provide your patients with options while still being experienced in the techniques that you use. The choice of implant material should be based on the location of the defect, potential for hypersensitivity reaction, desire for permanency, and the patient's feelings about the need for a "natural feel" of the implant. Safety should be the primary concern when using any implant material, not just in the short term but in the long run as well. Complications will inevitably occur if enough procedures are performed. Therefore, the physician must be completely honest with his or her patients, colleagues, and above all himself or herself. One of the most valuable lessons learned over the years by the authors is the following: It's not really what you use that is the most critical, it's how you use it.

SECTION TWO

Atlas of Surgical Procedures

PATIENT CONSIDERATIONS

An in-depth consultation prior to performing soft tissue augmentation is imperative. The patient's aesthetic goals and medical history must be carefully ascertained to ensure the appropriate choice of material and method. The patient must fully understand the limitations of the procedure and have realistic expectations for the short and long term. The appendixes following the chapter are useful in evaluating the patient and in preparing him or her for the procedure.

PROCEDURAL TECHNIQUES

Soft tissue augmentation procedures range in complexity from correcting a small subcutaneous furrow to reconstructing a patient with hemifacial atrophy or severe traumatic injury. Multiple tools are available, depending on the magnitude of the task, the depth of the defect, the amount of recuperation time a patient is willing to tolerate, and a physician's comfort level. Likewise, the techniques of soft tissue augmentation vary from physician to physician. The following illustrations are meant to demonstrate just a sampling of the materials available and methods that can be used with them. Videotapes as well as live seminars are often available from manufacturers to better assist the novice in developing his or her own technique and avoiding complications. Be certain to take photographs of front, side, and oblique views of patients prior to performing any surgical procedure.

Bovine Collagen

Indications for Zyderm Collagen I and II include horizontal forehead lines, glabellar lines, crow's-feet, shallow nasolabial and marionette lines, fine lip lines, shallow and distensible acne scars and excisional scars. Deep nasolabial and marionette grooves respond best to Zyplast with or without ZC I/ZC II overlay. ZP is also best suited to resurface the vermilion border between the lip and skin for lip enhancement. ZP is not recommended for use in glabellar frown lines.[110]

Zyplast Collagen Implant. For deeper defects such as nasolabial furrows, Zyplast (ZP) is the most robust form of bovine collagen. Cross-linked ZP may cause persistent beading and long-lasting overcorrection if placed too superficially. If Zyplast is placed too deeply, large amounts of material will be required for correction and improvement will be short lived. Correct placement is essential.

The rigid cross-linked structure of ZP accounts for the increased resistance upon injection and the decreased ability to smoothly flow this material. A 30-gauge needle is used with a serial puncture technique. The syringe of Zyplast is held at a 10- to 20-degree angle during the injection process, and the materials placed in the mid dermis, slightly deeper than Zyderm I or II (Fig. 16-1*A*). The resistance of the dermal matrix is felt against the injecting hand, and the plane of the injected site should elevate as the material is being placed (Fig. 16-1*B* and *C*).

Deliberate overcorrection should be avoided, as the material undergoes little syneresis or condensation upon implantation. Some individuals prefer a 90-degree angle for Zyplast implantation. If you use this method, only the needle tip should penetrate the skin with numerous serial punctures. The Adjustable Depth Gauge (ADG) is available to physicians to improve the accuracy of Zyplast implantation, though the authors have not found it to be useful. The practice of molding or massaging Zyplast after implantation for an improved cosmetic result remains unsubstantiated and may contribute to the loss of correction as the material is forced into the subdermal space.

Zyderm Collagen Implant. Although Zyderm I Collagen Implant is the most forgiving form of bovine collagen, it is also the most technique sensitive. As one's implantation techniques evolve, ZC I, rather than ZC II, will be the preferred filler for shallow defects. With very superficial placement, ZC II can be associated with persistent whiteness at the injection site. Many experienced practitioners limit the use of ZC II to deep acne scars unresponsive to ZC I and to deep glabellar furrows in patients who do not wish to be treated with Botox.

For fine defects, or the more superficial aspects of a deeper fold after Zyplast is used (as demonstrated here), Zyderm I is injected using a 30- to 32-gauge needle. The 32-gauge metal hub needle produces less trauma and ultimately a better cosmetic result. For extraordinarily fine defects, a 33-gauge needle may be employed. A 30-gauge needle is necessary when Zyderm II (ZC II) is used because of its increased viscosity over Zyderm I. Thirty percent of the injected ZC I volume is maintained, whereas 60% of ZC II volume persists during the correction period.

The physician prepares the treatment site by holding it taut between thumb and forefinger of the noninjecting hand. Next, the needle tip is guided horizontally with the bevel down along the skin surface until it barely penetrates the skin. The hub of the needle is then rocked gently over the thumb of the opposing hand, causing a tenting up of the skin with the needle tip (Fig. 16-2*A*). A flow of Zyderm I is created in the upper dermis as a smooth, yellowish mass that is both wide and flat and not three-dimensional in appearance (Fig. 16-2*B*). An upper dermal flow is created by applying each injection at the leading edge of the previously injected volume, generating a continuous flow of material that smoothly fills in defects (Fig. 16-2*C*). The continuous wide and flat flow of ZC I in the upper dermis smoothly augments the applicable soft tissue defect. Persistent beading and overcorrection are rarely associated with ZC I use (Fig. 16-2*D*).

Lip Augmentation with Bovine Collagen. The injection of bovine collagen in the circumoral area is the largest single indication for collagen. Even a small vol-

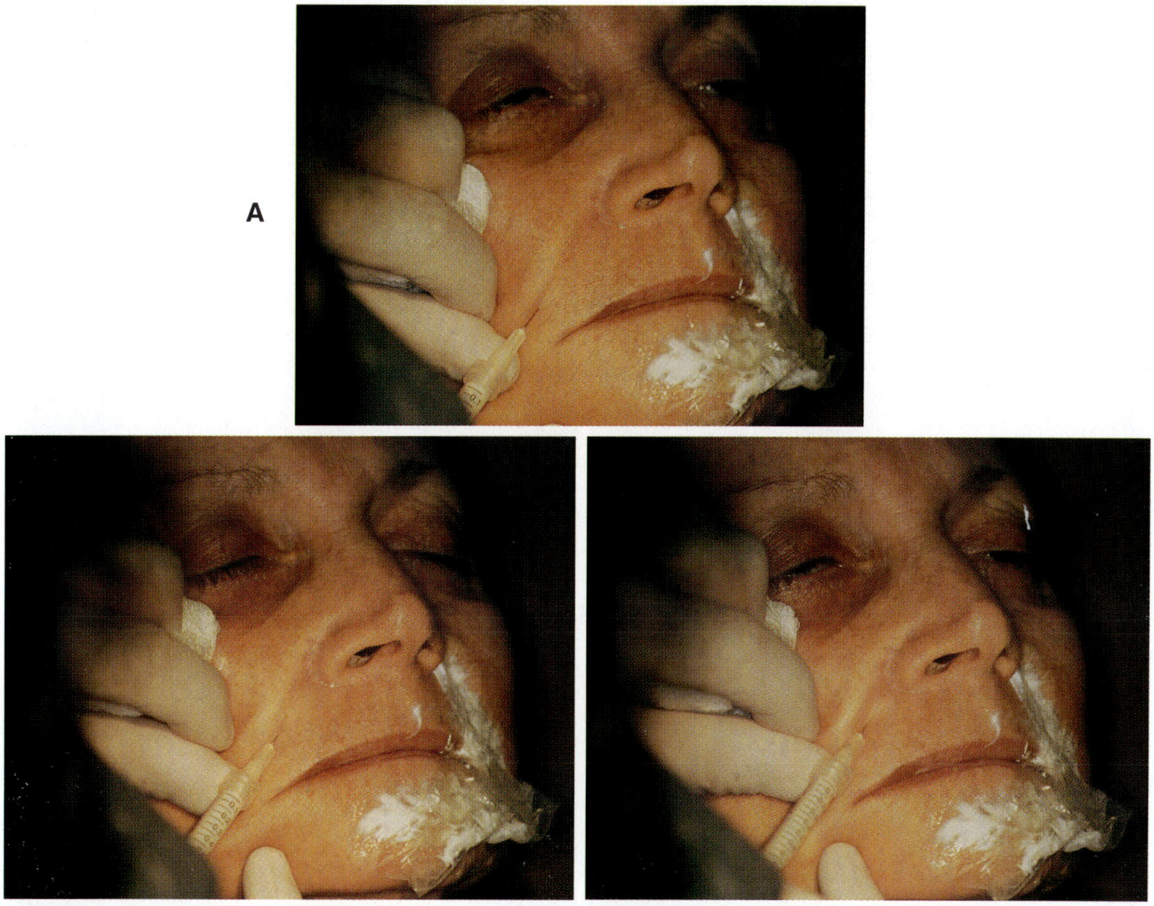

FIG. 16-1
A, The syringe of Zyplast is held at a 10- to 20-degree angle during the injection process, and the material is placed in the mid dermis slightly deeper than Zyderm I or II while the resistance of the dermal matrix is felt against the injecting hand. The plane of the injected site should elevate as the material is being placed (**B** and **C**).

umetric increase in the size of the lips in selected individuals can produce a most pleasing cosmetic result. Lip augmentation addresses age-related contour loss, enhances the vermilion border, and ameliorates radial grooves.

Injection into the glabrous skin surrounding the lips is an FDA-approved indication. Mucosal injection is an off-label use. A review of the procedure of lip augmentation by six investigators revealed that the best results were achieved by first injecting ZP into the potential space along the vermilion border in the upper and lower lip.[111] ZC I or ZP was then directly injected into the mucosa itself. The major vascular supply to the lips runs in the mucosa, and blind injections of ZP into this area occasionally will result in vascular events, especially after the lips are repeatedly treated. The ideal technique for lip enhancement and treatment of all soft tissue defects is variable and is certainly not uniform between physicians or even from patient to patient.

To enhance the perioral area, Zyplast is first placed in the potential space of the vermilion border. This is best accomplished by injecting right corner to center, then left corner to center (Fig. 16-3*A*). While injecting, the lip is held taut with the thumb of the opposing hand slightly stretching the lip posteriorly from the corner of the mouth. Anterior to the opposing thumb, the potential space at the corner is entered with a 30-gauge needle at about a 75-degree angle from the lip surface. The body of the syringe is held almost parallel to the lower lip. Once the physician feels the needle tip drop into the potential space, the injection angle is changed to about 45 degrees from the lip (Fig. 16-3*A*), and the flow of material is begun across the lower lip vermilion border.

If a spot is reached where the material will not easily advance, go to this location and inject onward. A smooth yellowish flow of Zyplast is desired in the potential space. White lumps are to be avoided. It is very important to place sufficient Zyplast in the lateral sites of the lower lip in order to "lift" the mouth.

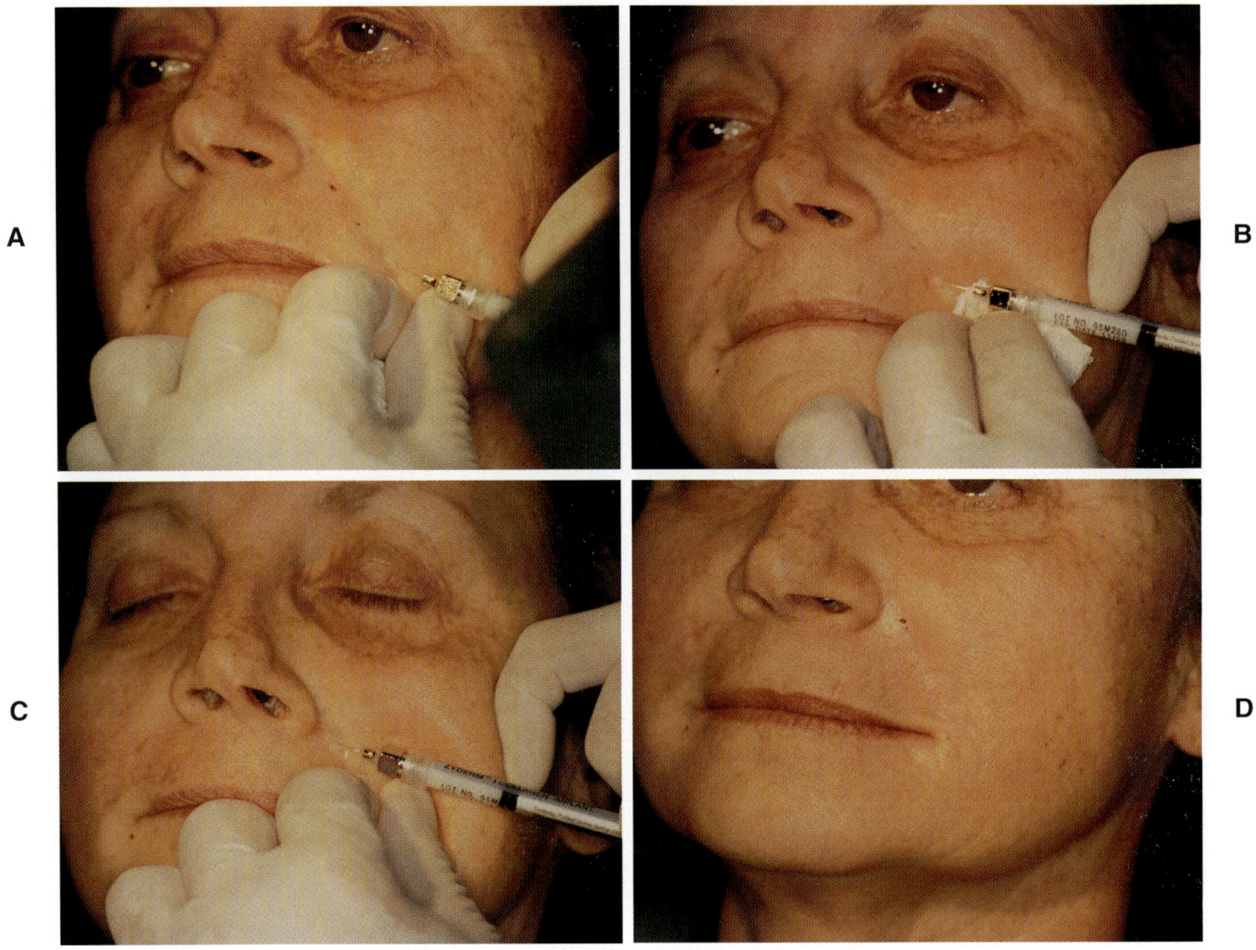

FIG. 16-2
A, With the treatment site held taut between thumb and forefinger of the noninjecting hand, the needle tip is guided horizontally with the bevel down along the skin surface until it barely penetrates the skin. **B,** The hub of the needle is then rocked gently over the thumb of the opposing hand, causing a tenting up of the skin with the needle tip while a flow of Zyderm I is created in the upper dermis as a smooth, yellowish mass that is both wide and flat and not three-dimensional in appearance **(C)**. **D,** The continuous wide and flat flow of Zyderm I Collagen Implant in the upper dermis smoothly augments the applicable soft tissue defect.

In the upper lip, the potential space can be entered from the corners as in the lower lip. Some physicians prefer to enter the space from the cupid's bow and move laterally to accentuate the central lip. Once outlined, the lip can be further enhanced by placing Zyplast, Zyderm I, or Zyderm II in the mucosa. Mucosal injection is an off-label use of these products. The collagen is flowed at this site in a manner similar to that used at other locations (Fig. 16-3*B*).

It has been author Klein's experience that frequency of injection in this area will decrease over time, possibly as a result of subtle fibroplasia. While various authors have advocated the use of nerve blocks in association with this augmentation, others have found implantation more difficult and the result aesthetically less pleasing when nerve blocks are performed.

Fascian

Fascian is an injectable form of preserved human fascia lata. Because it requires a larger-gauge needle than does bovine collagen and is injected subdermally, it is most appropriate for deeper defects such as nasolabial grooves. Smaller particle sizes of Fascian can be used for the vermilion border and smaller defects, although

A

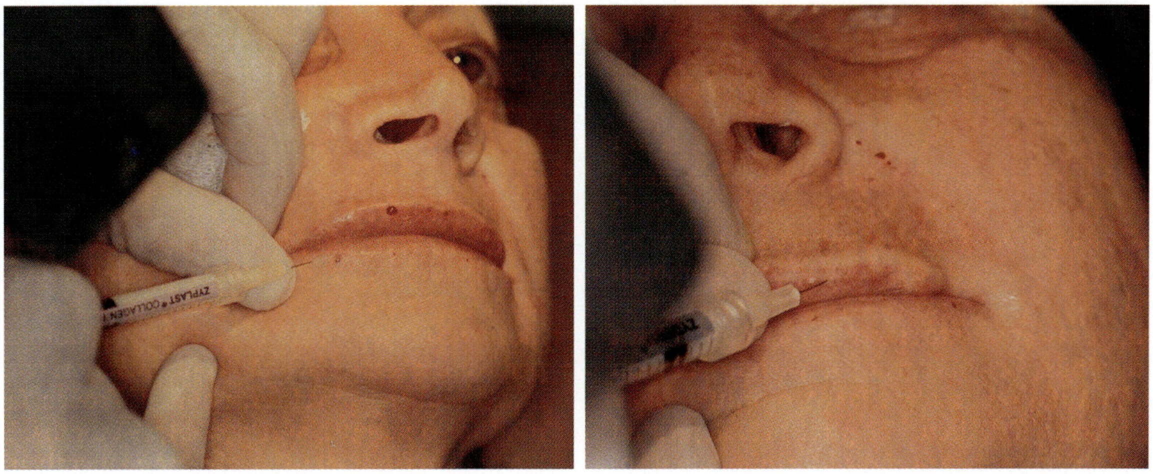

B

FIG. 16-3

A, To enhance the perioral area, Zyplast is first placed in the potential space of the vermilion border. **B,** Anterior to the opposing thumb, the potential space at the corner is entered with a 30-gauge needle at about a 75-degree angle from the lip surface.

the material is never as smooth nor as easy to inject as Zyplast collagen.

Fascian comes packaged as a powdery pellet in a sterile 3 cc syringe. It is reconstituted with up to 3 ml of 1% lidocaine, saline, or a combination of both. Over a period of 20 minutes, the rehydrated fascia lata can be passed multiple times through a sterile female-to-female adapter into another 3 cc syringe. The material is transferred back and forth to assist in the break-up of clumps and to later facilitate passage through a 16- to 22-gauge needle (Fig. 16-4). The size of needle used depends on particle size ordered from the manufacturer.

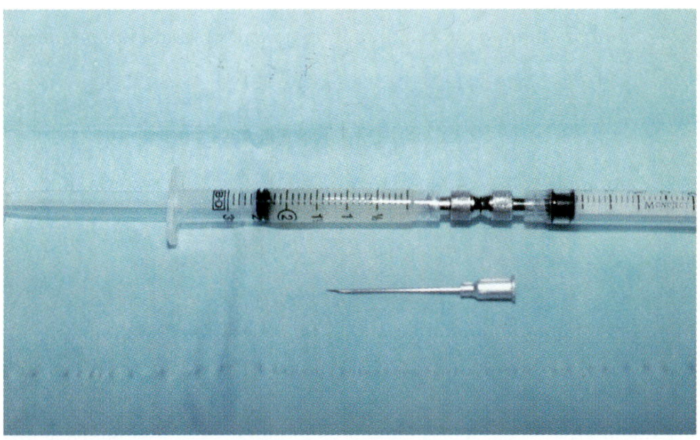

FIG. 16-4

Fascian comes packaged as a powdery pellet in a sterile 3 cc syringe. The size of needle used depends on particle size ordered from manufacturer.

While the Fascian is reconstituting, nerve blocks or local injection of lidocaine or both are performed to prepare the recipient sites. Utilizing sterile technique, scars or rhytides that are bound down may be undermined with an 18-gauge NoKor or beveled needle if desired. Fascian is then injected into the recipient site. If the needle becomes clogged, it is important not to increase force, as this increases the risk of intravascular injection. In the event of a blocked needle, the physician removes the needle from the patient; saline is drawn in through the clogged tip to clear, or the needle is changed if necessary. Antibiotic ointment is applied to entry sites. Steristrips or small Band-Aids may be used if desired, but they are often unnecessary.

Autologous Fat

The injection of autologous fat requires a harvesting procedure under sterile conditions. The material must be collected without contamination to decrease the risk of iatrogenic infection both for the injection of fresh fat and importantly for the injection of a patient's own thawed frozen fat at a later date.

The patient first washes both the recipient and harvest sites with Hibiclens solution. The areas to be augmented as well as the harvest sites are marked with the patient in an upright position. The harvest site is chosen depending on where the patient has excess adipose tissue and where the tissue is most resistant to weight loss. The harvest area is anesthetized with the tumescent technique after additional Betadine or Hibiclens prepping. See the chapter on tumescent liposuction for more information on techniques of anesthesia and suctioning. A 10 cc or larger syringe with a Luer-Lok is attached to a short spatula-tipped or Klein type cannula with a Luer-Lok base. The cannula is inserted into the anesthetized area, and the syringe plunger pulled back to create suction. Machine suction is not used, as this traumatizes adipocytes more than manual suction. Fat is harvested using a back and forth motion in a fan pattern from the entry site. This is repeated with fresh syringes until the required amount is obtained.

The syringe is allowed to stand in a rack for at least 20 minutes while the infranatant tumescent solution separates from the supernatant fat. A centrifuge may speed this process, if desired. The plunger is depressed gently, keeping the syringe upright. The infranatant solution is expressed until only pure fat remains in the syringe (Fig. 16-5). A female-to-female adapter is used to transfer the fat into 3 cc syringes.

During this time, the recipient areas should be anesthetized via the appropriate nerve blocks (infraorbital or mental blocks may be administered intraorally) and supplemented with local anesthesia as necessary. The recipient site is not tumesced, as this makes it more challenging to assess the appropriate amount of fat to inject. The area should be prepped with Betadine and draped prior to implantation. A blunt cannula (2 mm), spinal needle, or blunt introducer from a Potts spinal needle is attached to the 3 cc syringe containing pure fat (Fig. 16-6).

Through a tiny incision made with the tip of a No. 11 blade if necessary for entry, thin threads of adipocytes are injected while the cannula is repeatedly withdrawn. Injecting while advancing the cannula is avoided to minimize risk of intravascular injection. Using multiple levels and paths to inject thin threads of adipocytes maximizes the chance of survival of the autograft. For nasolabial folds, staying just medial to the fold leads to best results (Fig. 16-7). Steri-strips may be used to cover entry sites.

Unused syringes of fat are frozen by individually uncapping and submerging each in liquid nitrogen until it stops bubbling (Fig. 16-8). Syringes are capped, labeled with the patient's name, the date, and medical record number, and placed in a patient-labeled zip-lock bag or other specimen container, then transferred to a medical freezer. Ideally, the freezer should have a mechanism whereby any breaches in subfreezing temperatures risking bacterial contamination will be monitored and the physician notified. Frozen fat may be used for 3 months, and possibly 6 months, but is less likely than fresh fat to survive permanently after transplantation.

AlloDerm

AlloDerm is a solid material that, like Gore-Tex or SoftForm, requires a more extensive surgical procedure than injectable materials. It is excellent for patients desiring longer-term augmentation who are unwilling to tolerate a palpable implant. The implant may not be permanent, however. Its human cadaver derivation often leads to a more extensive discussion of long-term risks with the patient during consultation. There are many techniques for utilizing the material, one of which is described next. The manufacturer, LifeCell Corporation (The Woodlands, TX), provides useful videotapes for the practitioner to view prior to utilizing the material.

The patient is marked in an upright position (Fig. 16-9*A*). The length of the furrow to be corrected, or lip length, is measured to assess the size of implant required to enhance each area. Nerve blocks are admin-

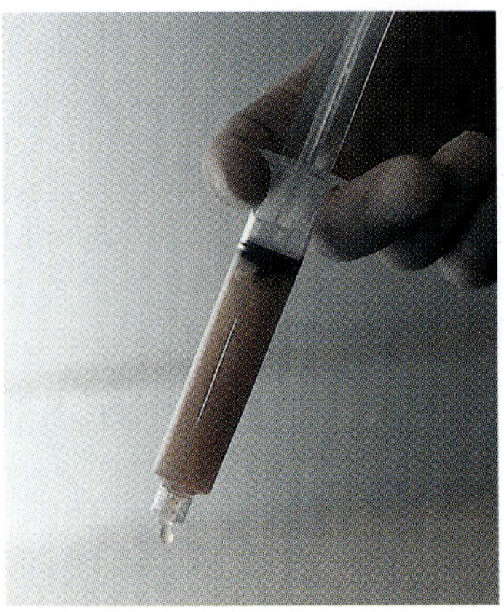

FIG. 16-5
The infranatant solution is expressed until only pure fat remains in syringe.

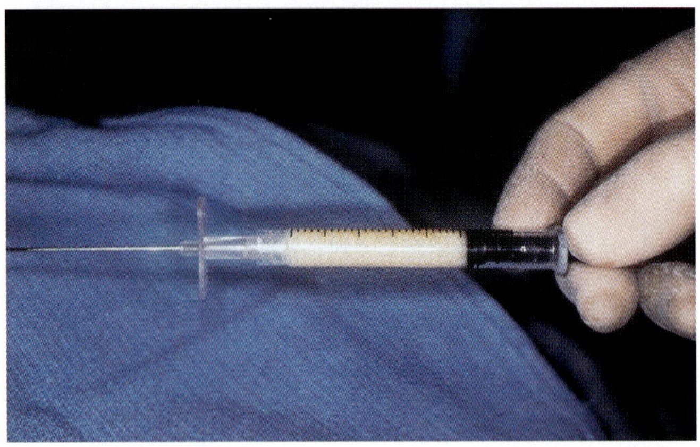

FIG. 16-6
A blunt cannula (2 mm), spinal needle, or blunt introducer from a Potts spinal needle is attached to the 3 cc syringe containing pure fat.

istered as necessary with 1% or 2% lidocaine with epinephrine. The patient may also receive oral or conscious sedation as needed. Local 1% lidocaine with epinephrine is used to augment anesthesia after the patient's blocks have taken effect. This is important for hemostasis, particularly in the vermilion border.

The nonsterile inner peel-pouch containing AlloDerm is removed from the outer foil packet (Fig. 16-9*B*). The inner peel-pouch is opened, and the physician or assistant sterilely removes the AlloDerm implant (e.g., using sterile forceps or by dropping onto a sterile field) (Fig. 16-9*C*). The implant may be cut now, prior to hydration, or after two hydration steps if preferred. The quantity of AlloDerm to be used and shape to be cut depend on the experience, preference, technique, and goals of the surgeon. For a modest upper and lower lip augmentation a single 1 mm thick 3 × 7 cm sheet can be cut as shown (Fig. 16-9*D*), although many surgeons routinely use more material. For deeper nasolabial furrows, one sheet for each side may be appropriate. Smaller pieces are available for scar revision and smaller defects.

The AlloDerm is placed into two consecutive baths containing at least 50 ml each of sterile saline, for a minimum of 5 minutes each (Fig. 16-9*E*). After the first bath the paper lining is removed from both sides of the implant and discarded. The AlloDerm can remain in the second bath for up to 4 hours. The implant may be rolled into a particular shape, stacked, and tacked with a plain gut suture if desired. This can be helpful if a large amount of material is to be used, such as in deep nasolabial folds.

After being prepped with Betadine solution and draped appropriately, the recipient site is prepared for implantation of AlloDerm. Acne scars may be undermined using an 18-gauge NoKor needle. Nasolabial folds require entry incisions made with a No. 11 blade in the alar crease or floor of the nares.

Lip vermilion augmentation, demonstrated here, requires bilateral incision sites within 5 mm of the oral commissures. A tunnel parallel to the vermilion border is initially begun with tenotomy scissors (Fig. 16-10*A*), then extended using a blunt liposuction cannula or Freer elevator (Fig. 16-10*B*). Tunneling too deeply can result in injury to the labial artery with resulting hematoma. Alligator forceps are then passed through the recipient site (Fig. 16-10*C*), the jaws of the forceps opened, and the implant grasped and pulled into position (Fig. 16-10*D*). The technique shown does not involve prerolling or tacking of the implant. Instead the implant is allowed to fold onto itself as it is pulled into the recipient site.

If the implant does not pass easily into the tunnel, the recipient site may need to be enlarged with passage of a slightly wider cannula or Freer, or the entry site may be too small. Once the implant is symmetrically in place (Fig. 16-10*E*), the lip is "milked" from the medial to lateral portions bilaterally to smooth out the implant. The ends of the implant are trimmed if necessary and tucked into the submucosa. The mucosal incision is closed with fast-absorbing gut suture (Fig. 16-10*F*). If any of the implant is included in this closure, the risk of infection is significantly increased. The instructions for postoperative care in the preceding section are followed to minimize pain and swelling. Prescription narcotic medication is indicated for this procedure.

SoftForm ePTFE

SoftForm and Gore-Tex are the appropriate implants for patients who will tolerate no resorption of material, do not mind palpability, and are willing to undergo a surgi-

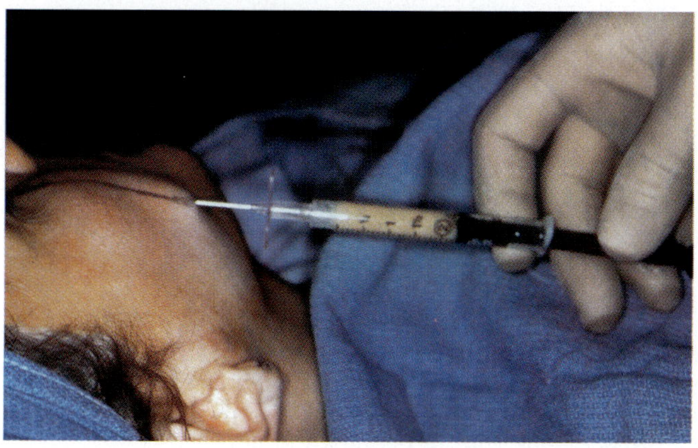

FIG. 16-7
Through a tiny incision made with the tip of a No. 11 blade if necessary for entry, thin threads of adipocytes are injected while the cannula is repeatedly withdrawn.

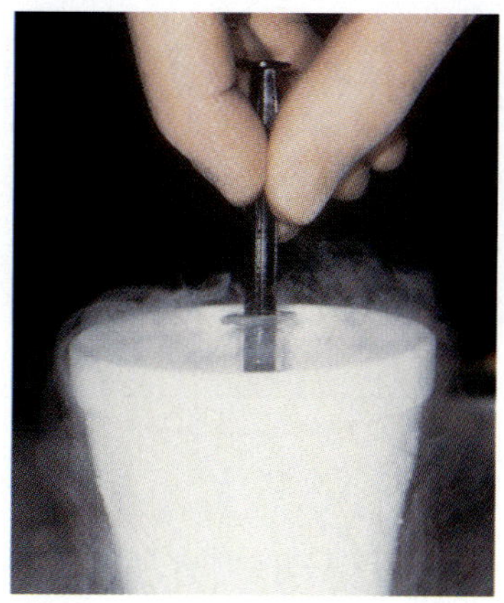

FIG. 16-8
Unused syringes of fat are frozen by individually uncapping and submerging each in liquid nitrogen until it stops bubbling.

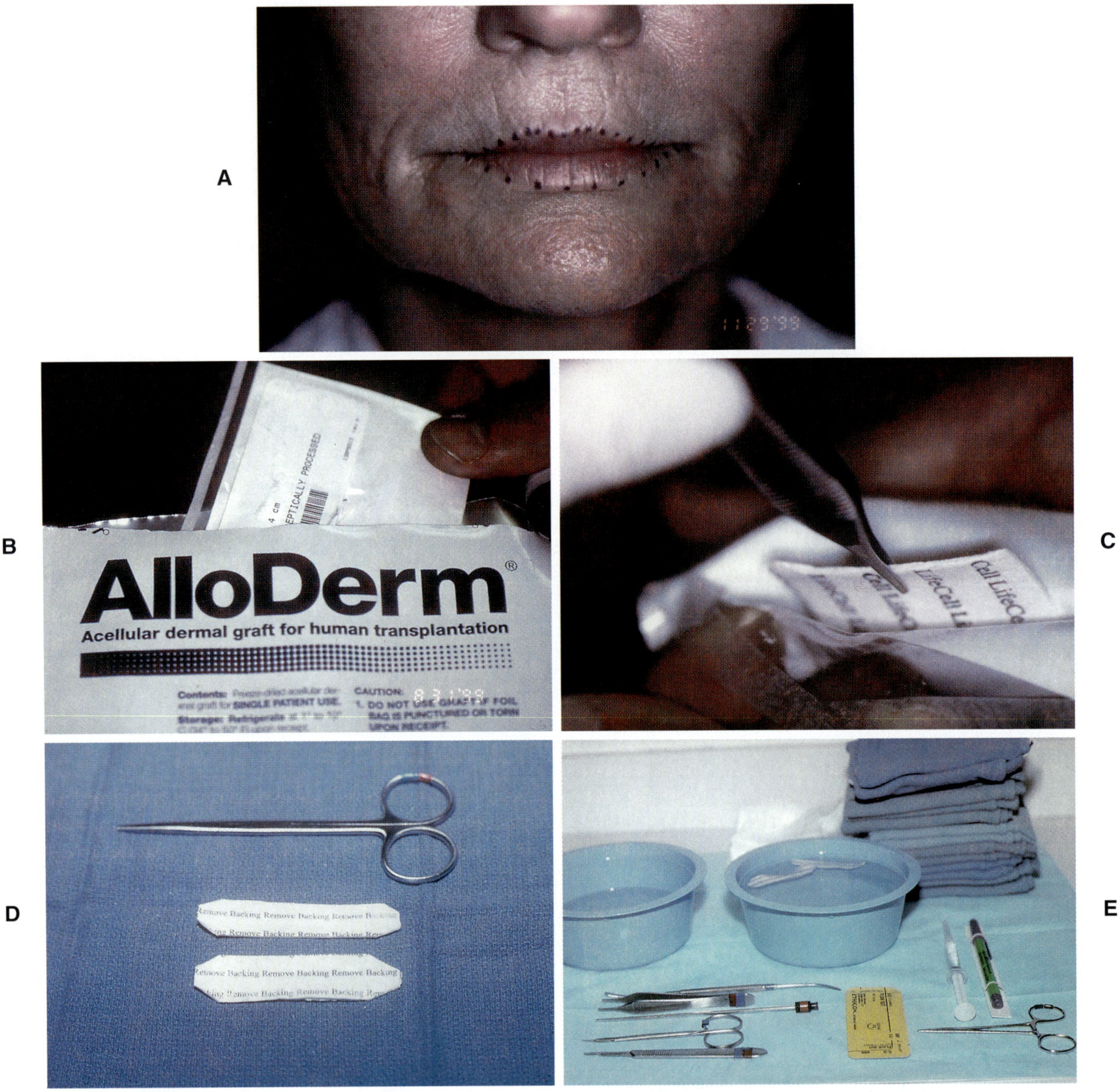

FIG. 16-9

A, The patient is marked in an upright position. **B,** The nonsterile inner peel-pouch containing AlloDerm is removed from the outer foil packet. **C,** The inner peel-pouch is opened, and the physician or assistant sterilely removes AlloDerm implant (e.g., with sterile forceps or by dropping onto a sterile field). **D,** The implant may be cut prior to hydration or after two hydration steps if preferred. **E,** The AlloDerm is placed into two consecutive baths containing at least 50 ml each of sterile saline.

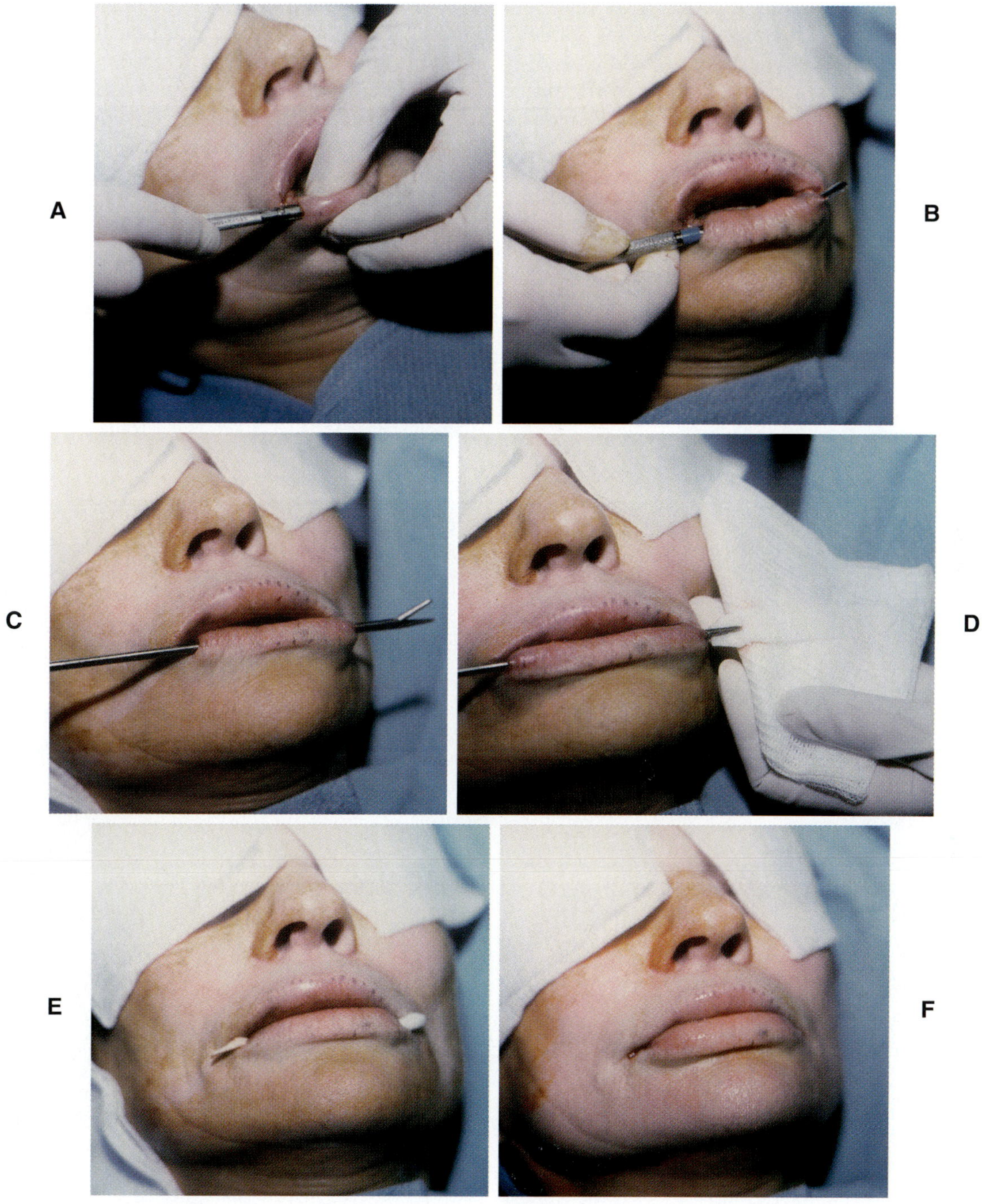

FIG. 16-10
A, Lip vermilion augmentation requires bilateral incision sites within 5 mm of the oral commissures. **B,** A tunnel parallel to the vermilion border is initially begun with tenotomy scissors, then extended with a blunt liposuction cannula or Freer elevator. **C,** Alligator forceps are then passed through the recipient site, the jaws of the forceps opened, and the implant grasped and pulled into position **(D)**. **E,** Once the implant is symmetrically in place, the lip is "milked" from the medial to lateral portions bilaterally to smooth out the implant. **F,** The mucosal incision is closed with fast-absorbing gut suture.

cal procedure rather than an injection. SoftForm's pliable texture allows it to be used in the lip vermilion with a natural result, but its benefits are limited by its manufactured cylindrical shape. This makes it less favorable for deeper nasolabial furrows. Many shapes and sizes of ePTFE are produced by W. L. Gore for use in the nasolabial folds and other subcutaneous defects. Instructional videos are available from the manufacturers.

Areas to be augmented with SoftForm are ideally straight, discrete, mild to moderate defects. After appropriate nerve blocks are obtained, 1% lidocaine with epinephrine is injected into the area to ensure anesthesia and improve hemostasis. For the nasolabial folds as demonstrated here, a No. 11 blade is used to create a 3 mm entry site for the trocar at the inferior pole of the furrow. An exit site is placed in the alar crease. These must be adequate to accommodate the trocar tip, or a stellate scar can develop if the skin tears.

The trocar is passed through the entry site, parallel to the skin surface in the subcutaneous fat (Fig. 16-11*A*). Probing too deeply in this area can injure the angular artery, resulting in a hematoma. Insertion within the dermis can result in skin irregularity and later extrusion. Placing the implant just medial to the nasolabial furrow maximizes results in this area. The trocar tip is gently eased out of the exit site (Fig. 16-11*B*). The tip is sharp and can damage the skin of the unanesthetized nose if pushed too vigorously. The trocar tip is held firmly with forceps while the plunger at the base of the trocar is depressed, releasing the metal tube from the inner spear within the ePTFE tube (Fig. 16-11*C*). The tube is withdrawn. Failing to hold the trocar tip firmly can result in injury to surrounding tissue and even to the eye, as the force of the release mechanism can be substantial. The spear is withdrawn, leaving the soft, tubular implant in place (Fig. 16-11*D*). The ends of the

A B C D

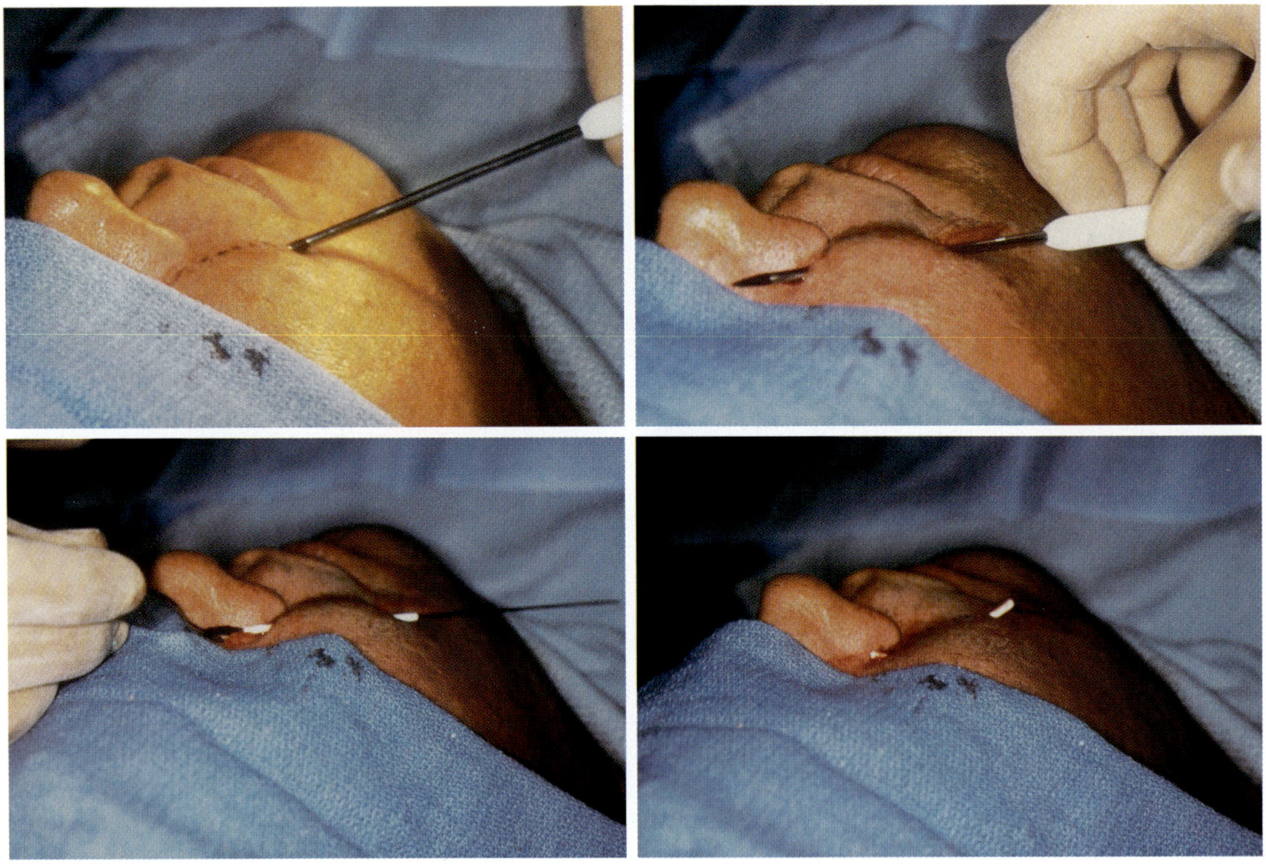

FIG. 16-11
A, The trocar is passed through the entry site, parallel to the skin surface in the subcutaneous fat. **B,** Placing the implant just medial to the nasolabial furrow maximizes results in this area. The trocar tip is gently eased out of the exit site. **C,** The trocar tip is held firmly with forceps while the plunger at the base of the trocar is depressed, releasing the metal tube from the inner spear within the ePTFE tube. **D,** The spear is withdrawn, leaving the soft, tubular implant in place.

implant are trimmed parallel with the skin, carefully tucked into the subcutaneous tissue to avoid later extrusion, and the entry and exit sites closed with fast-absorbing gut suture.

SUMMARY

Many options are available for soft tissue augmentation. Selection of the appropriate material rests on the goals of the patient and the skills of the physician. Adequate discussion and realistic expectations are important for success. The patient consent form should include possible complications in the short and long run. With proper preparation, soft tissue augmentation can be a wonderful experience for the patient and physician.

REFERENCES

1. Neuber F. Fettransplantation. Chir Kongr Verhandl Dsch Gesellch Chir 1893; 22:66.
2. Neuhof H. The Transplantation of Tissues. New York: Appleton & Company, 1923.
3. Stevenson TW. Fat grafts to the face. Plast Reconstr Surg 1949; 4:458.
4. Peer LA. The neglected "free fat graft," its behavior and clinical use. Am J Surg 1956; 92:40.
5. Gurney CE. Studies on the fate of free transplants of fat. Proc Staff Meet Mayo Clin 1937; 12:317.
6. Urback F, Wilne SS, Johnson WC, et al. Generalized paraffinoma (sclerosing lipogranuloma). Arch Dermatol 1971; 103:277-285.
7. Klein JA, Cole G, Burr RJ, et al. Paraffinomas of the scalp. Arch Dermatol 1985; 121:382-385.
8. Matton G, Amseeuw A, De Keyser F. The history of biomaterials and the biology of collagen. Aesthetic Plast Surg 1985; 9:133-140.
9. McDowell F. Complications with silicones—What grade of silicone? How do we know it was silicone? Plast Reconstr Surg 1978; 61:892-895.
10. Selmanowitz VJ, Orentreich N. Medical-grade fluid silicone: a monographic review. J Dermatol Surg Oncol 1977; 3:597-611.
11. Balkin SW. Treatment of painful scars on soles and digits with injections of fluid silicone. J Dermatol Surg Oncol 1977; 3:612.
12. Brozena SJ, Fenske NA, Cruse W, et al. Human adjuvant disease following augmentation mammoplasty. Arch Dermatol 1988; 124:1383-1386.
13. Spiera H. Scleroderma after silicone augmentation mammoplasty. JAMA 1988; 260:236-238.
14. Silver RM, Sahn EE, Allen JA, et al. Demonstration of silicon in sites of connective-tissue disease in patients with silicone-gel breast implants. Arch Dermatol 1993; 129:638.
15. Achauer BM. A serious complication following medical-grade silicone injection of the face. Plast Reconstr Surg 1983; 71:251-254.
16. Pearl RM, Laub DR, Kaplan EN. Complications following silicone injections for augmentation of the contours of the face. Plast Reconstr Surg 1978; 61:888-895.
17. Raszewski R, Guyuron B, Lash RH, et al. A severe fibrotic reaction after cosmetic liquid silicone injection. J Craniomaxillofac Surg 1990; 18:225-228.
18. Rae V, Pardo RJ, Blackwelder PL, et al. Leg ulcers following subcutaneous injection of a liquid silicone preparation. Arch Dermatol 1989; 125:670-673.
19. Mastruserio DN, Pasqueira MJ, Cobb MW. Severe granulomatous reaction and facial ulceration occurring after subcutaneous silicone injection. J Am Acad Dermatol 1996; 34:849-852.
20. Ellenbogen R, Ellenbogen R, Rubin L. Injectable fluid silicone therapy: human morbidity and mortality. JAMA 1975; 234:308-309.
21. Ousterhout DK, Stelnicki EJ. Plastic surgery's plastics. Clin Plast Surg 1996; 23:183-190.
22. Knapp TR, Kaplan EN, Daniels JR. Injectable collagen for soft tissue augmentation. Plast Reconstr Surg 1977; 60:389.
23. Kaminer M, Krauss M. Filler substances in the treatment of facial aging. Med Surg Dermatol 1998; 5:215-221.
24. Klein AW, Rish DC. Injectable collagen: an adjunct to facial plastic surgery. Facial Plast Surg 1987; 4:87.
25. Wainwright D, Madden M, Luterman A, et al. Clinical evaluation of an acellular allograft dermal matrix in full-thickness burns. J Burn Care Rehabil 1996; 17:124-136.
26. Lattari V, Jones LM, Varcelotti JR, et al. The use of a permanent dermal allograft in full-thickness burns of the hand and foot: a report of three cases. J Burn Care Rehabil 1997; 18:147-155.
27. Jones FR, Schwartz BM, Silverstein P. Use of a nonimmunogenic acellular dermal allograft for soft tissue augmentation: a preliminary report. Aesthetic Surg Q 1996; 16:196-201.
28. Achauer BM, VanderKam VM, Celikoz B, et al. Augmentation of facial soft-tissue defects with AlloDerm dermal graft. Ann Plast Surg 1998; 41:503-507.
29. Tobin HA, Karas ND. Lip augmentation using an Alloderm graft. J Oral Maxillofac Surg 1998; 56:722-727.
30. Castor SA, Wyatt CT, Papay FA. Lip augmentation with AlloDerm allogenic dermal graft and fat autograft: a comparison with autologous fat injection alone. Aesthetic Plast Surg 1999; 23:218-223.
31. Silverstein LH, Callan DP. An acellular dermal matrix allograft substitute for palatal donor tissue. Postgrad Dent 1996; 3:14-21.
32. Kridel RWH, Foda H, Lunde KC. Septal perforation repair with acellular human dermal allograft. Arch Otolaryngol Head Neck Surg 1998; 124:73-78.
33. Dalla Vecchia L, Engum S, Kogon B, et al. Evaluation of small intestine submucosa and acellular dermis as diaphragmatic prostheses. J Pediatr Surg 1999; 34:167-171.
34. Chaplin JM, Constantino PD, Wolpoe ME, et al. Use of an acellular dermal allograft for dural replacement: an experimental study. Neurosurg 1999; 45:320-327.
35. Griffey ES. Presentation. Congress on In Vitro Biology, May 20-24, 1995.
36. Bickenbach JR, Roop DR. Transduction of a preselected population of human epidermal stem cells: consequences for gene therapy. Proc Assoc Am Physicians 1999; 111:184-189.
37. Izumi K, Takacs G, Terashi H, et al. Ex vivo development of a composite human oral mucosal equivalent. J Oral Maxillofac Surg 1999; 57:571-577.
38. Lemperle G, Hazan-Gauthier N, Lemperle M. PMMA microspheres (Artecoll) for skin and soft tissue augmentation, part II: clinical investigations. Plast Reconstr Surg 1995; 96:627-634.
39. McClelland M, Egbert B, Hanko V, et al. Evaluation of Artecoll polymethylmethacrylate implant for soft-tissue augmentation: biocompatibility and chemical characterization. Plast Reconstr Surg 1997; 100:1466-1474.
40. Constantino PD, Friedman CD. Soft-tissue augmentation and replacement in the head and neck: general considerations. Otolaryngol Clin N Am 1994; 27:1-12.
41. Troilus C. Letter. Aesthetic Surg J 2000; 20:136-137.
42. Ersek RA. Letter. Aesthetic Surg J 2000; 20:135-136.
43. Sclafani AP. Micronized acellular tissue for soft tissue augmentation. Aesthetic Surg J 2000; 20:341-342.
44. Swinehart JM. Pocket grafting with dermal grafts: autologous collagen implants for permanent correction of cutaneous depression. Am J Cosmet Surg 1996; 12:321-331.
45. Goodman G. Laser-assisted dermal grafting for the correction of cutaneous contour defects. Dermatol Surg 1997; 23:95-99.

46. Nicolle FV, Chir M, Matti BA, et al. Dermal and facial autografts in facial aesthetic surgery. Aesthetic Plast Surg 1992; 16:219-225.
47. Davis RE, Guida RA, Cook TA. Autologous free dermal fat graft. Arch Otolaryngol Head Neck Surg 1995; 121:95-100.
48. Hinderer UT, Escalona J. Dermal and subdermal tissue filling with fetal connective tissue and cartilage, collagen and silicone: experimental study in the pig compared with clinical results: a new technique of dermis mini-autograft injections. Aesthetic Plast Surg 1990; 14:239-248.
49. Bright RW, Green WT. Freeze-dried fascia lata allografts: a review of 47 cases. J Pediatr Orthop 1981; 1:13-22.
50. Burres S. Recollagenation of acne scars. Dermatol Surg 1996; 22:364-367.
51. Burres S. Lip augmentation with preserved fascia lata. Dermatol Surg 1997; 23:459-462.
52. Orentreich DS, Orentreich N. Subcutaneous incisionless (subcision) surgery for correction of depressed scars and wrinkles. Dermatol Surg 1995; 21:543-549.
53. Moore JH, Kolaczynski JW, Morales LM, et al. Viability of fat obtained by syringe suction lipectomy: effects of local anesthesia with lidocaine. Aesthetic Plast Surg 1995; 19:335-339.
54. Lalikos JF, Li Y, Roth T, et al. Biochemical assessment of cellular damage after adipocyte harvest. J Surg Res 1997; 70:95-100.
55. Illouz Y. Present results of fat injection. Aesthetic Plast Surg 1988; 12:175-181.
56. Carpaneda CA, Ribeiro MT. Study of the histologic alterations and viability of the adipose graft in humans. Aesthetic Plast Surg 1993; 17:43-47.
57. Guerrerosantos J. Autologous fat grafting for body contouring. Clin Plast Surg 1996; 23:619-631.
58. Niechajev I, Sevcuk O. Long-term results of fat transplantation: clinical and histologic studies. Plast Reconstr Surg 1994; 94:496-506.
59. Matarasso A, Matarasso SL. Autologous fat transplantation. Plast Reconstr Surg 1995(letter); 95:933.
60. Coleman SR. Facial recontouring with lipostructure. Clin Plast Surg 1997; 24:347-367.
61. Fulton JE, Suarez M, Silverton K, et al. Small volume fat transfer. Dermatol Surg 1998; 24:857-865.
62. Pinski KS, Coleman WP. Microlipoinjection and autologous collagen. Cosmet Dermatol 1995; 13:339-351.
63. Eppley BL, Sidner RA, Platis JM, et al. Bioactivation of free-fat transfers: a potential new approach to improving graft survival. Plast Reconstr Surg 1992; 90:1022-1030.
64. Coleman WP, Lawrence N, Sherman RN, et al. Autologous collagen? Lipocytic dermal augmentation, a histopathologic study. J Dermatol Surg Oncol 1993; 19:1032-1040.
65. Field LM. Soft tissue augmentation by fibrosis: fat injections and other means. Dermatol Surg 1996(letter); 22:192-193.
66. Feinendegen DL, Baumgartner RW, Vuadens P, et al. Autologous fat injection for soft tissue augmentation in the face: a safe procedure? Aesthetic Plast Surg 1998; 22:163-167.
67. Egido JA, Arroyo R, Marcos A, et al. Middle cerebral artery embolism and unilateral visual loss after autologous fat injection into the glabellar area. Stroke 1993; 24:615-616.
68. Drommer RB, Mende U. Free fat transplantation in the face. J Craniomaxillofac Surg 1995; 23:228-232.
69. Castello JR, Barros J, Vazquez R. Giant liponecrotic pseudocyst after breast augmentation by fat injection. Plast Reconstr Surg 1999; 103:291.
70. Spangler AS. Treatment of depressed scars with Fibrin Foam—seventeen years of experience. J Dermatol Surg Oncol 1975; 1: 65-69.
71. Gottlieb S. "GAP repair technique." Poster exhibit. Annual meeting of the American Academy of Dermatology. December 1977; Dallas, TX.
72. Lassus C. Expanded PTFE in the treatment of facial wrinkles. Aesthetic Plast Surg 1991; 15:167-174.
73. Lassus C. A surgical solution to the deep nasolabial fold. Plast Reconstr Surg 1996; 97:1473-1478.
74. Walter C. Aspects of facial correction and reconstruction by using transplants (composite grafts and implants) with special reference to surgical membrane implants. Otolaryngol Head Neck Surg 1994; 110:524-529.
75. Cisneros JL, Singla R. Intradermal augmentation with expanded polytetrafluoroethylene (Gore-Tex) for facial lines and wrinkles. J Dermatol Surg Oncol 1993; 19:539-542.
76. Ellis DAF, Trimas SJ. Gore-Tex implants for the correction of thin lips. Laryngoscope 1995; 105:207-209.
77. Sherris DA, Larrabee WF Jr. Expanded polytetrafluoroethylene augmentation of the lower face. Laryngoscope 1996; 106:658-663.
78. Wolf DL. Complications following lip augmentation with Gore-Tex. Plast Reconstr Surg 1995(letter); 95:1334-1335.
79. Levet Y. Caveat regarding Gore-Tex. Plast Reconstr Surg 1995; 95:932-933.
80. Spira M, Liu B, Xu Z, et al. Human amnion collagen for soft tissue augmentation—biochemical characterizations and animal observations. J Biomed Mat Res 1994; 28:91-96.
81. Balazs EA, Leshchiner EA. Hyaluronan, its crosslinked derivative hylan, and their medical applications. In: Inagake H, Phillips GO, eds. Cellulosics Utilization: Research and Rewards in Cellulosics. New York: Elsevier Applied Science, 1989:233-241.
82. Piacquadio D. Crosslinked hyaluronic acid (hylan gel) as a soft tissue augmentation material: a preliminary assessment. In: Elson ML, ed. Evaluation and Treatment of the Aging Face. New York: Springer-Verlag, 1995:304-308.
83. Piacquadio D, Jarcho M, Goltz R. Evaluation of hylan b gel as a soft-tissue augmentation implant material. J Am Acad Dermatol 1997; 36:544-549.
84. West TB, Alster TS. Autologous human collagen and dermal fibroblasts for soft tissue augmentation. Dermatol Surg 1998; 24: 510-512.
85. Krajcik R, Orentreich DS, Orentreich N. Plasmagel: a novel injectable autologous material for soft tissue augmentation. J Aesthetic Derm Cosmet Surg 1999; 1:109-115.
86. Olenius M. The first clinical study using a new biodegradable implant for the treatment of lips, wrinkles and folds. Aesthetic Plast Surg 1998; 22:97-101.
87. Duranti F, Salti G, Bovani B, et al. Injectable hyaluronic acid gel for soft tissue augmentation: a clinical and histological study. Dermatol Surg 1998; 24:1317-1325.
88. Rofil Medical product literature, Rofil Medical Nederland B.V., Stadionstraat 1C, 4815 NC BREDA, The Netherlands. E-mail: RMI@rofil.nl
89. Achauer BM. A serious complication following medical-grade silicone injection of the face. Plast Reconstr Surg 1983; 71:251-254.
90. Selmanowitz VJ, Orentreich N. Medical-grade fluid silicone: a monographic review. J Dermatol Surg Oncol 1977; 3:597-611.
91. Maas CS, Eriksson T, McCalmont T, et al. Evaluation of ePTFE as a soft tissue filling substance: an analysis of design-related implant behavior employing the porcine skin model. Plast Reconstr Surg 1998; 101:1307-1314.
92. Kaminer M, Krauss M. Filler substances in the treatment of facial aging. Med Surg Dermatol 1998; 5:215-221.
93. Wallace DG, McPherson JJ, Ellingsworth LE, et al. Injectable collagen for tissue augmentation. In: Nimni ME, ed. Collagen, Vol. III, Biotechnology. Boca Raton: CRC Press, 1988:117-144.
94. Collagen Corporation, Bulletin re: Bovine spongiform encephalopathy.

95. McPherson JM, Ledger PW, Sawamura S, et al. The preparation and physiochemical characterization of an injectable form of reconstituted, glutaraldehyde crosslinked, bovine corium collagen. J Biomed Meter Res 1986; 20:79.
96. Klein AW. Indications and implantation techniques for the various formulations of injectable collagen. J Dermatol Surg Oncol 1988; 14(suppl 1):49.
97. Cooperman LS, Mackinnon V, Bechler G, et al. Injectable collagen: a six-year clinical investigation. Aesthetic Plast Surg 1985; 9:145.
98. Kamer FM, Churukian XM. The clinical use of injectable collagen: a three-year retrospective study. Arch Otolaryngol 1984; 110:93.
99. Klein AW. In favor of double testing. J Dermatol Surg Oncol 1989; 15:263.
100. Elson ML. The role of skin testing in the use of collagen injectable materials. J Dermatol Surg Oncol 1989; 15:301.
101. Klein AW, Rish DC. Injectable collagen update. J Dermatol Surg Oncol 1984; 10:519.
102. Hanke CW, Hingley HR, Jolivette DM, et al. Abscess formation and local necrosis after treatment with Zyderm or Zyplast collagen implant. J Am Acad Dermatol 1991; 25:319-326.
103. DeLustro F, Smith ST, Sundsmo J, et al. Reaction to injectable collagen: results in animal models and clinical use. Plast Reconstr Surg 1987; 79:581.
104. McGrew RN, Wilson RS, Havener WH. Sudden blindness secondary to injection of common drugs in the head and neck, part 1: clinical experiences. Otolaryngology 1978; 86:147.
105. McCoy JP Jr, Schade WJ, Siegle RJ, et al. Characterization of the humoral immune response to bovine collagen implants. Arch Dermatol 1985; 121:990.
106. Cooperman LS, Michaeli D. The immunogenicity of injectable collagen, part 2: a retrospective review of seventy-two tested and treated patients. J Dermatol Surg Oncol 1984; 10:647.
107. Siegle RJ, McCoy JP, Schade W, et al. Intradermal implantation of bovine collagen: humoral responses associated with clinical reaction. Arch Dermatol 1984; 120:183.
108. Kligman AM. Histologic responses to collagen implants in human volunteers: comparison of Zyderm collagen with Zyplast implant. J Dermatol Surg Oncol 1988; 14(suppl 1):35.
109. Stegman SJ, Chus S, Bensch K, et al. A light and electron microscopic evaluation of Zyderm collagen and Zyplast implants in aging human facial skin: a pilot study. Arch Dermatol 1987; 123: 1644.
110. Bailin PL, Bailin MD. Collagen implantation: clinical applications and lesion selection. J Dermatol Surg Oncol 1988; 14(suppl 1):49
111. Klein AW, Brandt FD, Grekin DA, et al. Collagen implants for lip augmentation. 1990; unpublished data on file at McGhan Medical, formerly the Collagen Corporation, Santa Barbara, CA.

APPENDIX A

Patient Evaluation: Aesthetic Goals

1. What are the patient's goals for soft tissue augmentation?
2. Does the patient have realistic expectations?
3. Is the patient willing to undergo skin testing with its necessary waiting period?
4. Are the aesthetic concerns appropriate for another modality (e.g., Botox for glabellar and forehead rhytides, or resurfacing for extensive photodamage)?
5. Are the rhytides or defects superficial, deep, or a combination of both?
6. Is the patient willing to achieve temporary or partial improvement that may require further treatment?
7. Is the patient willing to undergo a more extensive surgical procedure for greater longevity of correction (e.g., with AlloDerm or ePTFE)?
8. Is the patient willing to have a material implanted that may have temporary induration or permanent palpability?

APPENDIX B

Patient Evaluation: Medical

Assess if any of the following are present:
1. Bleeding disorders or anticoagulant use.
2. Allergies to bovine collagen or meat products, antibiotics, multiple severe allergies to a variety of substances, history of anaphylaxis to any substance.
3. Keloid formation or other scarring disorders.
4. Autoimmune disorders that may flare with implantation or cause abnormal destruction of implant.
5. Oral herpes simplex virus history.
6. Immunosuppression or increased risk of infection.
7. Any difficulties with local anesthesia, oral or conscious sedation (if pertinent), or pain medications in the past.

APPENDIX C

Preoperative Precautions and Instructions

1. Avoid aspirin and vitamin E for 10 days, NSAIDs such as ibuprofen (Advil) for 7 days, and alcohol for 3 days prior to any procedure to minimize bruising and swelling (with injectable treatment) and to avoid excessive bleeding and hematoma formation with solid implants.
2. Oral antibiotics such as Keflex, or Zithromax for patients allergic to penicillin, should begin 1 day before any solid implant or fat injection. The length of the course depends on the drug, procedure, and presence of complications but generally ranges from 3 to 7 days.
3. Antiviral prophylaxis (Valtrex 500 mg bid for 5 days beginning the day before the procedure) is recommended in all patients who will be undergoing a surgical augmentation in the vermilion (e.g., AlloDerm, SoftForm, Gore-Tex). It is also useful for those

patients with a history of oral HSV who will be undergoing augmentation with an injectable filler.

APPENDIX D

Postoperative Instructions for Surgical Augmentation (e.g., SoftForm or AlloDerm)

1. Ice packs (either conforming gel type or frozen peas in a zip-lock bag) should be applied for 15 minutes on, 15 minutes off during the first 24 to 48 hours while the patient is awake after surgical implantation procedures, particularly in the oral or perioral area.
2. The patient's head should be elevated as much as possible while he or she is sleeping or resting during the first 4 days to encourage resolution of edema.
3. Aspirin, NSAIDs, vitamin E, and alcohol should be avoided for the first week postoperatively. Tylenol or prescription narcotic analgesics (e.g., Percocet or Vicodin) should be used for pain control as needed.
4. For procedures involving the mouth, soft and easy-to-chew foods should be eaten during the first 2 days. The patient should not sip through a straw if lip augmentation was performed. Very hot foods should be avoided during the first 24 hours to avoid burns to the anesthetized area.
5. Talking, laughing, and exaggerated mouth movements should be minimized for the first few days after augmentation of the lips, nasolabial folds, and chin furrows (marionette lines).
6. The physician should be notified if there is significant bleeding, excessive pain, irregular swelling or dusky color to any area of the lips, eye pain, vision loss, headache, or other concerns.

CHAPTER 17

Botulinum A Exotoxin Injections for Photoaging and Hyperhidrosis

MICHAEL S. KAMINER
GEORGE J. HRUZA

SECTION ONE

History and Scientific Review

BACKGROUND AND HISTORY

Discovered in 1895 by E. Van Ermengem, *Clostridium botulinum* was found to be the causative organism of a fatal progressive paralysis known as botulism. Thirty-four Belgian citizens had become ill following ingestion of raw salted ham, and the toxin from *C. botulinum* was identified as the offending agent.

The first attempts at isolation and development of botulinum toxin began in 1920 with Dr. Herman Sommer. There are seven subtypes of botulinum toxin, identified as exotoxins A to G.[1] Type A, which was purified in 1946 by Dr. Edward Shantz, is the most potent of the seven subtypes and is also the most potent neurotoxin known.[2] Dr. Vernon Brooks first suggested its therapeutic use on hyperfunctional muscles in the 1950s. The initial batch of botulinum toxin A (BTX-A), made by Dr. Alan Scott, wasn't prepared for human experiments until 1979. That 150 mg batch, labeled 79-11, was the source for all BTX-A used in the United States until December 1997.[3] Since 1997 a new FDA-approved BTX-A source has been widely used in clinical practice (Allergan, Irvine, CA).

Botulinum A exotoxin (Botox, Allergan, Irvine, CA) is approved by the U.S. Food and Drug Administration (FDA) for the treatment of hyperfunctional muscles affected by conditions such as blepharospasm and spastic muscle activity. The cosmetic use of Botox dates to 1988 when Dr. Jean Carruthers noted resolution of periorbital wrinkles in patients treated with Botox for benign essential blepharospasm.[4] Since many rhytides are caused by muscle contraction, paralyzing or at least weakening the underlying muscles produces a smoother skin surface.

The work by Carruthers was seminal and has led to an expanded use of the toxin for cosmetic indications. Initially used for rhytides in the glabellar region, BTX-A is now used to treat the forehead, periorbital region, neck, and perioral areas. More recent work has led to its use in the treatment of headaches, as well as for palmar and axillary hyperhidrosis.

BASIC SCIENCE

BTX-A functions as an endoprotease inhibitor at the neuromuscular junction (NMJ) (Fig. 17-1).[5] The toxin is composed of two chains linked by disulfide bonds,[6] and it binds to specific cholinergic receptors on the presynaptic neuron. The toxin is then enveloped by the cell membrane and internalized through energy-dependent endocytosis. Once inside the cell, the disulfide bonds are broken and the light chain of BTX-A is released into the cytoplasm. It then inhibits acetylcholine release by acting as a zinc-dependent metalloendoprotease that deactivates specific components of the neuroexocytic mechanism.[7] Numerous proteins are required for the release of acetylcholine, and botulinum toxin cleaves one or more of these proteins as its mechanism of action. Botulinum toxins A, C, and E cleave the 25 kD synaptosomal associated protein SNAP-25. Types B, D, F, and G cleave a vesicle associated membrane protein.[6]

Striated muscle neuromuscular junctions are most sensitive to the toxin. Autonomic cholinergic ganglia are also inhibited by BTX-A, but to a much lesser degree. The toxin causes irreversible chemical denervation of striated muscle at the NMJ, and the effect is permanent at all NMJs exposed to the toxin. Recovery of muscle function is always seen after several weeks to several months because the muscle rapidly develops new NMJs through an amplification process that increases normal NMJ production by a factor of 10.[8] Clinically, muscle weakness becomes apparent 2 to 3 days following BTX-A injection, with complete paralysis seen after 8 to 10 days.[9] Histologically, the injected muscle atrophies with individual muscle fibers becoming smaller. After 1 month the atrophy stabilizes. Acetylcholinesterase spreads beyond the NMJ during the period of paralysis. After 3 to 6 months, with return of muscle activity, acetylcholinesterase again becomes localized to the NMJ.[10]

When ingested, BTX-A causes a progressive, often fatal paralysis with no known antidote. The lethal dose (LD_{50}) for BTX-A is approximately 2500 to 3000 U of toxin.[11] One unit of toxin is the amount needed to kill 50% of 18 to 20 g Swiss-Webster mice after intraperitoneal injection.[12]

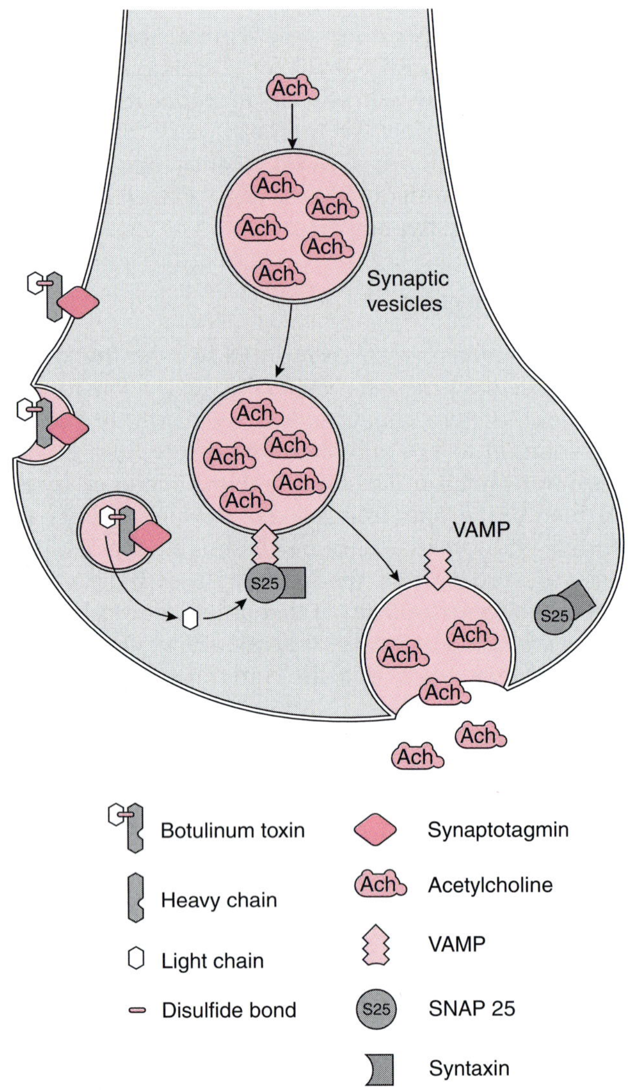

FIG. 17-1
Mechanism of action for botulinum toxin A at the presynaptic neuron.

BTX-A is capable of inducing the formation of neutralizing antibodies. Once formed, the antibodies make the patient relatively resistant to additional toxin injections. Antibody formation seems to be dose dependent. Patients receiving mean doses of ≥200 U are at increased risk for the development of neutralizing antibodies.[13] Such high doses are rarely used for the treatment of rhytides but may at times be used for the treatment of hyperhidrosis. Research is currently looking at the use of botulinum toxin subtypes B and F, which are only slightly less potent than subtype A. There is no cross-reactivity between the different subtypes, which would be an important clinical consideration for patients who have developed neutralizing antibodies to BTX-A.[14]

CLINICAL STUDIES

Each vial of Botox contains 100 U of lyophilized botulinum A exotoxin, 0.5 mg of human albumin, and 0.9 mg of sodium chloride (Box 17-1). It is kept freeze-dried at –4°C or colder until reconstitution with normal saline. Botox, which consists of a crystalline complex of the high molecular weight toxin protein and hemagglutinin protein, is easily denatured by shaking or allowing bubbles to percolate through the solution. Gentle handling is key to maintain potency. Once reconstituted, the material is supposed to be used within 4 hours, but Garcia and Fulton demonstrated continued potency of solution kept refrigerated up to 4 weeks after reconstitution.[15] However, there is a gradual loss of potency after 1 week. Lowe found that reconstituted Botox lost 50% of its potency after only 1 week.[16]

Botulinum toxin A is also marketed as Dysport (Speywood Pharmaceuticals, Maidenhead, Berkshire, United Kingdom) in Europe. Botox is 3 to 4 times more potent than Dysport, so that 3 to 4 times as many units of Dysport are needed to achieve equivalent clinical effects.[16,17]

Rhytides

Original work published by Alistair and Jean Carruthers[4,17-22] has opened the way for many other investigators to report their experience with Botox. Carruthers has found the most success with a relatively high Botox concentration of 10 U/ml, injecting small volumes into the targeted muscles. Hankins et al. performed a dose response study of Botox for glabellar rhytides in 46 subjects.[23] They found no statistically

BOX 17-1 Botox (Botulinum Exotoxin A, Allergan, Irvine, CA)

Botulinum A Exotoxin	100 U (lyophilized)
Human albumin	0.5 mg
Sodium chloride	0.9 mg

significant difference in efficacy using Botox doses from 12.5 to 50 U for the glabellar complex. They also found no difference between concentrations ranging from 200 down to 10 U/ml.

Matsudo reported his results of glabellar rhytide Botox injections using a concentration of 100 U/ml and injecting 10 to 20 U per patient. He saw muscle paralysis within 48 hours and the effect lasted approximately 6 months.[24] Guerrissi and Sarkissian used a Botox concentration of 25 U/ml for upper face rhytide correction in 54 patients. The onset of muscle paralysis commenced 3 to 5 days after injection. The muscles remained paralyzed for 6 to 8 months in all but four patients.[25] Guyuron and Huddelston found that they needed a Botox dose of 25 U per glabellar complex to achieve muscle paralysis lasting for several months.[26] Lower doses had an effect as short as 2 weeks.

In a collaborative study of 210 injection sites in 162 patients, Botox was injected under EMG guidance into various muscles of facial expression including the glabella (5 to 20 U), forehead (5 to 25 U), crow's feet (5 to 15 U), nasolabial folds (2.5 to 5 U), and platysma (10 to 20 U).[27] Effects of the toxin were usually seen within 1 to 3 days and lasted from 3 to 6 months. Seven patients experienced temporary weakness of nearby muscles including ptosis, eyebrow droop, and upper lip droop. In a study by Pribitkin et al. of 80 patients who had their glabellar complex injected with increasing doses of Botox under EMG guidance, the most effective dose of Botox was found to be 10 U per corrugator muscle.[28] Overall, 80% of the women but only 43% of the men achieved satisfactory improvement in their wrinkles. Lowe et al. have done the only double-blind placebo-controlled study of Botox for rhytides.[29] They injected 10 U of Botox or normal saline into each corrugator muscle of 30 subjects under EMG guidance. The subjects who received the Botox injection had a statistically significant reduction in their glabellar frown line depth and length compared with the placebo control 12 weeks after the injection.

Frankel and Kamer found, in a study of 30 patients, that injecting 20 U of Botox into the glabellar muscle complex achieved a modest brow elevation in 62% of patients.[30] In a collaborative study, 1500 patients were treated with Botox for platysmal bands and neck wrinkles.[31] Most patients were treated with 50 to 100 U of Botox. Among patients with mild to moderate platysmal bands and rhytides, 98.5% were judged to have achieved good to excellent results. The treatment of patients with severe platysmal bands was far less effective. One percent of patients reported temporary neck weakness, and one patient experienced dysphagia lasting 2 weeks.

Hyperhidrosis

Botox has also been used recently with success to treat axillary, palmar, and plantar hyperhidrosis. An initial report by Bushara et al. showed that injecting 50 U of Botox into the subdermal tissue of the axilla achieves anhidrosis lasting 6 to 8 months before wearing off.[32] Glogau reproduced these results in 10 patients with axillary hyperhidrosis, with the anhidrosis lasting 4 to 7 months in his patients.[33] Odderson blocked axillary sweating with 100 U per axilla in two patients; sweating started to return after 2 to 4 months.[34] In the only randomized, double-blind, placebo-controlled trial of botulinum A exotoxin for severe axillary hyperhidrosis, 13 patients received 200 U of Dysport into one axilla with the other one being injected with normal saline. Ninhydrin staining showed a 30% sweat reduction in the Dysport-treated side compared with the placebo-treated side at 3 months after injection. Subjectively the Dysport side had 60% less sweating compared with the placebo side.[35]

Shelley et al. achieved effective treatment of palmar hyperhidrosis in four patients by injecting 100 U of Botox into each palm, 50 subdermal injections of 2 U. The anhidrosis lasted from 4 to 12 months, and one patient experienced mild thumb weakness for 3 weeks after injection.[36] Naumann et al. injected 3 U of Botox per 4 cm^2 into the axillae, palms, or soles of 11 patients with hyperhidrosis of those areas. Hyperhidrosis was effectively blocked for the entire 5-month follow-up period.[37]

Frey's syndrome, or gustatory sweating onto the cheek, is a fairly common side effect of parotid gland surgery. Injecting Botox intracutaneously into the area of gustatory sweating has been shown to block the unwanted sweating. Bjerkhoel and Trobbe injected Botox into the cheeks of 15 patients with Frey's syndrome and found abolition of sweating for up to 13 months.[38] In another study of 45 patients, Botox injection blocked gustatory sweating during the entire 6-month follow-up period.[39] Laskawi treated 19 patients with severe Frey's syndrome and found the sweating effectively blocked with one Botox injection for a mean of 17 months.[40] Gustatory sweating recurs anywhere from 8 months to 30 months after Botox injection, but the recurrent sweating is always less severe than initially and responds to additional Botox injections. On the basis of these studies, Botox has become the nonsurgical treatment of choice for severe Frey's syndrome.[41]

Headaches

Botox injections into certain pericranial muscles has been associated with a reduction in tension as well as migraine-type headaches. Schulte-Mattler et al. injected a total of 200 U of Dysport into the frontal, temporal, occipital, and sternocleidomastoid muscles of nine patients with tension headaches.42 The frequency and severity of headaches was reduced by 50%. Wheeler achieved similar improvement in four patients suffering from tension headaches.43 Injecting Botox into only the temporal muscle does not seem to alleviate tension headaches.44 Recent anecdotal reports also link the use of BTX-A with the improvement or elimination of migraine headaches.

DISCUSSION

The use of botulinum A exotoxin has evolved dramatically over the past decade. Although it has been a fascinating molecule from both a historical and therapeutic standpoint, its evolution as a cosmetic surgical agent has been remarkable. Use of BTX-A in the treatment of hyperdynamic rhytides has literally revolutionized the practice of facial cosmetic surgery. Prior to the use of BTX-A, rejuvenation of the upper face was performed primarily with surgical interventions such as forehead lifts and face lift surgery. The morbidity of those procedures made them at times an unattractive alternative for those patients seeking a subtle enhancement in their appearance. With the advent of BTX-A, improvement in dynamic rhytides of the glabella, forehead, and periocular region became available to a much broader range of patients. In addition, the simplicity of the BTX-A procedure made it much more accessible to physicians. Doctors became comfortable treating rhytides with this injection technique due to its relative ease of use and superb safety margin.[45]

Early use of BTX-A in the dermatology community was greeted with cautious optimism. Patients were initially treated with a variety of techniques by a wide range of physicians, but a standard use and system of injections has begun to evolve. There continue to be many subtly different approaches to the clinical use of BTX-A, but the end goal is the same: elimination of wrinkles or sweating for a period of 3 to 6 months. It is generally accepted that BTX-A is a *temporary* solution for dynamic rhytides and hyperhidrosis, although opinions differ as to which concentration of toxin to use and how and where to inject. Some patients experience a prolonged period of clinical efficacy greater than the average 3 to 6 months, but that is the exception rather than the rule.

Recent advances in BTX-A use include the ability to achieve subtle brow elevation, a so-called nonsurgical browlift, as well as the reduction of infraorbital rhytides and lax skin. These advances have come in part because of the broad range of physicians who have gained experience with BTX-A injections, including plastic surgeons, facial plastic surgeons, dermatologists, and oculoplastic surgeons. Further additions to the use of BTX-A include treatment of neck rhytides as well as headaches. Injection techniques are similar regardless of the site being treated, but the important factor is the precise placement of BTX-A injections. Platysmal bands previously were treatable only through surgical platysmaplasty. In society's quest to achieve improvements in appearance with simple, low morbidity techniques, BTX-A was the right treatment at the right time. Platysmal bands, for example, can now be addressed for many patients in a 10-minute injection procedure instead of a 1- to 2-hour surgical procedure.[46] Surgical platysmaplasty is still the definitive treatment of choice, but clearly the recovery, cost, and risk profile for BTX-A can be much more attractive to the prospective patient.

Botulinum A exotoxin injection is a safe, reproducible, office-based method for treating hyperhidrosis and the aging face. Its role has evolved rapidly and will likely continue to do so. Newer uses for the toxin are almost certain to be explored, and physicians will continue to gain paradoxical comfort with utilizing the most potent neurotoxin known to medicine.

SECTION TWO

Atlas of Surgical Procedures

PREOPERATIVE CLINICAL CONSIDERATIONS

Botox is reconstituted with preservative-free normal saline immediately before injection. Several authors have explored the relationship of dose/dilution with clinical efficacy, but an industry-wide standard does not currently exist. Authors have used anywhere from 0.5 to 10 ml of saline to dilute the toxin, with no definitive difference in therapeutic efficacy demonstrated.[15,23] Concentrations ranging from 1 to 10 U of BTX-A per 0.1 ml have been employed with varying levels of success (Box 17-2), and there are many different individualized approaches to injection techniques and sites. The duration of action for BTX-A appears to lengthen to some degree in a dose dependent fashion. The higher the number of units injected per muscle, the longer the clinical effect. However, complication rates also tend to increase as dose increases.

We will describe a standardized injection technique to allow for reproducible results. We prefer to dilute the lyophilized toxin with 5 ml of normal saline, producing a concentration of 2 U of BTX-A per 0.1 ml, and to inject it in volumes of 0.1 ml per injection site (Box 17-3). Some authors have written that they inject volumes of 0.05 to 0.18 ml per site, but we have found this difficult

BOX 17-2 Dilution Options for Botox

Diluent (ml of 0.9% Saline)	Concentration (Units of Botox per 0.1 ml)
1	10
2	5
2.5	4
5	2 (our preferred dilution)

to reproduce from patient to patient because of the small volume injected. It would seem that injecting large volumes of Botox per injection site may increase the amount of edema and bruising as well as increasing the chance for the material to diffuse further away from the injection site and cause undesirable side effects. On the other hand, using very small amounts per injection site makes exact placement crucial in order to maintain efficacy. Therefore, it is important that one compare total dose (in units) as well as concentration of toxin (units per milliliter) when one is evaluating injection methods. In general, it is best to use up the entire vial during one treatment session, but we have found minimal deterioration of efficacy if the reconstituted BTX-A is refrigerated and used within 1 week of reconstitution (Box 17-4).

Injection for facial rhytides can usually be accomplished with significantly less than 50 U of BTX-A, which is well below the established LD_{50} for BTX-A. Injection of the palms, soles, or axillae for hyperhidrosis can require as much as 100 to 200 U per session, and physicians should exercise caution when deciding how many areas to treat at one time.

The issue of antibody development to the toxin has been raised in several publications, but to date, anti-BTX-A antibodies have not been identified when injections are performed at the recommended doses for rhytide improvement. It is advisable to remain under 200 U per session in order to reduce the risk of neutralizing antibody formation.[13] Also, it is recommended that reinjection be deferred for at least 30 days after the previous injection, and reinjection volume/concentration ratios should be kept to a minimum to avoid inducing antibody formation.[47] However, we routinely use 2 to 20 U of Botox for small touch-up procedures 1 to 2 weeks after the initial treatment session without any apparent antibody formation.

Pretreatment preparation is minimal, with patients asked to avoid aspirin, vitamin E, nonsteroidal anti-inflammatory drugs (NSAIDs), and alcohol before treatment (Box 17-5). However, BTX-A injection can safely be performed in individuals who have recently used agents that interfere with the coagulation cascade. In these individuals, care must be taken to apply firm pressure to the treated area for a minimum of 10 minutes following injection. BTX-A injection is contraindicated during pregnancy or nursing. It should be avoided in those with a known hypersensitivity to human albumin and in patients with neurological or muscular diseases such as amyotrophic lateral sclerosis. BTX-A injections should not be performed in patients receiving aminoglycoside antibiotics, which interfere with neuromuscular transmission.

PATIENT SELECTION

Hyperdynamic Rhytides

BTX-A is widely used to treat hyperdynamic wrinkles of the upper face. The forehead, glabella, and periorbital regions are especially well suited to this treatment modality (Box 17-6). Since BTX-A acts to inhibit the muscle actions that are the primary causes of wrinkles of the upper third of the face, it is particularly well suited to use in these locations. Other therapeutic op-

BOX 17-3 Dilution Technique

- Clean Botox bottle top with alcohol and allow to thoroughly dry before adding diluent.
- Use preservative-free 0.9% normal saline.
- Add diluent to Botox bottle through an 18- to 23-gauge needle
- Hold Botox bottle upside down when injecting diluent to ensure that no air is drawn into the bottle. Inject into the fluid level that is created with the initial saline flow.
- Air in the bottle can denature the toxin.
- Do not shake the bottle after dilution. Gently swirl it.

BOX 17-4 Botox Storage

- In freezer at –4°C or lower prior to reconstitution.
- In refrigerator after reconstitution. Package insert recommends use in less than 4 hours. Clinical experience suggests Botox can be stored and used for 7 days.

BOX 17-5 Pretreatment Instructions

- Avoid alcohol for 48 hours prior to treatment
- Avoid aspirin-containing products for 1 to 2 weeks before treatment
- Avoid NSAIDs for 3 days before treatment
- Contraindications to treatment
  - Neuromuscular disease
  - Aminoglycoside antibiotics
  - Allergy to human albumin
  - Pregnancy

BOX 17-6 Muscle Groups

■ Glabellar complex:	Corrugator supercilii, procerus, depressor supercilii
■ Forehead:	Frontalis
■ Crow's feet:	Lateral portion of orbicularis oculi

tions include bovine or human collagen injections, resurfacing techniques such as erbium or carbon dioxide lasers, as well as surgical muscular denervation or excision. While all of these options have selected advantages and disadvantages, BTX-A, in general, is superior to each when used to treat dynamic wrinkles. BTX-A can effectively treat large areas of the upper face with a few well-placed injection sites. It can also be performed on an outpatient basis with rapid recovery and very little associated morbidity, and patients can return to their normal activities almost immediately after treatment. This is in contrast to the numerous injections that are required with filler substances, and the prolonged recovery times associated with laser resurfacing and surgical therapy. Resurfacing is the treatment of choice when other signs of photoaging such as lentigenes, coarse texture, and mild rhytides are the patient's primary concern. Chemical (glycolic acid, trichloroacetic acid) or particulate resurfacing can also be an effective treatment for mild photoaging with minimal rhytides. The ideal patients for BTX-A injections are those with hyperdynamic wrinkles of the forehead, glabella, and crow's feet with little associated pigmentary or textural changes.

BTX-A injections have more recently been used to treat wrinkles of the upper lip and mental crease, as well as platysmal bands. Although laser resurfacing and dermabrasion continue to be the treatment of choice for perioral rhytides, BTX-A has a role in the treatment of mild upper lip rhytides for patients who prefer to avoid the morbidity associated with resurfacing. Vertical platysmal bands can be effectively treated with BTX-A injections, and some patients can achieve mild correction of horizontal rhytides as well. Patients with thin necks and well-defined muscular bands are likely to achieve better results than those with advanced photoaging, submental fat, and jowl formation. Those with advanced photoaging are likely to benefit more from liposuction of the neck and jowls with surgical repair of the platysma muscle. Full or partial face lift procedures are also options for treatment of the aging neck, as is laser resurfacing, according to recent reports.[48]

Hyperhidrosis

The axillae, palms, and soles are areas of the human body that are particularly susceptible to the problem of hyperhidrosis. Excessive sweating in these areas has clear social implications for those affected by it, and patients will often go to great lengths to try to improve it. Topical therapy such as 20% aluminum chloride hexahydrate (Drysol, Delasco, Council Bluffs, IA) has little associated morbidity, but patients often find this relatively ineffective. Iontophoresis acts by creating keratin plugs of eccrine gland ostia and can be effective in selected patients, but the improvement is relatively short lived, requiring continued iontophoresis. Surgical sympathectomy can achieve good results, but patients often are reluctant to expose themselves to the associated morbidity of the procedure. BTX-A injections can be performed on an outpatient basis with a high degree of efficacy for hyperhidrosis and therefore have quickly become the treatment of choice for excessive sweating of the palms, soles, and axillae.

While some patients experience sweating of just the palms, many have sweating that involves the fingers as well. This can be a debilitating problem for them, dramatically interfering with social interactions. These patients are typically reluctant to shake the physician's hand at the time of the initial consult due to being self-conscious about their sweating problem. While most patients are interested in having treatment of both hands, some are uneasy about the prospect of having injections into the hands, and we offer to them unilateral injection of the right hand. This allows them to experience the benefits of BTX-A injection during post-treatment social interactions, and many of these patients return to have the left hand treated in the future.

Headaches

It is estimated that 18% of women and 6% of men (approximately 23 million people) suffer from migraine headaches in the United States each year.[49] Although numerous treatments are available, none have proven to be the universal cure that so many patients who suffer from migraine or tension headaches are hoping for. As the use of BTX-A increased for hyperdynamic rhytides, an observation was made that some of these patients experienced a reduction in the frequency of headaches. Utilizing the standard treatment techniques for the forehead, glabella, and periocular region can reduce tension headaches. Migraine headaches can be improved with this technique as well, but some patients require additional injections placed into the belly of the temporalis muscle in the parietal region of the scalp. Clinical studies are currently in progress to assess the treatment parameters and clinical efficacy of BTX-A for the treatment of migraine headaches, but it is clear that BTX-A improves migraines and tension headaches in some patients.[42,43]

PROCEDURAL TECHNIQUES

Once reconstituted, BTX-A is injected directly into striated muscle to produce its effects for the treatment of dynamic rhytides of the face, and in the superficial subdermal subcutaneous space for hyperhidrosis. Some physicians choose to perform injections under electromyographic (EMG) guidance that indicates needle position within the muscle as an aid to injection, while others prefer to treat without it. Both methods

BOX 17-7 Injection Tools and Tips

- Allow the alcohol on the patient's skin to dry thoroughly before injection to prevent toxin denaturation.
- Use a 1 ml syringe with very clear 0.1 ml markings on the syringe barrel to allow easy visualization of injection volumes.
- Syringe should have a removable needle to allow change between needle for aspiration from bottle and injection needle.
- Use a 30-gauge ½-inch needle for injection.

allow for accurate placement of the toxin in experienced hands. We do not routinely use EMG. It can be a cumbersome technique and is not an exact and accurate predictor of efficacy. Although EMG is quite good at indicating intramuscular needle position, it does not tell the physician *which* muscle the needle is in. Therefore, a false sense of security can develop when using EMG. EMG is not indicated for the treatment of hyperhidrosis.

Injections are performed with 1 ml Luer-Lok syringes (Becton Dickinson, Franklin Lakes, NJ), which have clear markings on the barrel to allow easy observation of injection volumes (Box 17-7). The amount of BTX-A to be injected is calculated ahead of time, and the exact amount to be used is slowly drawn up into the syringe with an 18- to 23-gauge needle, taking care to prevent any bubbles from forming (which can denature the toxin). Upon removing the needle from the vial, the Botox left in the needle bevel is drawn into the syringe to reduce wasting any of this very expensive material. A 30-gauge, ½-inch needle is routinely used for injection, although some physicians prefer a 31- or 32-gauge needle.

Topical or local anesthesia is not required, nor are surgical markings. The area to be treated should be lightly cleaned with an alcohol wipe, and the alcohol allowed to completely dry before commencing therapy to prevent denaturation of the protein. While ice can be used as a pretreatment anesthetic, it may induce posttreatment headaches that can be quite troubling to the patient.

Glabellar Region

A thorough knowledge of the anatomy of the glabellar region is critical to understanding proper injection techniques for BTX-A (Fig. 17-2). The midline procerus muscle is a fingerlike muscle that originates on the superior nasal dorsum and inserts on the underside of the dermis in the inferior forehead just superior to the medial head of the eyebrows. Because procerus contraction depresses the medial head of the brows, it can be categorized as a brow depressor.

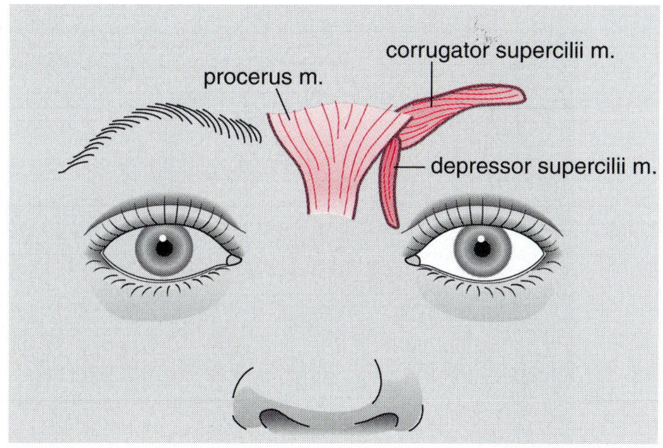

FIG. 17-2
Glabella anatomy. Procerus is a vertical midline muscle (light pink). Corrugator supercilii fibers are oriented horizontal/oblique bilaterally in a position at or just above the eyebrow. Depressor supercilii is a narrow bilateral muscle vertically oriented just lateral to procerus.

The corrugator supercilii muscle lies deep to the frontalis muscle and superficial to the periosteum, originates on the superior portion of the nasal dorsum, and inserts on the underside of the galea just above the medial head of the eyebrow bilaterally. Its course is approximately 30 degrees above horizontal. Due to its orientation, the corrugator muscle is categorized as both a brow apposer and depressor.

The depressor supercilii muscle is a thin muscle that lies superficial to the corrugator muscle bilaterally. It originates on the superior nasal dorsum and inserts on the underside of the galea in the region of the medial aspect of the corrugator muscle. Its vertical orientation and vector of action allows it to be categorized as a brow depressor.

Treatment of the glabellar complex must include inactivation of procerus, corrugator, and depressor supercilii to achieve the desired effects (Fig. 17-3). Failure to paralyze all three muscles leads to less-than-optimal results. Since the three muscles of the corrugator complex are the only known brow depressors, a positive effect of therapy, in addition to elimination of glabellar rhytides, can be elevation of the medial brow. This is due to unopposed action of the frontalis muscle, an elevator of the brow, along with the occipitalis muscle.

We use five injection sites to treat the glabellar complex and have standardized our patient positioning to allow for reproducible results. All five injections are performed with the needle and syringe barrel perpendicular to the skin surface. The patient is positioned so that she or he is very upright in the treatment chair, with the head resting comfortably but firmly against the headrest. The end result is a posture and needle position that allows for direct perpendicular injection into

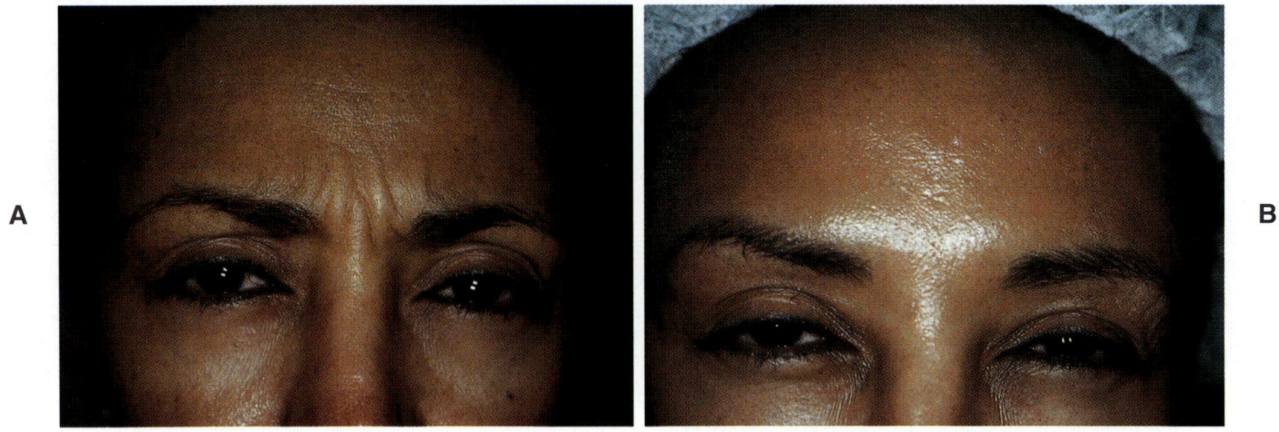

FIG. 17-3
A 41-year-old woman before **(A)** and 1 month after **(B)** BTX-A treatment of the glabella. Note inability to frown glabella region after treatment.

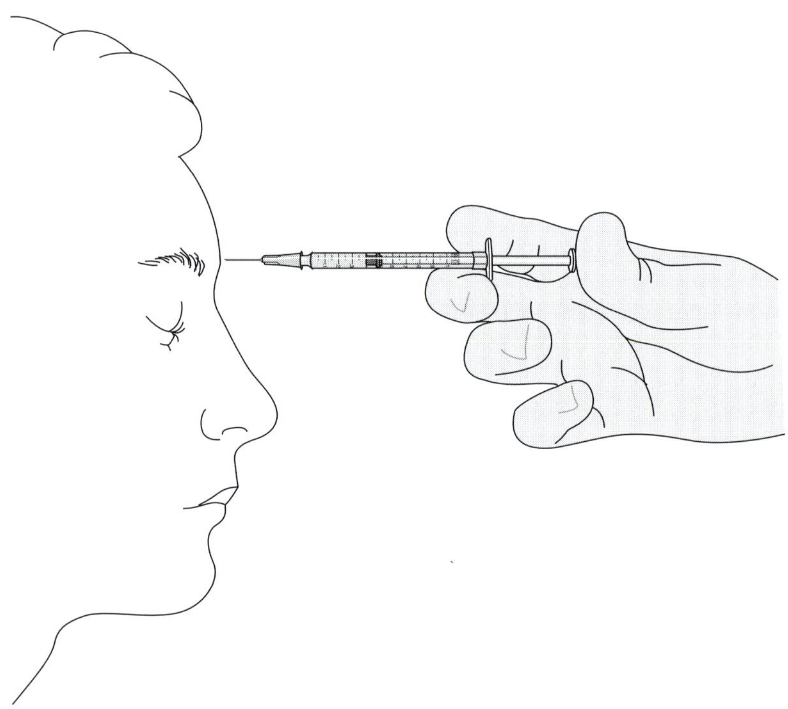

FIG. 17-4
Horizontal syringe position for BTX-A injection.

the skin (Fig. 17-4). All five injections are performed by advancing the needle to the periosteum and then withdrawing slightly before injecting 0.1 ml of BTX-A. Since each site receives 0.1 ml with 2 U of BTX-A per site, a total of 10 U is used to treat the corrugator complex. The patient is *not* asked to activate or contract the muscles at the time of injection of the glabellar region (Box 17-8).

The five injection sites are the following (Fig. 17-5):

1. Midline at the level of the medial head of the brows
2. Right side 1 to 2 mm above the brow along a vertical line drawn through the right medial canthus
3. A point 45 degrees lateral to injection site 2 approximately 1 cm lateral and 1 cm superior to site 2
4. Left side 1 to 2 mm above the brow along a vertical line drawn through the left medial canthus
5. A point 45 degrees lateral to injection site 4 approximately 1 cm lateral and 1 cm superior to site 4

Injection 1 inactivates the procerus muscle, and injections 2 through 5 inactivate the corrugator and depressor supercilii muscles. By advancing the needle down to the periosteum and withdrawing slightly, the physician ensures that the toxin is delivered directly to the muscle fibers. Some advocate injecting at an angle

BOX 17-8 Injection Techniques for Glabellar Complex

- Do not have patient contract muscles.
- Use five injection sites.
- Needle should remain parallel to floor and perpendicular to muscle groups/face.
- All injections of glabellar region are performed by inserting needle down to and touching periosteum, then withdrawing slightly prior to injecting 0.1 ml aliquot.
- Central injection is between medial head of eyebrows to treat procerus.
- Two symmetrical injections at medial head of brow, approximately 1 to 2 mm above brow in line drawn vertically up from medial canthus to treat depressor supercilii and medial portion of corrugator supercilii.
- Two symmetrical injections approximately 1 cm up and 1 cm out from medial brow injection (45-degree angle superior and lateral to medial brow head injection) to treat lateral portion of corrugator supercilii.

directed up or down along the corrugator, but we have found this to be unnecessary.[29] In addition, injecting at the level of the periosteum prevents inadvertently injecting the frontalis muscle, which lies just superficial to the corrugator and depressor supercilii muscles. With EMG-guided BTX-A injection, it is not possible to differentiate between corrugator and frontalis when advancing the needle. Frontalis muscle injection at the level of the medial brow produces an unnatural paralysis of the region.

Persistent muscle activity following Botox injection of the glabellar complex is not uncommon and can have one of several causes. There are some patients who need higher concentrations of BTX-A than 2 U/0.1 ml. For those patients, we will perform a trial at 4 U/0.1 ml and assess longevity. Concentrations as high as 10 U/0.1 ml can be used in an effort to produce longer-lasting results. Some individuals are able to furrow the glabellar area in the absence of corrugator or glabellar muscular activity by recruiting the lateral aspect of the orbicularis oculi muscle (Fig. 17-6). The horizontal superolateral portion of orbicularis oculi, when it contracts, can produce apposition of the medial head of the brows. To treat this, we employ symmetrical bilateral 0.1 ml injections of BTX-A approximately 2 mm inferior to the lateral portion of the eyebrow.

Proximal nose rhytides (so-called bunny lines) can also be effectively treated as part of the glabellar complex. The patient is asked to furrow the proximal nose and medial cheek, and bilateral 0.1 ml injections are placed into the proximal obliquely oriented nasal rhytides to weaken the muscles and produce the desired effect.

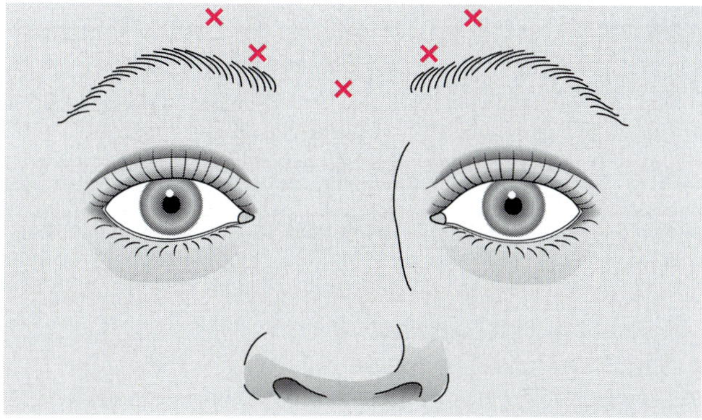

FIG. 17-5
Glabella injection sites. Pink "x" denotes individual 0.1 ml injection.

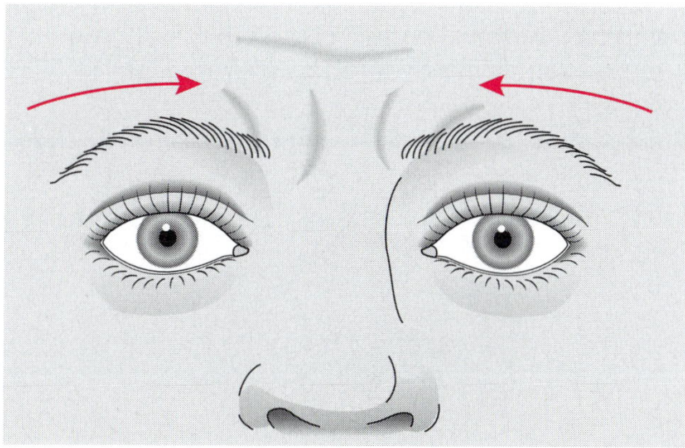

FIG. 17-6
Recruitment of lateral, horizontally oriented fibers of orbicularis oculi to frown glabella. Pink arrows denote motion vectors.

Periorbital Region

The lateral canthus region responds quite well to BTX-A injections, but in many patients the longevity of paralysis is slightly shorter than for other parts of the face. Three 0.1 ml injections are performed bilaterally to paralyze the lateral, vertically oriented fibers of the orbicularis oculi muscle (Box 17-9). The muscle lies deep to the subcutaneous tissue, but this layer is quite thin lateral to the eye. Therefore, injection of toxin can be performed in the deep subcutaneous plane near the muscle and still obtain good results. It is not necessary to use the periosteum as a guide as in glabellar injections. Needle angle can vary but is usually 45 degrees in the periorbital region. The three injection sites are spaced approximately 1 cm apart in an arcuate orientation around the crow's feet area approximately 1 cm lateral to the bony orbital rim (Fig. 17-7). It is helpful to

BOX 17-9 Injection Techniques for Lateral Canthus Region (Crow's Feet)

- Inject at approximately 45-degree angle directed away from the globe directly into the thin subcutaneous space.
- Have patient squint or smile slightly to accentuate the muscle.
- Inject total of 0.3 ml into each lateral canthus region in three 0.1 ml injections.
- Stay 1 cm lateral to the orbital rim.
- Stay lateral to an imaginary line drawn vertically through the lateral limbus of the iris.
- Avoid the vein that typically runs lateral to the lateral brow.
- The inferior injection site should be slightly medial and inferior to the lateral canthus at the prominence of the inferior rhytid.
- For patients with prominent infraorbital rhytides and crepelike skin, two 0.1 ml injections can be performed into the horizontal portion of the orbicularis oculi muscle approximately 5 to 10 mm below the lash line.

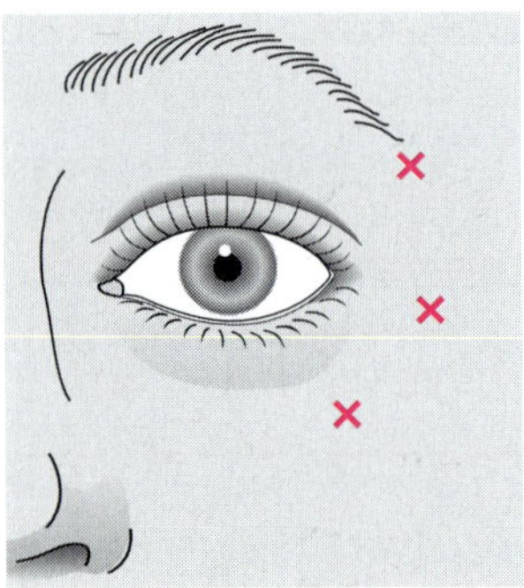

FIG. 17-7
Standard periorbital BTX-A injection sites. Pink "x" denotes individual 0.1 ml injection.

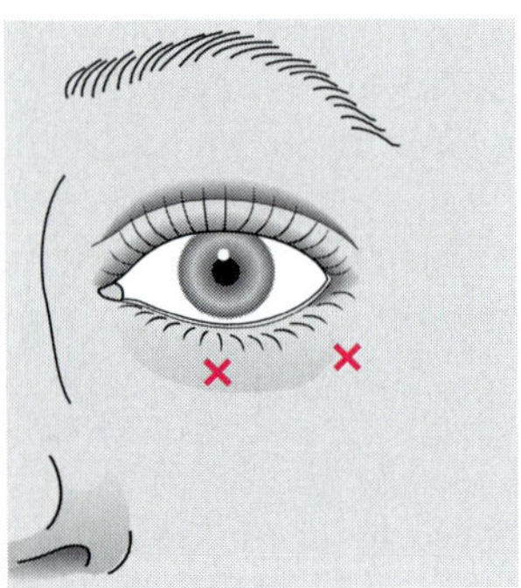

FIG. 17-8
Supplemental periorbital and infraorbital BTX-A injection sites. Pink "x" denotes individual 0.1 ml injection.

have the patient smile slightly at the time of injection to accentuate the rhytides and guide needle placement.

It is essential to examine the patient's lateral canthal region anatomy prior to injection, paying particular attention to the inferolateral region in the vicinity of the malar eminence. Many patients have very active muscle activity in this region and therefore produce rhytides inferior and medial to the lateral orbit. For this reason, we prefer to place our inferior injection site slightly medial to the others, approximately on a vertical line inferior to the lateral canthus itself. This helps to avoid the unnatural appearance some have following periorbital BTX-A injection due to the persistent muscle activity of the inferolateral orbicularis oculi muscle.

Recently, we have begun to inject small amounts of BTX-A into the inferior horizontal fibers of orbicularis oculi immediately below the lower eyelashes (Fig. 17-8). A single 0.1 ml injection totaling 2 U of BTX-A is placed in the superficial subcutaneous space approximately 0.5 cm below the lash line bilaterally in the vicinity of the midpupilary line. In some patients, this can help to improve fine lines and the "crepelike" texture of the skin in this region. A second 0.1 ml subdermal injection approximately 0.5 to 1 cm lateral and inferior to the lateral canthus can further improve and tighten contours of the infraorbital skin and muscle. Gentle massage of both of these injection points helps to spread the toxin and improve consistency and uniformity of results.

Brow Lift

For many patients, a subtle elevation of the mid and lateral eyebrow helps to improve the appearance of the upper one third of the face, and in particular the eyes. Patients comment that they look younger when the brow is elevated as little as 3 to 5 mm. Previous tech-

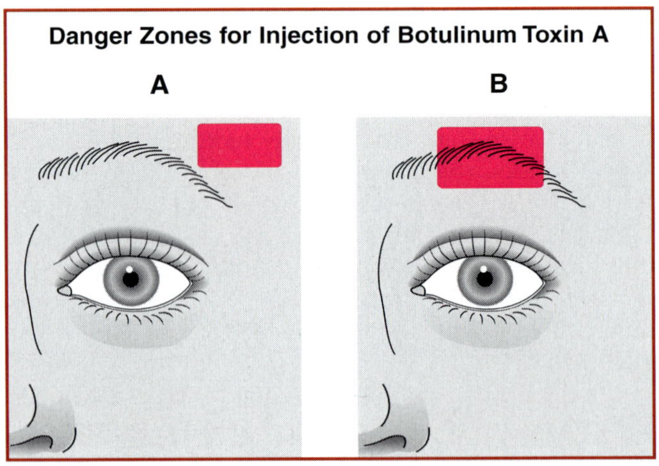

Figure **A** (shaded rectangle) denotes risk zone for eyebrow depression if this area is treated with BTX-A. Figure **B** (shaded rectangle) highlights risk zone for eyelid ptosis if this area is injected with BTX-A.

niques for brow elevation were cold steel surgery including coronal and endoscopic brow lifts. It is also possible to achieve a temporary, persistent, substantial elevation of the brows with BTX-A (Fig. 17-9).

Injection amounts of 0.1 ml of BTX-A are placed in the subdermal space in a horseshoelike shape around the lateral canthus. Injection points are placed at a distance of approximately 1 cm from the lateral canthus, and begin on a line drawn horizontally through the lateral canthus, then extend up for two injection points separated by 1 cm to include the lateral aspect of the eyebrow. A fourth injection is placed 1 cm inferior to the original injection that was placed at the mid lateral canthal region. It is useful to place the first injection point as described above, and then inject through the bleb raised from injection points to obtain a uniform treatment of the lateral canthus (Personal communication, Arnold Klein, MD, Cambridge, MA, 2000).

Additional treatment of the glabellar region to weaken the central brow depressors (corrugator, depressor supercilii, procerus) is also a useful adjunct to the BTX-A brow lift procedure. Treatment can be carried out the same as previously described for glabellar rhytides, or a single 0.1 ml injection point into the mid glabella will usually suffice to allow central brow elevation. Massage of this single injection point is helpful to facilitate even distribution of the toxin.

Carruthers has reported a technique for producing brow elevation chemically with BTX-A.[50] Three injection sites are used, all in an attempt to eliminate or reduce activity of the brow depressors (Fig. 17-10):

- Central glabella between the medial head of the brows
- Bilateral symmetrical injection sites approximately 0.5 cm below the lateral head of the brow (two injections, one on either side)

The central injection site is intended to paralyze or weaken the brow depressors procerus and depressor supercilii, with a minor effect on corrugator. The lateral injection sites are designed to weaken the lateral portion of orbicularis oculi, which is considered a brow depressor due to its vertically oriented muscle fibers.

Forehead

The forehead is one of the most challenging areas to inject with BTX-A. Although longevity of muscle paralysis can be longer in this region than with other areas of the face, technique flaws are readily apparent to even the casual observer. The area most prone to problems is the lateral forehead. Undertreatment can result in unnatural elevation of the lateral brow, producing a severe, angry, or surprised facial expression. Overtreatment of the lateral forehead can result in eyebrow depression and inability to elevate the brow, with a resultant sad, heavy appearance. In some patients, it is advisable to treat the forehead 2 to 3 weeks after the glabellar region. Although it is difficult to predict, some patients who have the glabella and forehead treated at the same time will develop 2 to 3 weeks of subtle, temporary medial brow depression. For these reasons, a careful inspection of the patient's forehead wrinkle pattern is essential prior to treatment.

The frontalis and occipitalis muscles are connected via the fibrous galea, and therefore both act as the only elevators of the eyebrows. However in many individuals the occipitalis contribution to eyebrow elevation is minimal to nonexistent, and we prefer to plan our surgical technique with the assumption that frontalis is the sole brow elevator. On exam, patients are asked to elevate their brows. There are basically two patterns of forehead elevation (Fig. 17-11). In the first, individuals

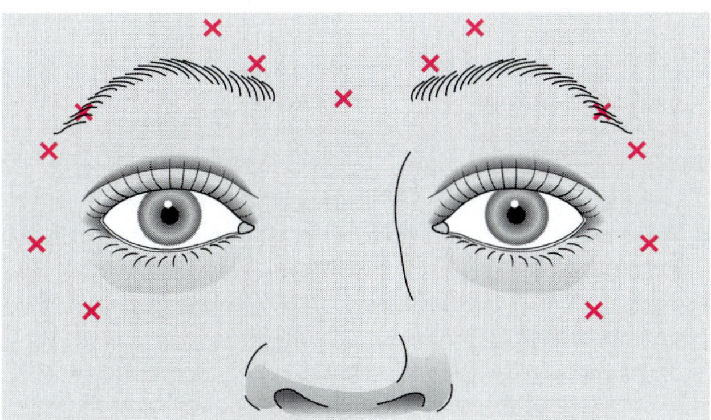

FIG. 17-9
Brow lift technique. Note treatment of lateral brow region, as well as glabella and standard periorbital injection sites. This technique treats the brow depressor muscles.

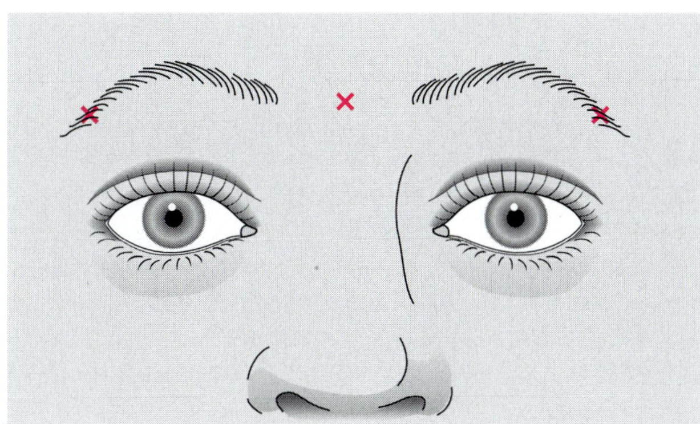

FIG. 17-10
Carruthers brow lift technique.

have muscle activity beyond the lateral limbus of the iris, and in some beyond the lateral head of the brows. In the second, patients have rhytides that remain central on the forehead between a vertical line drawn between the two pupils. In the latter group there is less of a concern with altering lateral brow shape and position with BTX-A, since there is little if any muscle activity in that region. However, the former group is at risk for alteration in eyebrow motion following BTX-A injection.

The frontalis muscle is a bifid, fan-shaped muscle that originates and merges with the galea superiorly and inserts into the skin of the eyebrow inferiorly (Fig. 17-12). In many patients, the midline fibers overlap considerably, so for practical purposes it is best to think of frontalis as a single muscular sheet across the forehead. Injection sites of 0.1 ml are placed approximately 1 cm apart into the body of the muscle, using caution to remain 1 cm above the eyebrows (Box 17-10). A good rule of thumb is to inject only above the inferior-most horizontal forehead rhytide and to have the patient contract frontalis and elevate the brows during treatment. In theory this is intended to prevent toxin migration into the upper lid, causing eyelid ptosis. An injection into the central forehead region should be performed for all patients when treating the forehead, as failure to

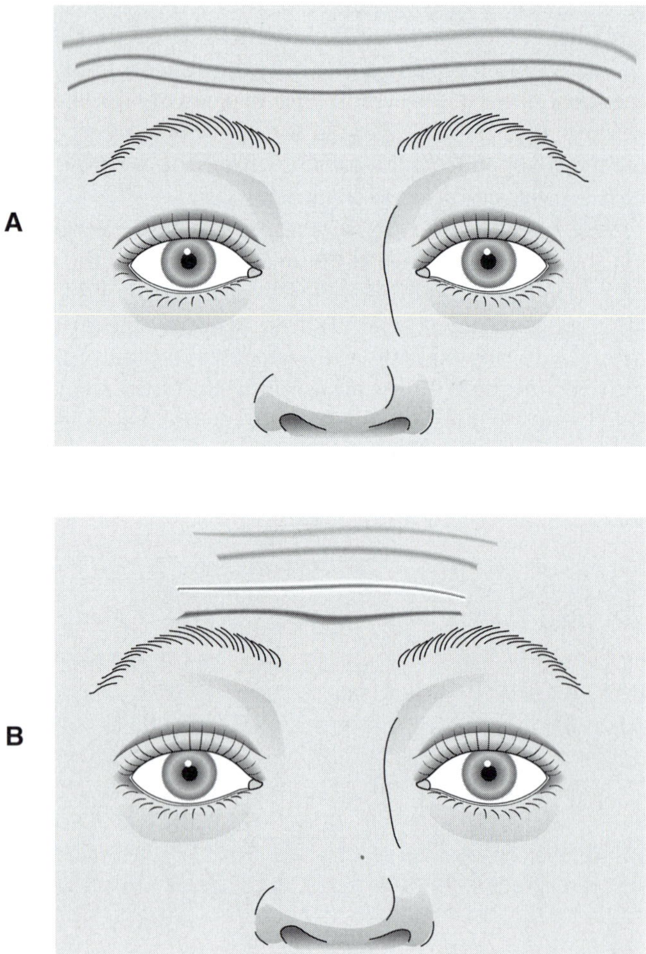

FIG. 17-11
Forehead elevation patterns. **A,** Rhytides extend beyond the lateral portion of the eyebrow. **B,** Rhytides remain central on the forehead.

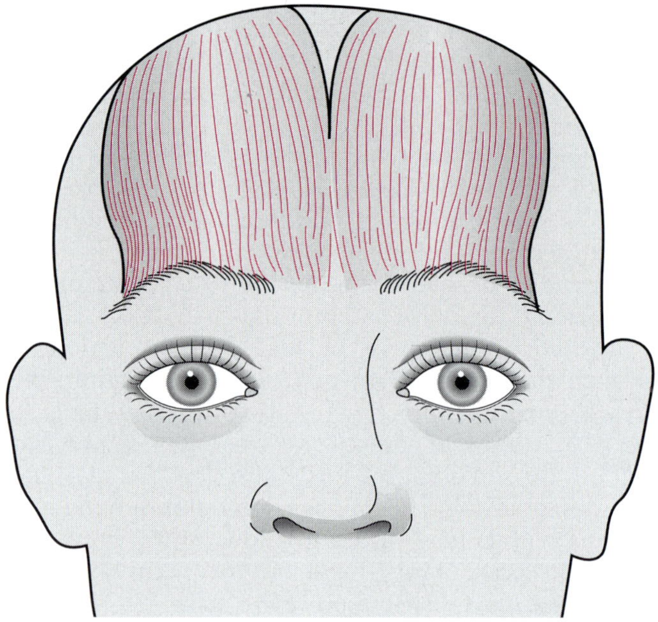

FIG. 17-12
Frontalis muscle anatomy and location.

BOX 17-10 Injection Techniques for Forehead

- Inject in 0.1 ml aliquots directly into the muscle belly.
- Have patient elevate brows to accentuate muscle belly.
- Inject approximately 0.6-0.8 ml total to treat the forehead.
- Avoid injection of lower lateral forehead.
- Maintain some frontalis muscle action to prevent eyebrow ptosis.
- Injection sites should be greater than 1 cm above the eyebrows. A good rule of thumb is to stay above the first horizontal forehead wrinkle.
- Try to stay medial to an imaginary line drawn vertically through the lateral limbus of the iris.
- You can treat the lateral forehead if you stay high (superior).
- The brow can be elevated laterally by leaving the lateral forehead untreated.
- If lateral brow elevation is too severe or unnatural following injection, add a small amount of Botox high on the lateral forehead.
- Consider treating the forehead 2 to 3 weeks after the glabella to decrease risk of medial brow ptosis occasionally seen when both areas are treated in one session.

perform this injection can lead to unnatural brow motion (Fig. 17-13).

The vertically oriented fibers of the frontalis muscle contract to elevate the brow. The lateral portion of the muscle, if left untreated, will continue to elevate the brow when contracted, but if the central frontalis is paralyzed, only the lateral brow will elevate. This can produce a dramatic change in eyebrow shape often referred to by patients as the "Jack Nicholson look" (Fig. 17-14), referring to a similarity with the eyebrow shape of the well-known actor. Some patients like and prefer this, but careful preoperative discussion and counseling are essential to determining the patient's objectives. Our main goal of treatment of the lateral forehead region is to always leave some frontalis muscle activity to prevent brow depression, which is universally unnatural in appearance (Fig. 17-15). To accomplish this, we tend to perform bilateral 0.1 ml BTX-A injections high on the lateral forehead 3 to 4 cm above the brow at the point of lateral-most frontalis muscle activity (assessed by having the patient contract the muscle). This helps to preserve activity of the inferior part of the lateral frontalis muscle and is sufficient to keep the brow elevated. In those patients who are interested in adding some arch to their brows, we will omit the high lateral forehead injection site. We tell our patients that they may not like the appearance of their brows when the BTX-A effect takes place in 3 to 4 days, and if so they can return for a small touch-up procedure where we will perform 0.1 ml injections to the high lateral forehead bilaterally.

There are a handful of patients who have extremely active lateral frontalis muscle fiber activity (Fig. 17-16). They note persistent arching of the lateral brow and will often return for retreatment despite the fact that we have already treated the high lateral forehead. For these patients, we perform additional 0.05 to 0.1 ml injections of BTX-A to the lower lateral forehead approximately 1 to 2 cm above the brow. We counsel these patients that they run the risk of developing eyebrow ptosis and depression with this technique. Some

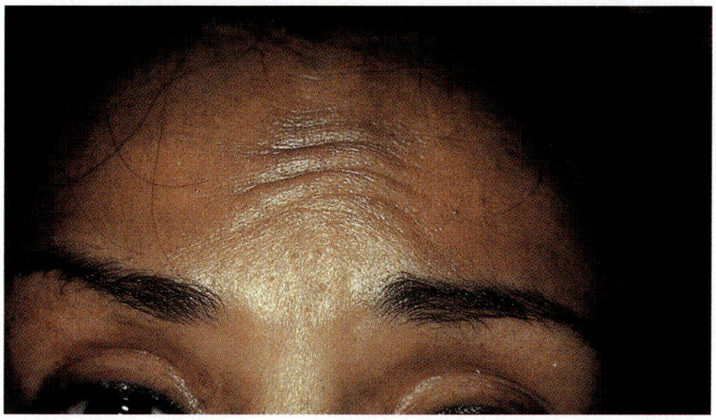

FIG. 17-13
Midline persistent forehead rhytides following BTX-A injection. This patient did not have the central forehead treated.

A

B

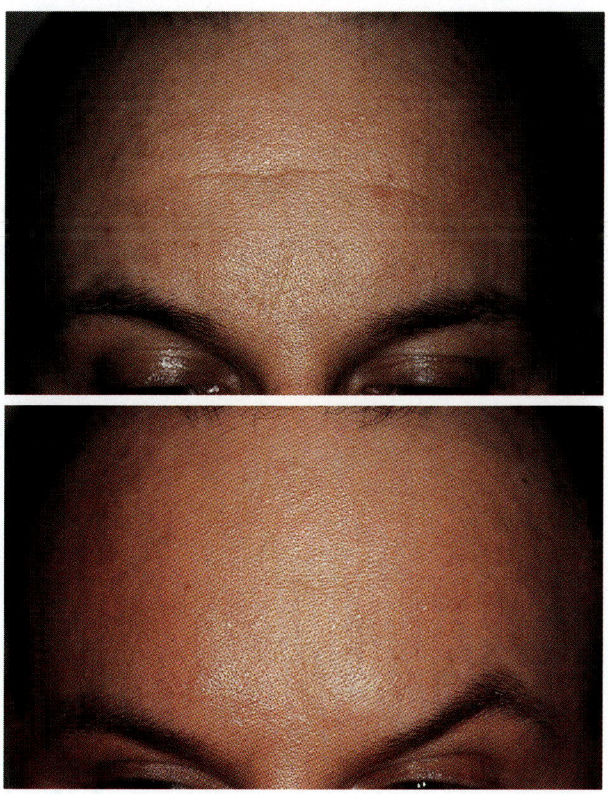

FIG. 17-14
A 31-year-old man before **(A)** and 2 months after **(B)** BTX-A injection of the forehead. Note improvement in horizontal rhytide at rest.

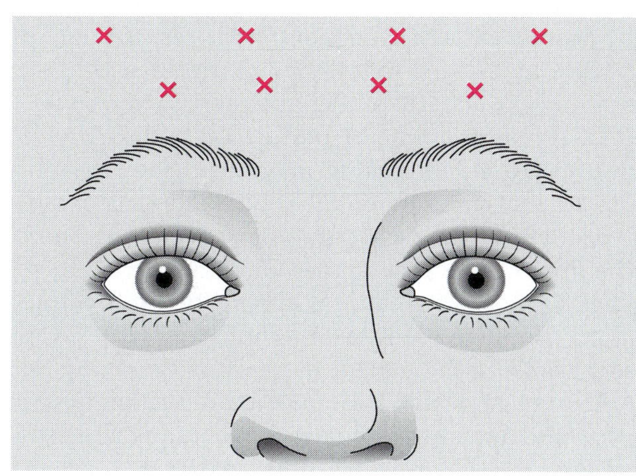

FIG. 17-15
Forehead injection technique. Pink "x" denotes individual 0.1 ml injection.

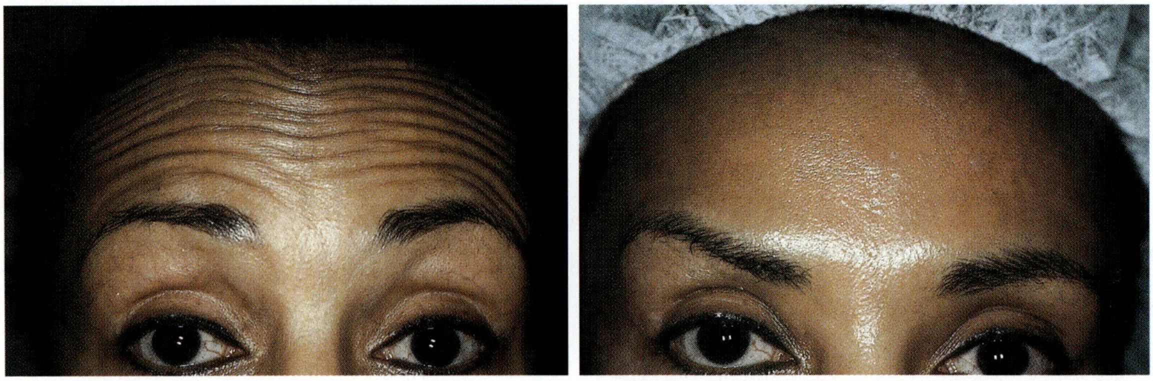

FIG. 17-16
A 41-year-old woman before **(A)** and 2 months after **(B)** BTX-A treatment of forehead. Note slight asymmetry when patient elevates brows after treatment. Right side persistent brow motion was minimized with 0.05 ml BTX-A touch-up injection 2 weeks after initial treatment.

choose to have the additional treatment performed, while others elect to forgo it. In many cases, persistent arching of the brows following high lateral forehead injection with BTX-A will soften with time as the treatment effect evolves, avoiding the need for lower lateral forehead injection.

Upper Lip

Vertical rhytides of the upper lip are currently treated with resurfacing techniques such as dermabrasion or laser skin resurfacing. However, both of these procedures carry with them significant morbidity, prompting some patients to seek alternative therapy. In addition, resurfacing is superb at eliminating cutaneous rhytides, but does not treat the muscle activity that can contribute to the formation of these wrinkles. Therefore, despite superb treatment with resurfacing, patients are at risk for redeveloping wrinkles with persistent muscle activity of the orbicularis oris muscle.

BTX-A injections can be performed to the upper lip region to reduce the ability to contract the horizontal fibers of the circumferential orbicularis oris muscle. The result of this muscle paralysis is decreased motion of the upper lip, with a limited or eliminated ability to pucker. Only mild weakness should be the treatment goal, as complete paralysis may interfere with normal speech, causing the patient to speak with an apparent lisp. The net gain from treatment is a reduction in wrinkle size and appearance. Injection technique varies, but in general three to four injections of 0.05 ml (or two to three of 0.1 ml) are performed 1 to 2 cm apart along the cutaneous upper lip at a distance of nearly 5 mm superior to the vermilion border. Injections should be placed within the muscle. EMG can help in this location, since the only muscle in the region that is treated is the orbicularis oris. In the absence of EMG, the practitioner can feel a decreased resistance to advancing the needle as he or she passes through the thick upper lip dermis and enters the subcutaneous space. Advancing 1 to 2 mm further will locate the needle in the vicinity of the muscle, where injection is performed.

Mental Crease

Injection of BTX-A of the lower lip region and mental crease is challenging at best. Overtreatment around the mouth can lead to quite unacceptable complications such as drooling, speech abnormalities, and inability to drink through a straw. The safety margin in this region is quite small, and for this reason the authors do not inject BTX-A into the chin or lower lip.

Neck

In the continuing quest for low-morbidity cosmetic surgical alternatives to the face lift, treatment of the aging neck with BTX-A has evolved. There are three primary features of the aging neck:

1. Cutaneous photoaging—rhytides, lentigenes, telangiectasias
2. Skin laxity
3. Muscle (platysmal) bands

BTX-A injections can be used to produce improvements in prominent platysmal banding. In addition, thorough treatment of the neck can yield an improvement in skin laxity and in some cases the horizontal rhytide component of photoaging. It will not change pigmented or vascular lesions that are seen with neck photoaging (poikiloderma of Civatte). Techniques of BTX-A injection differ depending on which aspects of neck aging are being treated. Therefore, the practitioner

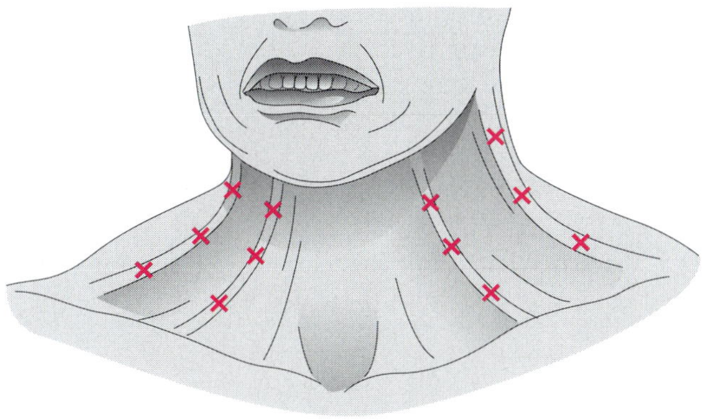

FIG. 17-17
Platysma muscle injection technique. Pink "x" denotes individual 0.1 ml injection.

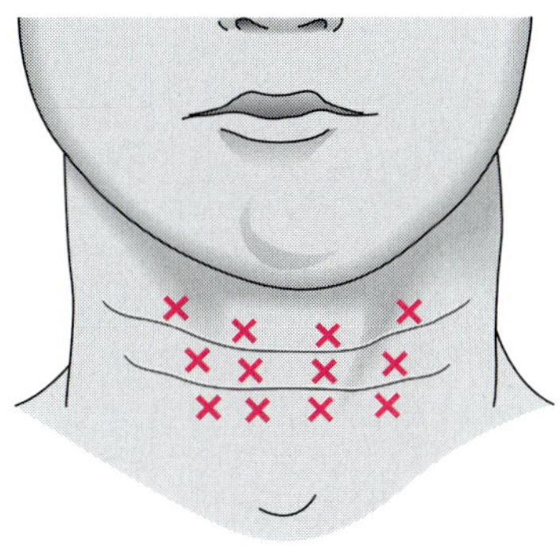

FIG. 17-18
Neck treatment technique to improve horizontal rhytides. Pink "x" denotes individual 0.1 ml injection.

must decide prior to treatment which of the three elements of the aging neck to treat.

Therapy of platysmal bands is a straightforward procedure (Fig. 17-17). Patients are asked to grimace and tighten the platysma muscle. The physician will then grasp the visible bands of muscle between the thumb and forefinger of the nondominant hand and inject two to four 0.1 ml aliquots of BTX-A directly into the muscle belly, approximately 1 cm apart. Most patients with platysmal bands have two distinct bands near the midline; however, some will have a broader, less distinct band lateral to the two central bands. All can be treated with BTX-A.

If the physician is attempting to improve skin laxity, jowls, and horizontal neck rhytides, then a more thorough and diffuse treatment of the neck is indicated. Many patients with cutaneous aging of the neck will have deep, prominent horizontal rhytides that are in part the result of years of contraction of the platysma muscle and motion of the neck. Treatment of the entire neck with 1 to 1.5 ml of BTX-A at 1 cm subcutaneous injection intervals surrounding the horizontal rhytides can substantially decrease activity of the platysma muscle (Fig. 17-18). Treatment of vertical platysmal bands is also performed in these patients as described above. The net effect is to produce unopposed action of the muscles of facial expression above the jawline and a tightening of the neck skin. This can produce a reduction in the appearance of fine and medium horizontal rhytides of the neck, as well as in some patients a tightening of skin along the jawline with resultant diminution of jowl appearance.

Neck results vary greatly from patient to patient, as well as physician to physician. Controlled trials documenting efficacy are lacking for BTX-A treatment of the neck, and further study is clearly needed to standardize treatment parameters and efficacy standards. Whereas therapy of the upper third of the face tends to produce uniform and predictable results, neck therapy with BTX-A is less predictable. For this reason, we counsel each of our patients that results may vary, and therefore we are unable to make any assurances as to outcomes following BTX-A therapy of the neck.

Nasolabial Fold

Scattered anecdotal and published reports have discussed treatment of nasolabial fold rhytides with BTX-A injection.[51] The intended targets of muscle paralysis are the zygomaticus major and minor muscles, which act to move the nasolabial fold and upper lip superior and lateral. Treatment of these muscles theoretically would reduce the appearance of nasolabial fold rhytides. However, our experience has been that on the rare occasion that the zygomaticus muscles are inadvertently treated during lateral canthus injection of BTX-A, patients are uniformly unhappy. They feel that their facial features have changed dramatically, and indeed they often have a noticeable change in their smile and mouth motion. Further study is therefore needed before this can be considered a standard use of BTX-A for facial rejuvenation.

THERAPY OF HYPERHIDROSIS

When used to treat hyperhidrosis, BTX-A is injected into the subdermal plane where it inhibits acetylcholine release from cholinergic nerve fibers associated with eccrine and apoeccrine sweat glands (Box 17-11). The subdermal plane of injection is the same for all areas of hyperhidrosis. Areas to be injected can be identified by one of several methods, but the overall goal is to inject areas of excess sweating. Because the areas to be injected are significantly larger in surface area than those injected for rhytides and the sweat gland nerve fibers are less sensitive to Botox, substantially larger amounts of toxin are used to treat hyperhidrosis in any given session.

Many patients with hyperhidrosis have only localized areas of increased sweating. The hyperactive areas can be localized with the starch-iodine test. An iodine solution is painted over the area and allowed to dry. At this point, starch powder is sprinkled on the area. Sweat causes the mixture to turn dark blue. By injecting only the positive areas, effective sweat reduction is achieved while reducing the total dose needed. The starch-iodine test can also be useful to quantitatively assess success of treatment.

Clinical effects begin to appear 2 to 4 days after injection, and longevity of sweat reduction varies from 2 to 8 months. We typically use a concentration of 2 U/0.1 ml, and inject 0.1 ml per needle site. If patients have persistent sweating after the BTX-A effects have begun, we will perform a small touch-up procedure to these areas. We ask the patient to wait at least 1 to 2 weeks following the initial session before we are able to fully assess efficacy of treatment.

A total of approximately 30 to 50 injections are done per hand or foot, for a total dose of 60 to 100 U of botulinum A exotoxin. We use a standard terminology of one hand, for example, being one hyperhidrosis "site." When either both hands or both feet are treated in one session, 120 to 200 U of toxin are injected. Similar doses are used to treat the axillae or feet as well. Therefore, we prefer to treat only two "sites" per session.

Topical anesthesia, such as eutectic mixture of local anesthetics (2.5% lidocaine with 2.5% prilocaine [EMLA, Astra USA, Westborough, MA]), is a useful adjunct to therapy and is routinely used. The patient is asked to place a thick layer of EMLA on the areas to be treated, and the area is occluded with a nonsterile medical glove or plastic wrap 1 to 2 hours before treatment. Application is repeated at 30-minute intervals until treatment is begun. At the time of treatment, ice cubes are used to preanesthetize the area about to be injected. An assistant holds an ice cube over the intended injection site for 10 to 15 seconds prior to needle insertion. We have found this technique to greatly improve patient comfort, particularly on the hands. Alternatively, the area can be briefly frozen with Fluro-Ethyl spray (Gebauer Pharmaceutical Preparations, Cleveland, OH) just prior to needle insertion. Occasionally, patients are unable to tolerate injections of the palms and soles with BTX-A using topical anesthesia. Regional anesthesia or nerve blocks can be used in these patients, but the morbidity associated with these forms of anesthesia may preclude their use in many patients.

BOX 17-11 Injection Techniques for Hyperhidrosis

- Inject at 1 to 2 cm intervals.
- Inject BTX-A in the immediate subdermal region.
- Be certain to inject lateral palms and soles when affected.
- Inject volar (palmar) interphalangeal joints of fingers, including fingertips.

Palms

Injection is accomplished with the needle held at approximately a 45-degree angle, and the needle advanced until a slight decrease in resistance is felt when it enters the subdermal plane. Injection sites are approximately 1 to 2 cm apart, since botulinum A exotoxin is thought to migrate nearly 1 cm from its site of injection (Fig. 17-19). A pattern of 12 to 16 injection sites can be marked on the palm with gentian violet when treating the first few patients, but this becomes less necessary as the physician gains experience. It is important to avoid injecting through the ink to prevent temporary

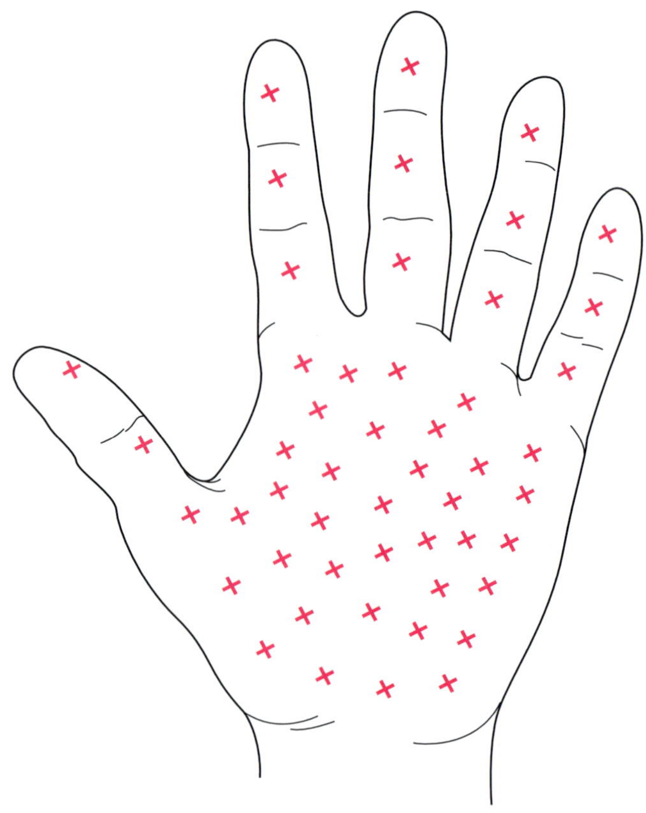

FIG. 17-19
Palm hyperhidrosis injection technique. A total of up to 50 sites are injected on each palm, with care to inject the lateral thenar and hypothenar eminences. Pink "x" denotes individual 0.1 ml injection.

tattooing. We also inject each palmar interphalangeal (IP) region, approximately midway between the IP creases, as well as the fingertips. There are a total of 14 IP and fingertip injection sites. Some patients have lateral palmar sweating as well, and therapy should be tailored to fit the individual patient.

Axillae

The axillae are treated by injecting 0.1 ml aliquots of subdermal BTX-A at 1 cm intervals. The area is inspected prior to treatment to define the extent of sweating, and the entire area is treated. Performing a ring of injections around the outer margin of the sweating areas is useful to delineate the extent of injections. Hair in the axilla does not need to be trimmed prior to treatment, but can obscure landmarks and previous injection sites. For this reason, care must be taken to use a consistent pattern within the axilla to maintain an efficient injection technique.

Plantar Foot

The plantar surface of the foot is a very challenging area to inject with BTX-A. Injection sites can be extremely painful, and many patients choose to avoid treatment of this area. For those who decide to have treatment performed, adequate anesthesia is essential. Topical anesthesia with EMLA and ice can be adequate for the minority of patients, but for the rest nerve blocks or other forms of regional anesthesia are essential. We have developed a system with our anesthesia colleagues to induce foot anesthesia with regional lidocaine anesthesia (Bier block) and conscious intravenous sedation. Sedation is achieved with standard agents such as intravenous propofol.

Regional anesthesia of the foot is obtained through the infusion of lidocaine intravascularly. An intravenous line is placed into a dorsal surface vein of both feet. Each foot is treated separately, with approximately a 10-minute wait between feet. The foot is exsanguinated with an elastic wrap, and a tourniquet is placed at the lower calf. Tourniquet pressure (with a blood pressure cuff) should be maintained between approximately 200 and 250 mm Hg. Once the tourniquet is inflated, local anesthesia, 25 ml of 0.5% lidocaine, is infused slowly into the foot. Anesthesia is obtained in approximately 5 minutes by diffusion of the anesthetic agent into the local tissue. Total tourniquet time should be less than approximately 15 minutes.

Injections are performed in a time-efficient manner at 1 cm intervals on the plantar surface of the foot, with care taken to inject the lateral soles. The toes are not injected. Once injections are completed, the tourniquet is deflated, and the foot massaged to decrease paresthesias. Posttourniquet hyperemia is to be expected and is transient. It is essential to have a physician who is skilled in obtaining regional anesthesia involved in the patient's care if the physician performing the BTX-A injections does not have significant experience with this form of regional anesthesia.

Alternatively, complete foot anesthesia can be achieved through posterior tibial, sural, peroneal, and saphenous nerve blocks. The tibial nerve, which innervates the heel and medial side of the foot is blocked by injecting anesthetic into the posterior groove of the medial malleolus near the posterior tibial artery. The sural nerve, which innervates the lateral side of the foot and the fifth toe, is blocked by injecting anesthetic between the Achilles tendon and the posterior surface of the lateral malleolus. The deep peroneal nerve innervates the space between the first and second toes. It is blocked by injecting anesthetic deep in the space immediately medial to the tendon of the hallucis longus muscle. Finally, the superficial peroneal and saphenous nerves innervate the spaces between the first to fifth toes and medial foot, respectively. The nerves are blocked by injecting anesthetic subcutaneously in a line anteriorly between the malleoli.

POSTOPERATIVE CLINICAL CONSIDERATIONS

Following injection, firm pressure is applied to the treated area for 5 to 10 minutes to prevent bruising. An added benefit of firm pressure held to the treated area appears to be even distribution and migration of the injected BTX-A within the locally treated area. This has the effect of improving results and producing a more uniform and even muscle paralysis or sweat reduction. The patient is instructed to remain upright for 3 to 4 hours to prevent migration of the toxin when the face is treated (Box 17-12). Whether this will in time prove to be unnecessary is unknown. Patients are also instructed to contract injected muscles several times per hour, in theory to increase presynaptic uptake of the toxin.

Clinical effects begin to appear within 2 to 3 days of injection, sometimes even sooner in patients who have had prior treatment (Box 17-13). Although clinical muscle paralysis is noted this early, true clinical improvement in rhytides often takes as long as 4 to 6 weeks to

BOX 17-12 Posttreatment Instructions

- Remain upright for 4 hours after treatment.
- Contract treated muscles for 30 to 60 seconds every 20 minutes for 4 hours after treatment.
- Avoid aspirin, nonsteroidal anti-inflammatory agents, alcohol, and vitamin E supplements for 24 hours after treatment.

become evident. Patients should be counseled to wait a minimum of 4 to 6 weeks after injection before assessing improvement in their rhytides. We have also observed that clinical wrinkle improvement continues to increase with subsequent injections.

The duration of clinical efficacy is related to several factors, including concentration of BTX-A, injection technique, and individual patient variation (Box 17-14). On average, the effects of BTX-A injection remain apparent for 3 to 4 months following injection. Clinical efficacy is in part dose related, so that the more toxin one uses, the greater the likelihood of inducing long-term effects. Therefore, in patients who do not achieve long-term correction at standard doses, the physician can choose to increase the concentration or dose of toxin injected at subsequent sessions to potentially increase therapeutic efficacy.

It remains unclear whether there is a point at which increasing concentration does not improve results but rather only serves to increase the risk of complications (Box 17-15). It appears that the more concentrated the toxin that is injected, the higher the risk of side effects. The most common complications are upper eyelid ptosis (Fig. 17-20) and ecchymosis. A rare side effect of BTX-A injection is diplopia. Both diplopia and ptosis are temporary and resolve spontaneously within 2 to 4 weeks. During this difficult time, patients are reassured that no intervention is warranted. In some instances of upper eyelid ptosis, midriatic agents such as apraclonidine hydrochloride 0.5% or phenylephrine can be used to temporarily elevate the upper eyelid by causing contraction of Müller's muscle.[52,53] More commonly, the so-called complications of Botox injection are not true complications at all, but rather cosmetic or efficacy-related concerns. These often take the form of persistent rhytides within days of treatment, persistence of muscle action, and change in eyebrow shape and position. These can often be addressed either by reassuring the patient or by a small touch-up procedure.

Patients on occasion will complain of a change in their facial expression and smile following injection of the periorbital region. In particular, they note that their mouth does not move the same as it did prior to treatment. Often this is due to inadvertent injection of the

BOX 17-13 Clinical Action

- Onset of effects is usually within 2 to 4 days.
- Initial injection for photoaging will last on average 3 months.
- Repeat injections will often last longer than 3 months.
- Injections for hyperhidrosis last on average 6 months.

BOX 17-14 Botox Longevity

- Forehead appears to last longer than other areas on the face.
- Periorbital Botox tends to wear off faster than other regions of the face.
- Palms and axillae will remain sweat-free for approximately 6 months.
- Our preferred dose of 2 U/ml can be increased to attempt to increase longevity if indicated.

BOX 17-15 Most Common Side Effects Following Therapy of Facial Hyperdynamic Rhytides

- Upper eyelid ptosis
- Diplopia
- Eyebrow ptosis
- Ecchymosis
- Alteration of facial expression
- Unnaturally arched eyebrows
- Change in motion of cheek with smile

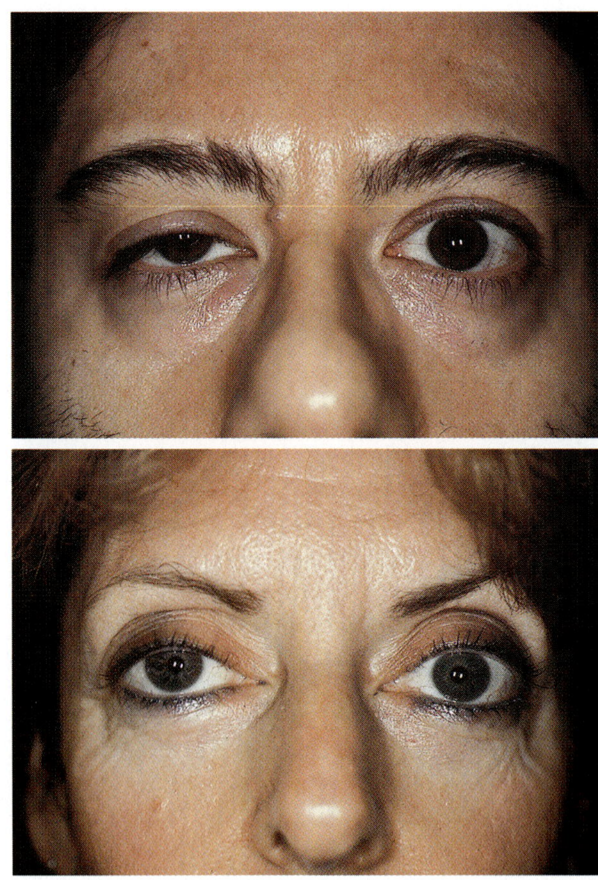

FIG. 17-20
Eyelid ptosis following BTX-A injection. **A,** Obvious right eyelid ptosis. **B,** Subtle right eyelid ptosis.

zygomaticus major or minor muscles that have their origin on the upper cheek near the malar eminence. When the crow's feet are injected with BTX-A, a medial injection site below the lateral limbus of the iris can be near the superior portion of the zygomaticus muscles. Toxin migration can affect these muscles and reduce the ability of the patient to elevate the corner of the mouth. There is no treatment for this condition, and patients must be reassured that this effect is temporary.

Complications are uncommon with Botox injection for hyperhidrosis. Sweating that continues 1 to 2 weeks after injection can be treated with additional BTX-A injected at a touch-up procedure. Patients are able to drive a car, write, and lift small objects without difficulty. Hand weakness can occur but is often mild and transient, lasting less than 3 to 4 weeks, and does not interfere with daily function. Weakness is likely due to action of the toxin on the thenar and hypothenar eminences and muscles, inhibiting apposition of the thumb and little finger. Intervention is not needed. Patients are instructed to use caution when lifting small objects with their hands. Finger weakness is very rare since, other than the lumbricals, the majority of the muscles that control finger motion are in the forearm, with only their tendinous insertions coursing through the palm. Similar concerns for the soles and axillae do not exist.

REFERENCES

1. Simpson LL. Molecular pharmacology of botulinum toxin and tetanus toxin. Ann Rev Pharmacol Toxicol 1986; 26:427-453.
2. Middlebrook JL. Cell surface receptors for protein toxins. In: Simpson LL, ed. Botulinum Neurotoxin and Tetanus Toxin. San Diego: Academic Press, 1989:95-119.
3. Schantz E, Scott A. Use of crystalline type A botulinum toxin in medical research. In: Lewis G, ed. Biomedical Aspects of Botulism. New York: Academic Press, 1981:143-150.
4. Carruthers A, Carruthers J. History of the cosmetic use of botulinum A exotoxin. Dermatol Surg 1998; 24:1168-1170.
5. Simpson LL. Peripheral actions of the botulinum toxins. In: Simpson LL, ed. Botulinum Neurotoxin and Tetanus Toxin. San Diego: Academic Press, 1989:153-178.
6. Hallett M. One man's poison—clinical applications of botulinum toxin. N Engl J Med 1999; 341:118-120.
7. Schmidt A, Dryer F, John C. At least three sequential steps are involved in tetanus toxin–induced block of neuromuscular transmission. Naunyn Schmiedebergs Arch Pharmacol 1981; 317:326-330.
8. Duchen L. Changes in motor innervation and cholinesterase localization induced by botulinum toxin in skeletal muscle of mouse: differences between fast and slow muscles. J Neurol Neurosurg Psychiatry 1970; 33:40-54.
9. Lange D. Systemic effects of botulinum toxin. In: Jankovic J, Hallett M, eds. Therapy with Botulinum Toxin. New York: Marcel Dekker, 1994:109-118.
10. Borodic G, Ferrante R, Pearce L, et al. Pharmacology and histology of the therapeutic application of botulinum toxin. In: Jankovic J, Hallett M, eds. Therapy with Botulinum Toxin. New York: Marcel Dekker, 1994:119-157.
11. Scott AB, Suzuki D. Systemic toxicity of botulinum toxin by intramuscular injection in the monkey. Mov Disord 1988; 3:333-335.
12. Schantz EJ, Kautter DA. Standardized assay for clostridium botulinum toxins. J Assoc Anal Chem 1978; 61:96-99.
13. Goschel H, Wohlfarth K, Frevert J, et al. Botulinum A toxin therapy: neutralizing and nonneutralizing antibodies—therapeutic consequences. Exp Neurol 1997; 147:96-102.
14. Moyer E, Settler P. Botulinum toxin type B: experimental and clinical experience. In: Jankovic J, Hallett M, eds. Therapy with Botulinum Toxin. New York: Marcel Dekker, 1994:71-85.
15. Garcia A, Fulton JEJ. Cosmetic denervation of the muscles of facial expression with botulinum toxin. Dermatol Surg 1996; 22: 39-43.
16. Lowe NJ. Botulinum A toxin type A for facial rejuvenation: United States and United Kingdom perspectives. Dermatol Surg 1998; 24:1216-1218.
17. Carruthers A, Carruthers J. Botulinum toxin used in the treatment of glabellar frown lines and other facial wrinkles. In: Jankovic J, Hallett M, eds. Therapy with Botulinum Toxin. New York: Marcel Dekker, 1994:577-595.
18. Carruthers JDA, Strubbs HA. Botulinum toxin for benign essential blepharospasm, hemifacial spasm and age-related lower eyelid entropion. Can J Neurol Sci 1987; 14:42-45.
19. Carruthers A, Kiene K, Carruthers J. Botulinum A exotoxin use in clinical dermatology. J Am Acad Dermatol 1996; 34:788-797.
20. Carruthers A, Carruthers J. Clinical indications and injection technique for the cosmetic use of botulinum A exotoxin. Dermatol Surg 1998; 24:1189-1194.
21. Carruthers J, Carruthers A. The adjunctive usage of botulinum toxin. Dermatol Surg 1998; 24:1244-1247.
22. Carruthers A, Carruthers J. Cosmetic uses of botulinum A exotoxin. In: Klein AW, ed. Tissue Augmentation in Clinical Practice: Procedures and Techniques. New York: Marcel Dekker, 1998:207-236.
23. Hankins CL, Strimling R, Rogers GS. Botulinum A toxin for glabellar wrinkles: dose and response. Dermatol Surg 1998; 24: 1181-1183.
24. Matsudo PKR. Botulinum toxin for correction of fronto-glabella wrinkles: preliminary evaluation. Aesthetic Plast Surg 1996; 20: 439-441.
25. Guerrissi J, Sarkissian P. Local injection into mimetic muscles of botulinum toxin A for the treatment of facial lines. Ann Plast Surg 1997; 39:447-453.
26. Guyuron B, Huddelston SW. Aesthetic indications for botulinum toxin injection. Plast Reconstr Surg 1994; 93:913-918.
27. Blitzer A, Binder WJ, Aviv JE, et al. The management of hyperfunctional facial lines with botulinum toxin: a collaborative study of 210 injection sites in 162 patients. Arch Otolaryngol Head Neck Surg 1997; 123:389-392.
28. Pribitkin EA, Greco TM, Goode RL, Keane WM. Patient selection in the treatment of glabellar wrinkles with botulinum toxin type A injection. Arch Otolaryngol Head Neck Surg 1997; 123:321-326.
29. Lowe NJ, Maxwell A, Harper H. Botulinum A exotoxin for glabellar folds: a double-blind, placebo-controlled study with an electromyographic injection technique. J Am Acad Dermatol 1996; 35:569-572.
30. Frankel AS, Kamer FM. Chemical browlift. Arch Otolaryngol Head Neck Surg 1998; 124:312-323.
31. Matarasso A, Matarasso SL, Brandt FS, Bellman B. Botulinum A exotoxin for the management of platysma bands. Plast Reconstr Surg 1999; 103:645-652.
32. Bushara KO, Park DM, Jones JC, Schutta HS. Botulinum toxin—a possible new treatment for axillary hyperhidrosis. Clin Exp Dermatol 1996; 21:276-278.
33. Glogau RG. Botulinum A neurotoxin for axillary hyperhidrosis: no sweat Botox. Dermatol Surg 1998; 24:817-819.
34. Odderson IR. Axillary hyperhidrosis: treatment with botulinum toxin A. Arch Phys Med Rehabil 1998; 79:350-352.
35. Schnider P, Binder M, Kittler H, et al. A randomized, double-blind, placebo-controlled trial of botulinum A toxin for severe axillary hyperhidrosis. Br J Dermatol 1999; 140:677-680.

36. Shelley WB, Talanin NY, Shelley ED. Botulinum toxin therapy for palmar hyperhidrosis [see comments]. J Am Acad Dermatol 1998; 38:227-229.
37. Naumann M, Hofmann U, Bergmann I, et al. Focal hyperhidrosis: effective treatment with intracutaneous botulinum toxin. Arch Dermatol 1998; 134:301-304.
38. Bjerkhoel A, Trobbe O. Frey's syndrome: treatment with botulinum toxin. J Laryngol Otol 1997; 111:839-844.
39. Naumann M, Zellner M, Toyka KV, Reiners K. Treatment of gustatory sweating with botulinum toxin. Ann Neurol 1997; 42:973-975.
40. Laskawi R, Drobik C, Schonebeck C. Up-to-date report of botulinum toxin type A treatment in patients with gustatory sweating (Frey's syndrome). Laryngoscope 1998; 108:381-384.
41. Laccourreye O, Muscatelo L, Naude C, et al. Botulinum toxin type A for Frey's syndrome: a preliminary prospective study. Ann Otol Rhinol Laryngol 1998; 107:52-55.
42. Schulte-Mattler WJ, Wieser T, Zierz S. Treatment of tension-type headaches with botulinum toxin: a pilot study. Eur J Med Res 1999; 26:183-186.
43. Wheeler AH. Botulinum toxin A, adjunctive therapy for refractory headaches associated with pericranial muscle tension. Headache 1998; 38:468-471.
44. Zwart JA, Bovim G, Sand T, Sjaastad O. Tension headache: botulinum toxin paralysis of temporal muscles. Headache 1994; 34:458-462.
45. Hruza GJ. Botulinum toxin. J Watch Dermatol 1999; 7:59-62.
46. Kane MA. Nonsurgical treatment of platysmal bands with injection of botulinum toxin A. Plast Reconstr Surg 1999; 103:656-665.
47. Scott A, Kennedy E, Stubbs H. Botulinum A toxin injection as a treatment for blepharospasm. Arch Ophthalmol 1985; 103:347-350.
48. Jimenez G, Spencer JM. Erbium:YAG laser resurfacing of the hands, arms, and neck. Dermatol Surg 1999; 25:831-835.
49. Lipton RB, Stewart WF. Migraine headaches: epidemiology and comorbidity. Clin Neurosci 1998; 5:2-9.
50. Huilgol SC, Carruthers A, Carruthers JDA. Raising eyebrows with botulinum toxin. Dermatol Surg 1999; 25:373-376.
51. Fagien S. Botox for the treatment of dynamic and hyperkinetic facial lines and furrows: adjunctive use in facial aesthetic surgery. Plast Reconstr Surg 1999; 103:701-713.
52. Edelstein C, Shorr N, Jacobs J, et al. Oculoplastic experience with the cosmetic use of botulinum A exotoxin. Dermatol Surg 1998; 24:1208-1212.
53. Matarasso SL. Complications of botulinum A exotoxin for hyperfunctional lines. Dermatol Surg 1998; 24:1249-1254.

APPENDIX A

Consent Form

CONSENT TO OPERATION, TREATMENT, OR OTHER PROCEDURE

PATIENT ______________________ AGE ____ DATE ___/___/___

1. I hereby authorize Dr. ______________ and those he may designate as his assistants to perform upon myself a Botox injection of the skin. I am aware that possible complications of Botox injection include, but are not limited to, need for touch-ups, as well as occasional temporary eyelid droop (for frown lines/forehead treatment), eyebrow droop (for forehead treatment), double vision (for crow's feet treatment), and grip weakness (for palm treatment).
2. The nature and purpose of the procedure has been explained to me. I am aware that the practice of medicine and surgery is not an exact science and I acknowledge that no guarantees have been made to me concerning the results of the operation, treatment, or procedure.
3. I understand and have been so informed there are risk(s) and consequences associated with the operation(s) described in Paragraph 1.
4. I hereby authorize Dr. ______________ to use my case materials, including photos and/or motion pictures, in teaching, medical publications, and exhibits.

I certify that I have read or have had read to me and fully understand the above consent to the procedure, that the explanations therein referred to were made, and that all blanks or statements requiring insertion or completion were filled in.

______________________________ ______________________________

Signature of Witness Signature of Patient

CHAPTER 18

Chemical Peels

ERIC F. BERNSTEIN

SECTION ONE

History and Scientific Review

CUTANEOUS BASIC SCIENCE, ANATOMY, AND PHYSIOLOGY

In order to understand the beneficial effects of topical treatments on photoaged skin, we must first gain an understanding of the alterations that occur as a result of chronic sun exposure. Most of the changes we attribute to chronological aging actually result from long-term sun exposure. To illustrate this fact, one can compare the pigmentary alterations, sallow color, fine lines, and wrinkles of sun-exposed skin to the smooth, supple sun-protected skin on the same individual. Our skin attempts to protect itself from the effects of chronic sun exposure via a number of mechanisms. These include our baseline melanin content that responds with an increase in synthesis and deposition of melanin in response to sun exposure, as well as our endogenous means of preventing oxidative damage. As much as half or more of the photodamage that occurs may result from oxidative mechanisms. Our natural defenses against oxidative damage include superoxide dismutase, glutathione-based systems, and the antioxidant vitamins C and E. As we age chronologically and gain cumulative damage from repeated sun exposure, these systems begin to fail. As a result of the decline in our defenses and repeated assaults on our cellular DNA from the sun, both the epidermis and dermis start to show signs of chronic photoaging.

The Epidermis

Clinically the epidermis in sun-damaged skin may demonstrate irregularities in pigmentation including ephelides and solar lentigenes. In addition, damage to keratinocytes leads to actinic keratoses. The viable epidermal layer in photoaged skin becomes hypertrophic compared with similar sites in the same individual. However, with severe photodamage, the epidermis will eventually become extremely atrophic. Although epidermal alterations resulting from chronic photodamage may be quite apparent due to the pigmentary changes that occur and their superficial location, the most striking alterations resulting from chronic sun damage occur in the dermis.

The Dermis

The dermis is composed of a number of extracellular matrix molecules that supply the stroma for the resident cells of the dermis and the dermal vasculature. The viable and nonviable components of the dermis interact extensively to maintain a healthy environment in the skin. The extracellular matrix includes collagen that provides strength to skin, elastic fibers that impart extensibility and resilience to skin, and the glycosaminoglycans (GAGs) and proteoglycans that serve a number of functions including maintaining the integrity of basement membrane zones and maintaining dermal hydration.

Collagen

The principal structural component of skin is collagen. Collagen composes approximately 80% of the dry weight of non-sun-damaged skin.[1,2] The triple helix configuration is characteristic of the collagen molecule and forms as a result of the amino acid sequence of the collagen chains. This sequence is the Gly-X-Y sequence where *Gly* represents the amino acid, glycine, and the X and Y positions are frequently the amino acids proline and hydroxyproline.[1,2] Together with vitamin C, hydroxyproline stabilizes the triple helical portion of the collagen molecule.[3,4]

The various collagens are named with roman numerals in order of their discovery. The most abundant type of collagen in adult skin is, by far, type I collagen. Type I collagen is the main structural protein in the entire body. The three-polypeptide chains that form the triple helix for collagen fibrils are two identical $\alpha 1(I)$

chains and a third distinct α2(I) chain. Collagen is deposited by the dermal fibroblasts, which are constantly breaking down and regenerating collagen, the steady state of which is the phenotype for skin. External factors such as wounding or sun exposure can alter the steady state amount and arrangement of collagen fibers.[2,5]

Collagen formation involves a number of steps. The first steps occur within the fibroblasts, with further refinement of the collagen molecule occurring in the extracellular space. Initially transcription factors bind to the promoter region of the collagen DNA. A mirror of the collagen DNA template is formed, resulting in collagen messenger RNA (mRNA). Following transcription, posttranscriptional modification of collagen mRNA takes place where introns are removed. Following this, procollagen molecules are synthesized and form the triple helix due to their Gly-X-Y structure. The procollagen molecules are then released from the cell to the extracellular space. These molecules contain nonhelical N-terminal and C-terminal domains. These domains are then cleaved from the procollagen molecule, resulting in the formation of more mature type I collagen. The fibrillar structure of a collagen molecule is quite characteristic when viewed by electron microscopy as a banding pattern that has a periodicity of 68 nm.[1-3,5] Lysyl oxidase then provides further strength to the collagen molecule by deamination of lysyl- and hydroxylysyl-residues.[6,7] Immunoperoxidase staining for the N-terminal and C-terminal domains of procollagen are often used as an indicator of new collagen production. Since the dermis is composed of 80% collagen, identifying new mature collagen can be difficult. Thus these components of the procollagen precursor molecule are often used as indicators of new collagen formation.

Type III collagen is the second most abundant type of collagen found in adult skin. Because it is present in large quantities in fetal skin, type III collagen is also known as *fetal collagen*.[8] Although abundant in fetal skin, it comprises only one seventh of the total collagen in adult skin. Type III collagen is composed of three identical chains referred to as α1(III) chains. As is typical for all collagen molecules, these chains arrange themselves in the prototypical triple helix configuration. Type III collagen is highly abundant in extensible tissues including the gastrointestinal tract, arteries, and skin.[2,5,9] Type III collagen fibers associate with type I collagen fibers and may play a role in the formation of the latter. Also possibly indicative of its role in assisting mature collagen fiber formation is its presence in early healing of wounds.[10] Type III collagen is the first type of collagen to appear in a healing wound.

In addition to serving as a structural protein in the dermis, collagen fibers also serve as components of the basement membrane zone separating the epidermis and dermis. Type IV collagen helps form the complex barrier that facilitates transportation of nutrients and waste products through the dermal-epidermal junction. Type IV collagen has interruptions in the triple helical domain that are thought to confer flexibility on the type IV collagen molecule. In addition, type IV collagen forms a scaffold for the incorporation of other extracellular matrix components.[11] Type VII collagen is also a major component of the basement membrane zone. Type VII collagen forms the anchoring fibers that help attach the epidermis to the underlying dermis.[12-14] The role of these fibers is well illustrated by the hereditary disorder dystrophic epidermolysis bullosa.[14] In this disorder blisters form deep in the basement membrane zone in persons with mutations of type VII collagen. Other collagens such as type VI collagen and the FACIT (Fibril-Associated Collagen with Interrupted Triple helices) may help form type I collagen fibers as well.[15-17] Decorin, a small chondroitin sulfate proteoglycan, is found in association with collagen fibers.[18,19] It is thought that decorin may contribute to the final arrangement of collagen fibers within skin.

Elastic Fibers

Elastic fibers confer the ability to stretch and recoil to skin and other organs (Fig. 18-1). Despite their prominent role as a structural component of skin, they compose only 1% to 2 % of the dry weight of non-sun-

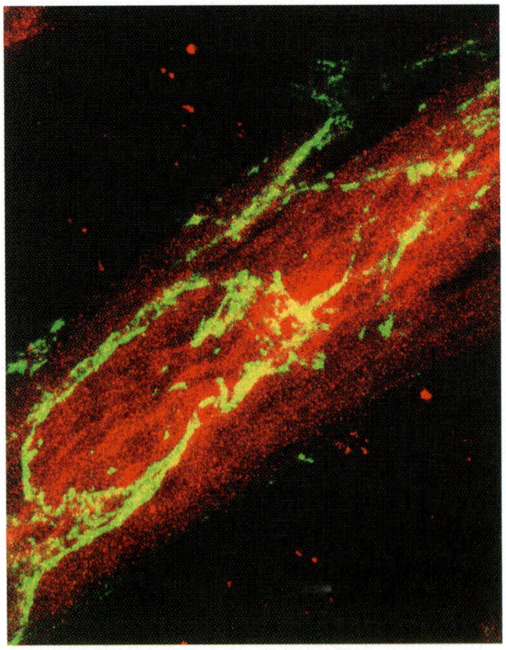

FIG. 18-1
Laser scanning confocal microscopy of immunoperoxidase-stained skin demonstrates the close association of a dermal collagen fiber (red) with elastic fibers (green).

damaged skin.[20,21] Elastic fibers are complex and are formed by a number of components, only one of which is the protein elastin. Elastic fibers can be compared to a bungee cord, which has a stretchy inner core and a more rigid outer string wrapping. The inner core may be compared to the protein elastin, while the outer wrapping is analogous to the protein fibrillin. The fibrillins comprise a family of highly insoluble proteins that are a component of elastic fibers.[22] In addition, the oxytalan fibers, which extend from the superficial dermis vertically to the dermal-epidermal junction, are composed solely of fibrillin.

Just as decorin is associated with collagen fibers, the proteoglycan versican is associated with elastic fibers.[23-25] However, in contrast to the small size of decorin, versican is a very large chondroitin sulfate proteoglycan. Versican may play a role in elastic fiber formation and arrangement within the dermis.

Glycosaminoglycans, Proteoglycans, and Fibronectin

Although GAGs comprise only a small portion of the dry weight of skin, they are critical to its proper functioning. They are widely distributed throughout skin as well as other tissues. Because GAGs bind a large amount of water, they help to regulate skin hydration and enable cell mobility within skin.[10,26,27] Hyaluronic acid may be found free in the dermis unattached to a protein, or associated with a protein by the terminal reducing sugar residue, thus forming a proteoglycan. Proteoglycans serve a number of functions, which include maintaining the integrity of basement membrane zones, regulating cell mobility and communication, and helping to form collagen and elastic fibers.

Decorin is a very small chondroitin sulfate proteoglycan that is distributed throughout the dermis in association with collagen fibers.[18,19] Decorin is composed of a core protein with only one attached chondroitin sulfate chain. Studies have demonstrated that decorin binds to specific areas on the collagen fibers, possibly helping to form the normal arrangement of collagen fibrils and thus determining collagen fiber diameter.[19] Decorin has also been found to bind transforming growth factor-β, and thus may regulate dermal remodeling during normal conditions, as well as during wound healing.[28] In contrast to the small size of decorin, versican is a very large chondroitin sulfate proteoglycan with many attached chondroitin sulfate chains. Versican is present diffusely throughout the superficial dermis as well as being found in association with elastic fibers throughout the dermis. Because versican has been found in association with elastic fibers, it is postulated that it may play a role in regulating elastic fiber formation in a manner similar to decorin.[25,28] Fibronectin is a glycoprotein that has an amino acid sequence, arg-gly-asp-ser (RGDS), that is known to serve as a binding site for cells. Fibronectin, therefore, aids in cell migration and thus may play a critical role in skin remodeling and wound healing.[29-31]

RESIDENT CELLS OF THE DERMIS

The cellular component of the dermis creates and maintains the dermal extracellular matrix. When wounding occurs, these cells respond with a healing response restoring dermal integrity. Fibroblasts are connective tissue cells that are responsible for the production of the majority of the extracellular matrix. They help maintain the dermis by constantly remodeling the dermal extracellular matrix. These cells respond with other blood-borne cells to the site of an injury and help restore the injured extracellular matrix.[2,10] A healing response may be stimulated without a break in the integrity of the skin by a variety of agents including α-hydroxy acids (AHAs), retinoids, and laser treatment.

Mast cells are bone marrow–derived cells residing in the dermis. These cells are capable of releasing vasoactive cytokines that can stimulate the production of dermal extracellular matrix. Mast cells are often clustered around blood vessels and thus respond quite rapidly to blood-borne stimuli. They are thus important participants in the wound-healing response.[32,33] Macrophages are also bone marrow–derived cells that develop from circulating monocytes. They function as phagocytes and produce large amounts of lysosomal enzymes. Thus they can help remove injured tissue and dead cells from the site of a wound and help with the normal remodeling of skin that occurs on an ongoing basis.[30,32,34]

CLINICAL STUDIES

Dermal Photoaging

Although most of us attribute an aged appearance to the passage of time, the majority of changes we commonly associate with aging are due to sun damage. Severely photodamaged skin has pigmentary alterations, wrinkles, a sallow color, and thick leathery appearance. Chronologically aged, sun-protected sites show few of the changes present in photodamaged skin. In addition, when compared under histopathologic examination, photoaged skin differs dramatically from chronologically aged skin taken from the same individual. In contrast, chronologically aged skin taken from sun-protected sites shows only minor changes when compared with skin taken from sun-protected sites of much younger individuals: the dermis taken from sun-protected aged skin has fewer cells, blood vessels, and elastic fibers. The reduction in the number of elastic fibers may be responsible for the fine wrinkling seen in sun-protected sites.[9,35-39]

The microscopic changes resulting from chronic photoaging are quite profound in comparison with the subtle changes in sun-protected sites. Sun-damaged skin demonstrates a massive accumulation of abnormally arranged elastic tissue, termed solar elastosis (Fig. 18-2).[40-42] Although the solar elastotic material is composed of the same constituents as normal elastic fibers, including elastin, fibrillin, versican, and hyaluronic acid, these constituents are arranged in a very disordered and haphazard manner.[25,40-44] The elastic fibers that normally extend vertically from the superficial dermis to the epidermis are partially destroyed or missing in severely sun-damaged skin. The fine elastic meshwork embedded in a rich dermal collagen matrix is replaced by large clumps of solar elastotic material. This elastotic material is intermixed with a decreased number of poorly organized collagen fibers.[44] Although abundant, the elastic tissue affected by solar elastosis is nonfunctional, and as a result sun-damaged skin loses its elasticity and resilience.

The zone of normal-appearing collagen that separates the solar elastotic material from the epidermis is referred to as a "grenz," or border zone. This border zone is critical to the maintenance of a healthy epidermis. Because the epidermis lacks its own vascular supply, it must depend on the underlying dermis for nutrients. Thus it is quite likely that the epidermal keratinocytes themselves secrete growth factors that maintain the underlying grenz zone. Many of the agents used to improve photodamaged skin exert their effects in this superficial grenz zone of normal-appearing collagen.

Dermal Wound Healing

After either an injury or a treatment that is able to stimulate the healing response in the absence of an injury such as AHA or retinoid treatment, the skin repairs itself with a distinct set of interrelated events. When a wound is created in the skin, one of the first events is formation of a fibrin clot. Following this there is an influx of circulating cells to the site of injury. In addition, circulating fibronectin accumulates at the wound site and provides a provisional matrix for cell migration and proliferation.[30,45,46] The first matrix to be formed by fibroblasts attracted to the wound site is rich in hyaluronic acid.[26] This matrix of hyaluronic acid allows cell migration to further occur, leading to the formation of granulation tissue and the first migration of keratinocytes to cover the wound surface. Granulation tissue is rich in blood vessels with their associated basement membrane zones and thus contains large amounts of chondroitin sulfate. Keratinocytes continue to migrate over the wound surface. The first type of collagen to be seen in a healing wound is type III collagen.[30] Following this, type I collagen is formed. Type I collagen continues to evolve and mature, giving the wound additional strength over the ensuing months. Although they are a component of normal skin, elastic fibers may not appear until very late in the healing cy-

A

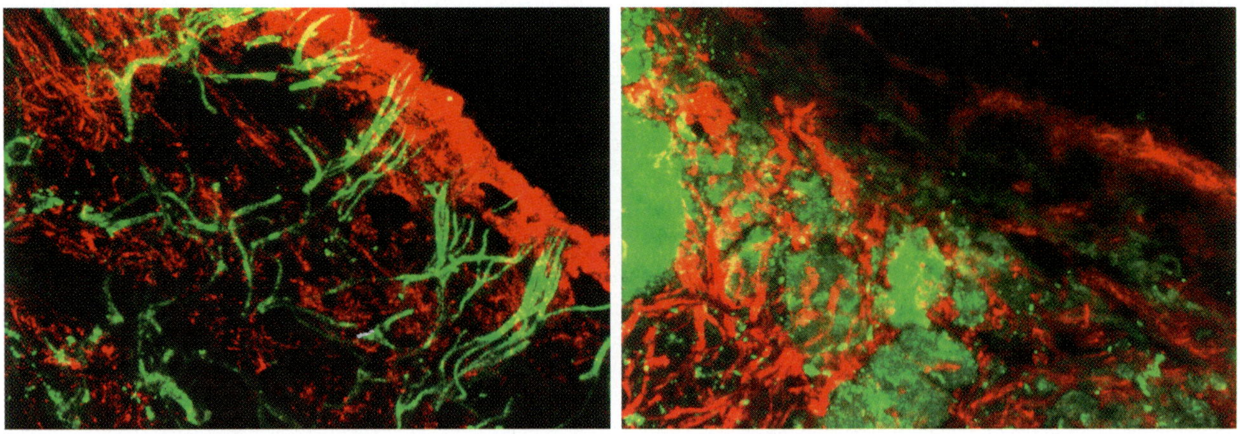

B

FIG. 18-2
A, Laser scanning confocal microscopy of immunoperoxidase-stained sun-protected skin reveals a dense collagen framework in red with a more intense red staining of the collagen just below the dermal-epidermal junction. The epidermis is to the upper right of this panel and is dark (unstained). The elastic fiber network is evident as green fibers forming a meshwork within the dense collagen network. **B,** Sun-damaged skin taken from the same individual reveals a dramatically altered morphology with a paucity of collagen fibers (red) intermixed with large clumps of abnormal elastic material (green). A faint red band of collagen is evident beneath the unstained epidermis in the upper right portion of this micrograph.

cle.[30] Agents used to treat photodamaged skin can stimulate this orderly sequence of extracellular matrix deposition even in the absence of an open wound.

CHEMICAL PEELS AS A TREATMENT FOR CUTANEOUS PHOTOAGING

Many patients are interested in obtaining a more youthful appearance to their skin, but they are not interested in the prospect of time away from work or looking unnatural. Since all patients will age in unique, subtle, but meaningfully different ways, it is useful to have a treatment option that can be custom fit to each individual patient. Chemical peels are just such an option.

With the ability to peel the skin to differing depths, physicians can choose peeling agents that take into account patient preference and risk tolerance, depth of cutaneous photoaging, amount of photoinjury to the epidermis, dermis, and dermal architecture, and the physician's skill with different techniques. It is possible to use chemical peels to treat from the most superficial aspect of the skin all the way to the deepest portion of the reticular dermis. The skill in chemical peeling comes not only from being able to master individual techniques but from learning how to custom fit the differing depths of chemical peels to the needs of the patient.

SECTION TWO

Atlas of Surgical Procedures

PREOPERATIVE PATIENT EVALUATION

Pretreatment evaluation is an important determinant of posttreatment results when utilizing chemical peels to rejuvenate photodamaged skin. Medical history must be obtained, with an emphasis on history of abnormal or keloid scarring, perioral herpes simplex virus (HSV) infection, past 13-*cis*-retinoic acid (Accutane) therapy, prior laser skin resurfacing, as well as medications that may photosensitize the patient. In addition, the patient's Fitzpatrick skin type must be assessed to help the physician determine the potential risks of postoperative pigment alteration.

Patients with a history of perioral HSV infection can be treated prophylactically with an oral antiviral medication, usually beginning 1 to 2 days prior to the procedure and continuing for 10 to 14 days after. Many physicians do not routinely use HSV prophylaxis for superficial chemical peels. Prior use of Accutane is not a contraindication to chemical peeling, but many physicians wait a minimum of 6 months after the last Accutane dose before performing a chemical peel. Although clinically unproven, the risk of abnormal scarring appears to increase in the posttreatment period with Accutane, and therefore a delay in injuring the skin is advisable.

Pigment alteration is a significant risk when one is using chemical peeling agents for skin rejuvenation. Patients with Fitzpatrick skin types I and II are unlikely to develop long-term pigment alteration from chemical peels, but patients with skin types III and IV often develop limited and transient (lasting less than 3 months) hyperpigmentation, particularly with deeper or more aggressive chemical peels (Table 18-1). Decisions to use a chemical peel for patients with Fitzpatrick skin types V and VI should be approached with great caution, as the risk of permanent pigment alteration is quite significant. Superficial chemical peels can be of significant value in these patients, but the risk of pigment alteration should be discussed with the patient in detail prior to proceeding with treatment.

Choosing the Proper Chemical Peeling Agent

There are three basic types of chemical peels: superficial, medium, and deep. This classification system is based on the achievable depth of penetration and clinical effect of the peeling agent used. Glycolic and salicylic acid peels are considered superficial, as are Jessner's-only peels. Trichloroacetic acid (TCA) peels are medium-depth peels, and phenol is used for deep peels. In general, superficial peels penetrate down through the epidermis and may reach as far as the papillary dermis. Medium-depth peels extend deeper, reaching the deep papillary dermis and often the superficial reticular dermis. Deep chemical peels are used to penetrate into the mid reticular dermis.

With this classification system in mind, the physician must assess the depth of photoaging and wrinkles the patient is interested in treating. Once the depth of photoaging has been determined, the physician can help the patient choose the proper peeling agent. As an example, it would be unwise to perform a deep phenol peel on a patient with limited superficial photodamage. The significant risks associated with the deeper peel

Table 18-1 Fitzpatrick Skin Types

Skin Type	Tanning Response
I	Always burns, never tans
II	Usually burns, tans with difficulty
III	Sometimes mild burn, tans average
IV	Rarely burns, tans with ease
V	Very rarely burns, tans very easily
VI	No burn, tans very easily

would not justify its use in this instance. However, patients with significant deep photodamage may benefit most from a deeper peel. Yet some patients may be unwilling to accept the risks or morbidity associated with a deeper peel and may elect to have a more superficial peel, knowing that the benefit may be less significant. In general, it is acceptable to perform a peel that is more superficial than the depth of photoaging as the physician factors in patient preferences, but it is unwise to perform a peel that penetrates deeper than the level of photodamage. The simple premise is that the deeper the peel the greater the risks and morbidity, and the physician should choose the peeling agent that most closely matches the patient's depth of photodamage.

ALPHA-HYDROXY ACIDS AND GLYCOLIC ACID CHEMICAL PEELS

The objective of AHA treatment and glycolic acid peels is to stimulate a healing response without ablating the epidermis or superficial dermis. The first report of a beneficial effect of AHAs applied to the skin was published over a quarter century ago.[47] Despite this initial report, AHAs have only recently been developed for widespread use. They have been used to treat a number of conditions including disorders of keratinization, xerosis, photoaging, acne, and pigmentary disorders, and to augment other topical preparations (Fig. 18-3). For example, AHAs have been shown to counteract the atrophogenic effects of topical corticosteroids on both the epidermis and the dermis.[48] They act by increasing viable epidermal thickness as well as by thickening the dermal compartment of skin.[48-50] Since both hyaluronic acid and chondroitin sulfate are among the first extracellular matrix components deposited in a healing wound, these may also be the first to be measured following AHA treatment. Indeed, application of AHAs increases not only epidermal thickness but also epidermal glycosaminoglycan deposition.[48-50] Specifically, hyaluronic acid has been shown to be increased in the epidermis of treated skin.[49] In addition, both hyaluronic acid and chondroitin sulfate have been shown to be increased in the dermis of AHA-treated skin.[49] Indirect evidence for the deposition of dermal collagen following AHA treatment has been demonstrated in human skin. Collagen mRNA expression has been shown to be increased in glycolic acid–treated skin.[51] In addition, in vitro data suggest that collagen production may be stimulated by application of glycolic acid.[52] This suggests that mature collagen may be measured after long treatment times with AHAs. Demonstrating increases in mature type I collagen is technically diffi-

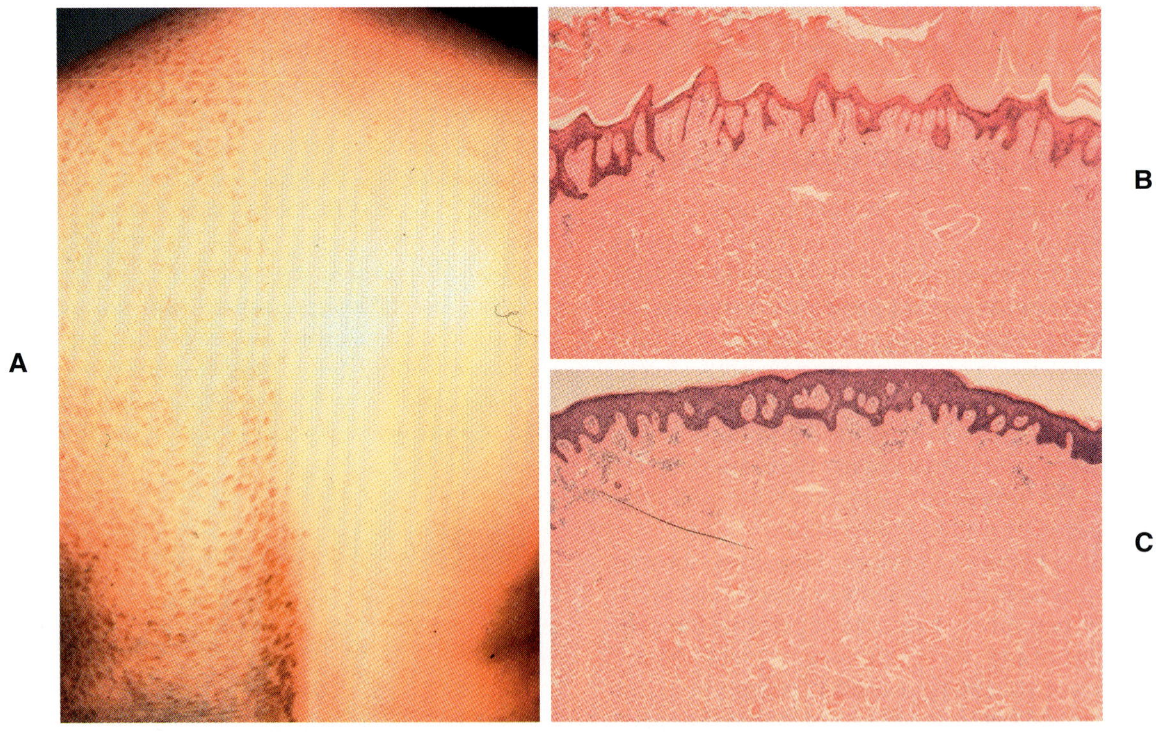

FIG. 18-3
A, An individual with lamellar ichthyosis has been treated on the right portion of his back with a combination of AHAs, while the left portion remains untreated. **B,** Histopathologic examination of a skin biopsy taken from untreated skin reveals a massively thickened stratum corneum **(C)** that is absent in treated skin.

cult, since the skin is normally composed largely of collagen. Since AHAs are applied topically, it is likely that they exert the majority of their effects superficially. The subepidermal grenz zone in sun-damaged skin is where the effect of AHAs and agents that rejuvenate skin is often demonstrated. This grenz zone has been shown to increase in thickness following deep chemical peels,[53] and ablative laser resurfacing,[54] treatments that rejuvenate photodamaged skin. The increase in thickness of the subepidermal grenz zone following deep chemical peels and laser resurfacing may indeed account for the clinical improvement that is seen following these treatments. It is quite probable that the epidermal keratinocytes play a significant role in the extracellular matrix formation following application of AHAs. These cells experience the highest concentrations of AHAs and may actively secrete growth factors to stimulate extracellular matrix production in the underlying grenz zone.

A number of AHAs have demonstrated the ability to increase both epidermal and dermal GAGs. Although GAGs make up only about 0.1% to 0.3% of the dry weight of normal skin, their ability to bind manyfold their weight in water increases their importance in maintaining skin hydration. As a result, small increases in the amount of epidermal and dermal GAGs may result in relatively large increases in epidermal and dermal hydration. This increase in dermal hydration may account for the increase in skin thickness measured after relatively short treatment periods with AHAs.[49,50] Skin treated with retinoids responds in a fashion nearly identical to AHA-treated skin. An increase in epidermal thickness and hyaluronic acid staining, nearly identical to that measured following AHA treatment, has been demonstrated after retinoic acid treatment.[55] In addition, dermal GAG staining is also increased following retinoid treatment.[56] The deposition of epidermal and dermal GAGs may in turn affect collagen and elastic fiber formation. Thus the early events associated with GAG deposition may lead to collagen formation that occurs much later. Indeed, procollagen formation has been demonstrated following 9 months of tretinoin treatment.[57] Just as altering one extracellular matrix component may affect many others subsequently, changes in epidermal thickness, stratum corneum morphology, and epidermal GAG content will have an effect on skin barrier function. Alterations in skin barrier function may, through a cascade of interrelated steps, affect the overall architecture of the dermal extracellular matrix. These changes in turn are capable of changing the structure, function, and appearance of skin.

Topical glycolic acid preparations in low concentrations have been shown to improve photodamaged skin.[58-60] Further improvement may be achieved by using high-concentration, short-duration applications of glycolic acid. Glycolic acid treatments, more commonly referred to as *peels,* are usually performed at weekly to monthly intervals. Improvement in skin texture, fine wrinkling, and actinic keratoses and lightening of solar keratoses have been demonstrated following glycolic acid peels with 50% glycolic acid.[61] Histopathologic examination of treated skin in these patients demonstrated increases in epidermal thickness and an increase in the thickness of the collagen layer of the dermis in some patients.[61] Recently, a new short-contact peel has been described utilizing glycolic acid with 5-fluorouracil for the treatment of actinic keratoses and other signs of cutaneous photodamage.[62] One study of these combination peels recorded the effect on actinic keratoses following eight weekly applications. The combination peel reduced more than 90% of actinic keratoses 6 months following cessation of the peels, as compared with less than 20% clearing using glycolic acid alone. This clearing occurred without the usual erythema and irritation associated with the daily use of 5-fluorouracil alone. In addition, patients showed improvement in the cosmetic appearance of their skin that typically results from glycolic acid treatments.[62] Thus patients utilizing this combination approach were able to derive the cosmetic benefits of an improvement in the appearance of photodamaged skin, while also dramatically reducing the number of actinic keratoses (Fig. 18-4).

Glycolic acid peels are also well suited for improving pigmentary alterations of the epidermis. They have been shown to increase epidermal cell turnover[63] and thus may hasten a return to normal pigmentation in hyperpigmented areas. Studies have demonstrated the efficacy of glycolic acid peels for improving postinflammatory hyperpigmentation in dark-complexioned individuals.[64-66] Melasma is one of the most common pigmentary abnormalities occurring in women. Glycolic acid products accompanied by glycolic acid peels can produce dramatic improvements in patients with melasma.[65,67] In addition, if corticosteroids are used as lightening agents, the ability of AHAs to negate the atrophogenic effect of topical corticosteroid preparations may permit them to be used for longer time intervals, even on the face.

Most of the claims regarding the ability of AHAs to improve acne focus only on improving postinflammatory hyperpigmentation, erythema, or scarring that arise secondary to acne. However, glycolic acid and glycolic acid peels are extensively used to improve acne quite successfully.[68] All types of acne have been shown to respond to glycolic acid peels. Comedonal acne improves most rapidly, followed by papulo-pustular acne, with nodular-cystic acne requiring the most treatments prior to significant improvement.[69] Glycolic acid peels are an effective treatment for the range of acne types and have the added benefit of improving acne-induced postinflammatory hyperpigmentation and erythema, as well as improving the depressed scars that often accompany severe acne. Daily application of topical glycolic acid preparations combined

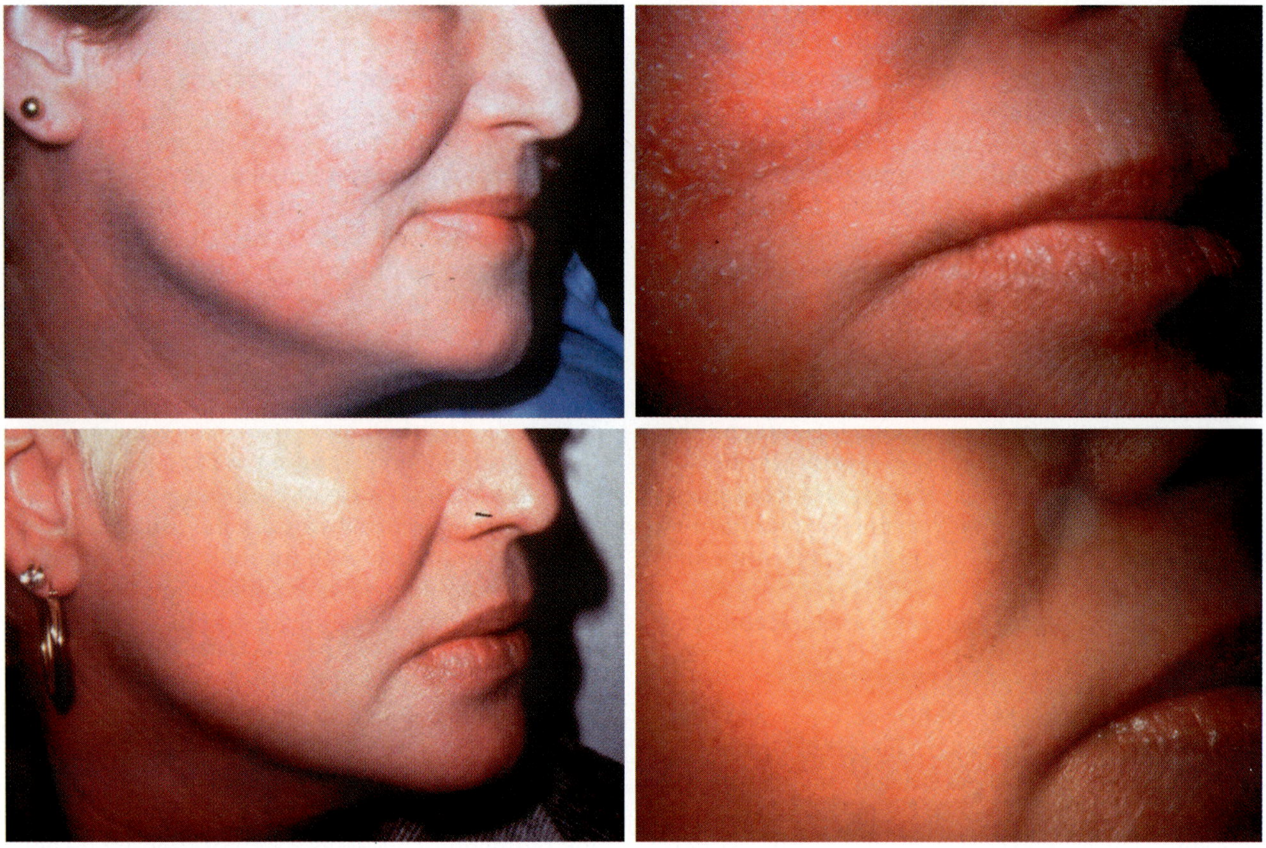

FIG. 18-4
A, Multiple actinic keratoses and other signs of sun damage are evident before glycolic acid/5-fluorouracil *pulse-peel.* **B,** Close-up of the area shown in **A. C,** Improvement of actinic keratoses and other signs of sun damage after pulse-peels. **D,** Close-up of the treated area shown in **B.** (Courtesy Dr. Bruce Katz.)

with glycolic acid peels is also quite effective for treating pseudofolliculitis barbae. In addition to improving the inflammatory papules associated with pseudofolliculitis barbae, glycolic acid peels may also help control the associated hyperpigmentation.[70] Although contrary to the popular opinion that glycolic acid treatment will aggravate rosacea, many individuals with rosacea respond quite well to glycolic acid treatment. Glycolic acid not only reduces the papular and pustular component of rosacea but may also decrease the associated erythema in many patients, despite fears that glycolic acid will increase associated erythema (Fig. 18-5).

Complications from lower-strength glycolic acid peels are predominantly limited to dryness and mild irritation. Irritation may also occur from application of products containing glycolic acid or tretinoin too soon following a glycolic peel. Transient hyperpigmentation may occur even following lower-strength peels in some darker-skinned or tanned individuals. This appears to be particularly true in Asian patients. Although glycolic acid is a weak peeling agent, 70% glycolic acid peel solutions may have a pH as low as 0.1.[71] The epidermis is normally left intact, in contrast to deeper peeling agents highlighted below, but significant epidermal damage evident as crusting can occur following a glycolic peel. Complications occasionally seen following medium-to-deep peels or laser resurfacing such as herpes simplex activation, bacterial infection, or scarring are rare following a glycolic acid peel; however, these complications can occur after significant epidermal damage from any therapy.

Glycolic Acid Treatment: Technique

The prepeel evaluation should go over the patient's medical history, paying particular attention to a history of perioral herpes virus infection (cold sores) or unusual tendency to scar; medication list, paying particular attention to current or previous 13-*cis*-retinoic acid (Accutane) therapy; medication allergies; and any sensitivity to AHAs or retinoids. Patients taking 13-*cis*-retinoic acid should not receive glycolic acid peels, and physicians may wish to delay starting glycolic acid peels until 6 months following a course of 13-*cis*-retinoic acid treatment. In addition, use of tretinoin cream may enhance penetration of a glycolic peel, and

A 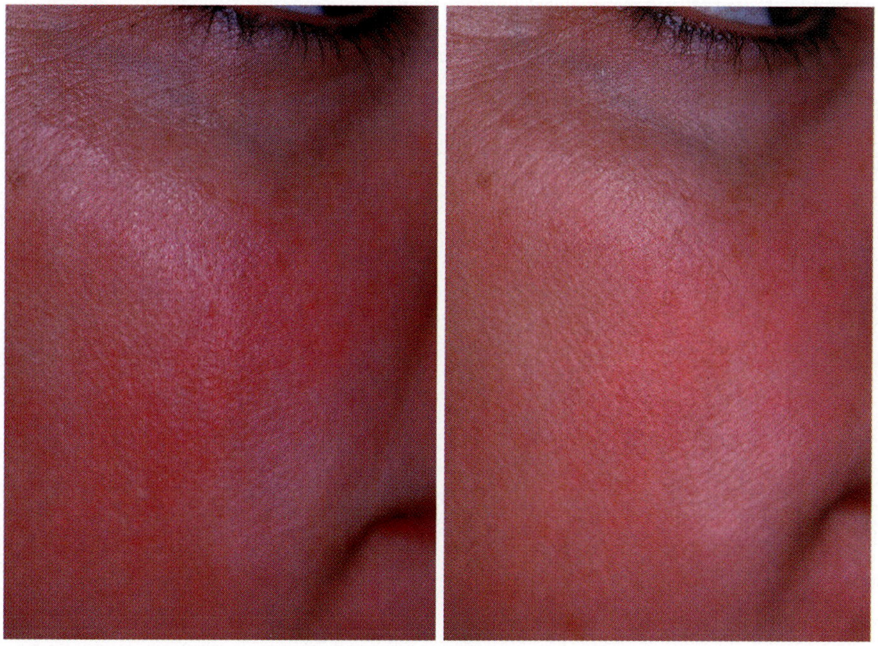 B

FIG. 18-5
The erythema associated with mild rosacea **(A)** is decreased following use of a 10% glycolic acid lotion for 6 weeks **(B).**

thus the person performing the peel should be aware of its use. The time a peel can be left on the skin without crusting or the risk of hyperpigmentation will shorten considerably if a patient begins using tretinoin during a course of glycolic peels. Concomitant administration of photosensitizing oral medications should also be noted and appropriate sun protection always used. It is also advisable to have the patient use a glycolic acid lotion for approximately 2 weeks prior to administering a glycolic acid peel. This helps create a more uniform stratum corneum barrier, ensuring a more uniform peel. In addition, it will identify patients who are sensitive to glycolic acid and who therefore may not be candidates for higher-strength glycolic acid peels. Asian patients are often found to be more sensitive to glycolic acid peels, and thus a lower concentration than is typically used should be administered. The use of a lower-strength glycolic acid preparation decreases the risk of inadvertent overtreatment.

Although glycolic acid treatments are referred to as glycolic acid peels, this moniker often gives patients the impression they are going to be peeling for a number of days. Thus it is more appropriate to refer to peels as glycolic acid *treatments.* Glycolic acid treatments not only help reverse the signs of cutaneous photodamage but also improve acne scarring, as well as dramatically improving acne itself. However, glycolic treatments for acne need to be administered at monthly intervals or the acne may recur. Thus, to control even severe acne in patients who may not tolerate 13-*cis*-retinoic acid, monthly glycolic peels are a viable alternative. Peels for photodamage may be administered at monthly intervals for 3 or more months and then spaced out less frequently according to the individual patient's skin response and lifestyle. As the skin responds to the glycolic treatments, the treatment time necessary to reach the desired end point of uniform erythema usually increases from session to session. This will not happen if the patient uses tretinoin for the first time during a course of glycolic treatments. Tretinoin use dramatically shortens the time to reach the desired end points. This effect may be exploited in patients whose treatment times exceed 5 minutes. Adding tretinoin will often shorten the treatment time significantly and allow continued clinical improvement without excessive treatment times. Administering peels at intervals less than 1 month will also result in a decrease in the treatment time, possibly because the epidermis and the stratum corneum have not had enough time to respond to the peel. In addition, during the drier winter months, treatments times may decrease, and a clinician should be aware of this potential in order to end a peel before skin whitening or epidermolysis takes place. Epidermolysis, or superficial whitening of the skin, is probably the clinical sign that low pH glycolic acid solution has reached the keratinocytes and is denaturing protein. This will result in superficial crusting of a small percentage of the whitened area.

Prior to performing a glycolic treatment, cleanse the skin with a nonirritating cleanser, followed by a mild degreasing agent (Fig. 18-6). A degreasing agent such as acetone that strips a considerable amount, perhaps

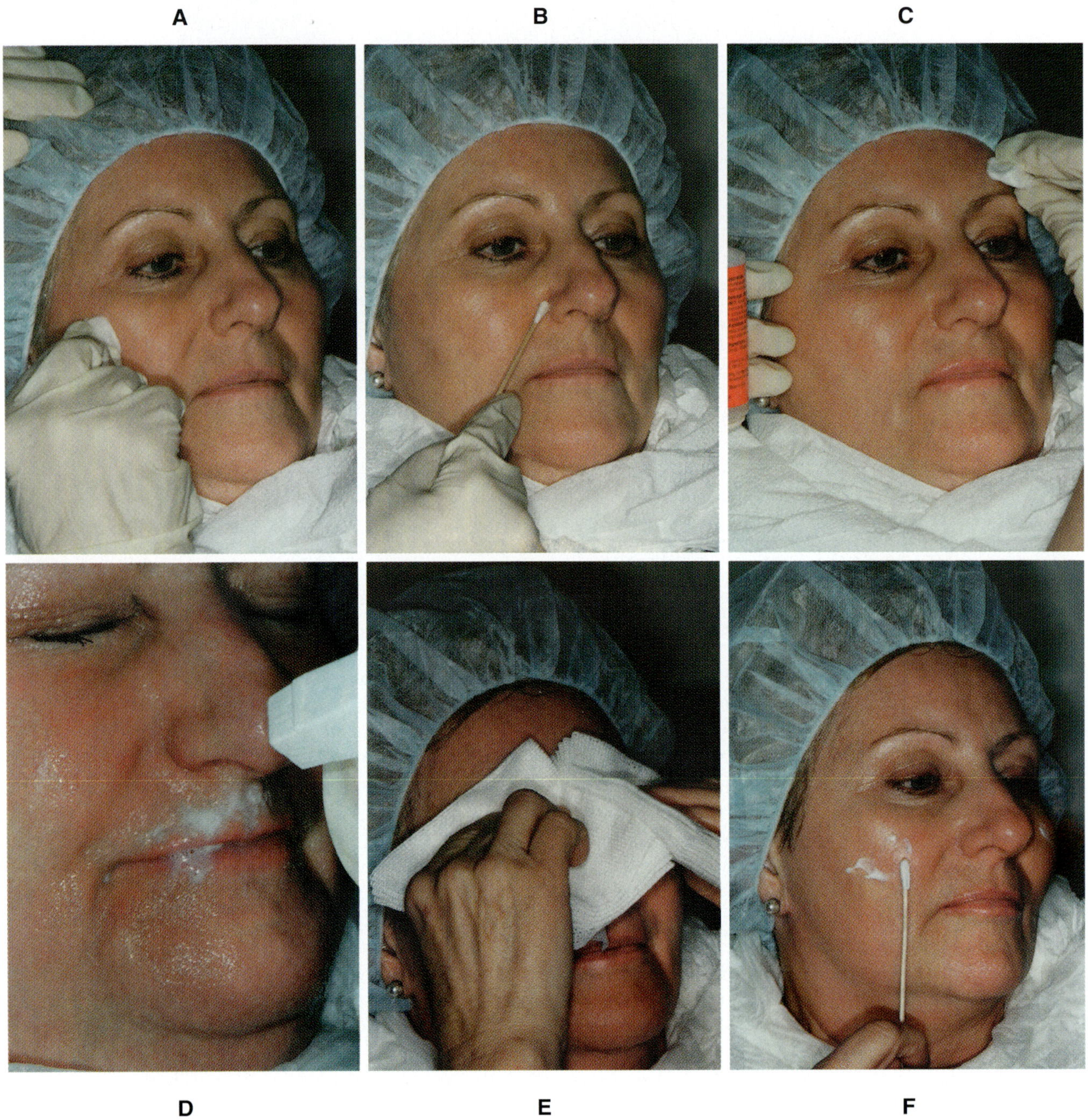

FIG. 18-6
A, Prior to performing a peel, the skin is cleansed and treated with a degreasing agent that gently removes surface oil. **B,** The lateral canthi, nasolabial folds, and lips are treated with petrolatum to prevent pooling of the peel solution and subsequent irritation. **C,** The peel solution is applied rapidly and evenly to ensure that the entire skin surface receives virtually the same contact time with the peel solution. **D,** The peel solution is neutralized to end the peel. The bubbles present on the lip are carbon dioxide bubbles, and cessation of bubbling signifies complete neutralization of the glycolic acid solution. Care should be taken to lift the cap to ensure no solution is left unneutralized. The neutralizing solution is patted dry **(E),** and an emollient postpeel cream is applied **(F).** The latter step may be avoided in acne-prone individuals.

too much, oil from the skin may result in an uneven glycolic treatment. Areas where glycolic acid can accumulate and cause irritation, such as the nasal ala, lips, and lateral canthal folds should be treated with petrolatum to prevent accumulation of glycolic acid and possible dryness or crusting. Once the skin is prepared, the glycolic acid is then applied. Low-strength peel solutions typically contain 20% to 35% glycolic acid, while higher-strength peels utilize 50% to 70% glycolic acid solutions. Especially when using a high concentration of glycolic acid, administer the solution evenly and rapidly. Rapid administration may be more easily accomplished using a cotton ball as opposed to a brush. The extra time it takes to cover the entire face using a brush may result in one portion of the face receiving an uneven peel relative to the other. At the sign of a diffuse erythematous glow, increased sensation or pain as reported by the patient, or immediately upon any evidence of epidermolysis (skin whitening), the peel should be neutralized. Often during a patient's first peel clinicians will neutralize the peel after a period of 2 minutes in the absence of any of these findings. A basic neutralizing solution containing sodium bicarbonate is preferable to water alone, especially when using a high-strength glycolic acid solution. Rapid neutralization often prevents progression of the peel during the neutralization phase, thus avoiding epidermolysis and subsequent crusting. Following a glycolic treatment, a bland emollient is administered to soothe the skin. In acne-prone individuals, this step should be avoided, since even noncomedogenic topicals can lead to the development of acne in such patients.

SALICYLIC ACID CHEMICAL PEELS

Salicylic acid has been used as a component of a number of peeling agents including Jessner's solution. In addition, it is a common component of numerous over-the-counter acne treatments. Recently, salicylic acid has been used in higher concentrations as a peeling agent, predominantly for the treatment of acne. A recent study investigated the effect of salicylic acid peels for treating acne, enlarged pores and oily skin, and pigmentary alterations in dark-skinned patients. Moderate to significant improvement was seen in 88% of patients. Side effects were minimal, occurring in only 16% of patients, and were limited to crusting and hypopigmentation, dryness, and hyperpigmentation.[72] Salicylic acid peels have been introduced relatively recently and may be increasingly used for the treatment of acne.

Salicylic Acid Treatment: Technique

Patients wash their skin before application of a pretreatment cleanser. Common solutions contain alcohol and witch hazel to remove surface oil and debris. Patients with very oily skin may be treated twice with the pretreatment solution, which is prepackaged on treated pads with one popular peel formulation. The salicylic acid peel is applied with a sponge, commonly using 20% to 30% concentrations of salicylic acid. Stinging and burning may be felt during the first minute, during which the skin begins to appear white. Mild discomfort may peak 2 to 3 minutes following application of the peel. Whitening of the skin is complete 4 to 5 minutes after application, when discomfort should be virtually gone. At this point the peel is finished without the need for neutralization. The skin is often washed again following treatment, and a mild lotion is applied to soothe the skin.

TRICHLOROACETIC ACID CHEMICAL PEELS

Trichloroacetic acid (TCA) has been widely used as a peeling agent for a quarter century. It has been used in concentrations ranging from 10% to 70%, most frequently as a light peel in concentrations of 15%, 20%, 25%, and 35%. TCA peels may be readministered after a period of weeks to months to enhance improvement or improve skin that has been continuously exposed to ultraviolet radiation. TCA peels have been found to be effective at treating a number of hyperkeratotic lesions including actinic keratoses, solar lentigenes, and the signs of photoaging.[73,74] In addition to improvement in epidermal and dermal signs of photoaging, tightening of lax photodamaged skin, as is often seen following laser resurfacing,[75] also occurs following surface wounding with TCA.[76] As is the case following laser resurfacing, it is unclear if skin tightening results from normal skin contraction during wound healing or the action of TCA on the partially damaged dermal collagen fibers that are not removed during the peel procedure. Attempts have been made to standardize the procedure of administering TCA peels to produce consistent results between patients, as well as to minimize potential side effects. As with glycolic peels, skin preparation is used to remove surface oil from the skin to allow even penetration of a TCA peel.[77] Because TCA may penetrate quite deeply if used in higher concentrations, skin preparation may be even more important than when administering a glycolic acid peel.

A number of agents have been combined with TCA peels to enhance penetration, ensure a more even peel, or promote faster healing following treatment. The addition of retinoic acid pretreatment to a TCA peel regimen may result in more rapid healing following the peel.[78] Jessner's solution consisting of resorcinol, salicylic acid, and lactic acid in ethanol has been used in combination with TCA to enhance the effectiveness of the peel while preserving its safety.[74,79,80] Jessner's solution is commonly combined with 35% TCA. Signs of photoaging as well as actinic keratoses have been successfully treated with this combination.[81] TCA has been combined with glycolic acid and used as a peeling agent for nonfacial skin. One group utilized glycolic acid gel augmented with TCA and neutralized the peel with sodium bicarbonate solution. Care was taken to prevent excessive skin damage by using a neutralizing solution. The combination improved both epidermal and dermal signs of cutaneous photoaging, with minimal complications.[82]

Because results may depend upon skin preparation, the TCA itself, and other characteristics of the patient and procedure, attempts have been made to standardize TCA peeling by providing indicators of peel depth. One of the more popular systems used is the Obagi TCA peel.[83,84] TCA is mixed with a solution containing glycerin, saponins, and a nonionic blue color base. This mixture is thought to slow penetration of the acid, resulting in a peel that is more easily controlled due to the extra time allowed to reach the desired depth of damage in the skin. The blue color base enables visualization of areas that have been adequately covered with the TCA solution, as opposed to using a colorless TCA solution where missed areas may not be visible. Areas receiving more TCA than others will appear darker blue in color. These investigators standardize the procedure of administering TCA peels to yield more consistently reproducible results. A specific concentration of TCA is used, 15% and 20%, and a standardized volume is administered to the skin with multiple coatings. Clinical signs of frost quality, even blue coloration, a background pink color, and excessive skin wrinkling when the skin is pinched are used to estimate the depth of the peel. These signs have been shown to correlate with healing time, and thus are presumed to correlate with the depth of the peel. The peel may be repeated two or three times 6 to 8 weeks apart.[83] TCA peeling of nonfacial skin may also improve signs of photodamage, although greater care must be taken to avoid scarring.[82,85]

TCA peels were introduced as a more superficial peeling agent than the long-popular phenol peel discussed below. Although more superficial than phenol peels as they are both most commonly used, TCA peels still are capable of producing necrosis of the superficial dermis.[86] When peeled to this level, herpes simplex virus activation, bacterial infection, pigmentary abnormalities, and even scarring due to poor wound healing are all possible. Hyperpigmentation when treating dark-skinned or tan patients is a greater risk with TCA than with glycolic acid.

Trichloroacetic Acid Peels: Technique

The skin is first thoroughly degreased with either an acetone scrub or hexachlorophene with alcohol (Septisol). For medium-depth peeling, Jessner's solution (Table 18-2) is first applied with either cotton-tipped applicators or 4 × 4 inch gauze. One coat is usually sufficient to produce a light, even frost. Some practitioners choose to use additional coats of Jessner's solution to increase the depth of penetration. The Jessner's frost is less intense than that produced with TCA and does not cause discomfort for most patients.

Table 18-2 Jessner's Solution

Resorcinol	14 g
Salicylic acid	14 g
Lactic acid	14 g
Ethanol	95% to total volume 100 ml

TCA 35% is then applied with either cotton-tipped applicators or 4 × 4 inch gauze, depending on the surgeon's preference. Even-handed application of the TCA is essential to produce a uniform and consistent depth of peel. The color and quality of the frost is the surgeon's guide to peel depth and uniformity. If inconsistencies are noted in the quality of the frost, as can be seen with numerous actinic keratoses, additional TCA application can be carefully performed to produce the desired end point. Experience and skill ultimately determine the end point of the procedure. Subtle color differences in the quality of the frost can be important clues to the surgeon, and careful inspection, as well as a detailed preoperative plan for peel depth, are imperative.

Iced saline compresses are applied immediately after completion of the procedure to provide comfort to the patient. Although iced saline does not neutralize the TCA, it is an important part of the procedure to soothe the patient's skin. Since TCA is not neutralized by water or saline, meticulous application of TCA is essential to prevent overtreatment, which can result in excessive peel depth and significant complications. Application of too much TCA or Jessner's solution can be major causes of morbidity from medium-depth chemical peeling. An emollient such as Aquaphor (Biersdorf) can be applied prior to discharge of the patient.

Erythema and edema are prominent for the first 48 to 72 hours after the procedure, as is the potential for discomfort. Crusting of the skin begins as the edema resolves, and continuous application of emollients is encouraged. Crust and exudate begin to separate from the skin with gentle washing 4 to 7 days after the procedure, and skin renewal is usually complete by postoperative day 10 to 14.

PHENOL CHEMICAL PEELS

Phenol is one of the longest used agents for medium-to-deep peels. It has been in use for over a century, and in widespread use for approximately a quarter century. Both epidermal and dermal signs of cutaneous photoaging have been treated with great success. In addition, phenol peels have been used to treat facial scarring, most commonly scars resulting from acne. Phenol has been used alone as a peeling agent, or in combination with other agents. Phenol is commonly combined with croton seed oil for peeling. Phenol alone in concentrations of less than 50% fails to produce significant peeling in the absence of occlusion.[87] The addition of croton oil of up to a maximum of 1% appears to result in the optimal clinical response. Greater concentrations can result in pigmentary alterations and other unwanted side effects.[87] The most popular formula is the Baker-Gordon phenol peel, in which phenol is combined with croton oil.[87-92]

Histopathologic examination of skin excised from phenol peel patients during face lift surgery was performed 1.5 to 20 years following their phenol peels. Treated and untreated skin were compared in the same specimens of excised skin. Examination of these specimens revealed a new band of collagen 2 to 3 mm thick beneath the epidermis, but above the abnormal solar elastotic tissue that characterizes the dermis of photoaged skin.[53] This border or grenz zone of normal collagen is often present beneath the epidermis of sun-damaged skin. An expansion of this zone results from regeneration of normal-appearing dermis, in this case due to the administration of a phenol peel. The presence of normal elastic fibers, often absent in healed wounds, attests to the normal architecture of this regenerated dermal extracellular matrix.[53] Similar changes are often demonstrated following other destructive treatments such as carbon dioxide laser resurfacing.[93] Because of their abilities to superficially damage surface skin, deep chemical peels and laser resurfacing both improve epidermal and dermal signs of chronic sun exposure including skin laxity.

Since phenol peels are most commonly used as medium-to-deep peels, side effects are more common than with the previously mentioned more superficial peeling agents. Hyperpigmentation, or more frequently permanent hypopigmentation, are among the most commonly encountered complications associated with phenol peeling (Fig. 18-7).[94] Since phenol is most commonly used as a medium-to-deep peel, herpes simplex activation,[95] bacterial infection,[96] and scarring[96] are seen following peels. In addition, post-peel erythema can persist for many weeks[97,98]; this phenomenon is commonly seen following carbon dioxide laser resurfacing. Phenol is absorbed systemically and associated with a significant risk of cardiac toxicity. This risk can be reduced by peeling portions of the face at a time interval of 20 minutes, to reduce the total surface area exposed to phenol at any one time.[99,100]

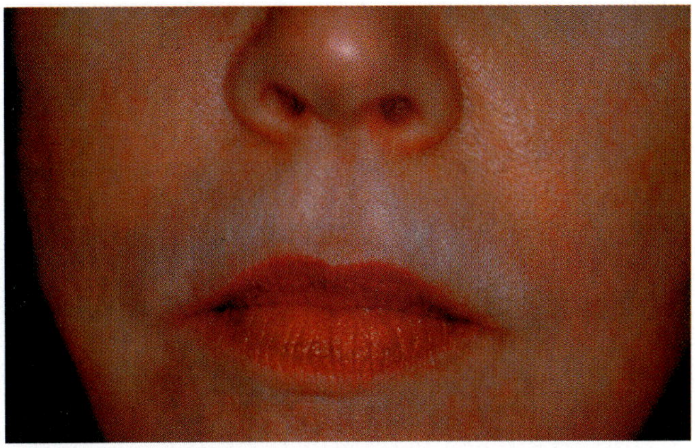

FIG. 18-7
This patient developed permanent hypopigmentation following a deep phenol peel. This may also occur following laser resurfacing and may be a late complication following laser treatment.

POSTOPERATIVE CONSIDERATIONS

Patients are instructed to maintain a moist environment on their skin to facilitate and enhance wound healing following chemical peels. The use of a bland petrolatum-based emollient is usually sufficient. Patients who have had superficial chemical peels may be able to use a medium to thick moisturizer in place of an emollient, but frequent application is essential to prevent drying of the skin. The duration of use for skin moisturizers depends on several factors, including the rate at which a given patient heals as well as the depth of the peel itself. In general, the deeper the peel, the longer the need for postoperative moisturizer use.

Crusting, if present, should be carefully removed by the patient or an assistant with gentle technique, including the use of cotton swabs soaked in warm water. Frequent application of moisturizers often helps to prevent crust formation. Once reepithelialization is complete, the use of a sunscreen is recommended as part of the moisturizing routine. Prior to complete reepithelialization, sun avoidance is essential. Although superficial peels can produce a small amount of crusting and epidermal loss, this is more an issue with medium and deep chemical peels.

Erythema can persist for days to weeks depending on the depth of the peel and the patient's skin type. Treatment of postoperative erythema is not necessary, but the physician should monitor carefully, as in some cases persistent erythema following deeper peels can be a sign of early hypertrophic scarring. If scarring is suspected, the physician should consider the use of a potent topical corticosteroid cream or ointment, as well as intralesional steroid injection if the scar begins to mature.

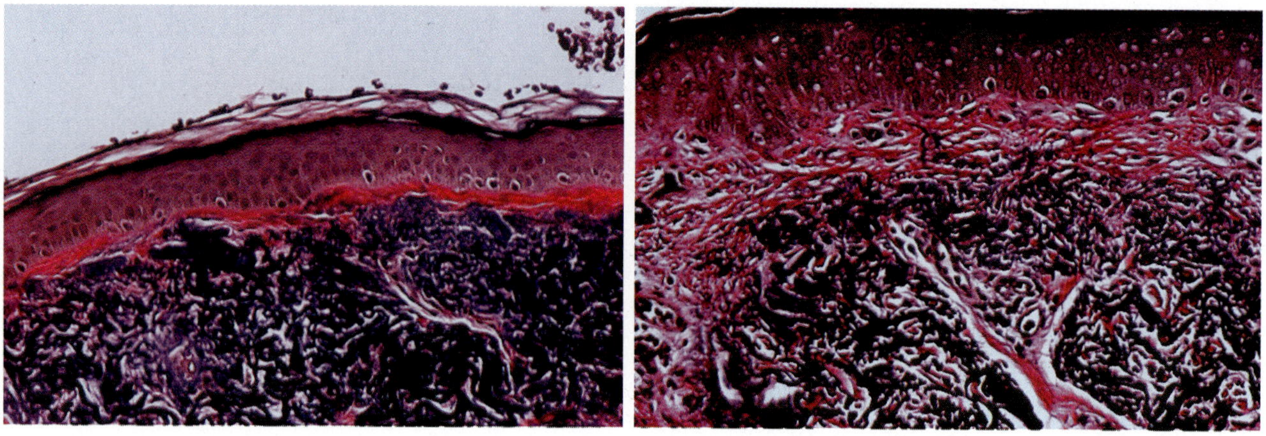

FIG. 18-8
A, Histopathologic examination of severely sun damaged skin demonstrates a thin band of collagen (pink) above massive clumps of abnormal solar elastotic material (black) that characterizes sun-damaged skin. **B,** Examination of a biopsy sample, taken from the same patient after carbon dioxide laser resurfacing, reveals an expanded zone of collagen beneath the epidermis (pink) due to laser treatment.

Postinflammatory hyperpigmentation is usually a transient element of healing following chemical peels but can be quite troubling to the patient. Early intervention with twice daily use of bleaching agents such as hydroquinone at a concentration of 3% to 4% is usually sufficient therapy. In some patients, the use of a product containing hydroquinone and glycolic acid may be of additional benefit. Topical agents such as tretinoin, sunscreens, and topical steroids can also be added to the regimen. However, the most important element of treating postinflammatory hyperpigmentation is avoiding it in the first place. Patients with Fitzpatrick skin types IV to VI are most at risk for developing pigment changes, and deeper peels are more likely to produce long-term pigment alteration. Carefully matching skin type with peel depth is an important determinant of posttreatment complications such as long-term hyperpigmentation.

FUTURE ADVANCES IN FACIAL RESURFACING AND REJUVENATION

The development of the short-pulsed and scanned carbon dioxide lasers and the pulsed erbium:YAG lasers has revolutionized facial resurfacing.[75,101-105] These lasers remove superficial layers of the epidermis or dermis while leaving behind very small amounts of residual thermal damage.[93,106,107] The treatment effect is quite reproducible from patient to patient, resulting in consistency and predictability of outcomes (Fig. 18-8). Peeling agents are often used in combination with laser resurfacing to diminish lines demarcating the site of laser treatment. Superficial peeling agents such as glycolic acid or topical tretinoin are often used prior to laser resurfacing in an attempt to reduce complications such as hyperpigmentation and possibly reduce healing time.

The recent popularity of nonablative resurfacing has added yet another modality of treatment for the signs of photoaging and superficial acne scarring.[108-111] This treatment exploits the ability of lasers or light sources commonly used to treat unwanted blood vessels to stimulate extracellular matrix deposition without ablation of the epidermis. These lasers are frequently combined with topical AHAs and glycolic acid peels or tretinoin. As our understanding of the effects of peeling agents increases, and the armamentarium of lasers for facial rejuvenation grows, the ability to combine these modalities should result in greater benefits for our patients.

REFERENCES

1. Uitto J. Collagen biosynthesis in human skin: a review with emphasis on scleroderma. Ann Clin Res 1971; 3:250-258.
2. Uitto J, Olsen DR, Fazio MJ. Extracellular matrix of the skin: 50 years of progress. J Invest Dermatol 1989; 92:61S-77S.
3. Uitto J. A method for studying collagen biosynthesis in human skin biopsies in vitro. Biochim Biophys Acta 1970; 201:438-445.
4. Booth BA, Uitto J. Collagen biosynthesis by human skin fibroblasts, III: the effects of ascorbic acid on procollagen production and prolyl hydroxylase activity. Biochim Biophys Acta 1981; 675:117-122.
5. Uitto J, Booth BA, Polak KL. Collagen biosynthesis by human skin fibroblasts, II: isolation and further characterization of type I and type III procollagens synthesized in culture. Biochim Biophys Acta 1980; 624:545-561.
6. Majamaa K, Sasaki T, Uitto J. Inhibition of prolyl hydroxylation during collagen biosynthesis in human skin fibroblast cultures by ethyl 3,4-dihydroxybenzoate. J Invest Dermatol 1987; 89:405-409.
7. Uitto J, Lichtenstein JR. Defects in the biochemistry of collagen in diseases of connective tissue. J Invest Dermatol 1976; 66:59-79.

8. Epstein EH Jr. (Alpha1(3))3 human skin collagen: release by pepsin digestion and preponderance in fetal life. J Biol Chem 1974; 249:3225-3231.
9. Uitto J, Fazio MJ, Olsen DR. Molecular mechanisms of cutaneous aging: age-associated connective tissue alterations in the dermis. J Am Acad Dermatol 1989; 21:614-622.
10. Clark RA. Biology of dermal wound repair. Dermatol Clin 1993; 11:647-666.
11. Timpl R. Structure and biological activity of basement membrane proteins. Eur J Biochem 1989; 180:487-502.
12. Ryynanen M, Knowlton RG, Parente MG, et al. Human type VII collagen: genetic linkage of the gene (COL7A1) on chromosome 3 to dominant dystrophic epidermolysis bullosa. Am J Hum Genet 1991; 49:797-803.
13. Ryynanen J, Sollberg S, Parente MG, et al. Type VII collagen gene expression by cultured human cells and in fetal skin: abundant mRNA and protein levels in epidermal keratinocytes. J Clin Invest 1992; 89:163-168.
14. Uitto J, Chung-Honet LC, Christiano AM. Molecular biology and pathology of type VII collagen. Exp Dermatol 1992; 1:2-11.
15. Castagnola P, Tavella S, Gerecke DR, et al. Tissue-specific expression of type XIV collagen—a member of the FACIT class of collagens. Eur J Cell Biol 1992; 59:340-347.
16. Yoshioka H, Zhang H, Ramirez F, et al. Synteny between the loci for a novel FACIT-like collagen locus (D6S228E) and alpha 1 (IX) collagen (COL9A1) on 6q12-q14 in humans. Genomics 1992; 13:884-886.
17. Shaw LM, Olsen BR. FACIT collagens: diverse molecular bridges in extracellular matrices. Trends Biochem Sci 1991; 16: 191-194.
18. Bianco P, Fisher LW, Young MF, et al. Expression and localization of the two small proteoglycans biglycan and decorin in developing human skeletal and non-skeletal tissues. J Histochem Cytochem 1990; 38:1549-1563.
19. Fleischmajer R, Fisher LW, MacDonald ED, et al. Decorin interacts with fibrillar collagen of embryonic and adult human skin. J Struct Biol 1991; 106:82-90.
20. Pasquali-Ronchetti I, Baccarani-Contri M. Elastic fiber during development and aging. Microsc Res Tech 1997; 38:428-435.
21. Frances C, Robert L. Elastin and elastic fibers in normal and pathologic skin. Int J Dermatol 1984; 23:166-179.
22. Dahlback K, Ljungquist A, Lofberg H, et al. Fibrillin immunoreactive fibers constitute a unique network in the human dermis: immunohistochemical comparison of the distributions of fibrillin, vitronectin, amyloid P component, and orcein stainable structures in normal skin and elastosis. J Invest Dermatol 1990; 94:284-291.
23. Tan EM, Hoffren J, Rouda S, et al. Decorin, versican, and biglycan gene expression by keloid and normal dermal fibroblasts: differential regulation by basic fibroblast growth factor. Exp Cell Res 1993; 209:200-207.
24. Zimmermann DR, Dours-Zimmermann MT, Schubert M, Bruckner-Tuderman L. Versican is expressed in the proliferating zone in the epidermis and in association with the elastic network of the dermis. J Cell Biol 1994; 124:817-825.
25. Bernstein EF, Fisher LW, Li K, et al. Differential expression of the versican and decorin genes in photoaged and sun-protected skin: comparison by immunohistochemical and northern analyses. Lab Invest 1995; 72:662-669.
26. Burd DA, Greco RM, Regauer S, et al. Hyaluronan and wound healing: a new perspective. Br J Plast Surg 1991; 44:579-584.
27. Carrino DA, Sorrell JM, Caplan AI. Age-related changes in the proteoglycans of human skin. Arch Biochem Biophys 2000; 373: 91-101.
28. Scott PG, Dodd CM, Tredget EE, et al. Immunohistochemical localization of the proteoglycans decorin, biglycan and versican and transforming growth factor-beta in human post-burn hypertrophic and mature scars. Histopathology 1995; 26:423-431.
29. Clark RA. Fibronectin in the skin. J Invest Dermatol 1983;81:475-479.
30. Clark RA. Cutaneous tissue repair: basic biologic considerations: I. J Am Acad Dermatol 1985; 13:701-725.
31. Kubo M, Kan M, Isemura M, et al. Effects of extracellular matrices on human keratinocyte adhesion and growth and on its secretion and deposition of fibronectin in culture. J Invest Dermatol 1987; 88:594-601.
32. Sueki H, Whitaker D, Buchsbaum M, Murphy GF. Novel interactions between dermal dendrocytes and mast cells in human skin: implications for hemostasis and matrix repair [see comments]. Lab Invest 1993; 69:160-172.
33. Trabucchi E, Radaelli E, Marazzi M, et al. The role of mast cells in wound healing. Int J Tissue React 1988; 10:367-372.
34. Schultz G, Rotatori DS, Clark W. EGF and TGF-alpha in wound healing and repair. J Cell Biochem 1991; 45:346-352.
35. Daly CH, Odland GF. Age-related changes in the mechanical properties of human skin. J Invest Dermatol 1979; 73:84-87.
36. Lavker RM, Kwong F, Kligman AM. Changes in skin surface patterns with age. J Gerontol 1980; 35:348-354.
37. Lavker RM, Zheng PS, Dong G. Aged skin: a study by light, transmission electron, and scanning electron microscopy. J Invest Dermatol 1987; 88:44s-51s.
38. Escoffier C, de Rigal J, Rochefort A, et al. Age-related mechanical properties of human skin: an in vivo study. J Invest Dermatol 1989; 93:353-357.
39. Lavker RM, Zheng PS, Dong G. Morphology of aged skin. Clin Geriatr Med 1989; 5:53-67.
40. Kligman AM, Zheng P, Lavker RM. The anatomy and pathogenesis of wrinkles. Br J Dermatol 1985; 113:37-42.
41. Oikarinen A, Karvonen J, Uitto J, Hannuksela M. Connective tissue alterations in skin exposed to natural and therapeutic UV-radiation. Photodermatol 1985; 2:15-26.
42. Bernstein EF, Uitto J. The effect of photodamage on dermal extracellular matrix. Clin Dermatol 1996; 14:143-151.
43. Bernstein EF, Underhill CB, Hahn PJ, et al. Chronic sun exposure alters both the content and distribution of dermal glycosaminoglycans. Br J Dermatol 1996; 135:255-262.
44. Bernstein EF, Chen YQ, Kopp JB, et al. Long-term sun exposure alters the collagen of the papillary dermis: comparison of sun-protected and photoaged skin by northern analysis, immunohistochemical staining, and confocal laser scanning microscopy. J Am Acad Dermatol 1996; 34:209-218.
45. Repesh LA, Fitzgerald TJ, Furcht LT. Fibronectin involvement in granulation tissue and wound healing in rabbits. J Histochem Cytochem 1982; 30:351-358.
46. Woodley DT, O'Keefe EJ, Prunieras M. Cutaneous wound healing: a model for cell-matrix interactions. J Am Acad Dermatol 1985; 12:420-433.
47. Van Scott EJ, Yu RJ. Control of keratinization with alpha-hydroxy acids and related compounds, I: topical treatment of ichthyotic disorders. Arch Dermatol 1974; 110:586-590.
48. Lavker RM, Kaidbey K, Leyden JJ. Effects of topical ammonium lactate on cutaneous atrophy from a potent topical corticosteroid. J Am Acad Dermatol 1992; 26:535-544.
49. Bernstein EF, Underhill CB, Lakkakorpi J, et al. Citric acid increases viable epidermal thickness and glycosaminoglycan content of sun-damaged skin. Dermatol Surg 1997; 23:689-694.
50. Ditre CM, Griffin TD, Murphy GF, et al. Effects of alpha-hydroxy acids on photoaged skin: a pilot clinical, histologic, and ultrastructural study [see comments]. J Am Acad Dermatol 1996; 34:187-195.
51. Bernstein EF, Lee J, Brown D, et al. Glycolic acid treatment increases type I collagen mRNA and hyaluronic acid content of human skin. Dermatol Surg 2001; 27:429-433.

52. Kim SJ, Won YH. The effect of glycolic acid on cultured human skin fibroblasts: cell proliferative effect and increased collagen synthesis. J Dermatol 1998; 25:85-89.
53. Kligman AM, Baker TJ, Gordon HL. Long-term histologic follow-up of phenol face peels. Plast Reconstr Surg 1985; 75:652-659.
54. Rubach BW, Schoenrock LD. Histological and clinical evaluation of facial resurfacing using a carbon dioxide laser with the computer pattern generator. Arch Otolaryngol Head Neck Surg 1997; 123:929-934.
55. Lundin A, Berne B, Michaelsson G. Topical retinoic acid treatment of photoaged skin: its effects on hyaluronan distribution in epidermis and on hyaluronan and retinoic acid in suction blister fluid. Acta Derm Venereol 1992; 72:423-427.
56. Kligman AM, Dogadkina D, Lavker RM. Effects of topical tretinoin on non-sun-exposed protected skin of the elderly. J Am Acad Dermatol 1993; 29:25-33.
57. Griffiths CE, Russman AN, Majmudar G, et al. Restoration of collagen formation in photodamaged human skin by tretinoin (retinoic acid) [see comments]. N Engl J Med 1993; 329:530-535.
58. Stiller MJ, Bartolone J, Stern R, et al. Topical 8% glycolic acid and 8% L-lactic acid creams for the treatment of photodamaged skin: a double-blind vehicle-controlled clinical trial. Arch Dermatol 1996; 132:631-636.
59. Van Scott EJ, Ditre CM, Yu RJ. Alpha-hydroxyacids in the treatment of signs of photoaging. Clin Dermatol 1996; 14:217-226.
60. Bergfeld W, Tung R, Vidimos A, et al. Improving the cosmetic appearance of photoaged skin with glycolic acid. J Am Acad Dermatol 1997; 36:1011-1013.
61. Newman N, Newman A, Moy LS, et al. Clinical improvement of photoaged skin with 50% glycolic acid: a double-blind vehicle-controlled study. Dermatol Surg 1996; 22:455-460.
62. Marrero GM, Katz BE. The new fluor-hydroxy pulse peel: a combination of 5-fluorouracil and glycolic acid. Dermatol Surg 1998; 24:973-978.
63. Effendy I, Kwangsukstith C, Lee JY, Maibach HI. Functional changes in human stratum corneum induced by topical glycolic acid: comparison with all-trans retinoic acid. Acta Derm Venereol 1995; 75:455-458.
64. Burns RL, Prevost-Blank PL, Lawry MA, et al. Glycolic acid peels for postinflammatory hyperpigmentation in black patients: a comparative study. Dermatol Surg 1997; 23:171-174; discussion 175.
65. Lim JT, Tham SN. Glycolic acid peels in the treatment of melasma among Asian women. Dermatol Surg 1997; 23:177-179.
66. Tsai TF, Paul BH, Jee SH, Maibach HI. Effects of glycolic acid on light-induced skin pigmentation in Asian and caucasian subjects. J Am Acad Dermatol 2000; 43:238-243.
67. Garcia A, Fulton JE Jr. The combination of glycolic acid and hydroquinone or kojic acid for the treatment of melasma and related conditions. Dermatol Surg 1996; 22:443-447.
68. Kim SW, Moon SE, Kim JA, Eun HC. Glycolic acid versus Jessner's solution: which is better for facial acne patients? A randomized prospective clinical trial of split-face model therapy. Dermatol Surg 1999; 25:270-273.
69. Atzori L, Brundu MA, Orru A, Biggio P. Glycolic acid peeling in the treatment of acne. J Eur Acad Dermatol Venereol 1999; 12: 119-122.
70. Perricone NV. Treatment of pseudofolliculitis barbae with topical glycolic acid: a report of two studies. Cutis 1993; 52:232-235.
71. Becker FF, Langford FP, Rubin MG, Speelman P. A histological comparison of 50% and 70% glycolic acid peels using solutions with various pHs. Dermatol Surg 1996; 22:463-465.
72. Grimes PE. The safety and efficacy of salicylic acid chemical peels in darker racial-ethnic groups. Dermatol Surg 1999; 25:18-22.
73. Brodland DG, Roenigk RK. Trichloroacetic acid chemexfoliation (chemical peel) for extensive premalignant actinic damage of the face and scalp [published erratum appears in Mayo Clin Proc 1988; 63:1122]. Mayo Clin Proc 1988; 63:887-896.
74. Lawrence N, Cox SE, Cockerell CJ, et al. A comparison of the efficacy and safety of Jessner's solution and 35% trichloroacetic acid vs 5% fluorouracil in the treatment of widespread facial actinic keratoses. Arch Dermatol 1995; 131:176-181.
75. Alster TS, Kauvar AN, Geronemus RG. Histology of high-energy pulsed CO_2 laser resurfacing. Semin Cutan Med Surg 1996; 15:189-193.
76. Morrow DM. Chemical peeling of eyelids and periorbital area. J Dermatol Surg Oncol 1992; 18:102-110.
77. Peikert JM, Krywonis NA, Rest EB, Zachary CB. The efficacy of various degreasing agents used in trichloroacetic acid peels. J Dermatol Surg Oncol 1994; 20:724-728.
78. Hevia O, Nemeth AJ, Taylor JR. Tretinoin accelerates healing after trichloroacetic acid chemical peel. Arch Dermatol 1991; 127: 678-682.
79. Monheit GD. The Jessner's-trichloroacetic acid peel: an enhanced medium-depth chemical peel. Dermatol Clin 1995; 13: 277-283.
80. Monheit GD. The Jessner's + TCA peel: a medium-depth chemical peel. J Dermatol Surg Oncol 1989; 15:945-950.
81. Witheiler DD, Lawrence N, Cox SE, et al. Long-term efficacy and safety of Jessner's solution and 35% trichloroacetic acid vs 5% fluorouracil in the treatment of widespread facial actinic keratoses. Dermatol Surg 1997; 23:191-196.
82. Cook KK, Cook WR. Chemical peel of nonfacial skin using glycolic acid gel augmented with TCA and neutralized based on visual staging. Dermatol Surg 2000; 26:994-999.
83. Obagi ZE, Obagi S, Alaiti S, Stevens MB. TCA-based blue peel: a standardized procedure with depth control. Dermatol Surg 1999; 25:773-780.
84. Johnson JB, Ichinose H, Obagi ZE, Laub DR. Obagi's modified trichloroacetic acid (TCA)-controlled variable-depth peel: a study of clinical signs correlating with histological findings [see comments]. Ann Plast Surg 1996; 36:225-237.
85. Fulton JE, Rahimi AD, Helton P, Dahlberg K. Neck rejuvenation by combining Jessner/TCA peel, dermasanding, and CO_2 laser resurfacing [see comments]. Dermatol Surg 1999; 25:745-750.
86. Dailey RA, Gray JF, Rubin MG, et al. Histopathologic changes of the eyelid skin following trichloroacetic acid chemical peel. Ophthal Plast Reconstr Surg 1998; 14:9-12.
87. Hetter GP. An examination of the phenol-croton oil peel, part IV: face peel results with different concentrations of phenol and croton oil. Plast Reconstr Surg 2000; 105:1061-1083; discussion 1084-1087.
88. Alt TH. Occluded Baker-Gordon chemical peel: review and update [see comments]. J Dermatol Surg Oncol 1989; 15:980-993.
89. Asken S. Unoccluded Baker-Gordon phenol peels—review and update. J Dermatol Surg Oncol 1989; 15:998-1008.
90. Hetter GP. An examination of the phenol-croton oil peel, part I: dissecting the formula. Plast Reconstr Surg 2000; 105:227-239; discussion 249-251.
91. Hetter GP. An examination of the phenol-croton oil peel, part II: the lay peelers and their croton oil formulas [published erratum appears in Plast Reconstr Surg 2000; 105:1083]. Plast Reconstr Surg 2000; 105:240-248; discussion 249-251.
92. Hetter GP. An examination of the phenol-croton oil peel, part III: the plastic surgeons' role. Plast Reconstr Surg 2000; 105:752-763.
93. Ross EV, Grossman MC, Duke D, Grevelink JM. Long-term results after CO_2 laser skin resurfacing: a comparison of scanned and pulsed systems. J Am Acad Dermatol 1997; 37:709-718.
94. Litton C, Trinidad G. Complications of chemical face peeling as evaluated by a questionnaire. Plast Reconstr Surg 1981; 67:738-744.
95. Perkins SW, Sklarew EC. Prevention of facial herpetic infections after chemical peel and dermabrasion: new treatment strategies

in the prophylaxis of patients undergoing procedures of the perioral area. Plast Reconstr Surg 1996; 98:427-433; discussion 434-435.
96. Korcok M. Untoward effect of a face peel: toxic shock syndrome [news]. JAMA 1982; 248:23.
97. Maloney BP, Millman B, Monheit G, McCollough EG. The etiology of prolonged erythema after chemical peel [see comments]. Dermatol Surg 1998; 24:337-341.
98. Rapaport MJ, Rapaport V. Prolonged erythema after facial laser resurfacing or phenol peel secondary to corticosteroid addiction. Dermatol Surg 1999; 25:781-784; discussion 785.
99. Gross BG. Cardiac arrhythmias during phenol face peeling. Plast Reconstr Surg 1984; 73:590-594.
100. Sorkin MJ. Cardiac arrhythmias during phenol face peel [letter]. J Dermatol Surg Oncol 1988; 14:477.
101. Fitzpatrick RE, Goldman MP, Satur NM, Tope WD. Pulsed carbon dioxide laser resurfacing of photo-aged facial skin [see comments]. Arch Dermatol 1996; 132:395-402.
102. Fitzpatrick RE, Rostan EF, Marchell N. Collagen tightening induced by carbon dioxide laser versus erbium:YAG laser. Lasers Surg Med 2000; 27:395-403.
103. Fitzpatrick RE, Smith SR, Sriprachya-Anunt S. Depth of vaporization and the effect of pulse stacking with a high-energy, pulsed carbon dioxide laser. J Am Acad Dermatol 1999; 40:615-622.
104. Alster TS. Cutaneous resurfacing with CO_2 and erbium:YAG lasers: preoperative, intraoperative, and postoperative considerations. Plast Reconstr Surg 1999; 103:619-632; discussion 633-634.
105. Alster TS, Garg S. Treatment of facial rhytides with a high-energy pulsed carbon dioxide laser. Plast Reconstr Surg 1996; 98: 791-794.
106. Bernstein EF, Brown DB, Kenkel J, Burns AJ. Residual thermal damage resulting from pulsed and scanned resurfacing lasers. Dermatol Surg 1999; 25:739-744.
107. Ross EV, Domankevitz Y, Skrobal M, Anderson RR. Effects of CO_2 laser pulse duration in ablation and residual thermal damage: implications for skin resurfacing. Lasers Surg Med 1996; 19: 123-129.
108. Goldberg DJ. Nonablative resurfacing. Clin Plast Surg 2000; 27: 287-292, xi.
109. Kelly KM, Nelson JS, Lask GP, et al. Cryogen spray cooling in combination with nonablative laser treatment of facial rhytides. Arch Dermatol 1999; 135:691-694.
110. Menaker GM, Wrone DA, Williams RM, Moy RL. Treatment of facial rhytids with a nonablative laser: a clinical and histologic study. Dermatol Surg 1999; 25:440-444.
111. Zelickson BD, Kilmer SL, Bernstein E, et al. Pulsed dye laser therapy for sun damaged skin. Lasers Surg Med 1999; 25:229-236.

CHAPTER 19

Lasers in Skin Resurfacing

GEORGE J. HRUZA
RICHARD E. FITZPATRICK
KENNETH A. ARNDT
JEFFREY S. DOVER

SECTION ONE

History and Scientific Review

BACKGROUND AND HISTORY

Laser skin resurfacing has revolutionized the approach to facial skin rejuvenation over the last decade. It has also added an approach to managing both atrophic and hypertrophic scars. There has always been a great interest in facial rejuvenation. For thousands of years, topical agents such as soured milk, vegetable extracts, and mudpacks have been used with limited success. More recently, prepared concentrations of topical agents have been used, including vitamin A derivatives (retinoic acid and retinol), antioxidants (vitamins C and E), and α-hydroxy and β-hydroxy acids. Public interest has been great, but the clinical effects only minimal.

In an effort to more effectively rejuvenate significantly photodamaged skin, a variety of chemical agents have been used to strip off a variable thickness of skin, expecting that reepithelialization will result in a more youthful skin appearance. Mechanically removing varying layers of dermis with dermabrasion can also improve wrinkles.

In the 1980s and early 1990s continuous wave carbon dioxide lasers were used in an effort to resurface photoaged skin.[1] Although the results of this procedure performed by a few were quite impressive, the risk/benefit ratio of the procedure was very high. Dwelling too long on a specific area led to excessive thermal diffusion and thermal damage resulting in scarring. The technique was never widely used for this specific reason. However, with the development of short-pulse high peak power and rapidly scanned focused beam carbon dioxide lasers and normal mode erbium:yttrium aluminum garnet (Er:YAG) lasers, the ability to remove photodamaged skin layer by layer in a precisely controlled manner while leaving behind a very narrow zone of thermal damage became possible.[2-9] There has been an explosion of interest in the use of this new technology to resurface photoaged skin, as well as for the treatment of scars.

BASIC SCIENCE

The use of lasers in dermatology is in general related to laser-induced heating. When this is accomplished with attention to the principles of selective photothermolysis, then very precise tissue effects can be achieved. The basic principles of this theory are that selective heating is achieved by preferential laser light absorption and heat production in the target chromophore, with heat being localized to the target by a pulse duration shorter than the target thermal relaxation time (or cooling time).[10]

The tissue chromophore that absorbs the 10,600 nm wavelength of the carbon dioxide laser is water. The depth of penetration of this wavelength into tissue depends only on water content; pigmentation and vascularity are irrelevant. The extinction length, or thickness of water that absorbs 90% of the radiant energy of the incident beam for the carbon dioxide laser, is approximately 30 μm.[11-13]

The vaporization or boiling temperature of water at 1 atmosphere pressure is 100°C. When the carbon dioxide laser is used in the continuous mode at modest powers for vaporization, the skin surface temperature fluctuates in cycles between about 120° and 200°C during ablation. Charring occurs because of extreme heating of desiccated tissue, which carbonizes. The immediate tissue effects are dependent on spot size and power as well as the speed with which the laser beam is moved across the tissue surface. When a very small beam diameter of 100 to 300 μm is used, very high irradiances may be achieved, resulting in rapid tissue vaporization. However, unless the beam is moved rapidly across the tissue surface, desiccation, charring and

Though other wrinkling and photodamage assessment scales exist, the need for a system related purely to visible wrinkling and visible textural changes secondary to solar elastosis was thought to be more relevant to the topic of wrinkle eradication.

Use of this scoring system allows broad classification into mild, moderate, and severe categories as well as a more objective numerical severity score. Assessing patients both before and after treatment in studies with an average follow-up of about 90 days revealed that the average patient's preoperative score decreased approximately 50% as a consequence of resurfacing.[3,8,37,38] This means that mild wrinkles generally resolve completely and moderate and severe wrinkles improve by one class. These are realistic expectations for the patient, though occasionally even severe wrinkles may completely resolve. The treated area continues to improve up to 18 months after laser resurfacing as collagen remodeling takes place.

In comparison to chemical peels, laser resurfacing is more effective in eradication of wrinkles while preserving normal skin texture and pigment (Figs. 19-1 to 19-3). Superficial chemical peels such as Jessner's solution and α-hydroxy acids remove only a partial thickness of the epidermis and have no appreciable effect on wrinkling.[39] Laser resurfacing is generally not done on such a superficial level. Medium-depth chemical peels done with solid carbon dioxide or Jessner's solution plus 35% trichloroacetic acid will improve textural irregularities and very superficial wrinkling, but rarely have a significant impact on clinically visible wrinkling.[40-42] This same level of resurfacing can be achieved with a single UltraPulse laser pass using a 250 to 350 mJ pulse and 3 mm spot size, one pass with the SilkTouch laser with a 200 mm handpiece at 15 to 18 watts, one pass with the FeatherTouch laser with a 200 mm handpiece at 34 watts, or two to three passes with an Er:YAG laser at 10 J/cm^2. Though this level of chem-

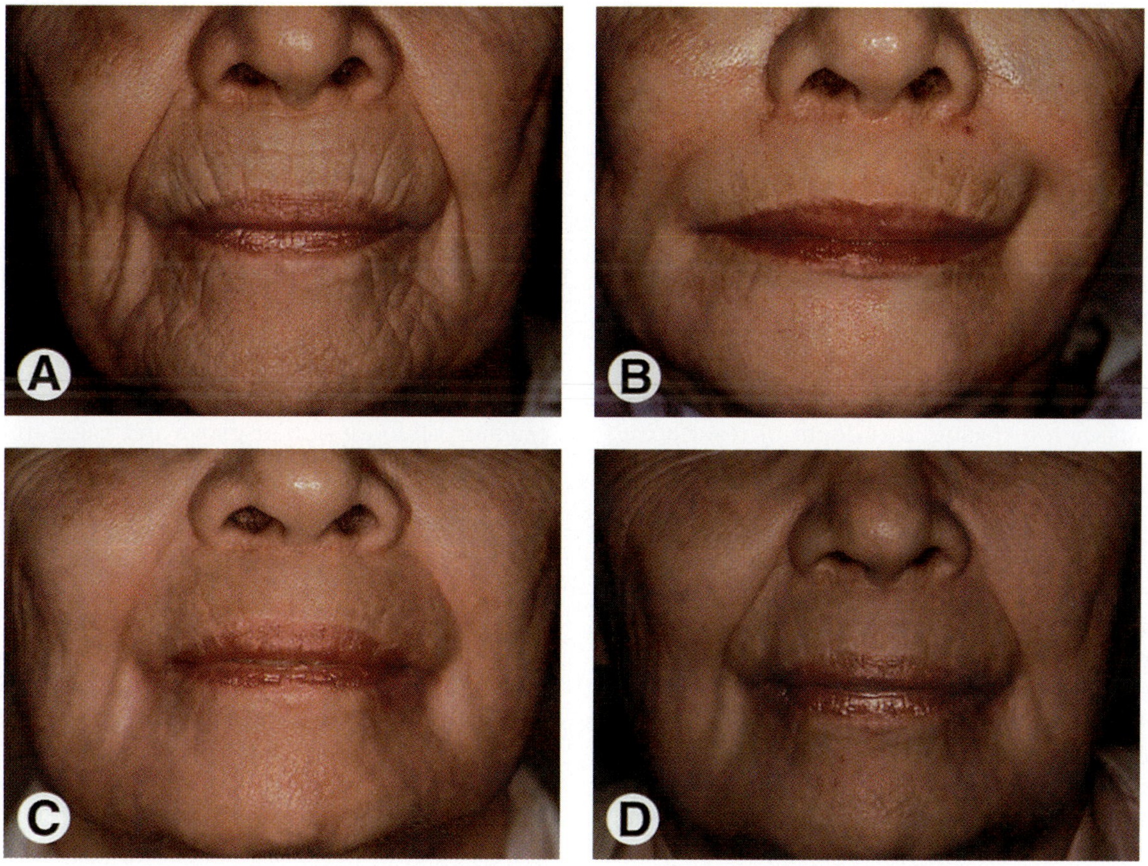

FIG. 19-2
A, A 72-year-old woman before perioral CO_2 laser skin resurfacing. **B,** Immediately after CO_2 laser skin resurfacing. **C,** Residual pink discoloration of the treated skin 6 weeks after CO_2 laser skin resurfacing. **D,** One year after perioral CO_2 laser skin resurfacing. (From Hruza GJ, Fitzpatrick RE, Dover JS. Laser skin resurfacing. In: Arndt KA, Dover JS, Olbricht SM, eds. Lasers in Cutaneous and Aesthetic Surgery. Philadelphia: Lippincott-Raven, 1997: 262-290.)

A

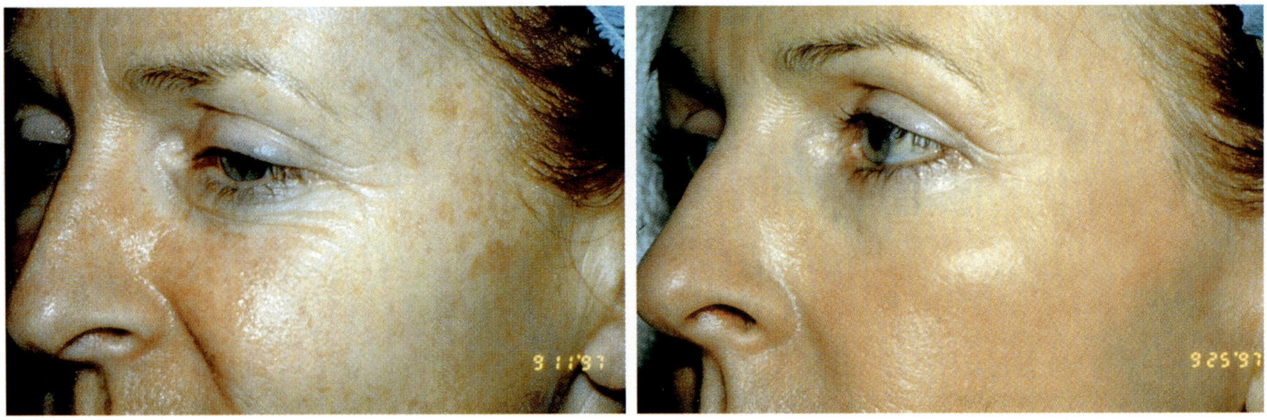

B

FIG. 19-3
A, Woman in her late thirties prior to Er:YAG laser skin resurfacing. (Courtesy Khalil Khatri, MD.) **B,** Six months after full face short-pulsed Er:YAG laser skin resurfacing for superficial early photoaging. (Courtesy Khalil Khatri, MD.) (From Dover JS, Arndt K, Geronemus R, Alora MB. Illustrated Cutaneous and Aesthetic Laser Surgery, 2nd ed. New York: McGraw-Hill, 2000.)

ical peeling is generally predictable and safe, there may be variable depth of penetration of acids, varying from patient to patient but also varying from one area to another within the same patient. This variation in depth of penetration may be related to the quantity of acid applied, the pressure exerted with rubbing the acid into the skin, the degree of cleansing and defatting of the skin surface, the degree of photodamage present, the number and density of adnexal structures, and other unidentifiable factors. Deeper than wanted penetration of the acid may cause scarring, hypopigmentation, and textural changes. When proper technique is used with laser resurfacing, this depth of resurfacing can be achieved with much greater predictability of depth and little risk of inadvertent deeper penetration with its associated risk.

Deep chemical peels with Baker's phenol solution will remove even deep lines and may result in dramatic clinical improvement, but virtually always results in hypopigmentation and an atrophically smooth, altered surface texture. It is difficult to obtain an even result on the upper lip. Lines present at the vermilion border often persist while the central area of the lip clears completely. In addition, because of the extreme depth of resurfacing, there is an extended period of erythema, often for 6 months or longer, and a significant risk of scarring. The postoperative course for phenol peeling is painful and requires at least 2 weeks for the skin surface to reconstitute itself.[43-46]

This depth of Baker's phenol chemical peel injury has not been reported with laser resurfacing, nor is it desired. Because of the combined effects of tissue removed, collagen contraction/skin tightening, and new collagen formation/remodeling, comparable degrees of improvement are often achieved with laser resurfacing without the unwanted side effects of hypopigmentation and altered surface texture that are seen with phenol. Virtually complete pigment loss (depigmentation), as occurs at times with phenol, is rarely seen with laser resurfacing.

Dermabrasion is significantly more difficult to perform from a technical viewpoint than laser resurfacing and carries with it additional risks of physician and assistant exposure to blood-borne infectious agents[47] and risks of trauma to the patient from accidental contact with a rapidly rotating wire brush or diamond fraise catching on loose skin or gauze and being thrown into an eyelid, lip, tooth, or other area.[48] To obliterate wrinkle lines with dermabrasion requires a degree of expertise not easily achieved and is always a challenge on the upper lip and the eyelids. Uneven results and hypopigmentation are common in the perioral area.[49] Often wrinkling is reduced centrally across the upper lip but persists at the vermilion border. The depth achieved in resurfacing with dermabrasion is usually comparable to that achieved with approximately two to four passes of the UltraPulse laser using 350 to 500 mJ per pulse, with two to three passes of the SilkTouch laser using a 200 mm handpiece at 15 to 18 watts, three to five passes with the FeatherTouch laser using a 200 mm handpiece at 34 to 36 watts, or six to eight passes with an Er:YAG laser at 10 J/cm^2.

In general, both wrinkling and photodamage of the epidermis and dermis are responsive to treatment. As far as epidermal pathology associated with aging is concerned, actinic keratoses, squamous cell carcinoma in situ, lentigenes, and seborrheic keratoses are all removed with stripping of the epidermal layer. Photodamage of the dermis results in fragmentation of elastin and collagen fibers, most profoundly in the papillary dermis. This is seen clinically as altered surface texture and pallor with crepelike changes progressing to those of severe photoaging with cream yellow discoloration and deep creases. These layers of altered dermal tissue may be removed by vaporization and thermal necrosis and replaced with new healthy collagen developed over a tightened matrix of shrunken collagen. The ability to change these tissues dramatically relates to the depth of damage, with the more superficial damage being more responsive. These dermal changes result in loose, sagging, or folded skin. These folds may be particularly visible under the eyes, on the medial lower cheeks, on the lateral cheeks anterior to the ears, and to a certain extent at the nasolabial folds. These areas tend to be very responsive to the tightening effects achieved with laser resurfacing (see Fig. 19-1).[3,6,8,50,51]

Other Indications

Laser skin resurfacing is used for a variety of other conditions apart from treating photoaged skin (Box 19-1). Acne scars traditionally have been treated with dermabrasion.[48,52] Moderate improvement can be achieved, but the procedure is quite bloody and the blood microdroplets can hang suspended in the air for several hours, posing a threat to the physician, staff, and other patients.[47] Laser resurfacing can achieve improvement in acne scars with much less risk to the surgical team (Fig. 19-4). In addition, the procedure is very precise. The edges of the scars can be sculpted. More tissue is vaporized in the areas of scar tissue while doing only superficial resurfacing in the rest of the cosmetic unit being treated. The procedure is most suited for distensible depressed or elevated acne scars.[53,54] Ice-pick and bound down scars should first be removed with subcision, punch excision, linear excision, punch elevation, or punch grafting before performing laser resurfacing 6 to 8 weeks later.[55] Alternatively, they may be performed at the time of the laser resurfacing either immediately before or after resurfacing. Any suturing is done immediately after resurfacing.[56] Crateriform varicella scars can be improved with spot laser resurfacing. The area around and over the scar is vaporized with one pass of the laser. Additional passes are concentrated along the edge of the scar crater until it has been completely effaced. When done 6 to 10 weeks after varicella, the scar can be almost totally effaced. Older scars respond, but less completely.[57] Postsurgical and traumatic scars can be dramatically improved, especially if resurfaced 6 to 10 weeks after the surgery or injury.[50,58] Immediate resurfacing after surgery of well-vascularized wound edges just prior to skin suture placement can be useful as well.[59]

Actinic cheilitis can be successfully treated by performing a laser vermilionectomy using one of the resurfacing lasers (Fig. 19-5).[50] Depending on its thickness, this usually requires one to several passes with the laser over the vermilion region. This has significantly reduced postlaser healing to approximately 10 days in contrast to the 4 weeks it took when the conventional carbon dioxide laser was used.[60-70] The risk of scarring seems to be greatly reduced, as the extent of thermal damage is much less. The end point of treatment is complete epidermal ablation with superficial submucosal coagulation. Ablating only the epidermis has resulted in frequent recurrence of actinic cheilitis. Actinic keratoses unresponsive to conventional treatment with liquid nitrogen and topical 5-fluorouracil can be removed by ablating the epidermis and superficially ablating the upper papillary dermis to remove follicular involvement using one of the resurfacing lasers. This is especially useful on the dorsal hands and scalp.

Pigmentation irregularities such as postinflammatory hyperpigmentation and dark circles under the eyes can sometimes be improved with laser resurfacing. It is important to use Retin-A and hydroquinones for an extended period of time before and after the procedure. Other lasers more specific for melanin or medium-depth chemical peels are often preferable, as they do not

BOX 19-1 Indications for Resurfacing CO_2 and Er:YAG Lasers

Benign Skin Lesions
- Dermatosis papulosa nigra
- Epidermal nevi
- Rhinophyma
- Rhytides, facial
- Rhytides, nonfacial (Er:YAG only)
- Atrophic acne scars
- Hypertrophic scars, facial
  - Acne
  - Surgical
  - Traumatic
  - Varicella
- Adenoma sebaceum
- Sebaceous hyperplasia
- Seborrheic keratoses
- Solar lentigenes, facial
- Syringoma
- Trichoepithelioma
- Xanthelasma

Premalignant and Malignant Skin Lesions
- Actinic cheilitis
- Actinic keratoses
- Bowen's disease (in-situ squamous cell carcinoma)
- Erythroplasia of Queyrat
- Superficial basal cell carcinoma

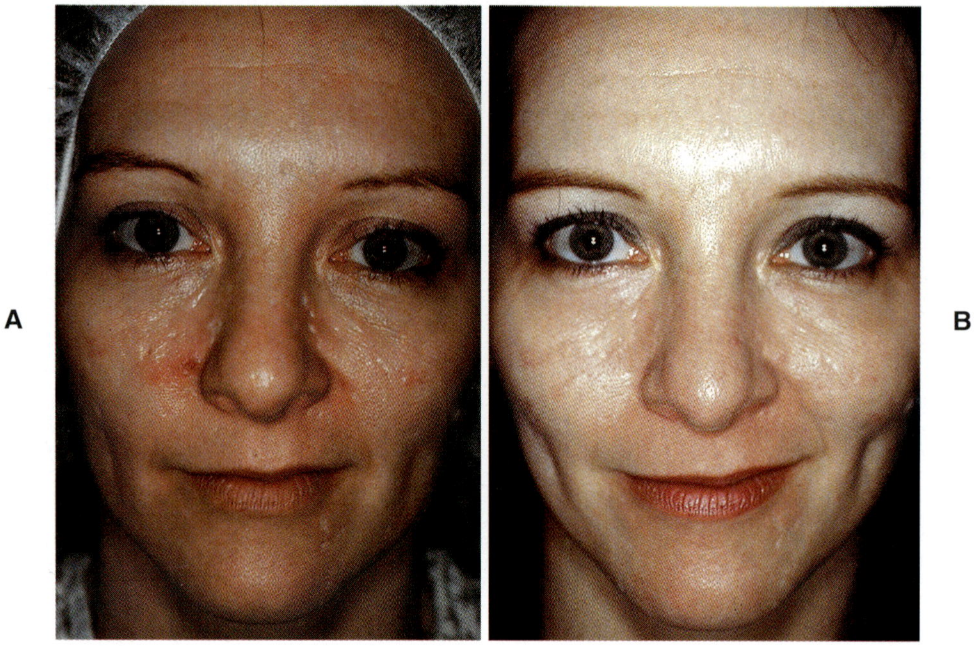

FIG. 19-4
A, A 42-year-old woman with acne scarring compounded by further scarring from years of excoriating and picking at the skin. **B,** One year after a series of punch excisions and linear scar excisions followed 3 months later by full face CO_2 and Er:YAG laser skin resurfacing.

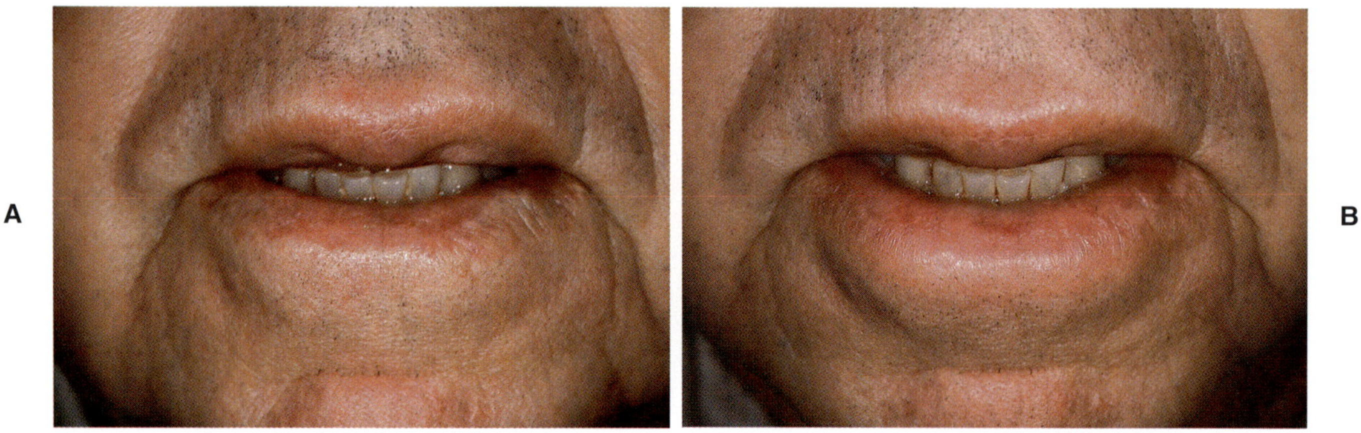

FIG. 19-5
A, Actinic cheilitis before treatment. **B,** Six weeks after SilkTouch laser treatment of the lower lip.

require anesthesia and the recovery time is much shorter.[41,42,71,72] Melasma responds variably, similar to its response to other modalities used for its treatment.[73]

Rhinophyma,[74,75] epidermal nevi,[76,77] and various small benign growths such as syringoma,[78] trichoepithelioma,[79] dermatosis papulosa nigra, xanthelasma,[80] adenoma sebaceum,[81] and sebaceous hyperplasia have traditionally been treated with the conventional carbon dioxide laser.[82] Using a resurfacing laser may reduce the healing time and risk of scarring by reducing the extent of unwanted thermal damage. Sometimes a combination approach can be employed. For example, a rhinophyma can be debulked using the carbon dioxide laser in the superpulse mode, and then removing the remaining rhinophyma with the resurfacing mode of the laser finishes the procedure. When treating epidermal nevi, it is important to cause damage into the papillary dermis with residual hypopigmentation expected. Failure to cause some degree of dermal fibrosis often results in nevus recurrence.[76,77]

Carbon dioxide resurfacing lasers should be used with great caution for rhytides off the face due to the very high risk of depigmentation and scarring.[83] Aggressive hydration of the skin with EMLA under occlusion seems to reduce the depth of thermal injury. This may allow a carbon dioxide resurfacing laser to be used for superficial treatment of the neck.[84] With the minimal residual thermal damage left behind by the Er:YAG laser, it is useful for the treatment of nonfacial photodamage and may have a role to play in the treatment of nonfacial rhytides, including the dorsal hands and neck.[85] Much more conservative settings and a smaller number of passes should be used. Only the epidermis should be ablated with the expectation that dyspigmentation of the skin will be improved while the associated rhytides are only minimally affected. The main indication for neck resurfacing is to reduce color mismatch between the laser resurfaced face and sundamaged bronze-color neck.

DISCUSSION

The Current State of Resurfacing

The choice of modalities for resurfacing procedures now include microdermabrasion, α-hydroxy and β-hydroxy acid peels, Jessner peels, trichloracetic acid peels, phenol peels, dermabrasion with wire brush, diamond fraise, or sandpaper, pulsed carbon dioxide laser, scanned carbon dioxide laser, erbium laser and long-pulsed erbium laser, electrical heating, and a variety of new modalities undergoing clinical testing.

The choice of technique is multifactorial. What depth of resurfacing is desired? What instruments and techniques are available and known to the clinician? What is the physician's experience and skill with the modalities? Does the device offer any unique features not seen with other approaches, for example, greater safety, fewer complications, different mechanisms of action, broader range of use?

All of the resurfacing modalities can bring about some positive changes, from improvement in skin texture and diminution of dyspigmentation and fine rhytides with procedures that affect more superficial epidermis and dermis, to remarkable decrease or elimination of the mild to severe changes associated with photoaging—deep lines and wrinkles, lentigines, dull yellowish complexion, and skin laxity—with laser resurfacing or other techniques that have greater depth of effects.

A mechanism unique to carbon dioxide laser and long-pulsed erbium laser is tissue tightening secondary to heat-induced collagen contraction. A more superficial laser resurfacing procedure may, therefore, be able to accomplish the same clinical results as a deeper, more-tightening resurfacing procedure. Hemostasis is unique to pulsed carbon dioxide and long-pulsed erbium laser resurfacing as well as the chemical peels, but is not seen with dermabrasion or short-pulsed erbium laser resurfacing. Postresurfacing healing, erythema, pigment loss, or scarring is directly proportional to the depth of resurfacing or prolongation of wound healing beyond the normal range. No mechanisms or unique sequelae are specific to any particular modality. Precise control of depth of resurfacing is therefore an important and significant advantage when comparing the different modalities.

Laser skin resurfacing has brought about dramatic changes in the approach to the treatment of photoaging and facial rejuvenation. It has significant advantages over many other resurfacing methods and has replaced dermabrasion and medium and deep chemical peels in many clinical settings. The best technique or combination of techniques for any given treatment, however, will depend on the judgment and experience of the skilled clinician.

Future Directions

Incisional Laser Surgery and Laser Hair Transplantation. Efforts have been made to assess the utility of using lasers to assist in hair transplantation. Carbon dioxide and Er:YAG laser–assisted hair transplantation has the potential benefit that a series of identical slits can be made at each session. Unlike making slits with cold steel, ablating tissue by laser has the added advantage of removing a small area of hairless skin with each slit, thus reducing the total hairless area at the same time as filling it with grafts. Potential disadvantages are residual thermal damage produced at the margin of the slit and the difficulty in grafting in areas that have been previously grafted without damaging already engrafted hairs. So far, there has been a lot of promise with limited success due to equipment limitations.[86-92]

Nonablative Resurfacing. New approaches to laser resurfacing include attempts at achieving selective dermal injury while keeping the remaining epidermis intact. The healing process in the dermis should lead to new collagen deposition and remodeling with the possibility of reducing rhytides. Several methods have been tried with variable results. Two methods have demonstrated moderate improvement of rhytides in small pilot studies: In the first a carbon-based topical suspension is applied to the skin followed by low-fluence Q-switched Nd:YAG laser irradiation[93]; the second combines a mid infrared (1.32 μm) pulsed (0.2 ms) laser to shrink the dermis with dynamic cooling to protect the epidermis.[94] Healing was faster than after carbon dioxide laser resurfacing, as there was no epidermal injury.

A bilateral comparison study of carbon dioxide laser resurfacing and nonablative resurfacing with a Q-switched Nd:YAG laser for the treatment of "crow's feet" demonstrated rhytide improvement in all carbon dioxide laser–treated sides and in 9 of 11 Nd:YAG laser–treated sides. On the Nd:YAG-treated side, the improvement in six patients was less than on the carbon dioxide laser–treated side, but in three patients the improvement was equivalent on both sides.[95] These three patients were the only Nd:YAG laser–treated patients who had prolonged erythema. The reproducibility of these results awaits larger patient series with long-term follow-up.

When pulsed dye laser at 585 nm and 0.5 ms pulse duration was used in 20 patients for sun-induced rhytides, 90% of the mild to moderate wrinkles showed objective improvement and 40% of the moderate to severe wrinkles showed improvement. Histologically, the treated areas showed a papillary dermal band of well-organized elastin and collagen fibers replacing pretreatment elastotic tissue.[96]

New Concepts. Lasers other than the carbon dioxide and Er:YAG may be worth considering for laser skin resurfacing. Using the free electron laser at wavelengths between 6 and 7.5 μm, specific molecular structures within tissue proteins can be targeted. By doing so, much greater contraction can be induced with no more tissue vaporization or residual thermal injury. This may result in greater improvement in tissue sagging while limiting the risks of excessive thermal injury, which results in scarring.

Conclusions

Because of its cosmetic implications, carbon dioxide and Er:YAG laser resurfacing has raised a huge amount of interest. Early treatment results have been impressive. As laser technology is refined, the side effect and complication profiles of laser resurfacing will improve. Many questions remain unanswered. How does carbon dioxide laser resurfacing work? Is more than one pass necessary? What is the optimal technique? Is thermal damage essential for beneficial results or is ablation the key to successful treatment? What role does collagen shrinkage and remodeling play? Is resurfacing of nonfacial skin, such as the neck or hands, safe and effective? The answers to these and many more questions are essential to better understanding of this rapidly evolving field.

SECTION TWO

Atlas of Surgical Procedures

PREOPERATIVE CLINICAL CONSIDERATIONS

Patient Selection

In evaluating the prospective patient and assessing the potential response to laser resurfacing, the two primary areas of attention are the perioral and periorbital regions. Wrinkling in these areas has been traditionally unresponsive to face-lifting procedures, as the laxity of skin removed and tightened by these techniques does not include these areas. Chemical peeling and dermabrasion, though helpful, have often been disappointing in their results in these locations. However, our experience in laser resurfacing has been very rewarding in achieving excellent results in these locations. Though any facial wrinkles may respond in an excellent manner to laser therapy, it is these locations that have defined the success of laser resurfacing, primarily because of their difficult response to treatment historically.[3,6,8,50,51]

On the other hand, lines of expression such as forehead creases, glabellar furrows, "crow's feet," and nasolabial folds may be responsive if superficial, but when present as deep folds or palpable deep creases they usually only soften. Even when these lines completely resolve, they recur much sooner because of the unavoidable effect of muscular contraction compressing and folding the skin with facial expression. This is true of certain perioral lines as well. Dynamic facial lines are best treated with additional modalities such as botulinum toxin muscle paralysis, bovine collagen injections, or other augmentation techniques.

As with any cosmetic procedure, patient expectations are the most important determinant of patient satisfaction. A patient must have realistic expectations as to the improvement that can be achieved. Laser resurfacing can improve but will not eliminate all or even most wrinkles. Showing before and after photographs may be helpful. However, photographs of rhytides can often be misleading due to changing light conditions, angle of camera, and patient facial expression. If photographs are used, both good and less than ideal results should be shown to the patient. A detailed discussion as to the potential complications and expected postoperative course is imperative to reduce patient anxiety as well as frequent calls from the patient in the immediate postlaser period.

Patients of any age who are in reasonably good health can undergo laser resurfacing. Screening laboratory tests are generally not necessary if the procedure is done under local anesthesia. Most full face resurfacing is done under deep IV sedation or general anesthesia and the choice of screening laboratory tests is up to the anesthesiologist depending on the patient's age and health status. Some laser surgeons screen for hepatitis B, hepatitis C, and HIV because of the potential infectivity of the laser plume. Contraindications for the procedure are similar to dermabrasion. Patients who are keloid formers should not undergo laser resurfacing. In situations where there is a reduction in the number of adnexal structures such as skin that has received prior x-ray treatment or patients with scleroderma, laser resurfacing should not be done, as a successful result relies on reepithelialization from normal and intact adnexal structures remaining after laser resurfacing.

Prior isotretinoin treatment has been reported to be associated with atypical scarring after dermabrasion or chemical peel even if the procedure was performed more than 1 year after isotretinoin treatment.[97] The frequency of this complication is unknown. Therefore, patients who have received isotretinoin should receive additional warnings about the possibility of scarring from laser resurfacing and the procedure should probably be done more conservatively. We recommend that the patient wait at least 1 to 2 years after isotretinoin treatment before undergoing laser resurfacing, because of the unknown effects on wound healing presented by isotretinoin.

Skin that has recently been undermined, as in a face lift or blepharoplasty, has an altered blood circulation for several months. Resurfacing procedures done at the same time as or soon after skin undermining increase the risk of skin necrosis with associated scarring.[98,99] We recommend that laser resurfacing of undermined skin be deferred for 6 months after the original surgical procedure. It is unknown how long after laser resurfacing a patient can safely undergo a procedure that undermines the resurfaced skin, but a wait of 3 to 6 months would seem prudent.

Medications

A number of medications are useful to make the procedure safer and more comfortable for the patient. Retin-A has been shown to speed reepithelialization after dermabrasion[100] and chemical peels, and it may work similarly after laser resurfacing. While there are no published controlled trials demonstrating the benefits of tretinoin, we encourage its use at the highest tolerable concentration daily for at least 6 weeks before the procedure.[101] We use α-hydroxy acids only in patients who are tretinoin intolerant.

Postinflammatory hyperpigmentation is a frequent occurrence after laser resurfacing. A majority of Fitzpatrick type IV patients will develop it, as will almost all darker skinned individuals.[3] To reduce the incidence of postinflammatory hyperpigmentation, all patients are encouraged to avoid having a suntan at the time of the procedure. While there is debate over whether preparing the skin with lightening agents prior to resurfacing decreases the risk of hyperpigmentation, many laser surgeons give skin type III to VI patients hydroquinone, kojic acid or azelaic acid.[101] To be effective, bleaching creams have to be used for a number of weeks before the procedure. The ideal time for laser resurfacing is late fall and winter.

In patients with a history of herpes labialis, laser resurfacing can trigger an outbreak that can spread to involve the entire denuded skin surface with resulting increased pain, prolonged healing, and an increased risk of scarring. We have encountered several instances in which patients who denied any history of herpes labialis developed severe herpes outbreaks after laser resurfacing. Therefore, all patients, regardless of cold sore or fever blister history, are prophylactically given either acyclovir 400 mg PO tid, valacyclovir 500 mg PO bid, or famcyclovir 250 mg PO bid starting up to 2 days before and continuing for at least 10 days after the procedure.

After laser resurfacing there is a layer of necrotic, thermally coagulated dermis that will slough over several days. This material serves as an ideal bacterial culture medium. Therefore patients are usually given prophylactic antibiotics such as dicloxacillin 500 mg PO bid or, in penicillin-allergic individuals, azithromycin 500 mg followed by 250 mg PO once daily starting up to 1 day prior to surgery and continuing for a total of 5 days.[101] Since introducing oral antibiotics, impetiginization of the treated areas has been almost totally eliminated.

A few laser surgeons recommend a dose of fluconazole on the day of resurfacing to reduce the risk of candidal infection in the treated area. Some prescribe a short, 3- to 4-day course of oral corticosteroids for the patient perioperatively to reduce the very significant edema that usually occurs during the first 72 hours after the procedure.

Anesthesia

Facial resurfacing with a laser requires the use of an anesthetic that effectively blocks the pain that results from vaporizing epidermal and dermal tissue. This is true for both carbon dioxide and Er:YAG laser resurfacing. Even though many physicians have attempted to perform carbon dioxide laser resurfacing using topical anesthetic agents alone, only a few have been successful because often only superficial anesthesia is achieved. However, one group does all resurfacing under only EMLA anesthesia with good success.[102] The occlusion necessary to induce deeper anesthesia with EMLA results in significant tissue hydration that may reduce the depth of thermal injury. This topical anesthesia approach has been found useful for enhancing the safety of neck carbon dioxide laser resurfacing.[84]

Local infiltration or regional nerve blocks are preferred for localized areas. Supraorbital, supratrochlear, infraorbital, and mental nerves are easily blocked, providing complete anesthesia of the central face, excluding the upper and lower eyelids, nasal tip, and oral commissures. These areas, as well as any locations on the lateral and inferior cheek, temple, and along the jawline must be anesthetized with local infiltration. The local anesthetic should be injected into the subcutaneous plane to minimize distortion of the surface rhytides. It may be helpful to mark out the rhytides prior to injecting the anesthetic. Sedatives and analgesics administered prior to performing these nerve blocks can be helpful.

Regional blocks are performed using 1% to 2% lidocaine with 1:100,000 epinephrine. With proper placement of the anesthetic, as little as 0.25 ml is needed to completely block the nerve. Because the procedure is relatively short, in general we have found no need to use longer-acting anesthetics such as bupivacaine. For local tissue infiltration, especially around the eyes and for the cheeks, we use a mixture of equal parts 2% lidocaine with 1:100,000 epinephrine, 0.5% bupivacaine, 1 part in 10 of 8.4% $NaHCO_3$, and 75 U of hyaluronidase in a 10 cc syringe. The bicarbonate neutralizes the pH and decreases the pain of injection, and the hyaluronidase improves tissue diffusion. When a large volume of anesthetic is needed, 0.5% lidocaine with 1:400,000 epinephrine can be used to minimize epinephrine-induced tachycardia and to stay within the 7 mg/kg total dose limitation for lidocaine.

When full face resurfacing is performed, several choices are available. While regional anesthesia augmented by local infiltration to the eyelids, corners of the mouth, and cheeks with some form of oral preoperative sedation may be used, we have found that this does not provide adequate sedation and that patients are uncomfortable during the procedure. Intravenous sedation performed by an anesthesiologist, using appropriate monitoring, is recommended. Versed and propofol are commonly used with some analgesic such as fentanyl. Use of a laryngeal mask, which allows delivery of inhalational anesthetic agents, enables us to perform full face resurfacing with intravenous agents alone without the need for regional and local infiltration. However, we will perform nerve blocks using 0.25% bupivacaine with 1:100,000 epinephrine at the conclusion of the procedure to reduce immediate postoperative pain.

PROCEDURAL TECHNIQUES

Technique for Resurfacing Wrinkled Skin[3,6,8,50,51]

The skin may be prepared with an antiseptic such as Betadine or Septisol. If alcohol antiseptics are used, they should be allowed to dry completely before starting the procedure. Chlorhexidine should be avoided because of its ocular toxicity, which might be aggravated by its vaporization with the laser. Extensive prepping of the skin prior to laser resurfacing is usually not necessary, as the laser sterilizes the surface as it vaporizes.[103]

Free-flowing oxygen should be kept away from the field to reduce the risk of fire. The treatment area is wrapped with wet towels. Depending on the area being treated, the patient's eyes are covered with opaque, metal, nonreflective shields, or wet eye pads.

The most commonly requested areas for laser resurfacing are the perioral, periorbital, and glabellar/forehead regions as isolated units. When treating any of these areas as an isolated treatment, it is important to follow the treated wrinkles out to their end rather than limit treatment to the cosmetic unit. That means, when treating the periorbital area, that the "crow's feet" of the lateral canthus area must be followed out to the temporal area as well as to their points over the superior lateral cheeks, and the medial lines over the nasal bridge.

When treating the perioral area alone, the wrinkle lines that often flare laterally off the lower nasolabial fold and the crescent lines of the medial lower cheek just lateral to the mouth should be treated as well. The treatment should be carried over the jawline to the level of the submental crease. We do not recommend treating across the vermilion border as it does not appear to enhance results but does increase discomfort and prolongs healing.

When these areas are treated in this manner, the treatment zone extends beyond what is commonly accepted as the anatomic unit of each area for cosmetic purposes. Because of this extension beyond the most visible anatomic markers such as the nasolabial fold and the orbital rim, it is important to use a feathering technique with the laser to blend into the untreated skin.

We do not recommend treating both the perioral and periorbital regions as isolated areas. It is far preferable to treat the entire face. When this is done, the treatment of the cheeks results in secondary improvement in the other two areas as well. In addition, the erythema and/or transient pigment changes are less visible when present in a more uniform distribution. Permanent hypopigmentation is far easier to camouflage when the entire face is treated.

Patients sometimes request treatment of only the glabellar lines. Though this may be done, it results in very visible erythema of only this location, making it difficult to conceal with makeup or other camouflage, and the results are not overly impressive. Furthermore, improvement is modest at best. It is preferable to continue the resurfacing across the entire forehead.

Carbon Dioxide Laser Resurfacing. The epidermis of the area to be treated is first removed using a confluent application of single vaporizing laser pulses with either an individual spot handpiece, scanner, or computer pattern generator (CPG). The spots are placed adjacent to each other with 10% or less overlap. Because of lateral heat spread at the dermoepidermal junction, small skip areas will be removed when wiping away the epidermal debris. These small skip areas in the dermis add a protective zone to help prevent heat accumulation that may occur with rapid pulse placement one on top of another. For these reasons, it is far preferable to leave small skip spaces during treatment rather than to overlap too much.[37] The desiccated proteinaceous debris that remains after laser application represents keratinous cellular remnants following intracellular vaporization (Fig. 19-6). In areas that receive only one laser pass, the debris can be left in place to act as a biologic dressing. Not wiping the debris seems to speed reepithelialization.[104] One-pass carbon dioxide laser resurfacing using the UltraPulse carbon dioxide laser with the CPG scanner and leaving the char intact without wiping is felt by Ruiz-Esparza and Barba Gomez to bring about near equivalent clinical results with lower risks of pigmentary change and scarring.[105] However, this debris must be wiped clear from areas that will receive more than one pass with the laser, as it blocks the laser light from penetrating into the skin because it no longer has water present as a target for the laser. Wiping this layer away with saline not

A B C D

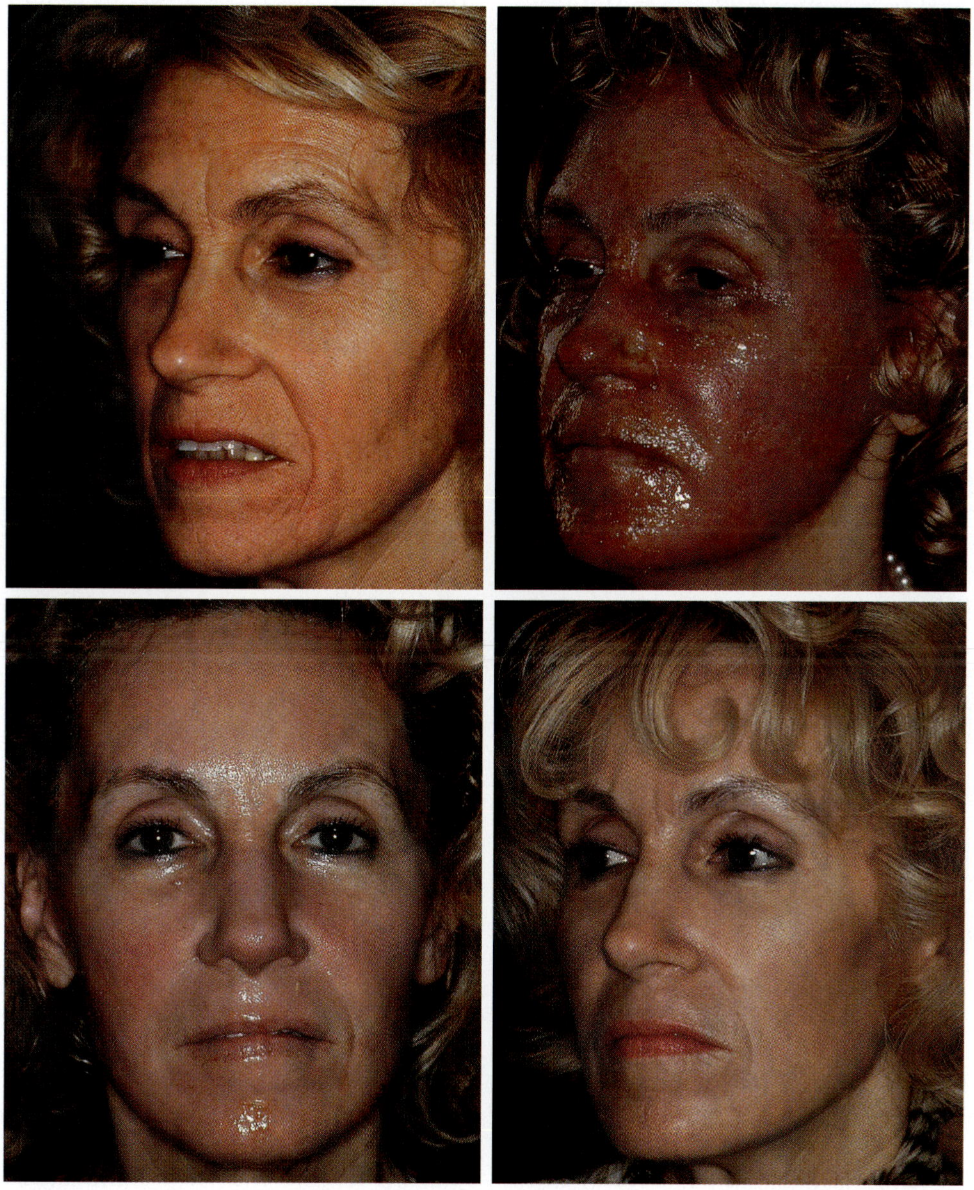

FIG. 19-6

A, A 58-year-old woman before CO_2 laser skin resurfacing. **B,** Three days after CO_2 laser skin resurfacing. **C,** Ten days after full face CO_2 laser skin resurfacing. **D,** Six weeks after full face CO_2 laser skin resurfacing. (From Dover JS, Arndt K, Geronemus R, Alora MB. Illustrated Cutaneous and Aesthetic Laser Surgery, 2nd ed. New York: McGraw-Hill, 2000.)

only removes this hurdle but also acts to rehydrate the underlying tissue. Once this debris has been wiped away, a dry gauze must be used to remove any water remaining on the skin surface, as this will absorb the laser energy and block its reaction with dermal tissue. A second laser pass is then performed over the entire area of photodamaged dermis. This is most easily performed in an even confluent application. However, as multiple passes are performed, the area treated with each pass generally becomes smaller as more superficially damaged areas are normalized with tissue vaporization. With each additional pass, there is further wrinkle smoothing as well as increased risk of complications due to the greater depth of tissue injury. The main end point of treatment is smoothing away tissue irregularities and visible wrinkle lines so that a smooth and even surface results. Bleeding is rarely encountered when resurfacing with carbon dioxide lasers.

There is rarely a reason to perform more than four passes with a carbon dioxide resurfacing laser in any given area, as studies have shown that with the energy fluences used, both vaporization and collagen tightening plateau at three to four passes, while residual thermal damage gradually increases with each additional pass.[22]

The tissue changes color as resurfacing proceeds deeper into the dermis. Entry into the papillary dermis is evident as a pink color of the surface. The color changes to gray with deeper papillary dermal ablation. With further ablation the tissue gets a yellowish hue that corresponds to ablation into the upper reticular dermis and is usually the end point of treatment. Additional passes cause a darker yellow to brown color. The color changes are probably related to the buildup of thermally denatured collagen rather than some intrinsic property of different dermal layers.

Lumenis UltraPulse. To achieve reproducible tissue effects, it is preferable to use the CPG scanner whenever possible and to use the 3 mm collimated spot for small areas or for edging. The CPG is preferable, because it precisely and rapidly places each laser spot within the pattern and thus is a faster, more uniform, and safer treatment.[106] However, any and all areas of the face may be treated using the 3 mm collimated beam handpiece and confluent single pulse vaporization with 10% or less overlap. Feathering with the laser is accomplished by decreasing both the pulse energy and the density of application of pulses. It is advisable to perform at least one peripheral zone with confluent application of pulse energy 100 to 150 mJ less than that used for treatment.

The initial CPG settings for treating large areas are pattern shape 2 (parallelogram) or 3 (square), pattern size 9 (largest), density 5, using 300 mJ per pulse, 60 watts, and repeat rate 1 to 1.5/s. Patterns are placed one next to the other in repetitive fashion with care to align each scan beside the adjacent one without skip areas or much overlapping (see Fig. 19-6). Coat hair-bearing areas such as the eyebrows and scalp margins with a water-based lubricant, such as Surgilube, prior to treatment to avoid vaporizing the hair shaft. When treating the forehead and temporal scalp margins, extend the treatment pattern onto the scalp for a few millimeters to produce uniform treatment of the entire face and to prevent a sharp visible edge of treatment before or at the edge of hair growth. The eyebrow margins can be protected with the burnished side of a Jaeger bone plate when treating this site in order to make a sharp margin and prevent inadvertent extension into the eyebrows. When treating the full face, extend treatment approximately 1 inch below the mandibular ramus. We routinely decrease the fluence to 250 mJ per pulse and the power to 50 watts in an effort to limit the amount of tissue damage at the edge of treatment to reduce the risk of unwanted pigmentary or textural changes and to help blend the treated skin into untreated skin.

Removing char and desiccated tissue after the first pass must be done with a saturated gauze pad in as gentle a fashion as possible, avoiding "scrubbing" the thermally altered epidermis, which induces additional, unnecessary friction and injury and perhaps prolongs posthealing erythema. Be sure to remove all desiccated tissue before proceeding to the second pass. Second or subsequent passes are carried out in the same fashion on moderately or severely photodamaged skin, except in periorbital skin and in areas that have only mild changes. In these areas "half passes" are recommended. By moving the scanner toward you very slightly as the scan is laid down, a zigzag or zippered pattern is produced. Zippering induces some tissue tightening while avoiding excessive or unnecessary thermal change. In the periorbital skin we recommend decreasing the pattern density to 4 on subsequent passes and decreasing the fluence to 250 mJ and the power to 50 watts. Shoulders of rhytides or edges of scars may be further sculpted using either a single or narrow pattern band (patterns) or by turning off the CPG and tracing borders with single repetitive pulses of the 2.25 mm spot from the CPG or 3 mm collimated hand piece at 350 to 500 mJ, wiping with moistened gauze or a Q-tip between passes.

Lumenis SilkLaser. For most resurfacing indications, the "start safe" default laser power settings are a good starting point. The laser parameters are set using a touchscreen. The surgeon selects the handpiece, mode (SilkTouch or FeatherTouch), scan size, and scan shape and the laser sets the correct scan time and suggests a power setting that is appropriate for most resurfacing cases. The time between scans is set by the surgeon to leave enough time to move the handpiece between scans and position it for the next scan, with intervals of 0.2 to 0.3 seconds appropriate for relatively short and small scans and 0.4 to 0.5 needed for long and large scans.[38]

The No. 1 determinant of safety and efficacy is the number of laser passes used. One pass with the SilkTouch mode approximates the depth of a medium-depth Jessner's solution plus 35% trichloroacetic acid chemical peel. Two to three passes approximate the depth of dermabrasion, and four or more passes approach the depth of a deep Baker's phenol peel. The FeatherTouch mode requires approximately twice as many laser passes as the SilkTouch mode for equivalent clinical results when the laser is set to the recommended start safe settings. Increasing the power (wattage) in the FeatherTouch mode will increase the amount of tissue vaporized per pass without significantly increasing the depth of thermal damage. Therefore, higher FeatherTouch power settings reduce the number of laser passes needed.

It is often helpful after the initial one to three passes to switch to a smaller scan size to treat the shoulder of each remaining rhytid. The edges of the treatment field receive only one pass to allow for feathering of the edges. Further feathering can be achieved by angling the handpiece away from perpendicular to the skin surface. This will space out the individual laser passes in the spiral scan farther apart at the edge of the treatment field.

The eyelids should receive a maximum of one pass with the SilkTouch mode or two passes with the FeatherTouch mode for an end point consisting of a pink to slightly gray surface. The temples, lateral cheeks, and jawline in women can receive a maximum of two SilkTouch passes or three FeatherTouch passes with a residual light yellow surface color. The skin of the rest of the face, including the forehead, glabella, medial cheeks, perioral region, and nose, is thicker and can usually tolerate up to three passes with the SilkTouch or five passes with the FeatherTouch when treating rhytides. Individual deep acne scars on the cheeks, especially in men, may require up to five SilkTouch or eight FeatherTouch passes in order to achieve even moderate improvement. After three SilkTouch or five FeatherTouch passes using standard resurfacing settings, there appears to be relatively little additional shrinkage, tissue vaporization, or added thermal damage.

Er:YAG Laser. In Er:YAG resurfacing, less tissue is removed per pass. The number of passes required to remove the epidermis depends on the fluence and spot size, ranging from one to as many as six. As many as two to ten passes may be needed to reach the desired end point. We recommend wiping away the proteinaceous material at least after the first pass. The end point of treatment is effacement of the rhytides and photoaged skin. As more passes are done and resurfacing enters the dermis, however, the amount of residual thermal damage is insufficient to coagulate medium-sized vessels, and bleeding may preclude further treatment.

Er:YAG resurfacing can be performed either freehand or with a scanner. Most Er:YAG lasers generate repetition rates from 1 to 10 Hz and spot sizes of 3 to 7 mm. The treatment field is covered with moderately overlapping laser pulses using spot sizes of 3 to 7 mm, or with most systems a pattern generator can lay down the spots in any shape desired. Approximately 4 μm of tissue is vaporized per J/cm^2 of energy.[31] Settings are adjusted depending on how much tissue you wish to ablate per pass. With a fluence of 5 J/cm^2, the epidermis is vaporized away in four passes. At 8 to 12 J/cm^2, the epidermis is vaporized away with two passes.[33] Additional passes are performed until the lesion or rhytide has been effaced, bleeding has been encountered, or a maximum safe number of laser passes has been completed. The number of passes depends on how deep the laser surgeon needs to go to remove the pathology while staying superficial enough to minimize the risk of scarring and permanent hypopigmentation. Wiping the tissue between passes, except when the epidermis is ablated, is not necessary. It is important to keep track of the number of laser passes to determine the level of ablation. Er:YAG laser ablation in the papillary dermis gives a smooth, glistening surface. Once the reticular dermis is entered, the surface becomes uneven, with sebaceous gland lobules becoming visible. At this point bleeding begins to interfere with deeper treatment.

Long-Pulsed Er:YAG Laser. When using one of the long-pulsed Er:YAG lasers, the end point of treatment is similar to that of the carbon dioxide laser. Namely, the rhytides are effaced and a yellowish tinge representing thermally coagulated collagen remains behind. However, the yellowish color is more subtle, as the thermal damage zone is intermediate in thickness between the short-pulsed Er:YAG and carbon dioxide lasers. In addition, rehydration by wiping will often eliminate any hint of yellowish color. Wiping is useful to assess the progress of resurfacing, including wrinkle effacement and depth of ablation.

When the long-pulsed mode is used, heat is delivered to tissue in a manner similar to that of the pulsed carbon dioxide laser. Therefore, this mode may be used to efficiently remove the epidermis, to induce collagen tightening, and to achieve coagulation of small dermal blood vessels. Short-pulsed mode may then be used for purely ablative functions such as fine sculpting of tissue irregularities and removal of the necrotic layer of thermal damage.

The settings used will be similar to the short-pulsed Er:YAG laser. A fluence of 10 J/cm^2 will remove 40 μm of tissue per pass. The ablation is done either with a scanner or freehand. Freehand ablation can be done efficiently by pulsing at 5 Hz or more and overlapping spots by 50% so that one pass achieves tissue ablation equivalent to two passes.

The variable pulse duration gives this laser added versatility. The pulse duration used will depend on the degree of thermal coagulation and visible shrinkage desired. Deeper wrinkles are best treated with the longest pulse durations available, and fine lines and minimal photodamage are treated with the short-pulsed option.

Combination Treatment. Combination treatment is performed to achieve the benefits of both carbon dioxide and Er:YAG lasers. The carbon dioxide resurfacing laser is usually used first. One to two passes are then performed at 5 to 10 J/cm^2 with an Er:YAG to remove some of the thermal damage left behind by the carbon dioxide laser. Patients appear to reepithelialize a little faster and the postlaser erythema is less intense and of shorter duration.[107] However, the difference may be quite subtle. It may not be worth the expense of using two different lasers unless the physician is adept at the technique. An alternative is to use a variable-pulsed Er:YAG laser, as both the "carbon dioxide" type effects (long pulse) and the "Er:YAG" type effects (short pulse) are found in one machine.

Using an Er:YAG laser followed by a carbon dioxide laser achieves deeper resurfacing as the self-limiting thermal damage feature of the carbon dioxide laser is bypassed. This sequence is useful when treating deep acne scars and should be done only on limited areas.

POSTOPERATIVE CLINICAL CONSIDERATIONS

Wound Care

During the first few days after laser resurfacing there is a significant amount of exudate with some sloughing of thermally denatured collagen. The variable amount of edema that develops in the first 48 hours can be controlled with ice packs, head elevation at night, and oral corticosteroids. Reepithelialization takes 3 to 10 days, increasing with the number of laser passes and decreasing if the patient's skin was primed with Retin-A or resurfaced with an Er:YAG laser. We encourage the use of bio-occlusive dressings such as Vigilon or Silon TSR during at least the first 24 to 72 hours, as this has been shown to speed reepithelialization after dermabrasion and laser skin resurfacing (Fig. 19-7). Continued moist wound healing is achieved with frequent 0.25% acetic acid, normal saline, or cool tap water soaks followed by Aquaphor healing ointment application. We have stopped using Polysporin and bacitracin ointment and petrolatum because Polysporin and bacitracin ointment frequently cause allergic contact dermatitis in these patients[108] and petrolatum may cause a folliculitis, especially if it is not stopped immediately after reepithelialization is complete.[101]

A

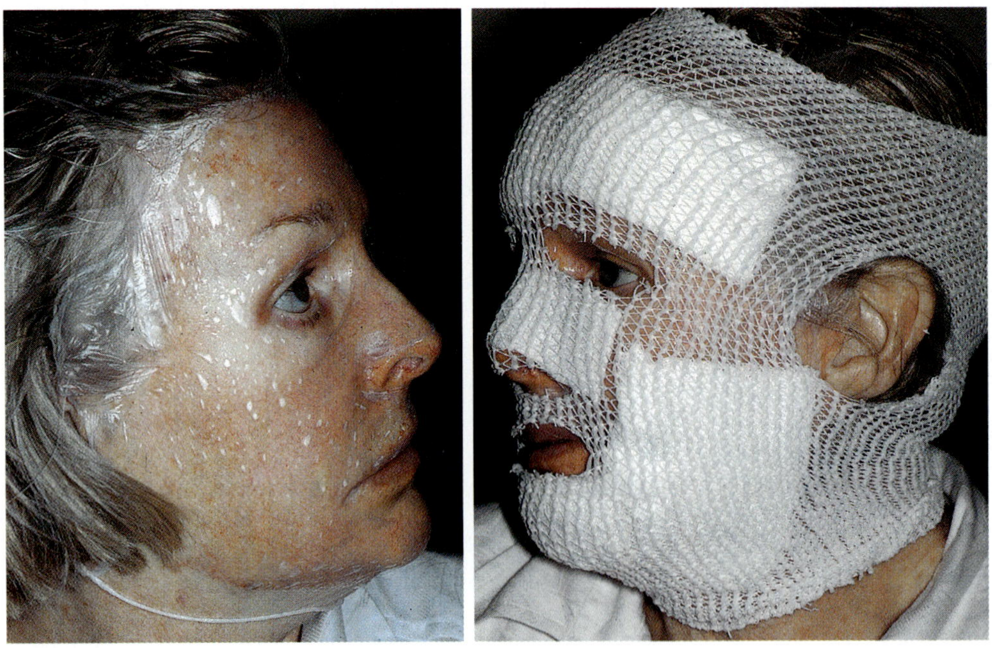

B

FIG. 19-7

A, Immediately after CO_2 and Er:YAG laser skin resurfacing. A Silon TSR in place prior to application of gauze followed by a flexinet dressing. **B,** Same patient after gauze and a flexinet dressing have been applied over the Silon TSR biologic skin dressing.

Moderate burning discomfort experienced by some patients during the first 24 hours after laser resurfacing is controlled most effectively with bio-occlusive dressings. In patients treated with the open technique, we recommend ice packs, cold compresses, and acetaminophen alone or with codeine. During the first few weeks after resurfacing, patients often develop pruritus that is usually self-limited and controlled with antihistamines or topical corticosteroids.

Patients almost universally experience a feeling of tightening of the treated skin that may last for several weeks to several months. This is generally thought to be a beneficial rather than an adverse effect of laser resurfacing.

After reepithelialization, there is a variable period of erythema ranging from 1 to 4 months in duration (Fig. 19-8). The erythema can be successfully camouflaged with makeup containing green foundation. We do not use topical steroids in the postoperative period except in cases of pruritus. Sun avoidance after laser resurfacing for the entire period of postlaser erythema should be stressed to the patient to reduce the risk of postinflammatory hyperpigmentation.

Occasionally, patients will develop milia 1 to 3 months after resurfacing. This is far less commonly seen than after dermabrasion. Retin-A pretreatment further reduces milia formation. The milia usually resolve spontaneously. Retin-A can speed their resolution, with milia extraction needed only on rare occasions.

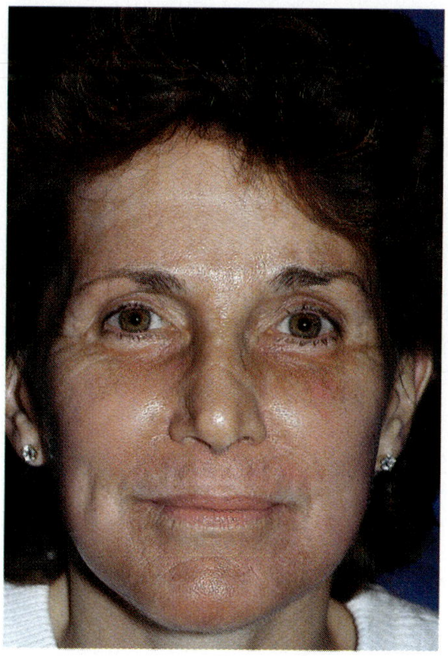

FIG. 19-8
Six weeks after CO_2 laser skin resurfacing this patient exhibits residual facial erythema.

Precautions

Nonadverse side effects following carbon dioxide laser resurfacing are frequent and predictable. Similar to those following chemical peels and dermabrasion, complications are less common and usually preventable if excellent technique is followed and postoperative management is fastidious. They can be divided into five categories: immediate and predictable; infectious; eczematous; follicular; scarring and pigmentary (Box 19-2).

Erythema lasting, on average, 6 to 12 weeks is universal and is considered part of the normal healing process (see Fig. 19-8). Erythema and flushing, which develop in the treated site with exertion or emotional upset, are frequent for a year after resurfacing. Some persons have persistent continual erythema lasting up to 12 months. This may be related to the depth of ablation.[8,37,38,109]

By far the most common adverse effect of laser resurfacing is postinflammatory hyperpigmentation (Fig. 19-9). Transient hyperpigmentation has been reported in up to 36% of patients.[54] It is most often seen in patients with Fitzpatrick's skin types III through VI. The hyperpigmentation is more frequent and severe during the summer months (year-round in southern areas such as Florida and Southern California). More recent studies demonstrate rates of hyperpigmentation as low as 2.8% in patients pretreated with bleaching creams and Retin-A.[110] At the first sign of hyperpigmentation,

BOX 19-2 Side Effects and Complications Associated with Laser Resurfacing

Predictable
Oozing, crusting, swelling (1-2 weeks)
Erythema, pruritus, skin tightness (1-4 months)

Infectious
Bacterial, viral, yeast (1-2 weeks)

Eczematous
Eczema (1-3 months)

Follicular
Acne, acneiform eruption, perioral dermatitis, milia (1-3 months)

Scarring
Atrophic, hypertrophic, keloidal (1+ months)

Pigmentary
Hyperpigmentation (1-6 months)
Permanent hypopigmentation (6+ months)

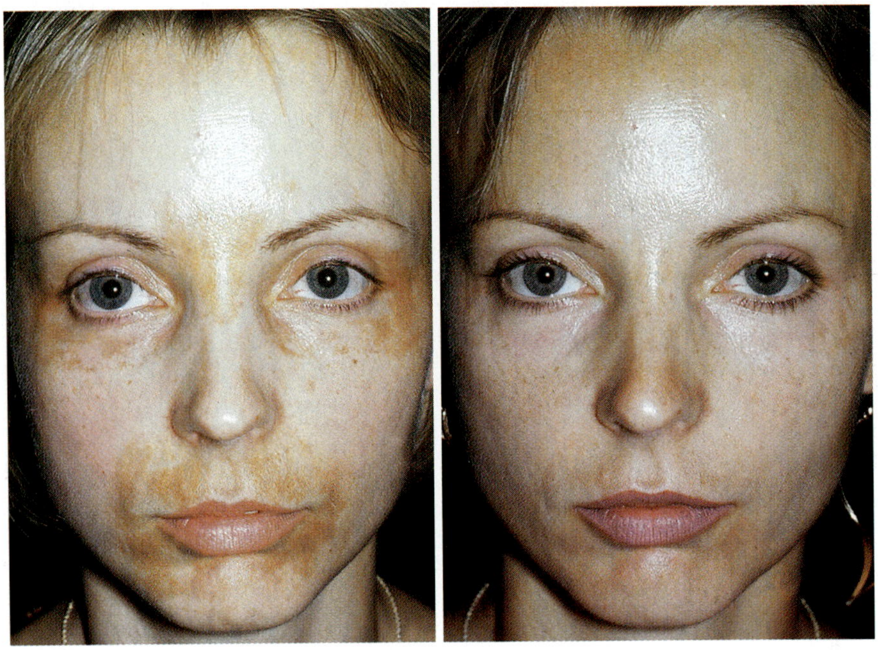

FIG. 19-9
A, Six weeks after CO_2 laser skin resurfacing of the glabella and periocular and perioral skin, this patient displays quite impressive hyperpigmentation. It started 3 weeks after the treatment. **B,** Three weeks after starting 4% hydroquinone with an SPF 15 sunscreen, the hyperpigmentation has completely cleared. (From Dover JS, Arndt K, Geronemus R, Alora MB. Illustrated Cutaneous and Aesthetic Laser Surgery, 2nd ed. New York: McGraw-Hill, 2000.)

bleaching creams and Retin-A are restarted.[101,111] Any sun exposure, even through window glass, at this time can be expected to prolong the period of hyperpigmentation as well as make it more severe. If treatment is started early enough, the hyperpigmentation usually resolves within a few months.[101,111]

Permanent hypopigmentation developing up to 12 months after resurfacing has been reported in 16% of patients and appears to be less frequent than after dermabrasion or deep chemical peels.[49,110] This hypopigmentation ranges from pale new "sun-protected" skin to white, depigmented skin (Fig. 19-10). Hypopigmentation is more common in patients who have previously been treated with dermabrasion.[54,112] Patients with significant actinic damage may develop a color mismatch between the pale new skin of the resurfaced area and the surrounding sun-damaged areas that may include ephelides and lentigenes.[113] This mismatch is minimized by resurfacing the entire face or at least entire cosmetic units and feathering the treatment into the surrounding areas. Rarely, a medium-depth chemical peel of the untreated areas will be needed to even out the skin color. Future sun exposure will also help to blend the resurfaced skin by developing new lentigines and ephelides.

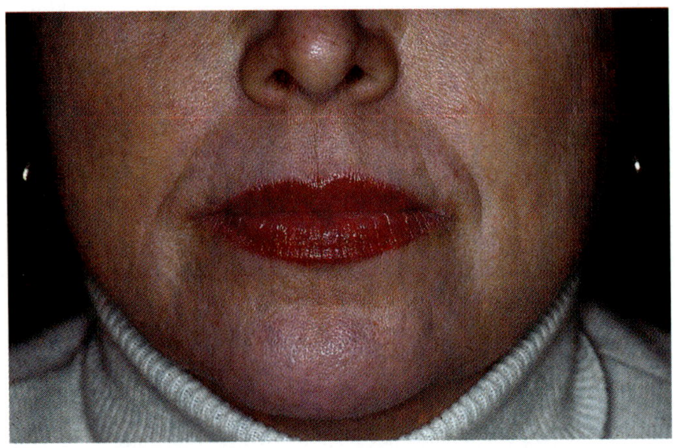

FIG. 19-10
Six months after perioral CO_2 laser skin resurfacing, this fair-skinned individual has subtle, but noticeable, hypopigmentation of the entire treated area. Without cover-up makeup, the hypopigmentation is noticeable.

Milia are a result of follicular reepithelialization compounded by the use of occlusive moisturizers. Acne is a frequent postoperative condition, especially in patients with a past history of acne. It usually develops in the first few weeks after resurfacing and responds to standard acne treatment.

Contact dermatitis, noted with the use of some topical anesthetic preparations, does not correspond with patch test findings but resolves with appropriate treatment.[3,8] This occurrence increases the chances of postoperative erythema and hyperpigmentation.[101] Spongiotic dermatitis occasionally develops in the first 4 weeks after treatment. It responds rapidly to moisturizers and topical midpotency corticosteroids. Infrequently, patients develop perioral dermatitis 1 to 3 months after resurfacing of the perioral region. This is easily controlled with tetracycline and is usually self-limited.

In a procedure that removes the epidermis and part of the dermis, infection is a concern.[8] Laser surgeons have learned from past experience with dermabrasion and have avoided bacterial infection through the judicious use of antibiotics. Antiviral chemoprophylaxis was originally confined to those with a history of herpes simplex infection, but results suggest that subjects with no past history of infection frequently develop herpes simplex activation in treated areas.[3,8,114] It is now standard practice to use antiviral prophylaxis in all laser resurfacing patients. Yeast infections have occurred but respond well to treatment.[3,114]

Hypertrophic scarring is seldom seen following laser resurfacing (Fig. 19-11). Scarring from laser resurfacing appears to be rare; proper patient selection, a conservative number of laser passes, and good post-laser wound care should further reduce the risk.[3,110,112] It may result from a large number of passes or use of excessive energy and from pulse stacking when a carbon dioxide laser is used (overlap of laser irradiated sites, especially after the first pass) resulting in excessive thermal damage.[22] It is better to do a touch-up procedure down the road than to go too deeply the first time in an attempt to totally eradicate the offending rhytides. Any areas that may be developing scar tissue should be promptly treated with topical and intralesional corticosteroids, Silastic gel sheeting, and pulsed dye laser photocoagulation.

The main advantages of the Er:YAG laser are thought to be the potential for an improved side effect profile. The procedure is less painful and, while some perform the procedure using only topical anesthesia, local or regional anesthesia with some form of sedation is usually recommended. There is less oozing and crusting and the subsequent erythema, although dependent on the number of passes, is shorter than that following carbon dioxide laser treatment.[9,33] While healing is slightly faster with Er:YAG laser resurfacing, the degree of improvement is not as impressive as with carbon dioxide resurfacing. It is too early to tell if the rate of permanent hypopigmentation and scarring will be any less after Er:YAG laser resurfacing. In treating superficial lesions, scarring and hypopigmentation would be unlikely to develop, as there is very little thermal damage left behind. However, the end point of treatment is often not clear-cut and the Er:YAG laser, unlike the carbon dioxide lasers, ablates additional tissue with each laser pass, making it possible to ablate all the way into the fat with resulting scarring. Therefore, it is important to keep track of the number of passes and energy fluence when using the Er:YAG laser.

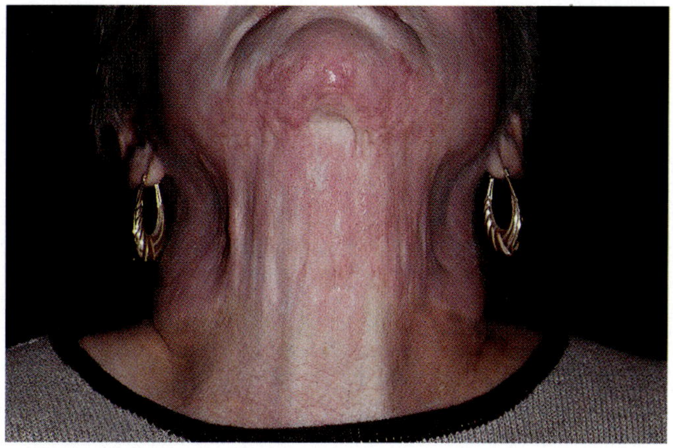

FIG. 19-11
A woman in her mid-sixties underwent CO_2 laser skin resurfacing with the SilkTouch CO_2 laser (Lumenis, Santa Clara, CA). Three passes were performed to the entire face and the neck. One year after the procedure the patient is left with impressive hypertrophic scarring of the neck, limiting mobility, and hypopigmentation as well as patchy erythema.

Other secondary events such as wound infection, allergic or irritant contact dermatitis, or inadequate protein intake by the patient (vegetarian) may extend the wound deeper than originally intended or prolong wound healing and result in scarring. There are also idiopathic episodes of scarring that defy explanation. Some of these cases may be related to collagen vascular disease or other systemic factors.

REFERENCES

1. David LM, Lask GP, Glassberg E, et al. Laser abrasion for cosmetic and medical treatment of facial actinic damage. Cutis 1989; 43:583-587.
2. Fitzpatrick RE, Goldman MP. Advances in carbon dioxide laser surgery. Clin Dermatol 1995; 13:35-47.
3. Fitzpatrick RE, Goldman MP, Satur NM, Tope WD. Pulsed carbon dioxide laser resurfacing of photo-aged facial skin. Arch Dermatol 1996; 132:395-402.
4. Fitzpatrick RE, Tope WD, Goldman MP, Satur NM. Pulsed carbon dioxide laser, trichloroacetic acid, Baker-Gordon phenol, and dermabrasion: a comparative clinical and histologic study of cutaneous resurfacing in a porcine model. Arch Dermatol 1996; 132:469-471.
5. Yang CC, Chai CY. Animal study of skin resurfacing using the ultrapulse carbon dioxide laser. Ann Plast Surg 1995; 35:154-158.
6. Chernoff WG, Schoenrock LD, Cramer H, Wand J. Cutaneous laser resurfacing. Int J Aesthetic Restorative Surg 1995; 3:57-68.
7. Chernoff G, Slatkine M, Zair E, Mead D. SilkTouch: a new technology for skin resurfacing in aesthetic surgery. J Clin Laser Med Surg 1995; 13:97-100.

8. Waldorf HA, Kauvar AN, Geronemus RG. Skin resurfacing of fine to deep rhytides using a char-free carbon dioxide laser in 47 patients. Dermatol Surg 1995; 21:940-946.
9. Teikemeier G, Goldberg DJ. Skin resurfacing with the erbium:YAG laser. Dermatol Surg 1997; 23:685-687.
10. Anderson RR, Parrish RR. Selective photothermolysis: precise microsurgery by selective absorption of pulsed radiation. Science 1983; 220:524-527.
11. Green HA, Domankevitz Y, Nishioka NS. Pulsed carbon dioxide laser ablation of burned skin: in vitro and in vivo analysis. Lasers Surg Med 1990; 10:476-484.
12. Green HA, Burd E, Nishioka NS, et al. Middermal wound healing: a comparison between dermatomal excision and pulsed carbon dioxide laser ablation. Arch Dermatol 1992; 128:639-645.
13. Walsh JJ, Deutsch TF. Pulsed CO_2 laser tissue ablation: measurement of the ablation rate. Lasers Surg Med 1988; 8:264-275.
14. Schenk P, Ehrenberger K. Effect of CO_2 laser on skin lymphatics: an ultrastructural study. Langenbecks Arch Chir 1980; 350:145-150.
15. Slutzki S, Shafir R, Bornstein LA. Use of the carbon dioxide laser for large excisions with minimal blood loss. Plast Reconstr Surg 1977; 60:250-255.
16. Walsh JJ, Flotte TJ, Anderson RR, Deutsch TF. Pulsed CO_2 laser tissue ablation: effect of tissue type and pulse duration on thermal damage. Lasers Surg Med 1988; 8:108-118.
17. Hobbs ER, Bailin PL, Wheeland RG, Ratz JL. Superpulsed lasers: minimizing thermal damage with short duration, high irradiance pulses. J Dermatol Surg Oncol 1987; 13:955-964.
18. Fitzpatrick RE, Ruiz EJ, Goldman MP. The depth of thermal necrosis using the CO_2 laser: a comparison of the superpulsed mode and conventional mode. J Dermatol Surg Oncol 1991; 17: 340-344.
19. Fitzpatrick RE, Goldman MP, Ruiz-Esparza J. Clinical advantage of the CO_2 laser superpulsed mode: treatment of verruca vulgaris, seborrheic keratoses, lentigines, and actinic cheilitis. J Dermatol Surg Oncol 1994; 20:449-456.
20. Brugmans MJP, Kemper J, Gijsbers GHM, et al. Temperature response of biological materials to pulsed non-ablative CO_2 laser irradiation. Lasers Surg Med 1991; 11:587-594.
21. Ross EV, Barnette DJ, Glatter RD, Grevelink JM. Effects of overlap and pass number in CO_2 laser skin resurfacing: a study of residual thermal damage, cell death, and wound healing. Lasers Surg Med 1999; 24:103-112.
22. Fitzpatrick RE, Smith SR, Sriprachya-Anunt S. Depth of vaporization and the effect of pulse stacking with a high-energy, pulsed carbon dioxide laser. J Am Acad Dermatol 1999; 40:615-622.
23. Kauvar AN, Waldorf HA, Geronemus RG. A histopathological comparison of "char-free" carbon dioxide lasers. Dermatol Surg 1996; 22:343-348.
24. Ross EV, Naseef GS, McKinlay JR, et al. Comparison of carbon dioxide laser, erbium:YAG laser, dermabrasion, and dermatome: a study of thermal damage, wound contraction, and wound healing in a live pig model: implications for skin resurfacing. J Am Acad Dermatol 2000; 42:92-105.
25. Duke D, Khatri K, Grevelink J, Anderson RR. The comparison of a 60 μs pulse duration to a 1 ms pulse duration CO_2 laser system in laser resurfacing. Lasers Surg Med 1997; 20(suppl 9):30-31.
26. Hale GM, Querry MR. Optical constants of water in the 200-nm to 200-m wavelength region. Applied Optics 1973; 12:555-563.
27. Vogler K, Reindl M. Erbium laser parameters for new medical applications. Biophotonics Int 1996; Nov/Dec:40-47.
28. Walsh JT, Deutsch TF. Er:YAG laser ablation of tissue: measurement of ablation rates. Lasers Surg Med 1989; 9:327-337.
29. Walsh JJ, Flotte TJ, Deutsch TF. Er:YAG laser ablation of tissue: effect of pulse duration and tissue type on thermal damage. Lasers Surg Med 1989; 9:314-326.
30. Hohenleutner U, Hohenleutner S, Baumler W, Landthaler M. Fast and effective skin ablation with an Er:YAG laser: determination of ablation rates and thermal damage zones. Lasers Surg Med 1997; 20:242-247.
31. Kaufmann R, Hibst R. Pulsed erbium:YAG laser ablation in cutaneous surgery. Lasers Surg Med 1996; 19:324-330.
32. Stuzin JM, Baker TJ, Baker TM. CO_2 and erbium:YAG laser resurfacing: current status and personal perspective. Plast Reconstr Surg 1999; 103:588-591.
33. Ziering CL. Cutaneous laser resurfacing with the erbium:YAG laser and the char-free carbon dioxide laser: a clinical comparison of 100 patients. Int J Aesthetic Reconstr Surg 1997; 5:29-37.
34. Khatri KA, Ross V, Grevelink JM, et al. Comparison of erbium: YAG and carbon dioxide lasers in resurfacing of facial rhytides. Arch Dermatol 1999; 135:391-397.
35. Pozner JN, Lombardo AA. Histological and clinical study of a new variable pulsewidth erbium:YAG laser. Lasers Surg Med 1999; 24(suppl 11):27.
36. Adrian MA. Pulsed carbon dioxide and long pulse 10-ms erbium-YAG laser resurfacing: a comparative clinical and histologic study. J Cutaneous Laser Ther 2000; 1:197-202.
37. Lowe NJ, Lask G, Griffin ME, et al. Skin resurfacing with the Ultrapulse carbon dioxide laser: observations on 100 patients. Dermatol Surg 1995; 21:1025-1029.
38. Lask G, Keller G, Lowe N, Gormley D. Laser skin resurfacing with the SilkTouch flashscanner for facial rhytides. Dermatol Surg 1995; 21:1021-1024.
39. Stagnone JJ. Superficial peeling. J Dermatol Surg Oncol 1989; 15:924-930.
40. Brody HJ. Variations and comparisons in medium-depth chemical peeling. J Dermatol Surg Oncol 1989; 15:953-963.
41. Brody HJ, Hailey CW. Medium-depth chemical peeling of the skin: a variation of superficial chemosurgery. J Dermatol Surg Oncol 1986; 12:1268-1275.
42. Monheit GD. The Jessner's + TCA peel: a medium-depth chemical peel. J Dermatol Surg Oncol 1989; 15:945-950.
43. Stegman SJ. A comparative histologic study of the effects of three peeling agents and dermabrasion on normal and sun-damaged skin. Aesthetic Plast Surg 1982; 6:123-135.
44. Alt TH. Occluded Baker-Gordon chemical peel: review and update. J Dermatol Surg Oncol 1989; 15:980-993.
45. Asken S. Unoccluded Baker-Gordon phenol peels—review and update. J Dermatol Surg Oncol 1989; 15:998-1008.
46. Baker TJ, Gordon HL. Chemical peeling as a practical method for removing rhytides of the upper lip. Ann Plast Surg 1979; 2: 209-212.
47. Wentzell JM, Robinson JK, Wentzell JMJ, et al. Physical properties of aerosols produced by dermabrasion. Arch Dermatol 1989; 15:1637-1643.
48. Yarborough JM Jr. Dermabrasion by wire brush. J Dermatol Surg Oncol 1987; 13:610-615.
49. Falabella R. Postdermabrasion leukoderma. J Dermatol Surg Oncol 1987; 13:44-48.
50. Hruza GJ. Skin resurfacing with lasers. Fitzpatrick's J Clin Dermatol 1995; 3:38-41.
51. Schoenrock LD, Chernoff WG, Rubach BW. Cutaneous UltraPulse laser resurfacing of the eyelids. Int J Aesthetic Restorative Surg 1995; 3:31-36.
52. Yarborough JM Jr, Beeson WH. Dermabrasion. In: Beeson WH, McCollough EG, eds. Aesthetic Surgery of the Aging Face. St. Louis: Mosby, 1986:142-181.
53. Apfelberg DB. A critical appraisal of high-energy pulsed carbon dioxide laser facial resurfacing for acne scars. Ann Plast Surg 1997; 38:95-100.
54. Alster TS, West TB. Resurfacing of atrophic facial acne scars with a high-energy, pulsed carbon dioxide laser. Dermatol Surg 1996; 22:151-154.

55. Abergel RP, Dahlman CM. The CO_2 laser approach to the treatment of acne scarring. Cosmet Dermatol 1995; 8:33-36.
56. Grevelink JM, White VR. Concurrent use of laser skin resurfacing and punch excision in the treatment of facial acne scarring [see comments]. Dermatol Surg 1998; 24:527-530.
57. Young CK. Resurfacing of pitted facial scars with a pulsed Er:YAG laser. Dermatol Surg 1997; 23:880-883.
58. Wheeland RG. Revision of full-thickness skin grafts using the carbon dioxide laser. J Dermatol Surg Oncol 1988; 14:130-134.
59. Greenbaum SS, Rubin MG. Surgical pearl: the high-energy pulsed carbon dioxide laser for immediate scar resurfacing. J Am Acad Dermatol 1999; 40:988-990.
60. Alamillos-Granados FJ, Naval-Gias L, Dean-Ferrer A, Alonso del Hoyo JR. Carbon dioxide laser vermilionectomy for actinic cheilitis. J Oral Maxillofac Surg 1993; 51:118-121.
61. Stanley RJ, Roenigk RK. Actinic cheilitis: treatment with the carbon dioxide laser. Mayo Clin Proc 1988; 63:230-235.
62. Robinson JK. Actinic cheilitis: a prospective study comparing four treatment methods. Arch Otolaryngol Head Neck Surg 1989; 115:848-852.
63. Zelickson BD, Roenigk RK. Actinic cheilitis: treatment with the carbon dioxide laser. Cancer 1990; 65:1307-1311.
64. Dufresne RJ, Garrett AB, Bailin PL, Ratz JL. Carbon dioxide laser treatment of chronic actinic cheilitis. J Am Acad Dermatol 1988; 19:876-878.
65. Johnson TM, Sebastien TS, Lowe L, Nelson BR. Carbon dioxide laser treatment of actinic cheilitis: clinicohistopathologic correlation to determine the optimal depth of destruction. J Am Acad Dermatol 1992; 27:737-740.
66. Ries WR, Duncavage JA, Ossoff RH. Carbon dioxide laser treatment of actinic cheilitis. Mayo Clin Proc 1988; 63:294-296.
67. Scheinberg RS. Carbon dioxide laser treatment of actinic cheilitis. West J Med 1992; 156:192-193.
68. Whitaker DC. Microscopically proven cure of actinic cheilitis by CO_2 laser. Lasers Surg Med 1987; 7:520-523.
69. Frankel DH. Carbon dioxide laser vermilionectomy for chronic actinic cheilitis. Facial Plast Surg 1989; 6:158-161.
70. David LM. Laser vermilion ablation for actinic cheilitis. J Dermatol Surg Oncol 1985; 11:605-608.
71. Brauner GJ, Schliftman AB. Treatment of pigmented lesions of the skin with alexandrite laser. Lasers Surg Med 1992; 12(suppl 4):72.
72. Goldberg D. Benign pigmented lesions of the skin: treatment with the Q-switched ruby laser. J Dermatol Surg Oncol 1993; 19: 376-379.
73. Taylor CR, Anderson RR. Ineffective treatment of refractory melasma and postinflammatory hyperpigmentation by Q-switched ruby laser. J Dermatol Surg Oncol 1994; 20:592-597.
74. Greenbaum SS, Krull EA, Watnich K. Comparison of CO_2 laser and electrosurgery in the treatment of rhinophyma. J Am Acad Dermatol 1988; 18:363-368.
75. Wheeland RG, Bailin PL, Ratz JL. Combined carbon dioxide laser excision and vaporization in the treatment of rhinophyma. J Dermatol Surg Oncol 1987; 13:172-177.
76. Ratz JL, Bailin PL, Wheeland RG. Carbon dioxide laser treatment of epidermal nevi. J Dermatol Surg Oncol 1986; 12:567-570.
77. Hohenleutner U, Wlotzke U, Konz B, Landthaler M. Carbon dioxide laser therapy of a widespread epidermal nevus. Lasers Surg Med 1995; 16:288-291.
78. Apfelberg DB, Maser MR, Lash H, et al. Superpulse CO_2 laser treatment of facial syringomata. Lasers Surg Med 1987; 7:533-537.
79. Wheeland RG, Bailin PL, Kronberg E. Carbon dioxide (CO_2) laser vaporization for the treatment of multiple trichoepithelioma. J Dermatol Surg Oncol 1984; 10:470-475.
80. Apfelberg DB, Maser MR, Lash H, White DN. Treatment of xanthelasma palpebrum with the carbon dioxide laser. J Dermatol Surg Oncol 1987; 13:149-151.
81. Wheeland RG, Bailin PL, Kantor GR, et al. Treatment of adenoma sebaceum with carbon dioxide laser vaporization. J Dermatol Surg Oncol 1985; 11:861-864.
82. Olbricht SM. Use of the carbon dioxide laser in dermatologic surgery: a clinically relevant update. J Dermatol Surg Oncol 1993; 19:364-369.
83. Fitzpatrick RE, Goldman MP. Resurfacing of photodamage of the neck using the UltraPulse CO_2 laser. Lasers Surg Med 1997; 20(suppl 9):33.
84. Kilmer SL, Chotzen V, Calkin J, et al. Resurfacing of the neck with the CO_2 UltraPulse. Lasers Surg Med 1999; 24(suppl 11):24.
85. Goldberg DJ, Meine JG. Treatment of photoaged neck skin with the pulsed erbium:YAG laser. Dermatol Surg 1998; 24:619-621.
86. Unger WP, David LM. Laser hair transplantation. J Dermatol Surg Oncol 1994; 20:515-521.
87. Fitzpatrick RE. Laser hair transplantation: tissue effects of laser parameters. Dermatol Surg 1995; 21:1042-1046.
88. Unger WP. Laser hair transplantation, part III: computer-assisted laser transplanting. Dermatol Surg 1995; 21:1047-1055.
89. Ho C, Nguyen Q, Lask G, Lowe N. Mini-slit graft hair transplantation using the Ultrapulse carbon dioxide laser handpiece. Dermatol Surg 1995; 21:1056-1059.
90. Hitzig GS, Schwinning JP, Handler SL. Linear grafting using a modified slot method: introducing the linear punch. Dermatol Surg 1996; 22:788-792.
91. Unger WP. Laser hair transplantation, part II. Dermatol Surg 1995; 21:759-765.
92. Unger WP. Laser hair transplantation, part I. Dermatol Surg 1995; 21:186-187.
93. Goldberg DJ. Topical carbon suspension potentiated Q-switched Nd:YAG laser resurfacing of rhytides. Lasers Surg Med 1997; 20(suppl 9):31.
94. Nelson JS, Milner TE, Dave D, et al. Clinical study of non-ablative laser treatment of facial rhytides. Lasers Surg Med 1997; 20(suppl 9):32.
95. Goldberg DJ, Whitworth J. Laser skin resurfacing with the Q-switched Nd:YAG laser. Dermatol Surg 1997; 23:903-907.
96. Zelickson BD, Kilmer SL, Bernstein E, et al. Pulsed dye laser therapy for sun damaged skin. Lasers Surg Med 1999; 25:229-236.
97. Rubenstein R, Roenigk HH Jr, Stegman SJ, Hanke WC. Atypical keloids after dermabrasion of patients taking isotretinoin. J Am Acad Dermatol 1986; 15:280-285.
98. Hayes DK, Stambaugh KI. Viability of skin flaps subjected to simultaneous chemical peel with occlusive taping. Laryngoscope 1989; 99:1016-1019.
99. Hayes DK, Berkland ME, Stambaugh KI. Dermal healing after local skin flaps and chemical peel. Arch Otolaryngol Head Neck Surg 1990; 116:794-797.
100. Alt TH. Technical aids for dermabrasion. J Dermatol Surg Oncol 1987; 13:638-648.
101. Lowe NJ, Lask G, Griffin ME. Laser skin resurfacing: pre- and posttreatment guidelines. Dermatol Surg 1995; 21:1017-1019.
102. Kilmer SL, Chotzen V, Calkin J, et al. Full face laser resurfacing utilizing topical anesthesia alone. Lasers Surg Med 1999; 24(suppl 11):30.
103. Mullarky MB, Norris CW, Goldberg ID. The efficacy of the CO_2 laser in the sterilization of skin seeded with bacteria: survival at the skin surface and in the plume emissions. Laryngoscope 1985; 95:186-187.
104. Ross EV, Mowlavi A, Barnette D, et al. The effect of wiping on skin resurfacing in a pig model using a high energy pulsed CO_2 laser system. Dermatol Surg 1999; 25:81-88.
105. Ruiz-Esparza J, Barba Gomez JM. Long-term effects of one general pass laser resurfacing: a look at dermal tightening and skin quality. Dermatol Surg 1999; 25:169-173; discussion 174.
106. David LM, Sarne AJ, Unger WP. Rapid laser scanning for facial resurfacing. Dermatol Surg 1995; 21:1031-1033.

107. Goldman MP, Manuskiatti W. Combined laser resurfacing with the 950-microsec pulsed CO_2 + Er:YAG lasers. Dermatol Surg 1999; 25:160-163.
108. Fitzpatrick RE, Williams B, Goldman MP. Preoperative anesthesia and postoperative considerations in laser resurfacing. Semin Cutan Med Surg 1996; 15:170-176.
109. Alster TS, Garg S. Treatment of facial rhytides with a high-energy pulsed carbon dioxide laser. Plast Reconstr Surg 1996; 98: 791-794.
110. Bernstein LJ, Kauvar ANB, Grossman MC. The short- and long-term side effects of carbon dioxide laser resurfacing. Dermatol Surg 1997; 23:519-525.
111. Ho C, Nguyen Q, Lowe NJ, et al. Laser resurfacing in pigmented skin. Dermatol Surg 1995; 21:1035-1037.
112. Weinstein C. Ultrapulse carbon dioxide laser removal of periocular wrinkles in association with laser blepharoplasty. J Clin Laser Med Surg 1994; 12:205-209.
113. Manuskiatti W, Fitzpatrick RE, Goldman MP. Long-term effectiveness and side effects of carbon dioxide laser resurfacing for photoaged facial skin. J Am Acad Dermatol 1999; 40:401-411.
114. Sriprachya-Anunt S, Fitzpatrick RE, Goldman MP, Smith SR. Infections complicating pulsed carbon dioxide laser resurfacing for photoaged facial skin. Dermatol Surg 1997; 23:527-535.

CHAPTER 20

Blepharoplasty

BRIAN S. BIESMAN
MAMI AIELLO IWAMOTO

SECTION ONE

History and Scientific Review

DEFINITIONS

Blepharoplasty refers to the excision of excessive eyelid skin and muscle, with or without the removal or repositioning of orbital fat, performed for functional or cosmetic reasons. The procedure is designed to improve conditions such as steatochalasis, or steatoblepharon, referring to prominence of periocular fatty tissue, or dermatochalasis, a term describing age-associated development of excess eyelid skin. Dermatochalasis should be differentiated from blepharochalasis, a familial, idiopathic condition characterized by recurrent, transient episodes of eyelid edema. This rare condition, occurring more often in younger women, may lead to dermatochalasis if the lid skin becomes stretched and redundant following repeated bouts of edema. Blepharoptosis, or ptosis, refers to an abnormally low upper eyelid position relative to the superior edge of the cornea (corneoscleral limbus) when the eye is in a straight-ahead position (primary gaze). Normally, the upper eyelid margin rests 2 mm below the superior corneal limbus. Ptosis is classified by onset (congenital or acquired) and by etiologies: myogenic (affecting levator muscle and superior tarsal, or Müller's muscle), aponeurotic (such as dehiscence of the levator muscle aponeurosis), neurogenic (conditions such as myasthenia gravis, abnormalities of the sympathetic nerves to Müller's muscle or of the oculomotor nerve to levator muscle), mechanical (neoplasms weighing down the lid), or traumatic (injury to the levator muscle or tendon).

The lower lid margin normally rests at or 1 mm above the inferior corneal limbus and protects the inferior ocular surface when the eyes are in primary gaze. Inferior scleral show refers to the condition where the white sclera is visible between the inferior limbus and the lower eyelid margin. Such a finding suggests the presence of horizontal lid laxity, orbicularis muscle denervation (as in facial nerve paresis), prominent globes, shallow orbits, or internal eyelid scarring and contraction due to trauma or prior surgery. This condition should be differentiated from ectropion, a term used to refer to the rotation of the lid margin away from the globe. Ectropion may occur as a result of involutional horizontal eyelid laxity, contraction from postsurgical scarring, excessive resection of lower eyelid skin, injury to the zygomatic branch of the facial nerve, and other etiologies.

BACKGROUND AND HISTORY

The medical literature from the first century AD contains references to excess upper lid skin and its surgical treatment. Aulus Cornelius Celsus (25 BC to AD 50), Roman philosopher in the first century, described the treatment of a "relaxed eyelid" *(palpebrae laxioris)*.[1] Although he had not distinguished between ptosis and dermatochalasis, portions of the surgery described are quite similar to that of modern blepharoplasty.[2,3] Von Graefe in 1809 performed an eyelid reconstruction termed *blepharoplastik* (*blepharon,* Greek, meaning eyelid; *plastos,* Greek, meaning formed).[4] He is credited with having introduced the meaning of *plastic* into the surgical literature.[2]

A.W. Sichel, in 1844, was the first to describe eyelid "herniated orbital fat," but did not suggest surgical treatment.[5] Indeed, in an era prior to the 1840s when operations were performed with only alcohol or opium for anesthesia, surgery was undertaken for mostly functional indications. Nitrous oxide was introduced by H. Wells in 1844 for use in dentistry, and ether by C.W. Long in 1849 for use during surgery.[5] In 1867, J. Lister published his landmark article "On the Antiseptic Principle in the Practice of Surgery."[6] Charles Conrad Miller is credited with having published the first book on cosmetic surgery in 1907,[7] which in a revised version[8] contained diagrams of incisions in the upper lid crease and subciliary region for upper and lower lid transcutaneous blepharoplasty, respectively. One of the first women to contribute to cosmetic surgery was Suzanne Noël, who in 1926 published a book enriched with photodocumentation, thereby introducing the critical role of photography in the practice of cosmetic surgery.[5] Interest in cosmetic surgery occurred not only in Europe and America, but also in Asia. Methods for cosmetically altering the Asian upper eyelid crease were proposed by Sayoc in 1954 and Pang in 1961.[9,10]

The continued evolution of blepharoplasty techniques over the subsequent seven decades is well documented.[2,3] The 1970s were noted for the awareness of potential complications associated with blepharoplasty, including dry eye syndrome and lower eyelid malposition. Techniques incorporating concurrent horizontal lower lid tightening and later transconjunctival approaches were introduced subsequently.

Carbon dioxide laser technology has also been applied to blepharoplasty since 1980.[11] The prevailing opinion in the 1980s was that carbon dioxide lasers produced too much thermal damage to be useful in cutaneous surgical procedures.[12] Interest in laser-assisted blepharoplasty was restored with the introduction of newer lasers in the 1990s. Surgery could be performed quickly and efficiently and yielded equally satisfactory results, leading to more widespread acceptance of laser incisional surgery as a viable technique in certain clinical settings. With the availability of a variety or incisional devices, such as cold steel, radiofrequency knife, monopolar cautery, long-pulsed Er:YAG laser, and carbon dioxide laser, the instrumentation becomes a personal choice made by each surgeon.

Until recently, blepharoplasty was characterized as a subtractive surgery, consisting primarily of removing skin, muscle, or fat. A greater emphasis on fat preservation and the conceptualization of the eyelid as an integral part of the upper face or mid face are part of the newest trends in blepharoplasty techniques.[13,14] The role of carbon dioxide laser resurfacing as an adjunct to blepharoplasty was first introduced in 1994 by Weinstein.[15] This underscored the concept that a combination of procedures may be necessary to achieve a more comprehensive facial rejuvenation effect and that incisional surgery established the "foundation" in creating structural improvements. Chemical peeling and laser resurfacing achieve skin quality improvements that cannot otherwise be attained with surgery alone. Chemical peels and laser resurfacing techniques are reviewed elsewhere in this book. Elements critical in optimizing results after blepharoplasty include careful preoperative patient evaluation, comprehensive discussion of potential treatment options, emphasis of the benefits and limitations of blepharoplasty surgery, attention to those anatomic factors that may predispose an unsatisfactory outcome, and execution of a well-planned and technically sound procedure.

BASIC SCIENCE

An understanding of the topographic anatomy of the periocular, upper, and mid facial regions and the anatomy of involutional changes is of paramount importance in planning blepharoplasty surgery. Knowledge of surgical anatomy of the eyelids, anterior orbit, upper face, and mid face is fundamental in performing blepharoplasty effectively and safely.

Topographic Anatomy: Features of Youth and Age, Signals of Expression

The impression of aging is conveyed by changes in both the skin and soft tissue structures overlying the bony skeleton. The dynamic configuration of periorbital skin and soft tissue structures imparts expression to the face in general, and the eyes in particular.

Skin. Aging changes in the skin are characterized by development of rhytides, pigmentary or textural abnormalities, and loss of elasticity.16 Because skin quality is not altered by blepharoplasty surgery, adjunctive therapies such as dermabrasion, chemical peeling, or laser skin resurfacing may need to be incorporated into rejuvenation strategies.

Forehead and Eyebrows. The forehead (from the hairline to the eyebrow) has an approximate vertical span of 51 m in women and 58 mm in men.[17,18] Dynamic horizontal forehead rhytides may indicate compensatory eyebrow elevation and should be relaxed to properly evaluate the forehead and eyebrow anatomy. The eyebrows normally rest at or above the superior orbital rim. In the upper third of the face (from the hairline to the upper lid), soft tissue aging changes manifest as forehead rhytides, glabellar furrows, or eyebrow descent.[19] Since the eyebrow is contiguous with the upper eyelid skin, brow ptosis will affect the eyelid folds.

There are several gender specific characteristics in the eyebrows. For example, the male brow normally has a flatter configuration than the arched female brow. Cilia in the male brow are typically thicker and more numerous than in the female brow. The subbrow fat pad, also known as submuscular fibroadipose layer or retro-orbicularis oculi fat (ROOF), may be more pronounced in males, although the size and position of this fat pad differs with gender and age. In general, fullness of eyebrow soft tissue tends to be a more masculine feature. Excessive prominence in the temporal aspect of the eyebrow and upper lid region is characteristic of Grave's disease, but may simply reflect involutional descent of the ROOF fat into the upper lid within the plane between the orbicularis muscle and the orbital septum (Fig. 20-1).

Eyebrow configuration is a powerful communicator of moods. Raising the eyebrows produces a surprised look, while lowering of the medial eyebrow may give the impression of anger or sternness, particularly when accompanied by visible glabellar frown lines. Generalized drooping of the eyebrows may signal sadness or fatigue, especially when the downward displacement aggravates hooding of upper eyelid skin.

There is no single "correct" resting position or shape of the eyebrow, and concepts of "normal" vary with gender and race. In general the male eyebrow rests at the level of the orbital rim and the female eyebrow lies superior to the orbital rim. The eyebrows tend to be more arched in women, peaking between the lateral limbus and lateral canthus meridians. Eyebrows positioned below the superior rim are considered to be ptotic. Another frame of reference is the distance from the inferior border of the eyebrow cilia to the upper eyelid margin, which centrally should be 10 mm. Any amount less than this suggests eyebrow ptosis. Aesthetically acceptable exceptions to this rule are common.[20] In eyebrow ptosis the upper eyelid skin is compressed downward, producing the impression of dermatochalasis. Eyebrow lift alone may correct the apparent skin excess or may need to be combined with upper lid blepharoplasty. Blepharoplasty without correcting significant coexistent eyebrow ptosis only drags the eyebrow further downward, worsening the upper lid crowding and resulting in a cosmetically unacceptable outcome.

Upper Eyelid and Palpebral Dimensions. The upper eyelid edge normally rests 2 mm below the superior corneal limbus. The maximal distance between the upper and lower eyelids (vertical palpebral dimension) with the eyes in primary (straight ahead) position is 9 to 12 mm. Abnormalities in the upper eyelid position should be recognized, since underlying etiologies may need to be evaluated or the conditions corrected. In individuals with eyelid retraction, the lid margin rests higher than normal and simulates "staring" or signals "surprise" (Fig. 20-1). Those individuals with ptosis have a narrowing of the vertical palpebral dimension, imparting a "sleepy" appearance.

The upper eyelid crease is usually 9 to 12 mm above the central lid margin in adult Occidental women and 8 to 10 mm above the lid margin in adult Occidental men[21] (Fig. 20-2). The upper lid crease in Asian individuals is lower, usually in the range of 2 to 5 mm from the eyelid margin. There are additional anatomic differences between Asian and Occidental eyelids.[22,23] The lid crease is created by the anterior insertion of the levator aponeurosis into the orbicularis and dermis. The distance from the eyelid crease to the inferior border of the eyebrow should be approximately twice the distance from the eyelid margin to the eyelid crease.

The lid fold represents the skin and orbicularis muscle that drape over and obscure the lid crease when the eye is in primary position. Excessive folding or hooding may result from dermatochalasis, brow ptosis, or both. Affected individuals may perceive a sensation of lid "heaviness," early fatigue with reading or watching television, and even loss of peripheral vision, a finding easily demonstrated on visual field testing.

The superior sulcus is the region between the superior orbital rim and the eye. In young or thin individuals, the sulcus may be flat or concave. Sulcus fullness may be due to orbital fat herniation or generalized lid edema. In patients with both concave and convex sulcus areas, liposculpting or fat distribution should be performed to even the sulcus definition and avoid exacerbating a peaked appearance.

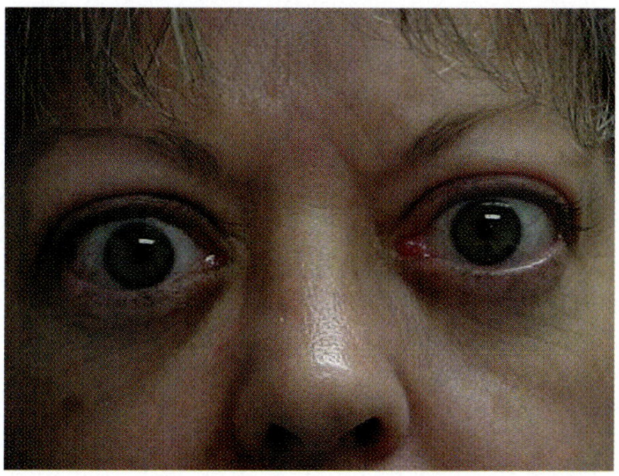

FIG. 20-1
Bilateral upper eyelid retraction caused by dysthyroid orbitopathy.

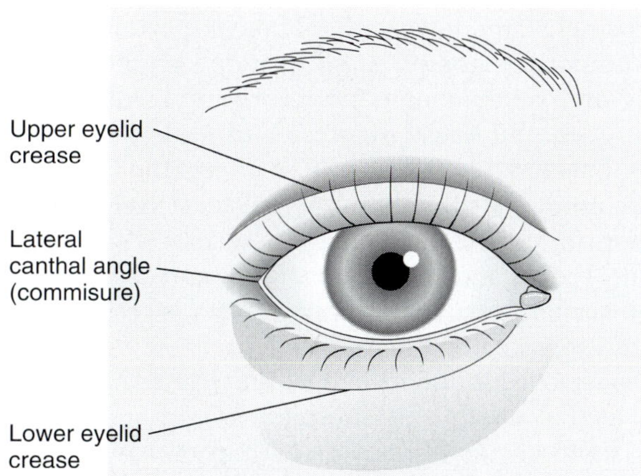

FIG. 20-2
Topographical features of the eyelids. The lateral canthus approximately 2 mm higher than the medial canthus.

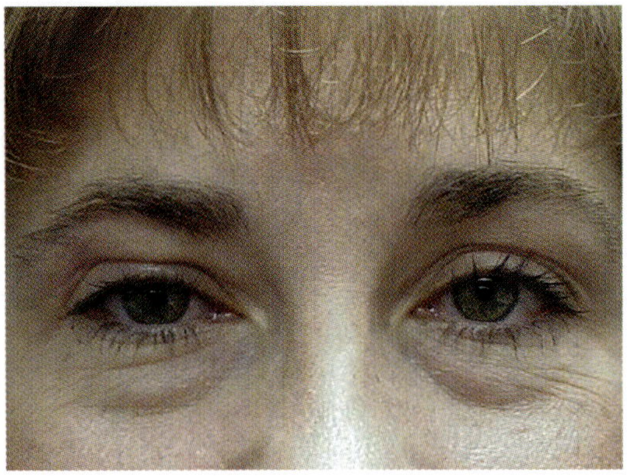

FIG. 20-3
Prominent inferior orbital fat in a 45-year-old woman.

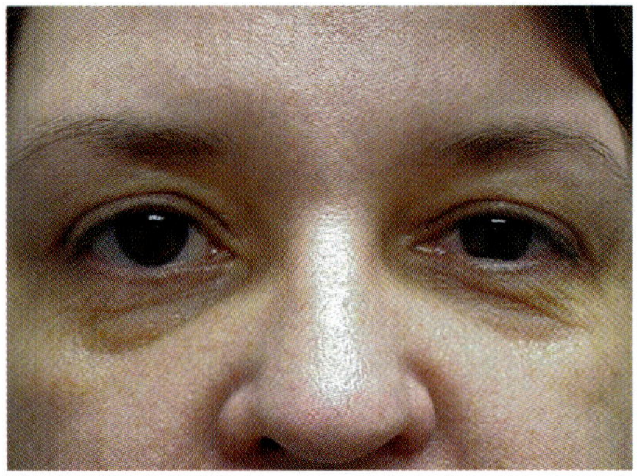

FIG. 20-4
A 40-year-old woman with a prominent nasojugal tear trough deformity.

The horizontal width of the palpebral fissure from medial to lateral canthi is approximately 28 to 30 mm.[24] The lateral canthal angle is situated approximately 2 mm higher than the horizontal meridian of the medial canthal angle. Involutional lowering of the lateral canthal angle can produce a "sad" look.

Lower Eyelid and Mid Face. Normally, the lower lid margin covers the inferior corneal limbus. With increasing age, there is a tendency for the lid to bow downward and rest at a lower position, sometimes resulting in scleral show.[25] In youth, the lower lid contour is generally flat or concave. Over time, the lower lid fatty tissue may protrude anteriorly, resulting in steatoblepharon and creating the impression of "bags under the eyes" that may signal "fatigue" (Fig. 20-3). The lower eyelid fatty tissue appears clinically to protrude in three zones, conceptualized as medial, central, and temporal compartments.[26] However, anatomic studies indicate that there is actually no division and there exists a single large lower orbital fat compartment.[27,28]

Additional signs of aging include progressive skin laxity and subcutaneous fat resorption leading to descent of the midfacial structures (middle third of the face). This downward migration affects the lower eyelid anatomy, creating a nasojugal tear trough, malar festoon, or a decrease in cheek projection (Fig. 20-4). In profile, the lid and cheek lose the smooth contour transition seen in youth and adopt a "double convex" configuration, discussed in detail later.

Dark circles in the nasojugal areas of the lower lids and medial canthus (periorbital hyperpigmentation) may represent epidermal or dermal melanin deposition.[29] These dark circles give a strong impression of "fatigue." In the presence of steatoblepharon, the shadow from the convex lid contour often worsens the appearance of periorbital hyperpigmentation. The fatty prominence and thus only the shadowing can be eliminated with appropriate lower eyelid blepharoplasty techniques, but the dark circles will remain. The areas of skin discoloration may occasionally be surgically removed.[30] Treatment with combinations of lasers offers additional potential options.[31] Makeup concealers are an acceptable remedy, the efficacy of which is further enhanced by improving the lower lid contour surgically or improving the quality of skin with resurfacing techniques.

SURGICAL ANATOMY

Eyebrows and Upper Eyelids

The eyebrows are composed of four layers: skin, muscle, fat, and aponeurosis. The skin is thick and glandular and contains prominent cilia in a characteristic distribution. Medially, the cilia are directed superiorly. In the central upper region the cilia become oriented inferotemporally (30 degrees from the vertical meridian), and in the lower half of the brow, they are directed superotemporally (30 degrees upward from the vertical meridian).[32]

Eyebrow movement is controlled by the occipitofrontalis, orbicularis oculi, corrugator supracilii, depressor supercilii, and procerus muscles. The frontalis muscle has vertically oriented fibers and is the primary brow elevator. Its fibers interdigitate with the orbital orbicularis muscle laterally, with the procerus muscle medially, and with the corrugator and depressor supracilii muscles inferiorly. It inserts into the skin at the level of the brow cilia.[33,34] The eyebrow depressors include the obliquely oriented corrugator supracilii muscle, which lies posterior to the frontalis and orbicularis muscles, originates from the superior-medial orbital rim, and inserts into the skin where fibers of all three muscle fibers interdigitate. Contraction of the corrugator supracilii alone results in elevation of the head of the brow; as the corrugator usually cocon-

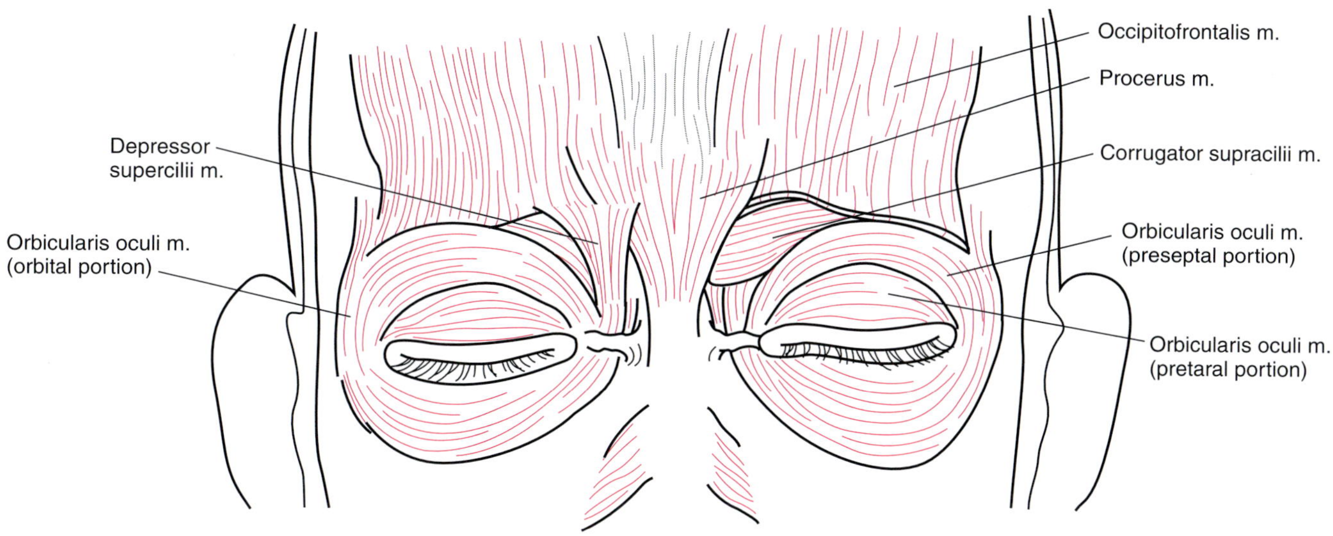

FIG. 20-5
Muscles controlling eyebrow movements. These muscles may be modified during blepharoplasty or brow lift surgery.

tracts with the depressor supracilii, with the net result being downward movement of the medial portion of the brow, it is generally considered a brow depressor. Contraction of the corrugator contributes to the development of vertical glabellar furrows. The procerus—a pyramid-shaped muscle arising from tendinous fibers and fascia overlying the inferior portion of the nasal bone and the superior lateral portion of the nasal cartilage—inserts into the skin and subcutaneous tissue between the eyebrows. The procerus lies in the same plane as the occipitofrontalis muscle, and its contraction pulls down the medial eyebrows and wrinkles the nasal skin in a transverse fashion. The depressor supracilii is a powerful brow depressor that arises from the medial portion of the orbicularis muscle. As mentioned previously, its fibers interdigitate with those of the corrugator supracilii prior to their insertion in the subcutaneous tissue subjacent to the head of the brow (Fig. 20-5).

The central aponeurotic layer of the scalp, the galea aponeurotica, splits into two layers to envelop the occipitofrontalis muscle. The superficial layer forms the anterior sheath and a deep layer forms the posterior sheath of the frontalis muscle. This deep layer splits again to envelop the eyebrow fat. The posterior layer is firmly attached along the medial half to two thirds of the superior orbital rim but is loosely attached laterally. For this reason, eyebrow ptosis is more common temporally.

The presence of a fat layer along the inferior and lateral portions of the eyebrow enhances eyebrow mobility.[33] With aging, this fat may descend into the upper eyelid, where it is referred to as the submuscular fibroadipose layer[34] or the ROOF (Fig. 20-6). This fat prolapses anterior to the orbital septum and thus can be distinguished from preaponeurotic or retroseptal fat. During surgery to reduce this fat pad, great care must be taken to preserve a layer above the periosteum and below the dermis. Failure to do so will fix the brow to the periosteum, producing a depression that is prominent and difficult to repair.

Upper Eyelid Anatomy

The upper eyelid skin is the thinnest in the body and overlies a minimal layer of subcutaneous tissue. Deep to this is found the orbicularis oculi muscle, a strong, circular sphincter with concentrically arranged fibers whose primary function is to close the eyelids. The orbicularis muscle is divided into three regions: orbital, preseptal, and pretarsal. Superiorly, the orbital portion blends with the frontalis, procerus, and corrugator supraciliaris muscles (see Fig. 20-5). Laterally the orbicularis overlies the superficial temporalis fascia. Inferiorly the fibers cover the origins of the muscles that elevate the nasal ala and upper lip. Medially the orbital orbicularis fibers arise from the superomedial orbital rim and nasal bones. The preseptal orbicularis fibers originate from the medial canthal tendon and arc laterally, overlying the orbital septum in the upper and lower eyelids before joining to form the lateral canthal tendon. The pretarsal orbicularis muscle is located immediately anterior to the tarsal plate, a firm structure formed by compressed collagen fibers. The eyelids are suspended by derivatives of the orbicularis muscle, the medial and lateral canthal tendons. Disruption or

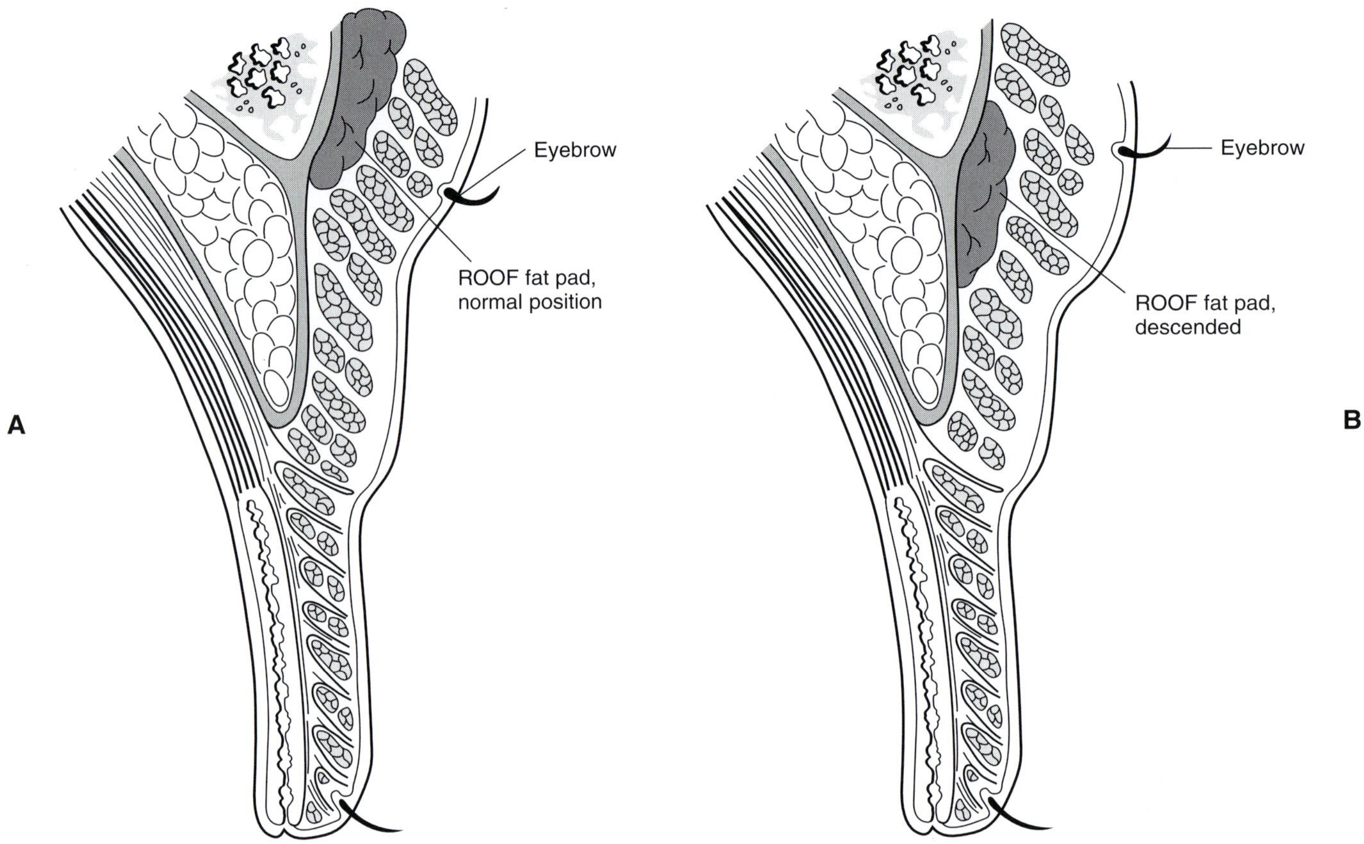

FIG. 20-6
A, Normal position of retro-orbicularis oculi fat (ROOF) pad. **B,** With the onset of involutional changes the ROOF fat may descend into the upper eyelid.

marked laxity of either of these structures will result in eyelid malposition or canthal deformities.

The orbital septum, a firm, fibrous structure found deep to the preseptal orbicularis oculi muscle, arises from a thickened region of the orbital rim periosteum known as the arcus marginalis and extends toward the tarsal plates where it fuses with the levator aponeurosis (Fig. 20-7). The location of this fusion varies between Asian and Occidental eyelids.[35] The orbital septum acts as a divider between intraorbital and extraorbital structures. Laterally, the septum is contiguous with the lateral canthal tendon and the lateral horn of the levator aponeurosis. The septum ordinarily serves as a barrier that keeps the orbital fat in a posterior position relative to the orbital rim. The surgical importance of the septum is that it should be distinguished from the levator aponeurosis in the upper lid. If opened surgically or found to be naturally dehisced, the orbital septum should not be sutured closed. Trapping the orbital septum into a wound can lead to vertical contraction and restriction of eyelid excursion.

Immediately posterior to the orbital septum in the upper eyelid lies the central or preaponeurotic fat pocket, one of two upper eyelid fat pads. This fat pocket is an extremely useful landmark in eyelid surgery, as it always lies anterior to the levator muscle and its aponeurosis. The anterior-posterior separation between the orbital septum and the levator aponeurosis is greatest just below the superior orbital rim, and it is at this location that the septum should be opened during eyelid surgery if the risk of injury to deeper structures is to be minimized. The preaponeurotic fat pad (located posterior to the orbital septum) should be distinguished from fat found anterior to the septum (submuscular fat) in Asians or ROOF fat descended into the eyelid, an involutional change. The yellow preaponeurotic fat is separated from the pale yellow or white nasal fat by the interpad septum. The nasal fat pad is located medial and inferior to the trochlea of the superior oblique muscle and care should be taken when dissecting in this portion of the eyelid (Fig. 20-8).

The levator muscle arises from the greater wing of the sphenoid and, through its tendinous aponeurosis, is the primary retractor of the upper eyelid (Fig. 20-9). Damage to or dehiscence of the levator tendon will result in ptosis. The levator complex exerts its effect via two insertions, a broad band that fuses onto the anterior-superior third of the upper eyelid tarsal plate, and

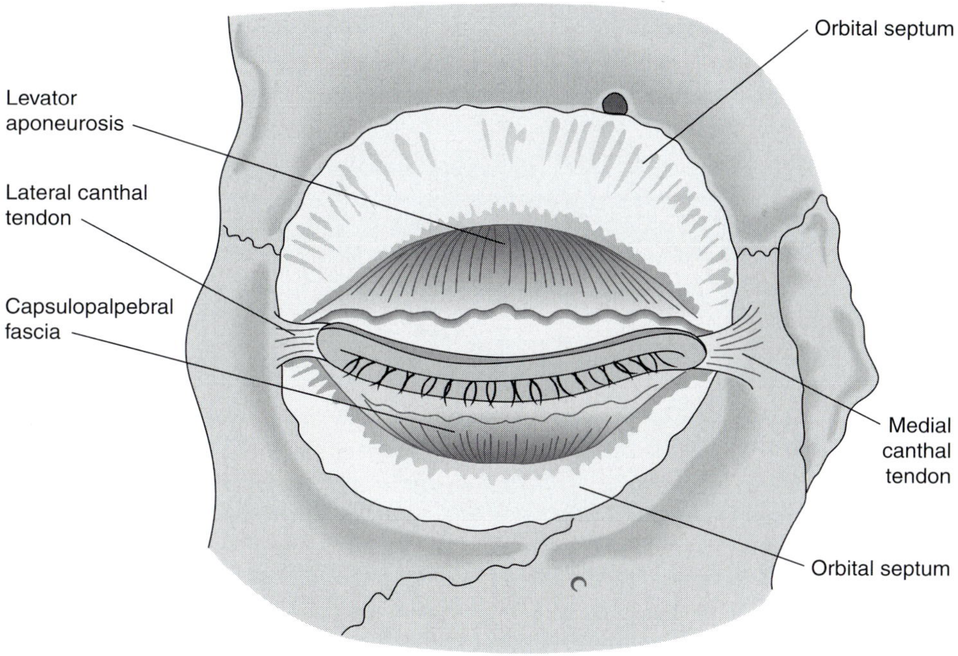

FIG. 20-7
Anatomy of the orbital septum. Note that the septum fuses with the levator aponeurosis in the upper eyelid and the capsulopalpebral fascia in the lower eyelid.

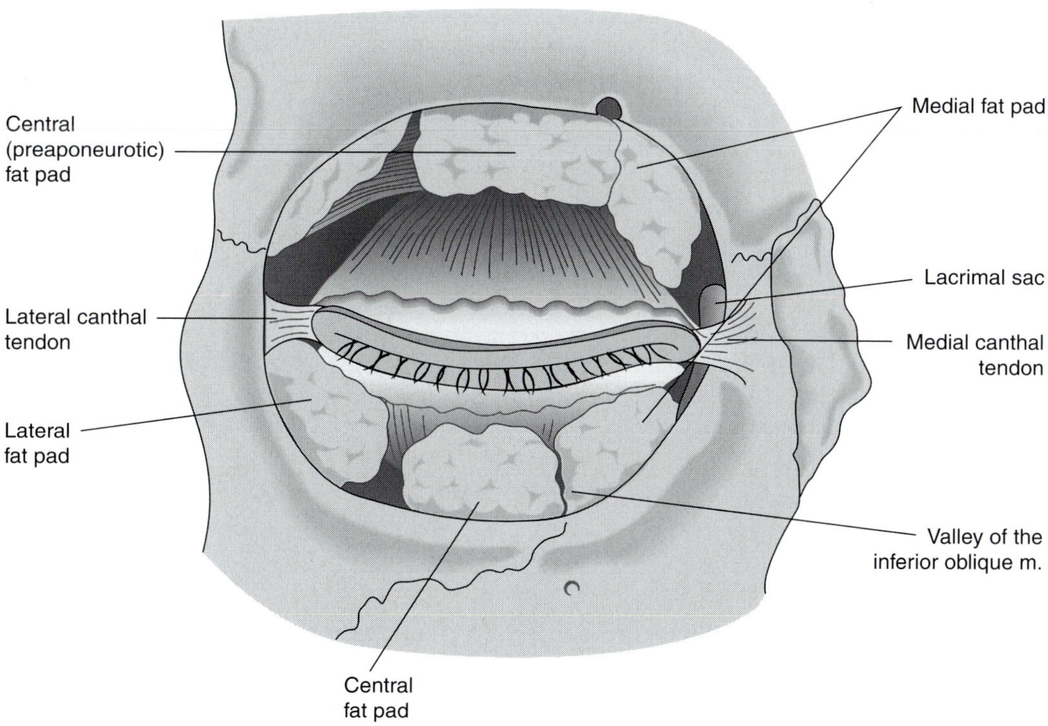

FIG. 20-8
Distribution of the anterior orbital fat pads. There are two pads in the upper eyelid and three in the lower lid.

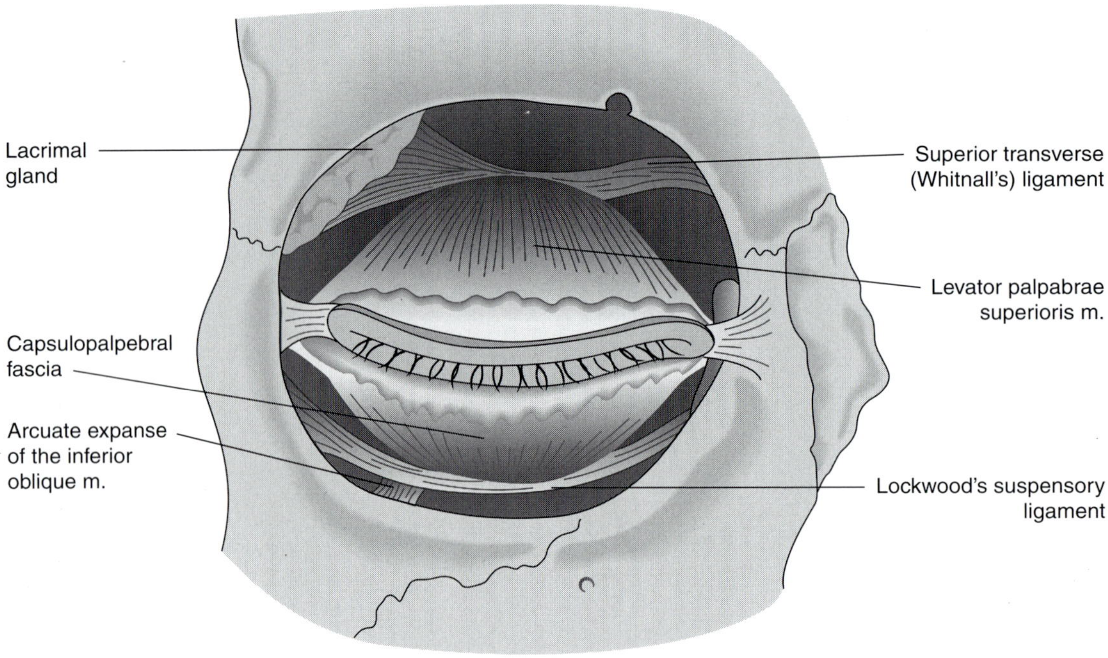

FIG. 20-9
Anatomy of the primary upper and lower eyelid retractors and their suspensory ligaments.

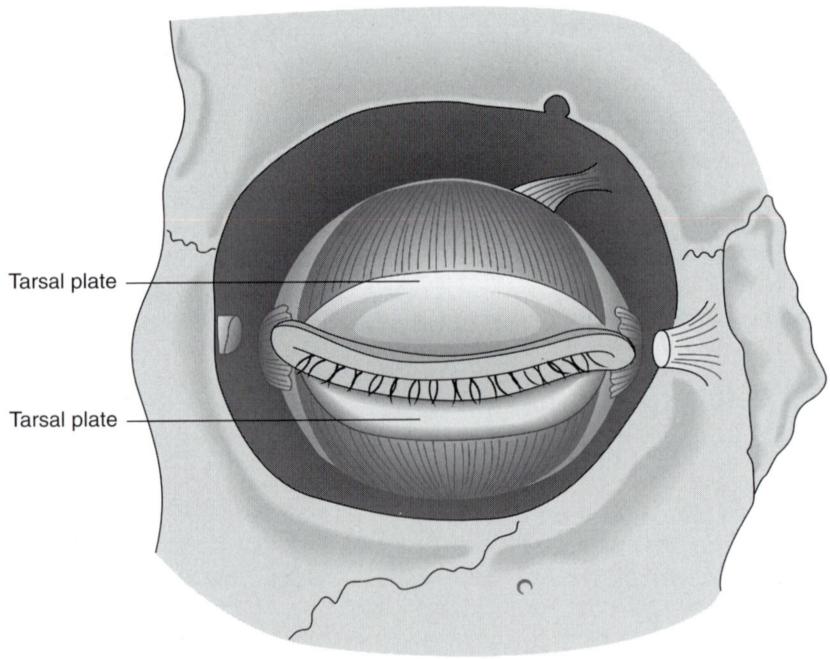

FIG. 20-10
The upper and lower tarsal plates are collagenous structures that provide mechanical support to the eyelids.

a series of fine leaflets extending through the orbicularis oculi muscle that insert onto the skin approximately 8 to 10 mm above the eyelid margin. These attachments result in close approximation of the skin to the tarsal plate and form a clearly visible line known as the upper eyelid crease. This is the usual position of the inferior border of a blepharoplasty incision. The tarsal plates themselves are collagenous structures that serve to provide mechanical support to the eyelids. The upper lid tarsus has a greater vertical dimension than its lower lid counterpart (10 vs. 4 mm) (Fig. 20-10). Müller's muscle is a sympathetically innervated smooth muscle that originates high in the orbit beneath the levator aponeurosis and inserts onto the superior tarsal border (Fig. 20-11). It is a secondary elevator of the eyelid whose effect can be most easily appreciated

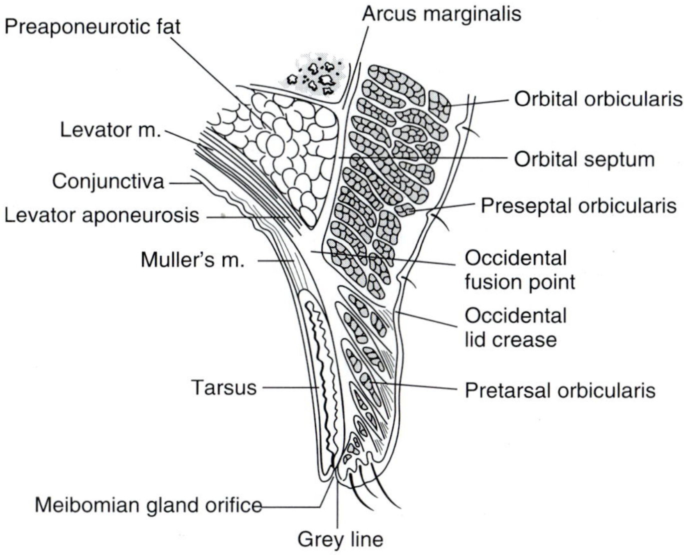

FIG. 20-11
Sagittal view of an occidental upper eyelid. Note position of Müller's muscle and the anteriorly directed leaflets of the levator aponeurosis that insert into the skin to form the upper eyelid crease.

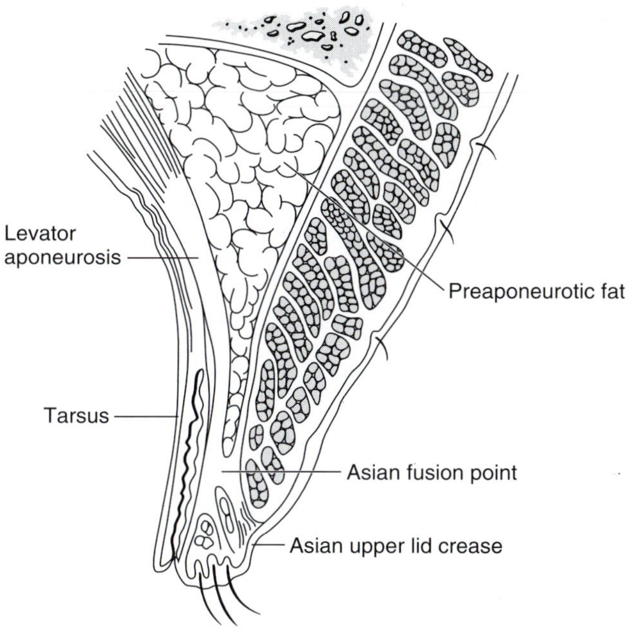

FIG. 20-12
Sagittal view of an Asian upper eyelid. Note the low position at which the orbital septum fuses with the levator aponeurosis, the preaponeurotic fat anterior to the tarsus, and the low position of the eyelid crease.

in patients with Horner's syndrome in which the sympathetic innervation to the orbit is interrupted due to a lesion in the superior cervical spine, apex of the lung, or the neck. The upper and lower eyelids are lined by a thin, transparent membranous structure known as the conjunctiva. The conjunctiva functions to protect, lubricate, and support the ocular surface.

The difference in appearance between Occidental and Asian eyelids is primarily a reflection of anatomic differences between the orbital septum and its relationship to the levator aponeurosis and the location and distribution of fat. These differences between the Asian and Occidental upper eyelids can be appreciated in cross-section. In the Asian lid, the orbital septum fuses with the levator aponeurosis at a location often well below the superior tarsal border and anterior to the tarsal plate (Fig. 20-12). It is for this reason that some Asian lids have low or even absent eyelid creases.[36,37] Necessarily following from the low fusion of the septum and levator, the preaponeurotic fat pad lies nearer the lid margin in the Asian lid imparting an appearance of greater fullness.[37] Further contributing to this "thickened" appearance is a submuscular fat pad that often spans the upper lid above the superior tarsal border. This fat pad is not found in Occidental lids and is well known as a source of confusion to surgeons not accustomed to operating on Asian lids.

Lower Eyelid Anatomy

The upper and lower eyelids are analogous structures. That is, each structure found in the upper eyelid has a counterpart in the lower eyelid. For example, Müller's muscle in the upper eyelid is analogous to a sympathetically innervated smooth muscle in the lower lid known as the inferior tarsal muscle. Similarly, the levator complex is the primary elevator of the upper eyelid and has as its lower lid counterpart the capsulopalpebral fascia (CPF), a thick fibrous tissue that is the primary lower eyelid retractor (see Fig. 20-9). As the levator aponeurosis and orbital septum fuse before inserting into the tarsal plate on the upper eyelid, the CPF and septum fuse prior to inserting into the lower lid tarsus.

The capsulopalpebral head emanates from the inferior rectus muscle and divides to envelop the inferior oblique muscle. After rejoining anteriorly as Lockwood's suspensory ligament, further extension anteriorly and superiorly from this point is known as the capsulopalpebral fascia. Lockwood's ligament is attached to the medial orbital wall and to the lateral orbital wall, where it forms part of the lateral retinaculum, consisting of the lateral horn of the levator aponeurosis, lateral canthal tendon, Lockwood's ligament, and the check ligament of the lateral rectus muscle. A portion of the capsulopalpebral fascia inserts onto the inferior tarsal border and the conjunctival fornix (suspensory ligament of the fornix), and at a level ranging from 3 to 5 mm inferior to the tarsus is fused with the orbital septum. The inferior tarsal muscle is found between the capsulopalpebral fascia and conjunctiva.

The inferior orbital fat pads appear clinically to be three distinct pads, a white or light-colored nasal pad, and more typical yellow central and lateral fat pockets (see Fig. 20-8). In fact, the lateral fat pocket seems to be subdivided into two pads, one adjacent to the central fat and the other located more posterior and lateral to the first. Interestingly, dye injection studies fail to demonstrate these divisions and suggest that anatomically the inferior orbital fat lies in one large compartment.[26,27] The inferior oblique muscle separates medial and central fat pads. This muscle originates from the anterior medial orbital floor, just posterior to the lacrimal sac fossa and passes laterally and posteriorly to insert onto the inferolateral globe. The arcuate expansion of the inferior oblique muscle is a fascial band extending from the inferior oblique muscle to the inferolateral orbital rim and appears to separate the central from the lateral fat areas. This structure may be surgically divided during transconjunctival lower lid blepharoplasty to facilitate exposure of the lateral fat compartments. The lateral fat pad is thought to consist of a more obvious anterior portion and another slightly posterior and lateral fat pad.[38]

Midfacial Region Superficial Muscular Aponeurotic System

The midfacial region is bordered above by the inferior orbital rim and below by the mouth.[39] The superficial muscular aponeurotic system (SMAS), a distinct fibromuscular layer contiguous throughout the head and neck, is thought to transmit contractions of the facial muscles to the skin, thus facilitating facial expression. The SMAS is stabilized by its attachments to the orbital rim superiorly and the body of the zygoma and the zygomatic arch laterally.[40] Inferiorly the SMAS is continuous with the platysma muscle and in the medial portion of the midface it is less well defined.[41,42] Attenuation of the SMAS itself and the connections between the SMAS and its overlying skin are believed to account for some of the involutional changes occurring in the aging face.

The malar and nasojugal folds have been described, indicating a region where a fascial extension attaches the orbital rim through the orbicularis muscle to the skin.[43] The orbitomalar ligament represents the collagen and elastin fiber attachments extending from periosteum along the inferior orbital rim, through the submuscular fat and orbicularis oculi muscle, and inserting into the skin.[40,44] The orbitomalar ligament has been noted to elongate with age, contributing to the sagging appearance of malar folds commonly known as festoons with advancing age. In addition, the descent of midfacial soft tissue exposes the contour of inferior orbital rim, leading to a nasojugal "tear trough" deformity.

Subcutaneous fat is found both anterior and posterior to the SMAS (Fig. 20-13). The pre-SMAS fat is more prominent in the buccal and malar regions and less thick in the forehead. The malar fat pad is an area of thickened subcutaneous (pre-SMAS) fat shaped like a triangle with its base along the nasolabial fold and the

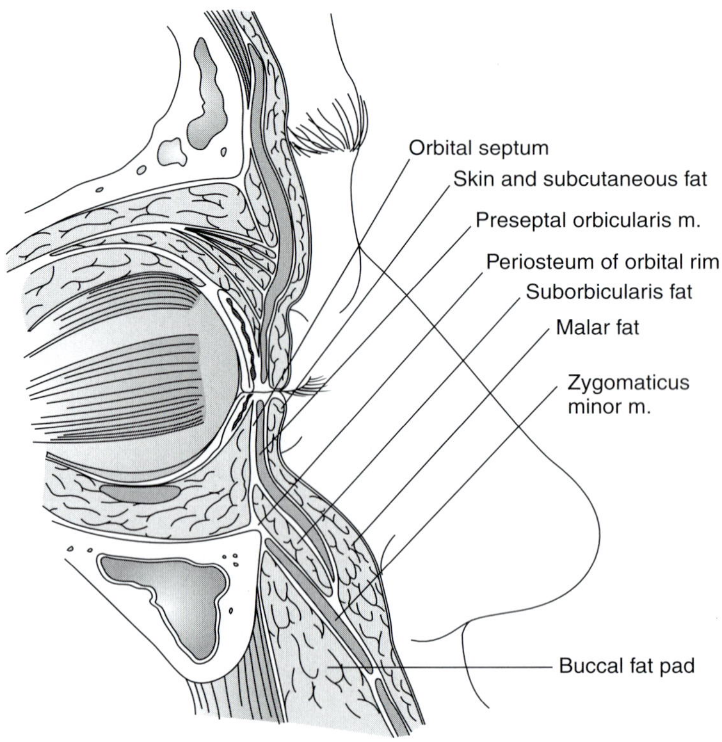

FIG. 20-13
Schematic drawing of midfacial anatomy.

apex pointing toward the zygoma.[45] This fat pad is adherent to the overlying skin and underlying SMAS in youth. The sub-SMAS adipose tissue is also pronounced in the malar region. Of note, anatomic studies have demonstrated continuity of sub-SMAS fat such that the ROOF and SOOF (see next paragraph) are site-specific terms for a contiguous anatomic layer.[40]

Age-related changes in the lower eyelid and midfacial regions have been described by various terms suggesting downward migration, including festoons, mounds, and bags[46] (Fig. 20-14). With the effects of time and gravity, elastic fibers in both the dermis and the SMAS degenerate and weaken. The malar fat pad remains more closely adherent to the overlying skin and thus descends in a plane anterior to and independent of the SMAS.[47] A similar phenomenon occurs in a deeper, sub-SMAS fat layer known as the suborbicularis oculi fat pads (SOOF).[48] Both the SMAS and SOOF attach to the inferior border of the orbicularis oculi muscle, and when they migrate inferiorly the orbicularis muscle is stretched inferotemporally, resulting in a redundant fold below the inferior orbital rim known as a malar festoon or malar bag.[42] Festoons must be differentiated from prominence of the orbital fat, as these conditions often coexist. When viewed sagitally, orbital fat produces a bulge above the inferior orbital rim while malar festoons create a bulge below the rim. When these findings are present simultaneously, a "double convexity" deformity results.[49] Involutional changes in the midface must be recognized and addressed so as to permit adequate rejuvenation at the time of blepharoplasty surgery.

VASCULATURE

Internal and External Carotid Artery Supply

The arterial supply to the eyelids and face is composed of anastomosing branches from the internal and external carotid arteries. The internal carotid artery, through its ophthalmic artery branch and then terminal branches (dorsal nasal, supratrochlear, supraorbital, and lacrimal arteries), contributes to the blood supply of the eyelids. Important branches from the external carotid artery include the facial, the superficial temporal, and the internal maxillary arteries. The facial artery courses along the nasolabial fold and is called the angular artery in the medial canthal area. The artery then perforates the orbital septum and anastomoses with branches of the ophthalmic artery. The superficial temporal artery supplies many of the collateral vessels in the scalp. As the artery courses in a plane anterior to the temporalis muscle, it gives rise to three branches: the frontal, the zygomaticofacial, and the transverse facial arteries, which anastomose with the lacrimal and supratrochlear branches of the facial artery in the lower eyelid. The internal maxillary artery becomes the infraorbital artery and exits the infraorbital foramen to supply blood to the lower eyelid and anastomose with terminal branches of the dorsal nasal artery.

Eyelid Vascular Arcades

In the upper eyelid, the peripheral arcade, located at the upper tarsal border, and the marginal arcade, coursing

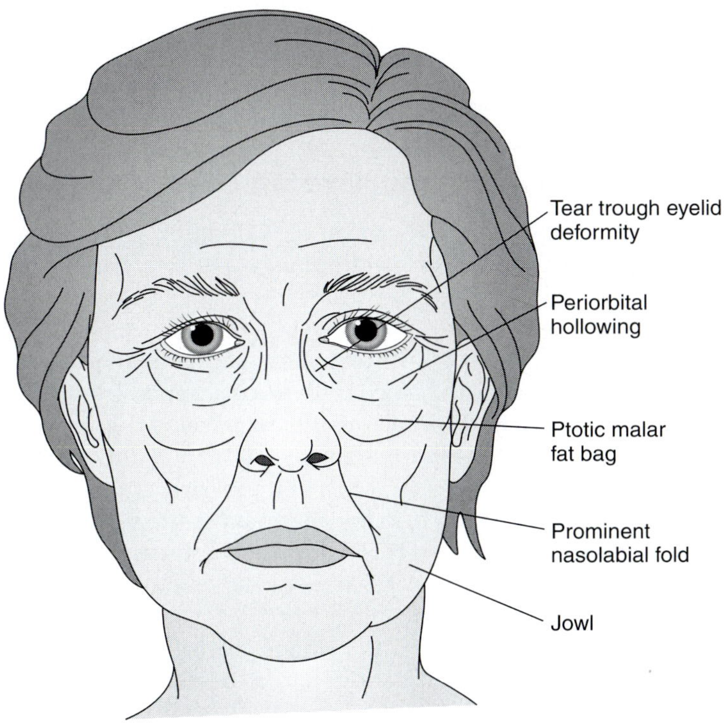

FIG. 20-14
Typical age-related changes as manifest in the periorbital region, mid face, and lower face.

anterior to the tarsus 2 to 3 mm from the eyelid margin, are supplied medially by the medial palpebral artery and laterally by the lacrimal artery. In the lower eyelid, the inferior palpebral artery is located at the inferior border and anterior surface of the tarsus. Medially the arcade is supplied primarily by the angular artery branch of the facial artery in addition to branches of the infraorbital artery, and laterally there are anastomoses with the lacrimal and zygomaticofacial branch of the anterior deep temporal artery.[50]

Veins

The venous system also forms superficial and deep orbital anastomoses in the periocular region. The anterior facial vein, comprising the main superficial venous system, roughly parallels but lies superficial and lateral to the course of the facial artery. In the medial canthal region, it is called the angular vein, which then becomes the supratrochlear vein, forming deeper anastomoses in the superonasal orbital region with the supraorbital vein. The angular, supraorbital, and supratrochlear veins join to form the superior ophthalmic vein, which continues posterolaterally in the orbit through the superior orbital fissure to enter the cavernous sinus.[51] Since the orbital veins lack valves, facial infections can potentially spread posteriorly into the cavernous sinus through these venous communications.

Lymphatics

In the eyelid, the lymphatic channels are composed of deep and superficial systems. The deep lymphatic plexuses along the tarsal borders drain the tarsal and conjunctival areas. The superficial lymphatics drain the eyelid skin and orbicularis oculi muscle. Lymphatics drain from the medial aspect of both upper and lower eyelids and medial conjunctiva into the submandibular lymph nodes through channels that course along the angular and facial arteries. Most of the upper eyelid and the lateral half of the lower eyelid and the lateral half of the conjunctiva drain into the superficial preauricular nodes and into the deeper cervical nodes. There are no lymph nodes or vessels in the orbit itself.

Nerves

The eyelids are innervated by the facial (cranial nerve VII), trigeminal (CN V), and sympathetic nerves. The ophthalmic and maxillary divisions of CN V provide cutaneous and deep sensory innervation to the upper two thirds of the face and orbit. The ophthalmic division divides into three main branches (frontal, lacrimal, and nasociliary nerves), which enter the orbit through the superior orbital fissure. The lacrimal nerve innervates the lacrimal gland, conjunctiva, and lateral upper lid. The frontal branch divides into the supraorbital and supratrochlear nerves. The supratrochlear nerve supplies the trochlear, medial upper lid, and forehead regions. The supraorbital nerve exits the orbit through the supraorbital notch and innervates most of the forehead. The nasociliary branch divides into the posterior and anterior ethmoidal nerves to the ethmoid sinuses, long ciliary nerves to the iris, cornea, and ciliary muscle, a sensory root to the ciliary ganglion, and the infratrochlear nerve to the medial upper lid skin.

The maxillary division of the trigeminal nerve is divided into the infraorbital, zygomatic, sphenopalatine, and posteriosuperior alveolar nerves. The zygomatic branch divides into the zygomaticofacial nerve to the cheek skin and the zygomaticotemporal nerve to the lateral forehead. The infraorbital nerve supplies the lower lid skin and conjunctiva, nasal skin and septum, and upper lip skin and mucosa.

The facial nerve supplies motor innervation to the muscles of facial expression, including the orbicularis oculi, procerus, corrugator supercilii, and frontalis muscles. The facial nerve branches into the temporal, zygomatic, buccal, mandibular, and cervical divisions. The temporal division gives rise to the frontal branch innervating the frontalis muscle. This nerve courses in a predictable plane within the temporoparietal fascia.[52] The temporal, zygomatic and buccal divisions overlap in innervation to the orbicularis oculi muscle.

The sympathetic nerves to the orbit are responsible for pupillary dilation, vasoconstriction, and hidrosis. Branches also innervate the infratarsal muscle of the lower lid and Müller's muscle of the upper lid. The parasympathetic nerves enter the eye as the short posterior ciliary nerves after synapsing in the ciliary ganglion. The innervation is responsible for accommodation (ciliary muscle) and pupillary constriction (pupillomotor fibers).

CLINICAL STUDIES

Historical Perspective on Laser Surgery

Cutaneous incisional carbon dioxide laser surgery was first performed with continuous wave lasers that produced a 1 mm diameter beam some three decades ago. The wounds produced by these early devices had decreased tensile strength, an increased rate of dehiscence, and in many cases healed with an unacceptable appearance. These undesirable results were related in part to the broad zone of thermal injury (200 to 500 μm) created at the wound edges.[53,54] Most of these early studies evaluated incisions made in the abdomen or the extremities, regions in which the blood supply is limited relative to the head and neck. Subsequent experience identified areas of rich blood supply as those best suited to use of carbon dioxide lasers as cutaneous incisional devices. Superpulsed carbon dioxide lasers produced a smaller zone of thermal injury than their continuous wave counterparts, and some of the higher-powered superpulsed lasers are used today for a variety of incisional applications including cutaneous surgery. Despite the availability of superpulsed lasers in the late 1980s, few surgeons used the carbon dioxide laser to perform cutaneous incisional surgery until the mid-1990s.

Interest in cutaneous carbon dioxide laser incisional surgery reemerged in the early 1990s, in part because of the introduction of a carbon dioxide laser that used a radiofrequency pulsing technique to produce a beam with a peak power of approximately 500 watts, far greater than earlier devices. This device, known by the trade name UltraPulse (Lumenis, Santa Clara, CA), produced a high-frequency pulsed beam that made incisions with a smaller zone of thermal injury than was previously possible. This laser cut soft tissue with a pulsed beam whose frequency and energy could be independently varied to achieve the ideal blend of cutting and coagulation. Even when operated in "continuous wave" mode this laser produced a pulsed beam with a frequency of 1000 to 3000 Hz. The UltraPulse also produced a small (0.2 mm) diameter beam that made it more useful for working in the periorbital region. When it was used properly, surgery could be performed quickly, intraoperative hemostasis and visualization of delicate anatomic structures were dramatically improved, and the zone of thermal injury surrounding the laser incisions was only about 115 μm.[55] Consequently, when these wounds healed, they were usually indistinguishable in appearance from cold steel wounds. In an effort to further reduce the risk of complications, in 1998 Sciton (Palo Alto, CA) began adapting an Er:YAG laser to produce soft tissue incisions. This device, known as the Contour, cuts soft tissue by alternately firing two laser heads. A short-duration (<1 ms) ablative pulse is followed immediately by a long-duration (up to 8 ms) coagulative pulse, producing a beam 0.25 mm in diameter. This device produces a relatively hemostatic incision with a surrounding zone of thermal injury measuring approximately 70 μm, some 40% smaller than that produced by carbon dioxide lasers.[56] The disadvantage of the Contour as an incisional device is that it cannot operate with the high frequency of the UltraPulse laser and thus cuts tissue much more slowly. It also produces so much tissue splatter that the lens in the distal portion of the handpiece often requires cleaning during surgery. Efforts remain under way to improve these deficiencies.

Clinical Perspective

Proponents of laser incisional surgery find that soft tissue surgery may be performed more efficiently and, in some cases, more effectively with lasers than with standard techniques. There are several reasons for this. First, when used properly, the laser handpiece acts as three instruments: a cutting tool, a cautery, and a blunt dissection device. The intraoperative transfer of instruments and therefore total operating time are thus decreased. Second, intraoperative efficiency is increased further by the near absolute hemostasis that is often achieved when working in areas such as the periorbital region, where most blood vessels have an internal diameter of 0.5 mm or less. For this reason, the carbon dioxide laser has found its greatest incisional applications in the periorbital region. Third, dissection with the carbon dioxide laser in the eyelids and periorbital region allows surgery to be performed on delicate vascular structures such as the levator palpebrae superioris and the superior tarsal (Müller's) muscle with a lower risk of tissue distortion, functional impairment, or hematoma formation. Consequently, the use of lasers allows certain incisional procedures such as blepharoptosis repair or correction of eyelid retraction to be performed with greater precision.

One of the most important questions is whether using lasers to perform incisional procedures benefits the surgeon, the patient, both, or neither. The literature is decidedly unclear in attempts to answer this question. Anecdotal reports and small unmasked studies offer conflicting conclusions as to the benefit of lasers in blepharoplasty, the aesthetic procedure performed most often with lasers rather than traditional instrumentation.[57-60] Some authors report that the carbon dioxide laser offers little advantage over the scalpel,[61] whereas a survey comparing scalpel versus carbon dioxide laser blepharoplasty indicated benefits of using a laser, including quicker recovery time to usual activities (6.3 vs. 9.1 days) and shorter operating times (four-eyelid blepharoplasty times of 58 vs. 94 minutes).[62] Biesman, Buerger, Flaherty and colleagues have performed the only prospective, multicenter, double-masked study to address this issue. Ophthalmic plastic surgeons experienced in both laser-assisted and traditional techniques (at least 100 cases of each over the preceding 2 years) performed blepharoplasty procedures on 35 patients using laser on one side and cold steel on the other. The side treated with laser was randomly selected, and the patients were blinded to the surgeon's choice. Patients were examined 1, 2, and 4 weeks after surgery. Results were assessed by patient questionnaire and by evaluation of photographs by a skilled, masked observer. Two weeks after surgery there was no significant difference in the amount of swelling, discoloration, or wound appearance. This study did not evaluate surgical times (Biesman BS, Buerger DE, Yeatts P, et al., unpublished data).

Laser Incision Histology and Its Clinical Correlates

The carbon dioxide laser produces a zone of irreversible thermal injury (coagulative necrosis) along the wound edge, an observation that has been correlated with the well-recognized delay in the rate of laser wound healing, postoperative wound dehiscence, and unacceptable scarring (Fig. 20-15). As long as these tissue effects are recognized and understood, postoperative problems can be avoided. For example, laser incisions should be made parallel to relaxed skin tension lines. This will allow wounds to be closed with the least amount of tension, thus reducing the risk of unacceptable scarring. Similarly, cutaneous laser incisions should be placed in areas such as the head and neck that have a rich blood supply. When closing cutaneous laser wounds, absorbable suture materials should be avoided, as the coagulative necrosis produced by the laser, in conjunction with the inflammation stimulated by the suture material, can produce wounds with an unacceptable appearance. Nonreactive sutures, such as nylon or polypropylene, should be left in place for 7 to 10 days.

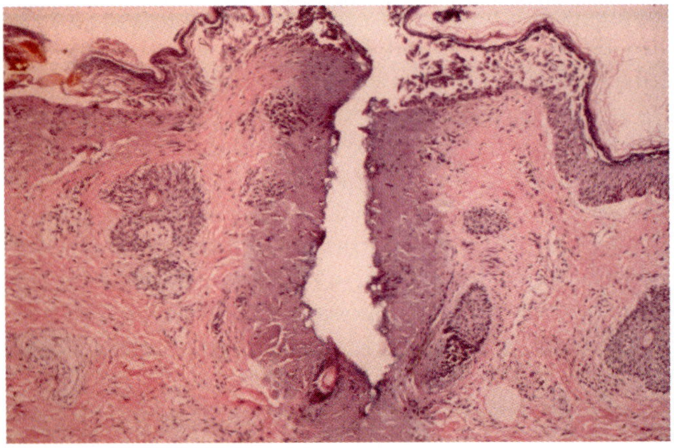

FIG. 20-15
A zone of thermal injury measuring approximately 115 μm is created by a high-frequency pulsed carbon dioxide laser when used to cut human eyelid skin.

Soft-tissue effects can vary widely with the type of laser system used (Table 20-1). High-frequency pulsed lasers such as the Nidek UniPulse or Lumenis UltraPulse, when used with a 0.2 mm focused handpiece, produce a zone of thermal injury measuring approximately 110 μm. The long-pulsed Er:YAG laser maintains good hemostasis with an even smaller zone of thermal injury (about 70 μm), but this advantage is offset by a slower rate of cutting. Critics of laser incisional surgery have argued that using cold steel avoids thermal damage entirely. This approach requires use of bipolar cautery or other means of achieving hemostasis, all of which produce thermal injury.

Table 20-1 Relative Zones of Thermal Injury Associated with Various Incisional Devices

Device	Settings	Injury Zone (μm)	Comment
Scalpel	n/a	0	Various studies
UltraPulse CO_2, 0.2 mm focused spot (Biesman)	5 watts, 15 mJ, 333 pulse/s, 1 cm/s speed	110	Human eyelid skin
UltraPulse CO_2 in CW mode, 0.2 mm focused spot (Biesman)	6 watts, CW mode (i.e., 3000 Hz), 1 cm/s speed	115	Human eyelid skin
Microneedle electrocautery (Farnworth)	Valley Lab, blend 1, 40 watts	180	Rat skin necrosis
Superpulse CO_2, 0.22 mm focused spot (Schroder)	10 watts, 500-700 Hz, 150 μs pulse	200	Pig skin thermal injury
Standard needle electrocautery (Farnworth)	Valley Lab, blend 1, 40 watts	250	Rat skin necrosis
Shaw scalpel (Farnworth)	220°F	250	Rat skin necrosis
Standard needle electrocautery (Schroder)	Valley Lab, blend 2, 50 watts	250	Pig skin thermal injury
True CW CO_2 (Schroder)	10 watts, 0.22 mm focused spot	300	Pig skin thermal injury
Contact Nd:YAG (Schroder)	14 watts, CW mode, 0.2 mm frosted tip sapphire	350	Pig skin thermal injury
Contact CW CO_2 (Fuller)	Nonfrosted tip sapphire	300-500	Manufacturer data

Note: All measurements are for one side of the incision only.

From Khan J, Biesman BS. Laser incisional surgery. In: Biesman BS, ed. Lasers in Facial Aesthetic and Reconstructive Surgery. Philadelphia: Lippincott Williams & Wilkins, 1999.

COMPLICATIONS OF BLEPHAROPLASTY

Understanding the potential complications associated with blepharoplasty will allow the surgeon to more effectively reduce the risk of adverse sequelae. A more comprehensive discussion of such complications is published in review articles.[63] The following is a summary of the important problems and the mechanisms by which they exert their effect.

Vision Loss

Surgeons should be aware of the catastrophic potential for vision loss following blepharoplasty surgery. While one survey estimated this complication to occur in 0.04% of all blepharoplasties,[64] the exact frequency in not known. In the English language literature, more than 75 cases of postblepharoplasty blindness, mostly associated with lower lid surgeries, have been reported.[63]

The mechanism for vision loss is often related to orbital hemorrhage (Fig. 20-16). The compressive effect of hemorrhage in the orbit causes increased intraorbital and intraocular pressure, which compromises the vascular supply to the eye, specifically the retina, and optic nerve. The source of the hemorrhage is controversial and is traditionally believed to be due to excessive manipulation of anterior orbital fat with subsequent transmission of force to posterior orbital vessels.[65] Systemic risk factors for uncontrolled hemorrhage include hypertension, atherosclerosis, use of anticoagulants or aspirin, and bleeding dyscrasias. Postoperative hematomas develop usually within 24 hours of surgery.[66] Activity restrictions should be emphasized especially during the immediate postoperative period. Patients may note significant pain, asymmetric swelling, proptosis, and visual dimming. Vision loss from hemorrhage is an ophthalmic emergency and warrants urgent referral for ophthalmic intervention.

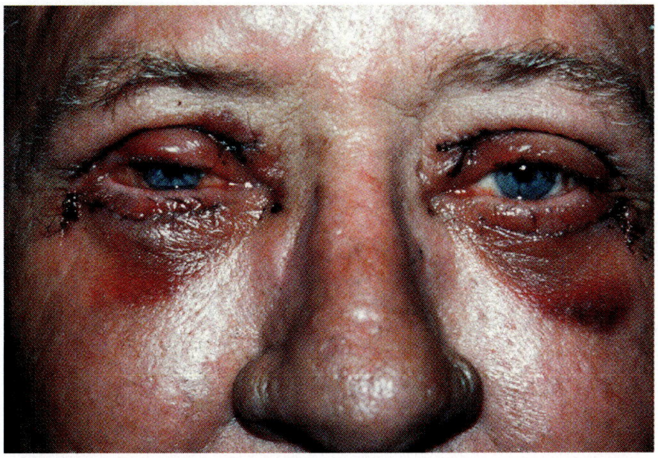

FIG. 20-16
Orbital hemorrhage following blepharoplasty surgery. Vision was not lost. (Courtesy Sterling Baker, MD.)

Mechanisms of visual injury other than hemorrhage include excessive vasospasm from epinephrine in the local anesthetic injection[67] and inadvertent globe injury during administration of local anesthesia[68] or laser-assisted surgery.[69]

Diplopia

Diplopia, or double vision, may be a transient or persistent complication resulting from interference with extraocular muscle function. The occurrence is rare, estimated to be 0.03% in one study,[70] and should be avoidable. Temporary diplopia may be caused by edema or local anesthetic injection effects on the extraocular muscles.[71,72] Often improvement is spontaneous and should be monitored by an ophthalmologist.

Persistent motility disturbances may result from direct or indirect injury to extraocular muscles or their innervation. The inferior oblique[70,73] is the muscle most frequently injured during blepharoplasty as it courses between the nasal and central fat compartments in the anterior orbit. By identifying the muscle, dissection and fat removal can be performed safely.[74] Damage to the superior oblique muscle, tendon, or trochlea may occur during aggressive liposculpting of the nasal fat pad in upper lid blepharoplasty.[73,75,76] Less common is surgical trauma to the inferior rectus muscle.[77]

Upper Lid Malposition

Temporary ptosis may result from postoperative edema. Persistent ptosis as a direct result of surgery is infrequent and may involve injury to the levator tendon,[78] levator muscle anesthetic toxicity,[71] or internal scarring that restricts lid mobility. If significant ptosis develops immediately after upper blepharoplasty, the wound should be explored and the levator muscle and its aponeurosis should be carefully inspected for disinsertion or transection.

Lagophthalmos, or incomplete eyelid closure, can be a temporary or permanent sequela of blepharoplasty. When related to postoperative edema or decline in orbicularis muscle tone, the condition should improve spontaneously within the first 1 to 2 weeks after surgery. The mechanism involved in persistent lagophthalmos may be vertical shortening from excess skin removal, inadvertent trapping of the orbital septum into the wound, or septal adhesions, all of which can limit eyelid excursion. As a result of the poor eyelid closure, the cornea and eye surface may become dry. Symptoms may include foreign body sensation, blurred vision, and tearing, which may accompany clinical findings of ocular injection or lid swelling. Topical artificial tear supplements in drop, gel, or ointment form may be necessary to protect the cornea. Massage or forced orbicularis closure may reduce mild postoperative lagophthalmos. Severe conditions may require surgical intervention, such as skin grafting or midface lifting.

Lower Lid Malpositions

Malposition of the lower eyelid is one of the most common postblepharoplasty complications[63] (Fig. 20-17). Findings may range from downward bowing with inferior scleral show to frank ectropion. Ectropion after blepharoplasty surgery occurs only when a transcutaneous approach has been employed. The most common etiology of postblepharoplasty lower eyelid ectropion is over resection of skin such that the downward vector created overrides the ability of the horizontal force vectors generated at the canthi to maintain an appropriate eyelid position.[79] This problem can largely be avoided by resecting eyelid skin only when the patient gazes upward with the mouth open, thus placing the lower lid skin on maximum stretch. Other etiologies include closure of the orbital septum within the wound, excessive cauterization of the septum or eyelid, hypertrophic scarring, and injury to the facial nerve. Temporary lower lid displacement may result from edema, hematoma, or reduced orbicularis muscle tone.[79,80] Conservative measures such as lid massage, orbicularis contraction exercises,[81] and artificial tear supplements and lubricants can be instituted. If the lids do not close completely and the eye is exposed, an ophthalmologist should monitor the patient and determine the need for corrective interventions.

If the lower eyelid does become ectropic after blepharoplasty surgery, it should be assessed for the presence of horizontal laxity. If present, the lid can usually be repaired by a simple tightening procedure performed at the lateral canthus. If the lid is not horizontally lax, then vertical lengthening of the lid will be required. Identifying the need for horizontal lid tightening and performing prophylactic measures before or at the time of blepharoplasty should reduce the risk of these secondary complications.

Incision Irregularities and Webbing

Eyelid crease asymmetries or improper placement of the incision are unsatisfactory results of blepharoplasty that should be avoided with careful preoperative planning. Webbing in the medial canthal region resembles an epicanthal fold and results from excessive medial skin excision or from vertical cicatrix if the upper lid incision extends too far inferomedially. In the lateral canthal region, webbing is the result of inadequate separation between the upper and lower blepharoplasty incisions (Fig. 20-18). If the conditions do not improve spontaneously or with conservative measures, then surgical intervention is indicated.

Incision line suture tracts or hypertrophic scarring may be avoided by careful skin closure using monofilament sutures and by removing sutures 3 to 5 days after surgery. Tissue adhesives, such as autologous fibrin glue[82] or *N*-butyl-2-cyanoacrylate,[83] may also reduce development of incision irregularities by eliminating the need for sutures. While this concept is appealing, tissue glue is not practical in most cases of cosmetic blepharoplasty due to discomfort, wound dehiscence, and possible failure to evert the wound edges. Suture milia are cystic elevations at the sites where suture passes into the skin; they emerge 1 week postsurgery and often remit spontaneously over a period of months.[84] Milia can occur with most sutures, including silk, mild chromic gut, and polypropylene. Subcuticular closure or early suture removal may reduce the occurrences.

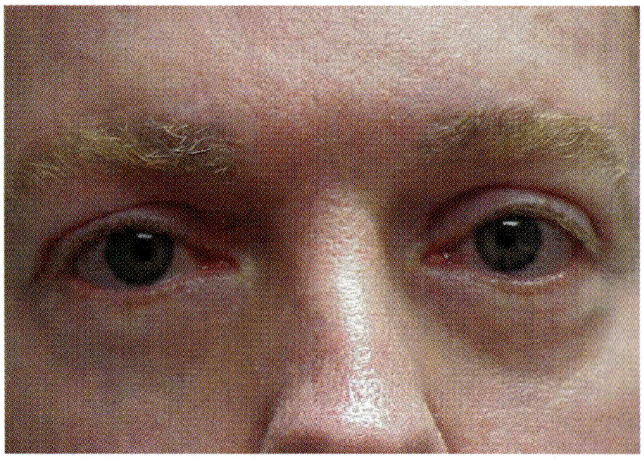

FIG. 20-17
Lower eyelid retraction and inferior scleral show following lower transcutaneous blepharoplasty.

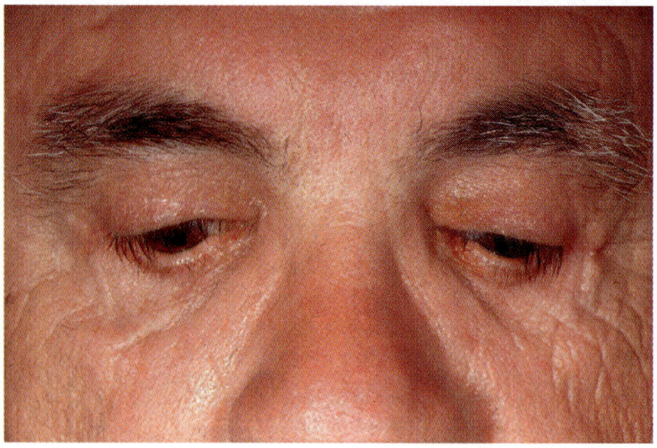

FIG. 20-18
Left lateral canthal webbing resulting from inadequate separation between upper and lower blepharoplasty incisions.

Overcorrection and Undercorrection

Aggressive removal of orbital fat in the upper lid may lead to a sunken superior sulcus. This is particularly undesirable in males as it imparts a feminine look. When fat is unevenly sculpted, the sulcus may have an irregular contour. Excessive excision of fat from the lower lids may result in undesirable lower lid concavity and can exaggerate visible contour of the orbital rim and nasojugal tear trough deformities. Free fat grafts have been used to correct the volume deficit, but variable degrees of fat absorption is common. Overcorrection of dermatochalasis by excessive skin or muscle removal was discussed earlier.

While possibly disappointing to the patient, undercorrection (referring to inadequate skin, muscle, or fat removal) has far fewer adverse sequelae and may be improved with carefully planned "touch-up" surgery. If there is apparent undercorrection of steatoblepharon, it is advisable to wait at least 3 months for complete resolution of tissue edema before proceeding with revisions.

Lacrimal Gland Prolapse and Injury

An estimated 10% to 15% of young individuals undergoing blepharoplasty have symmetrically or asymmetrically displaced lacrimal glands, although prolapse is considered an involutional process.[85] If a prolapsed lacrimal gland is not repositioned during upper lid blepharoplasty, residual lateral lid fullness will produce an unsatisfactory result. While a few surgeons routinely resect the prolapsed portion of the lacrimal gland, this practice should be avoided to reduce the risk of producing a pathologically dry eye.[26]

SECTION TWO

Atlas of Surgical Procedures

PREOPERATIVE CLINICAL CONSIDERATIONS FOR BLEPHAROPLASTY

Patient Communication and Counseling

The first step in evaluating a potential candidate for aesthetic surgery is establishing the patient's specific concerns, motivations, and ultimate expectations. The combination of a hand mirror and old photographs is the best way to demonstrate to a patient the involutional changes that have occurred in the periorbital region. Surgery should be avoided on those patients who are unable to describe their goals or expectations, whose expectations are unattainable or unrealistic, or who complain bitterly about other surgeons while heaping praise upon the examiner. The goal of the initial consultation is not only to determine whether a patient's concerns can appropriately be addressed via surgery, but also to allow the patient and surgeon to build rapport and to help the surgeon gain insight into the patient's personality and motivation for seeking aesthetic surgery.

Careful counseling of patients prior to blepharoplasty or other aesthetic procedures will help reduce postoperative confusion, misunderstandings, disappointment, or frustration. A careful discussion about the preparation for surgery, the relative risks and benefits of the contemplated procedure, and the expected postoperative recovery period is extremely important. The potential complications of surgery should be discussed openly and not minimized. Surgical consent forms may be given to patients for review at their leisure. Patients should be given realistic estimates of anticipated length of recovery time. Overestimations are better received than underestimations.

Preoperative Medical History

Patients should be asked about their general state of health, use of medications, and allergies. Medical conditions can affect eyelid appearance or may be associated with dry eye syndromes. Lid retraction, periocular fatty prolapse, and eyelid edema are commonly seen in Graves' disease. These individuals may undergo blepharoplasty as long as they have no orbital or ocular discomfort, decreased vision, conjunctival injection, or other symptoms of ocular disease, and their eyelid position and systemic thyroid state have been stable for at least 6 to 12 months. Abnormalities in eyelid position such as retraction may be addressed at the time of blepharoplasty surgery but must be carefully discussed during the preoperative consultation. Environmental allergies may induce periocular edema and therefore should be controlled prior to blepharoplasty surgery. Transient episodes of unilateral or bilateral eyelid swelling in younger individuals may suggest a relatively uncommon condition called blepharochalasis, a variant of hereditary angioedema.[86] Recurrent bouts may result in stretching and wrinkling of skin that ultimately leads to dermatochalasis. A history of rheumatoid arthritis or autoimmune disease may be associated with coexisting dry eye syndrome.

Every patient should be questioned about bleeding disorders or tendencies, use of aspirin, nonsteroidal anti-inflammatory agents, anticoagulants, chronic oral steroids, vitamin E, St. John's Wort, or garlic supplements in order to assess the relative risk for excessive intraoperative or postoperative bleeding (Box 20-1). The decision to discontinue blood-thinning agents at least 11 to 14 days preoperatively through the early postoperative period should be made in conjunction with the prescribing physician.

BOX 20-1 Aspirin and Aspirinlike Agents to Be Avoided Preoperatively

A.P.C.	Indocin
Advil	Measurin
Aleve	Meclomen
Alka Seltzer	Midol
Anacin	Monacet and Codeine
Ascodeen-30	Motrin
Ascriptin	Nalfon
Aspirin Suppositories	Naprosyn
Bayer Aspirin	Norgesic
BC Powders	Nuprin
Buff-A-Comp	Orudis
Buffadyne	Pabirin Buffered Tabs
Bufferin	Panalgesic
Butalbital	Percodan
Butazolidin	Persantine
Cama-Inlay Tabs	Persistine
Ceracol Capsules	Robaxisal
Clinoril	Sine-Off
Congespirin	SK-65 Compound Caps
Cope	St. John's Wort
Coricidin	Stendin
Darvon Compound	Stero-Darvon and A.S.A.
Dolobid	Supac
Dristan	Synalgos Capsules
Duragesic	Synalgos D. C.
Ecotrin	Tolectin
Emprazil	Triaminicin
Equagesic	Vanquish
Excedrin	Vitamin E
Feldene	Voltaren
Fiorinal	Zomac
Garlic Supplements	

Preoperative Ophthalmic History and Screening

Surgical candidates should be questioned about preexisting ocular diseases and the use of ophthalmic medications. Individuals with visual complaints (blurred vision, diplopia) or any ocular symptoms (including foreign body sensation, pain, itching, dryness, discharge) should be referred to an ophthalmologist before considering periocular surgery. In patients with an underlying dry eye condition, blepharoplasty should be approached conservatively with judicious removal of skin and orbicularis muscle so as to minimize impairment of eyelid closure. Patients should be warned of possible exacerbation of dry eye symptoms and temporary contact lens intolerance that may occur after any blepharoplasty procedure.[87]

Even in the absence of symptoms, basic assessment of vision (with a pocket eye chart), pupils (for size, reaction, and symmetry), and eye movement should be included for all patients. Certain findings should alert the surgeon to the potential for postoperative ocular complications. Redness or crusting of eyelid margins may indicate infection or inflammation and should be controlled preoperatively. Abnormalities in blink frequency or completeness of lid closure may increase the risk of corneal exposure problems after blepharoplasty surgery.

Surgical Goals and Planning

One of the objectives in a preoperative examination is to assess which anatomic features can or should be surgically altered to achieve the desired objective. Techniques in upper lid blepharoplasty are designed to excise and tailor redundant skin and orbicularis muscle and reduce contour fullness from herniated fat or other soft tissue. The lid crease can be defined or redefined, the pretarsal skin made more apparent, and the superior sulcus deepened. Eyelid edema from systemic causes or rhytidosis will not be eliminated surgically. In addition, abnormalities in upper eyelid position are not corrected by blepharoplasty.

Lower lid blepharoplasty traditionally has been regarded as a means of removing excess skin, orbicularis muscle, and fat. A younger individual demonstrating significant steatochalasis with good skin quality and no skin excess is well suited for a transconjunctival approach with the objective of reducing the excess projection of fat in profile view. In some individuals with a flat midface contour, even a relatively small amount of steatochalasis will be cosmetically unacceptable because of the shadowing from the lid convexity. The transconjunctival approach would be suitable in this situation. Even younger individuals may display a nasojugal tear trough deformity with a visible contour indentation along the inferior orbital rim. In these situations, fat removal alone would risk accentuating a sunken appearance, and fat-repositioning techniques can be employed through a transconjunctival incision.

Lower lid steatochalasis may be associated with skin redundancy, in which case a transcutaneous approach will permit horizontal tightening of the skin in addition to providing access to the fat for liposculpting. The presence of orbicularis hypertrophy, most apparent with an exaggerated smile, will require selective surgical or electrosurgical reduction of orbicularis prominence with or without skin removal. Older patients may demonstrate dermatochalasis, steatochalasis, and a nasojugal tear trough deformity created by involutional descent of midfacial structures. The transcutaneous approach will address the excess skin while fat repositioning and liposculpting will improve the transitional contour of the lower lid into the mid face.

A proptotic appearance may be due to large globes associated with high myopia, shallow or hypoplastic orbits, or true proptosis (exophthalmos, or anterior displacement of the globe) from orbital disorders such as thyroid disease, tumors, or inflammatory conditions. Although individuals with this appearance may also have steatochalasis or dermatochalasis, blepharoplasty must be considered with great caution; fat removal alone may exacerbate the "bulging eye" appearance, and excision of skin and orbicularis muscle may induce significant lower lid malposition or impair eyelids' ability to close. In certain situations, proptosis from thyroid disease may be addressed by orbital decompression or bony orbital advancement.

As discussed earlier, malar festoons must be distinguished from dermatochalasis and steatochalasis as blepharoplasty alone does not adequately address this problem. Malar festoons provide a challenging clinical problem. Direct excision techniques are effective but often leave objectionable scars. Aggressive resurfacing with the carbon dioxide laser, SOOF lifting, and midface lifting techniques have all been used with variable success to reduce festoons.

When planning blepharoplasty the surgeon should remain cognizant of the need to maintain a balanced overall appearance. Overly aggressive blepharoplasty performed on an elderly patient with full facial involutional changes may produce an unnatural postoperative appearance. When patients with aging stigmata of the upper and lower face seek blepharoplasty alone, they should be given the option of conservative blepharoplasty alone versus more aggressive blepharoplasty combined with other techniques such as upper and lower face lifting, chemical peeling, or laser skin resurfacing.

Photodocumentation

Photographs are important tools for preoperative documentation. Photographs will be required in order to obtain insurance compensation when surgery is being considered for improvement in visual function. Preoperative photographs are useful illustrative tools in preoperative discussions with patients. Intraoperatively they are useful as references to a patient's appearance in the upright position. Postoperative photographs are valuable for purposes of comparison. They are particularly helpful when patients are convinced that surgery produced particular findings that in fact were preexisting. Many patients become more attentive to their eyelid appearance after surgery and have forgotten their presurgical appearance.

The preoperative photographic series includes several different views. Typically, the patient is photographed in a full-face view (looking directly at the viewer with eyes opened naturally) incorporating the full face, "raccoon view" that includes both eyes, oblique or three-quarter angles, and a profile view. Front view images with the patient looking up or to the sides may illustrate areas of prominent fatty protrusion. Oblique or three-quarter angles may better capture the extent of temporal brow ptosis, upper lid dermatochalasis, or nasojugal troughs. Profile views are useful in illustrating globe prominence, upper lid hooding, lower lid steatochalasis, or double convexity deformity.

Preoperative Examination and Considerations in Upper Eyelid Blepharoplasty

The rigorous and systematic examination in preparation for upper eyelid blepharoplasty should include studying the forehead, orbital rim, brows, subbrow fat, lacrimal gland, fatty prolapse, upper lid crease, and upper lid position. The objective is to identify any features or abnormalities that may predispose an individual to unsatisfactory outcome. Such preexisting conditions may need to be addressed in order to safely and effectively proceed with blepharoplasty. Surgical plan should be formulated in the preoperative evaluation.

Upper Face and Lid Examination. The forehead, brows, and upper lids are assessed as a unit with the patient sitting upright. Particular attention should be directed to brow position, symmetry, and presence of horizontal forehead dynamic rhytides or frontalis muscle weakness. Old photographs of the patient may reveal acquired involutional changes that will be helpful in selecting the appropriateness of brow lifting. When assessing the forehead-brow area, the frontalis muscle should be relaxed to determine the resting height of the brows; compensatory brow recruitment, manifested by forehead furrowing from frontalis muscle contraction, may mask an underlying brow ptosis, dermatochalasis, or upper eyelid ptosis.

To determine the amount of brow ptosis that may need to be corrected, the brow is held at a desired position and the distance the brow falls to its relaxed level is measured. The brow position is not usually altered by blepharoplasty,[88] although postoperative brow relaxation may occur. If there is preexisting brow ptosis and the blepharoplasty candidate does not desire brow correction, a conservative skin and muscle excision should be performed to avoid downward traction of the brow toward the eyelid crease. If a brow elevation is necessary to optimize the blepharoplasty results, the brow lift should be conducted first, before or at the time of blepharoplasty.

Lateral brow fullness due to excessive bony orbital rim projection may be altered by surgically reducing the bony contour. Fullness from soft-tissue thickening from ROOF prominence is sculpted through the upper lid blepharoplasty incision. Superotemporal eyelid fullness inferior to the ROOF may represent dermatochalasis from lateral brow ptosis or involutional lacrimal gland prolapse. A prolapsed lacrimal gland presents as a palpable, discreet, somewhat mobile mass located just below the superotemporal orbital rim. If gland repositioning is overlooked at the time of blepharoplasty, there will remain undesirable residual lateral lid fullness. Diffuse lid edema should be differentiated from steatochalasis. Orbital fat will protrude when pressure is gently applied against closed eyelids or when eyes are directed to the sides or upward. In contrast, the fullness from lid edema will appear stable with these maneuvers. Lid edema may be a response to ocular allergies or systemic abnormalities such as thyroid disease.

A patient's gender and cultural background must be considered when planning eyelid surgery. For example, a strategy that effectively achieves the impression of rejuvenation for a female may not be appropriate for a male. Likewise, aesthetically pleasing features of the Occidental eyelid may not be desirable to an Asian individual. Elderly patients with generalized signs of facial aging may not wish to have aggressive blepharoplasty and seek only age-appropriate improvements. The preoperative discussion must include clear communication of anticipated anatomic modifications in a manner that reduces ambiguity of expectations.

Preoperative Clinical Considerations for Lower Lid Blepharoplasty

Planning lower eyelid blepharoplasty requires recognition of various anatomic associations and of the typical involutional changes that occur in the mid face. The evaluation should be attentive to lower lid skin quality, quantity, and pigmentation, contour of the eyelid relative to the globe and mid face, lower lid margin position, and horizontal laxity.

Skin and Orbicularis Oculi Muscle. Hypertrophy of the orbicularis oculi muscle will cause a bunching effect that is particularly prominent when an individual smiles. The lower lid should thus be evaluated in both the relaxed state and with a forced smile in order to determine the relative contributions of skin, muscle, and fat to the eyelid's overall appearance. This maneuver also helps determine if excess skin is present in the lids and provides valuable information about the skin's elasticity (Fig. 20-19).

Lower Lid Contour and Midfacial Anatomy. It is important to assess the bony support of the lower eyelid prior to performing lower blepharoplasty. If the lower lid does not have adequate bony support, following blepharoplasty the lid may "slide down" the globe, producing an aesthetically and possibly a functionally unsatisfactory result. A helpful test to evaluate the bony support for the lower lid is to view the patients in profile as they hold their heads level and gaze straight ahead. An imaginary coronal plane is drawn through the anterior-most projection of the malar eminence and the position of the globe relative to this plane is noted (Fig. 20-20). If the plane passes anterior to the cornea, the lid has adequate support; if the plane

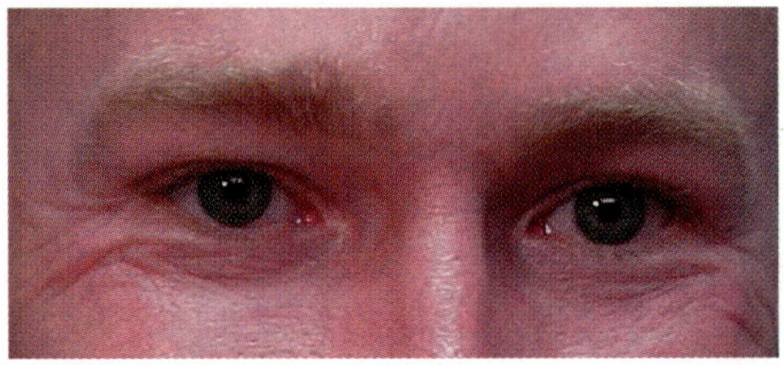

FIG. 20-19
"Hypertrophic" orbicularis oculi muscle.

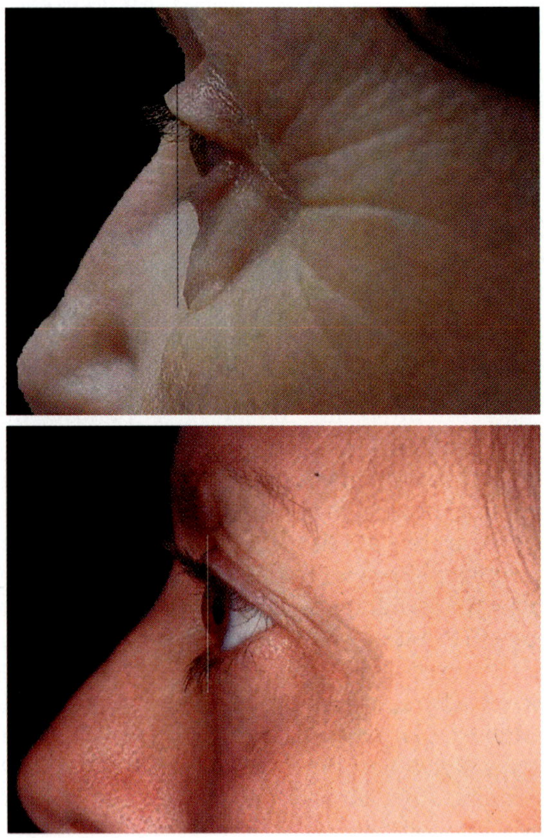

A

B

FIG. 20-20
A, A coronal plane drawn through the anterior-most projection of the zygoma passes anterior to the cornea. There is adequate bony support for the eyelid. **B,** The same plane passes through the eye indicating insufficient bony support for the lower eyelid.

passes through the globe itself, midfacial elevation, cheek implants, or other maneuvers may be considered at the time of blepharoplasty surgery.

Lower Lid Laxity and Position. If a transcutaneous approach is being considered, the lower lid position and degree of horizontal laxity must be assessed. Preexisting lower lid retraction, scleral show, or laxity may require correction prior to or in conjunction with blepharoplasty to avoid postoperative lid malpositions and corneal exposure complications. The snap test is performed by pulling the lower lid inferiorly and observing for a normal quick resumption of its position against the globe prior to the next blink. A lid that fails to return to position briskly demonstrates lower lid laxity and the snap test is interpreted to be positive. The distraction test is performed by gently grasping the lower lid skin horizontally and pulling away from the globe to determine how far the lid can be stretched. If this distance is greater than 6 mm, there is laxity and the test is considered positive.[89]

If lower lid laxity is identified, skin removal should be conservative and concurrent lower lid tightening measures should performed. Involutional eyelid laxity results more often from weakness of the lateral canthal tendon rather than medial canthal weakening or tarsal lengthening.[90-93] The surgical correction usually entails lateral tightening procedures.

PROCEDURAL TECHNIQUES FOR UPPER LID BLEPHAROPLASTY

Skin Marking

Marking of the skin incisions is perhaps the most important step in blepharoplasty surgery; if the initial marking is not performed well, the ultimate surgical outcome will be suboptimal. Skin markings may be made with the patient in an upright or supine position. If the initial markings are made with the patient supine, it is helpful to recheck the marks with the patient upright to assess changes that may occur due to gravitational effects on the eyelid or eyebrow. Calipers or a ruler are useful for achieving greater symmetry. One can use a fine-point marking pen, a standard surgical marking pen sharpened to a point with a No. 15 blade, or a sterile toothpick dipped in dye such as brilliant green or methylene blue. Eyelid marking is usually performed in the holding area prior to administration of sedative agents.

The inferior border of the blepharoplasty incision should be placed at the desired height of the eyelid crease. In Occidental patients the central portion of the crease is highest while the temporal and nasal ends are lower. In the Asian lid, the crease is more often less arched.[23] Nasally, the incision should extend no closer than 5 mm from the superior punctum and, in general, should not extend more medially than an imaginary line drawn vertically through the upper punctum. Extending the incision too far nasally can induce cicatricial band formation, or "webbing." The lateral portion of the upper eyelid incision is flared temporally and usually does not extend beyond the tail of the brow (the lateral-most portion of the brow cilia). If concurrent transcutaneous lower blepharoplasty is planned, the upper and lower eyelid incisions should be separated by at least 5 mm so as to diminish the risk of lateral canthal webbing and chronic lymphedema.[94-96]

To estimate the amount of eyelid skin to be removed, begin with the patient's eyes gently closed. One arm of a smooth forceps is placed in the eyelid crease while the other pinches the redundant skin until the eyelashes just begin to rotate. This marks the maximum amount of skin that may be safely removed. In men, skin excision is often performed more conservatively than in women, as lids with minimal folds may appear "feminized." In general, the superior border of the incision should pass no closer than 1 cm from the inferior border of the eyebrow cilia (Fig. 20-21). This approximates the zone where the thicker skin of the eyebrow transitions into the thinner skin of the eyelid.

Upper eyelid blepharoplasty should be planned carefully. The surgeon will do well to always remember the axiom that "form should follow function." That is to say, normal eyelid functions such as blinking and closing must not be compromised in an effort to improve appearance. To underscore this point, the surgeon should view the planned excision in terms of how much skin needs to remain to ensure proper function rather than how much should be excised. Some suggest that 20 mm of upper lid skin must be preserved in order to retain normal eyelid function. Failure to follow this principle may result in an inability to maintain ad-

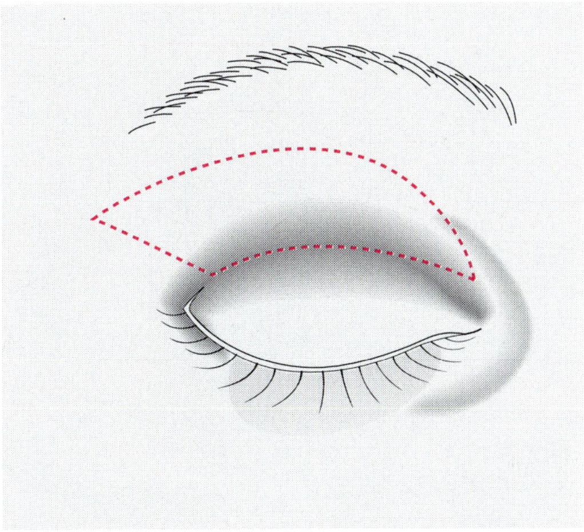

FIG. 20-21
Typical appearance of upper blepharoplasty incision, right eye, frontal view.

equate protection of the ocular surface, dry eye syndrome, and even corneal scarring and vision loss.

If brow ptosis is present and is not to be corrected at the time of blepharoplasty, the brow may be manually elevated to an appropriate position when the eyelids are marked. Failure to do this may result in resection of an excessive amount of skin such that if the patient subsequently decides to undergo brow lifting, lagophthalmos will result.[88]

One drop of topical anesthetic (such as proparacaine) is instilled in each eye and protective plastic scleral shells lubricated with ophthalmic ointment are placed behind the lids. A No. 15 Bard-Parker blade is used to incise along the skin markings (Fig. 20-22). Hemostasis is achieved and a skin-muscle flap is then elevated, taking care to stay in the plane deep to the orbicularis muscle, as failure to do so will result in excessive bleeding. Sharp dissection of skin and muscle in the plane anterior to the septum is facilitated by countertraction. Once the skin-muscle flap is removed, the orbital septum should be visible (Fig. 20-23). The preaponeurotic fat pad, a useful landmark, should be visualized beneath

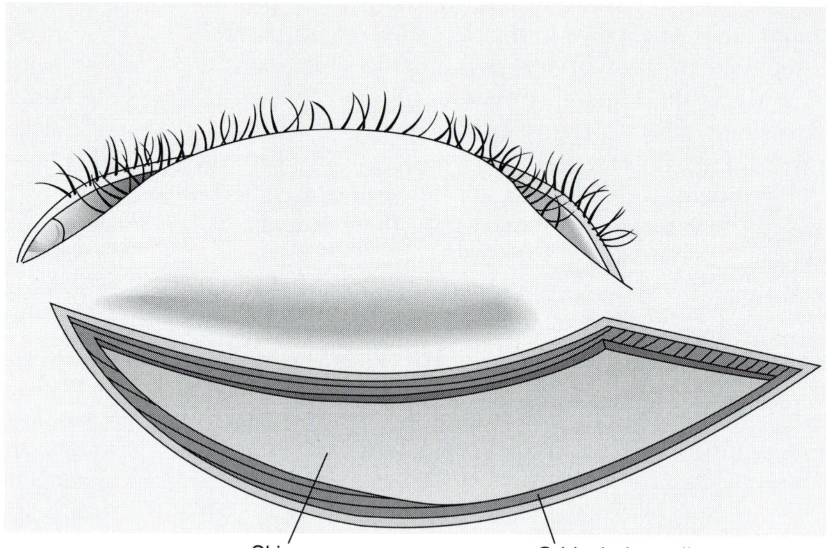

FIG. 20-22
Upper blepharoplasty, right eye, surgeon's view. Appearance of the wound upon completing the skin incision.

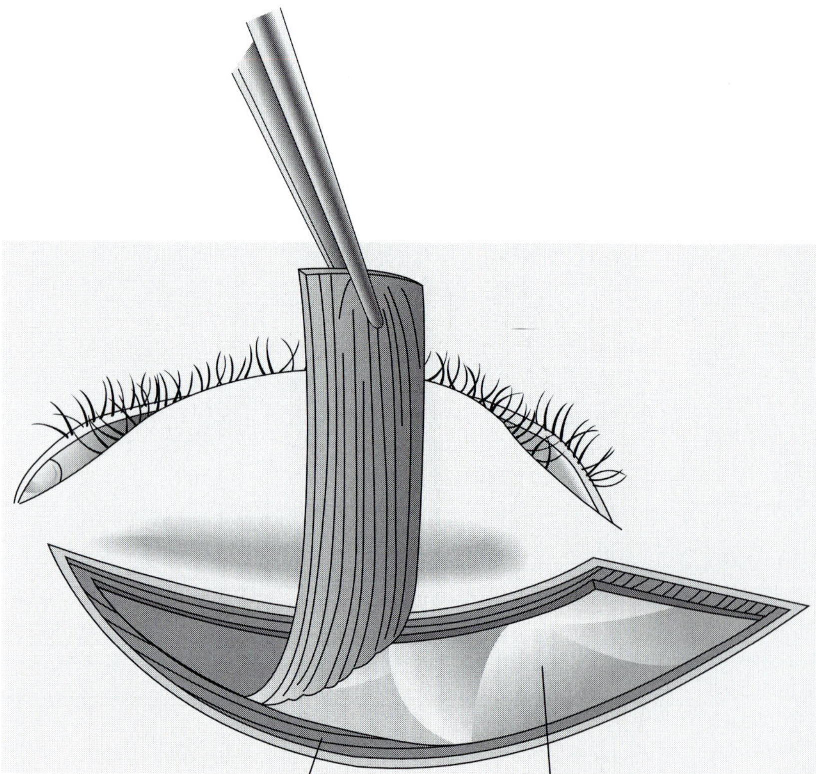

FIG. 20-23
Upper blepharoplasty, right eye, surgeon's view. A skin-muscle flap is elevated, exposing the underlying orbital septum. Care is taken not to dissect within the muscle itself.

the septum, as it will protrude anteriorly when pressure is gently applied to the globe. If there is still uncertainty as to the septum's identity, the edge of the tissue should be grasped with a forceps to verify the septum's firm attachment to the orbital rim, thus distinguishing it from the levator aponeurosis, which moves freely.

The septum is opened horizontally in the area overlying the orbital fat, allowing the fat to prolapse into the wound (Fig. 20-24). The preaponeurotic fat is yellow; the nasal fat appears whiter. The nasal fat pad may be divided into two seemingly separate pockets by a fibrous septum.[97] Therefore, this area should be dissected carefully yet thoroughly. Traction on the fat pads should be avoided to prevent rupturing of deeper orbital blood vessels. It is preferable to allow the fatty tissue to emerge into view by gently applying pressure to the globe with a cotton tip applicator. Bipolar cauterization is used to maintain hemostasis. Fat removal requires exquisite control of bleeding. Fat lobules can be cauterized or clamped in advance of cutting. The removed fat may be set aside for comparison with quantity anticipated preoperatively and for comparison between the left and right lids. Undercorrection is far easier to correct than the hollow deformities resulting from excessive fat removal. While sculpting the nasal fat pad, it is imperative to avoid injury to the medial canthal tendon and the trochlea of the superior oblique muscle (Fig. 20-25).

Lacrimal gland tissue is normally firm and whitish as opposed to the soft texture and yellow of the fat of

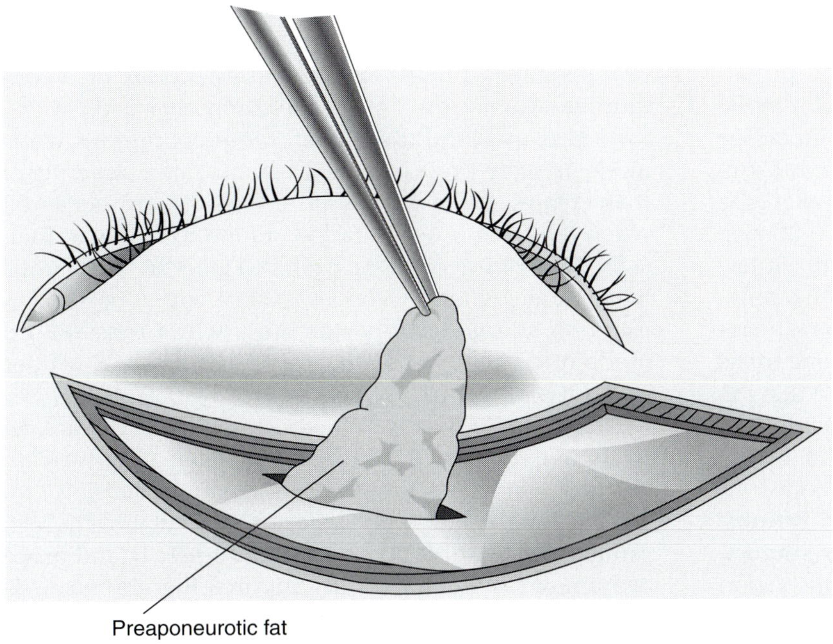

FIG. 20-24
Upper blepharoplasty, right eye, surgeon's view. The preaponeurotic fat pad is prolapsed into the surgical field after the orbital septum is opened near the superior orbital rim.

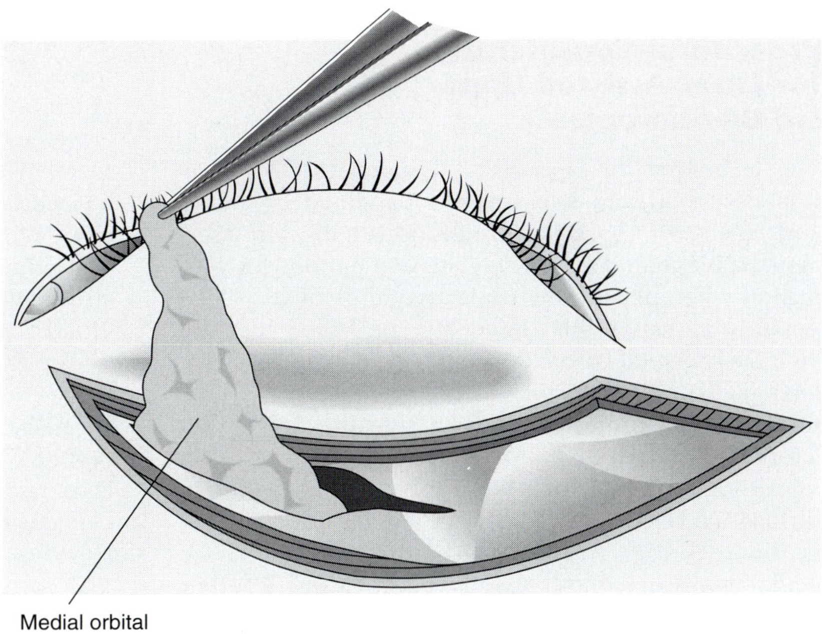

FIG. 20-25
Upper blepharoplasty, right eye, surgeon's view. The nasal fat pad is examined, taking care to avoid injury to the superior oblique muscle tendon or the trochlea.

the central fat pad. A prolapsed gland should be suspended and repositioned behind the orbital rim using 5-0 or 6-0 absorbable or permanent sutures. Abnormal lacrimal gland appearance or friable texture of the adjacent periosteum is an indication for biopsy.

If the ROOF is to be sculpted, dissection in the suborbicularis muscle plane extends 10 to 15 mm above the lateral portion of the superior rim, avoiding injury to the lacrimal nerve. The fat pad is reduced in the lateral third to half of the brow in an en bloc fashion, tapering the perimeters to avoid abrupt disparities in thickness. The dissection should not extend medial to the central brow to avoid damaging the supraorbital neurovascular complex. A layer of fat should be preserved between the orbicularis oculi muscle and rim periosteum as excision of the entire ROOF complex may result in surface irregularities, skin adhesions producing brow immobility, or a combination of these problems.

Excess orbicularis or septum in the wound may be trimmed to further improve lid contour. If the lid crease is to be re-formed, a maneuver known as supratarsal fixation may be performed. With this maneuver, the wound edges are sutured to the superior tarsal border. Supratarsal fixation may be performed with interrupted or running absorbable sutures such as 7-0 polyglactin or chromic gut. Alternating superficial skin closure and deep passes to engage the levator aponeurosis can also be used to define the new lid crease. When the wound is aligned in preparation for skin closure and excess skin is encountered at the medial end of the wound, a Burow's triangle can be excised. The resultant wound should be closed with interrupted sutures. Ice compresses are applied immediately after surgery. Occlusive dressings are avoided so that abrupt vision changes or excessive bleeding from the wound will be apparent.

Procedural Considerations for Laser-Assisted Upper Lid Blepharoplasty

The technique for laser-assisted blepharoplasty was first described and subsequently modified by Baker and others.[11,58,98,99] Ocular protection is critical in laser-assisted blepharoplasty. There are two options for protection when performing upper eyelid blepharoplasty. A study at Vanderbilt University concluded that the Stefanosky metal corneal protectors offer the best protection currently available for preventing injury.[100] Although these protectors have a metallic finish that lends itself to reflected laser beams that could result in injuries, the manufacturer will apply a Teflon coating to diffuse the laser beam. Metal eye shields are available in different sizes and ideally should cover the entire ocular surface without readily decentering. Another option for laser-safe eye protection is the David-Baker clamp, a metal clamp with a large blade that extends the entire width and length of the superior fornix.[101] This device offers superior eye protection relative to a contact lens, but has the disadvantage of causing crush injury to the upper eyelid. When applied properly this is not a significant problem. The David-Baker clamp offers the additional advantage of stabilization of the upper eyelid, a useful feature when incisions are made.

A carbon dioxide laser is positioned in such a fashion that there is no counter pull on the handpiece as the surgeon holds it lightly. This may require proper positioning of the laser or adjustment of weights or springs. The laser used for incisional periorbital surgery should produce the smallest possible beam diameter, ideally no more than 0.2 mm. The laser may be operated in continuous wave or high-frequency pulse mode. As one would anticipate, less lateral thermal damage is produced by a pulsed laser than one producing a continuous wave beam. One of the commonly used lasers, the Lumenis UltraPulse, when set in continuous wave mode actually produces a high-frequency pulsed beam that creates the same tissue effects as are achieved when the laser is set in pulsed mode to make an incision. Those surgeons who prefer to work in continuous wave mode generally choose to start with a power setting of 5 to 8 watts, whereas those who prefer pulsed mode often begin with an energy setting of 25 mJ per pulse at a power of 5 watts.

The depth to which an incision extends correlates directly with the power setting on the laser and inversely with the surgeon's hand speed. A single incision created through skin and anterior orbicularis muscle, rather than multiple passes, will minimize lateral propagation of laser energy with minimal thermal necrosis while achieving excellent incisional hemostasis. During laser dissection, careful techniques will avoid injury to deeper layers. The orbital septum is opened at the level just below the superior orbital rim, where there is greatest separation of septum from levator aponeurosis. Once an opening in the septum is created, a wet cotton-tipped applicator or specially designed metal instrument (Oculoplastik, Montreal, Canada) can be inserted beneath the septum and used as a backstop along which a laser incision can be extended. The fat is excised by draping the tissue over an antireflective instrument such as an anodized bone plate and is divided with the laser.

The ROOF complex is contoured with a continuous wave energy setting of 10 watts. Higher energy is used because of the more fibrous and vascular nature of this tissue. When the ROOF complex is being excised, the laser handpiece should be held in a focused position. Defocusing the beam to "shrink" the fat is relatively ineffective and significantly increases the amount of thermal damage. Significant bleeding from larger-caliber vessels may be encountered in the ROOF complex, and bipolar cautery should be readily available. The beginning aesthetic laser surgeon should approach this area conservatively.

In performing the initial skin incision in Asian patients, the laser may produce inconsistent results with regard to the epicanthal fold areas. Unacceptable scarring of the upper eyelid incision site has been reported.[12] The risk of this problem may be minimized by limiting the amount of inflammation at the wound edges or avoided by using a No. 15 Bard-Parker blade for the initial incision. If laser is used to create the initial skin incision, slightly slower wound healing is anticipated and permanent suture material used for closure should not be removed before 7 to 10 days to avoid wound dehiscence.

PROCEDURAL TECHNIQUES FOR LOWER LID BLEPHAROPLASTY

Selecting the approach to lower lid blepharoplasty depends upon whether there is excess skin, excess orbicularis muscle, excess herniated fat, or malar descent. When there is fat herniation in the absence of excessive lower lid skin, then a transconjunctival approach is favored. When there is moderately excessive lower lid skin, herniated orbital fat, or hypertrophy of the orbicularis muscle, a skin-muscle flap approach is used.

Transconjunctival Blepharoplasty

Areas of prominent fat protrusion should be marked with the patient sitting upright; when the patient is in a supine position the fat falls posteriorly into the orbit and is difficult to assess. Topical anesthetic is administered and scleral shields lubricated with an ophthalmic ointment are inserted to protect the eye. Local anesthetic is injected subconjunctivally, into the fatty tissue compartments (posterior to the rim where the septum originates) and along the inferior orbital rim, near the infraorbital nerve. If anesthetic is injected into the inferior oblique muscle, temporary pupillary dilation and diplopia may result. The lower lid is retracted inferiorly using a Desmarres retractor, which should rest against the maxilla anterior to the inferior orbital rim. A lid plate or malleable retractor is placed in the fornix and over the protected globe to ballot the eye so as to induce protrusion of orbital fat. The incision is created horizontally through conjunctiva and lid retractors overlying the area of fat herniation, usually half way between the inferior fornix and inferior tarsal border (Fig. 20-26). Since the lower lid retractors may fuse with the orbital septum as low as 2 to 3 mm below the inferior tarsal border, the orbital fat does not extend superiorly beyond this point and the incision should be made below this level. A battery-operated disposable hot cautery, Colorado needle, radiofrequency device, or carbon dioxide laser may be used to achieve hemostatic cutting. Once the conjunctiva and lower eyelid retractors have been divided, the anterior orbital fat becomes visible within its fibrous sheath (Fig. 20-27). While the wound edges are retracted with scleral hooks, dissection is extended through the capsulopalpebral fascia until the central fat pad is visualized (Fig. 20-28). The incision is extended laterally to the lateral canthal angle and medially to a point just lateral to the plica semilunaris.

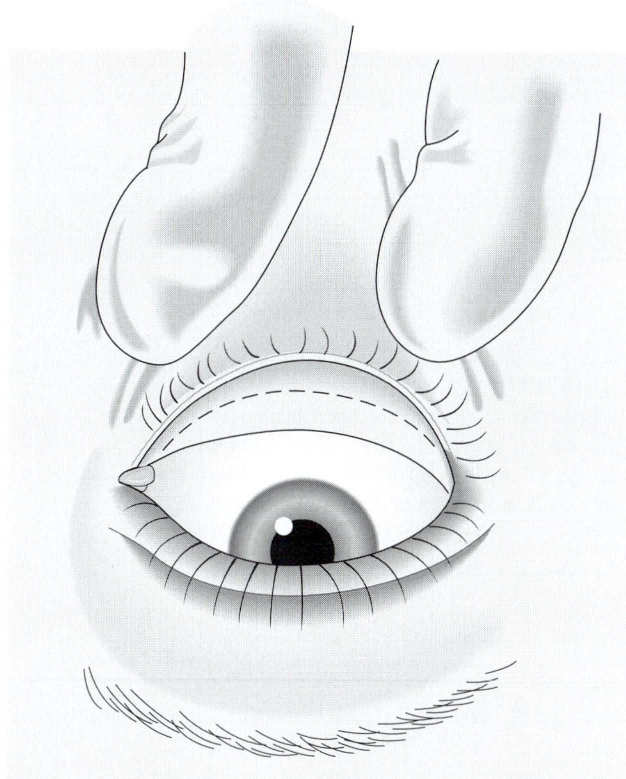

FIG. 20-26
Lower eyelid transconjunctival blepharoplasty, right eye, surgeon's view. The dashed line indicates the recommended placement of the incision.

The amount of anticipated fat removal is determined in the preoperative evaluation, the goal being to eliminate the fatty tissue prominence while avoiding a "hollow" appearance. A Desmarres retractor can be placed within the wound to retract and expose the orbital fat. If the fat is not transected with a hemostatic device, it should be carefully clamped with a hemostat prior to division. If a carbon dioxide laser is used to transect the fat, clamping is not necessary. Fat excision should proceed in a systematic fashion and only that fat herniating anterior to the level of the orbital rim is removed. Care must be taken to avoid injury to the inferior oblique muscle when working in the medial and

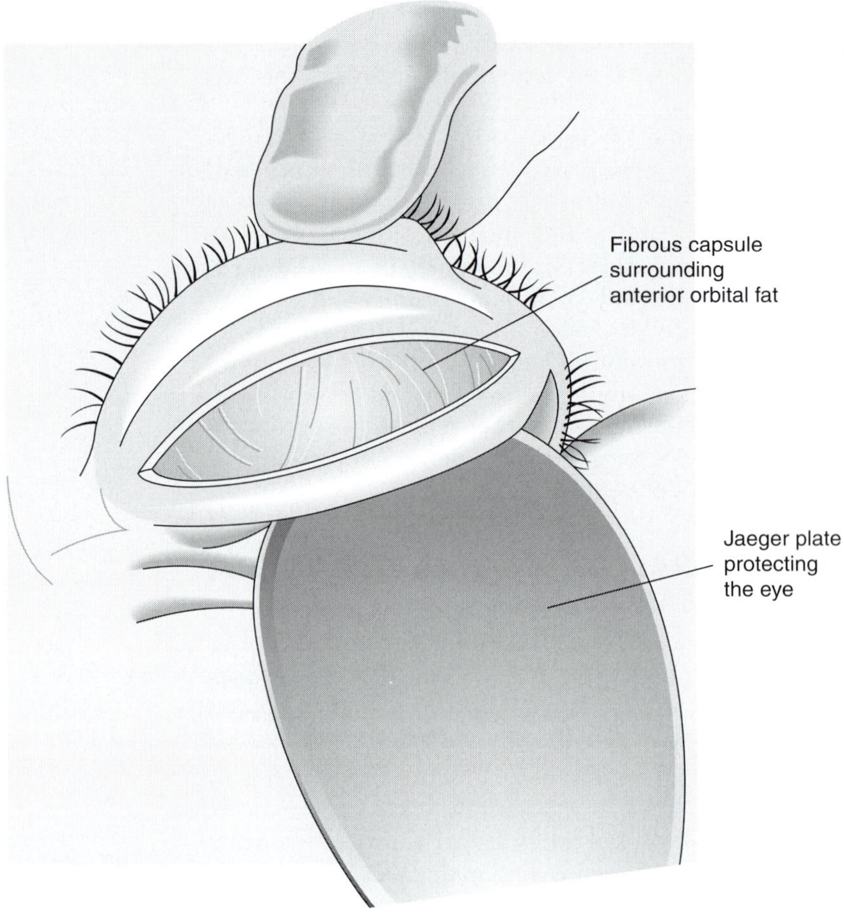

FIG. 20-27
Lower eyelid transconjunctival blepharoplasty, right eye, surgeon's view. The conjunctiva and lower eyelid retractors have been divided, exposing the fibrous capsule surrounding the anterior orbital fat.

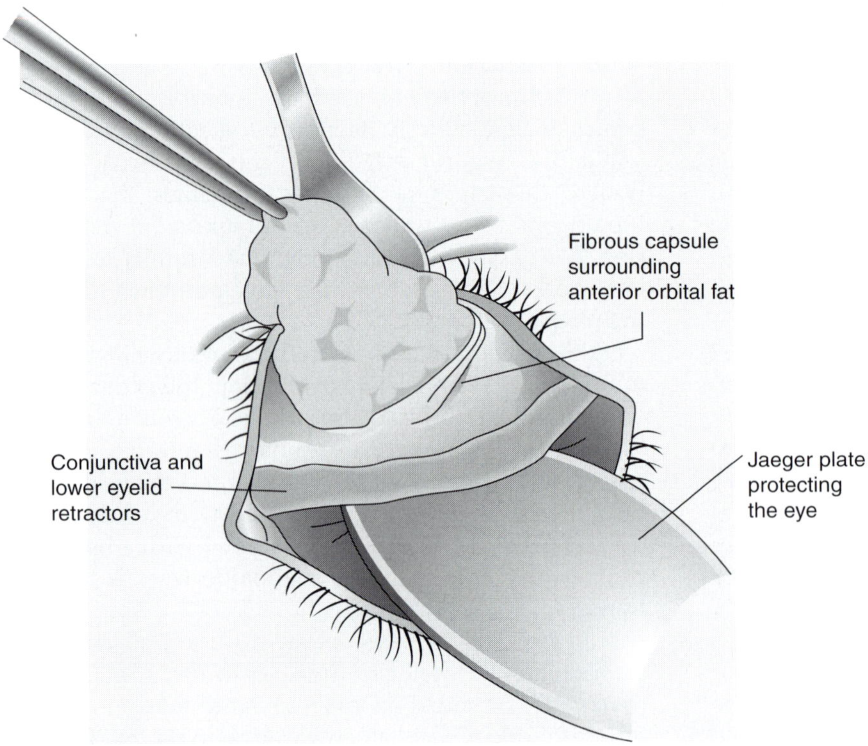

FIG. 20-28
Lower eyelid transconjunctival blepharoplasty, right eye, surgeon's view. The central fat pad has been prolapsed into the surgical field where it may be resected or repositioned.

central portions of the lower eyelid (Fig. 20-29). The lateral fat pad is usually divided into two compartments, one adjacent to the central fat pad and another located more posteriorly and laterally.[38] To adequately expose these lateral fat lobules, the arcuate expanse of the inferior oblique may be divided. The inferior oblique muscle divides the central and nasal fat compartments and should be recognized by its horizontal orientation in the anterior-inferior orbit. Injury to this muscle or its sheath may result in double vision. The presence of prominent vessels associated with the medial fat compartment should be anticipated. Medial fat repositioning can be performed with the transconjunctival approach. The orbital septum remains intact and the periosteum can be incised at the arcus marginalis in order to access the subperiosteal space (see below).

The patient may be assisted to the sitting position to assess symmetry and effectiveness of the fat reduction. The wounds are irrigated and hemostasis is ascertained. The conjunctival incision is under little tension and may be left to close spontaneously or sutured with one or two buried interrupted 7-0 chromic gut stitches. The retractors do not require closure. The scleral shells are removed and a combination antibiotic-steroid drop (such as Tobradex, Alcon, TX) is instilled. Because of the frequency of adverse reactions, products containing neomycin should be avoided.

Procedural Considerations for Laser-Assisted Transconjunctival Lower Lid Blepharoplasty

Lower eyelid blepharoplasty is readily accomplished using the carbon dioxide laser as an incisional device. Standard laser safety precautions are observed at all times. The laser set at 6 to 8 watts continuous wave or 15 to 25 mJ per pulse, 5 to 8 watts pulsed mode with a 0.2 mm focused handpiece is used to make an incision directly into the orbital fat, posterior to the orbital septum. The laser is held in a focused position and directed anteriorly and inferiorly, aiming toward the inferior orbital rim as the conjunctiva and lower eyelid retractors are divided. After two to three passes in the same incision, the orbital fat should present itself into the wound. The assistant holds the retractor in one hand and the Jaeger plate in the other, taking care to maintain the plate's position while applying gentle posterior pressure on the globe. The surgeon holds the laser in one hand and a toothed forceps in the other while the fat pads are exposed. The central fat pocket with its surrounding fascial investments is exposed in the midportion of the wound. The fibrous septae surrounding the fat should be carefully stripped away from the fat pad itself using blunt dissection with the laser handpiece or a cotton-tipped applicator. Once the

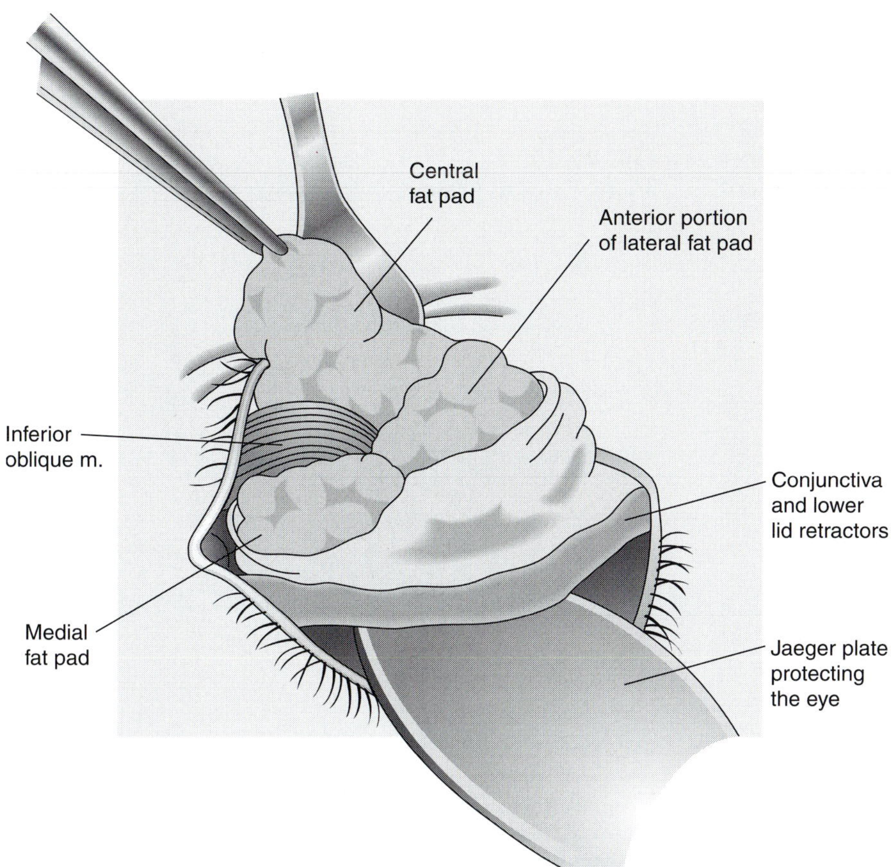

FIG. 20-29
Lower eyelid transconjunctival blepharoplasty, right eye, surgeon's view. The inferior oblique muscle passes between the nasal and central fat pads. It should be identified but not manipulated during blepharoplasty surgery.

entire pocket has been isolated, it is held against the Desmarres retractor and transected with the carbon dioxide laser at the level of the orbital rim. Inadvertent laser burns are avoided if the laser is directed against the metal retractor and held stationary while the fat pad is grasped with a forceps and moved slowly from side to side. If large vessels are apparent within the fat these should be closed with bipolar electrocautery prior to division of the pad with the laser. Every effort should be made to avoid piecemeal removal of the fat so as to reduce the total amount of laser energy applied to the orbit.

The laser should never be directed posteriorly, as the globe or extraocular muscles may be inadvertently divided or damaged.[99]

Transcutaneous Lower Lid Blepharoplasty With or Without Fat Repositioning

Skin Marking. Preoperative markings should be drawn with the patient sitting upright. It is helpful to delineate the nasojugal tear trough, specific location and severity of fatty prolapse, and the extent of orbicularis muscle hypertrophy when applicable. Using forceps to gently pinch the lower lid, determine the maximum amount of skin that can be removed from the subciliary area without inducing downward lower lid margin bowing. This mark will remind the surgeon of the upper limit of vertical shortening when skin is actually removed in subsequent steps. Preoperative photographs are useful for intraoperative reference. Topical anesthetic is instilled in both eyes and protective scleral shields lubricated with artificial tear ointment are placed behind the lids. Local anesthetic for subcutaneous injection, consisting of 2% lidocaine with 1:100,000 epinephrine in a 1:1 mixture with 0.75% bupivacaine with 1:200,000 epinephrine, provides analgesia and hemostasis.

Incision and Dissection. A standard subciliary incision placed 1.5 mm below the cilia can be initiated laterally with a No. 15 Bard-Parker blade (Fig. 20-30). The incision is extended medially to within 2 mm of the lacrimal punctum using sharp Wescott scissors or a No. 15 Bard-Parker blade. Lateral to the lateral canthal angle, the incision is directed inferotemporally along a natural laugh line. This lateral portion of the lower lid incision is extended if more skin needs to be removed, but initially, the length need only facilitate skin and muscle dissection inferiorly. A 6-0 polypropylene or silk suture placed partial thickness through the tarsus centrally and just at the subciliary incision (avoiding skin puncture) is useful for providing countertraction.

Generally, a combined skin and muscle flap method is used. However, it may be advantageous to elevate skin only in the pretarsal orbicularis area, since keeping the muscle layer undisturbed may decrease the chance of developing a depressed subciliary scar (Fig. 20-31). Once the orbicularis muscle has been exposed, a blunt-tipped scissors is used to button-hole the preseptal muscle (Fig. 20-32). The muscle is then opened across the full extent of the wound and dissection is performed inferiorly in the suborbicularis oculi plane until the inferior orbital rim is exposed. Meticulous hemostasis is maintained during this dissection.

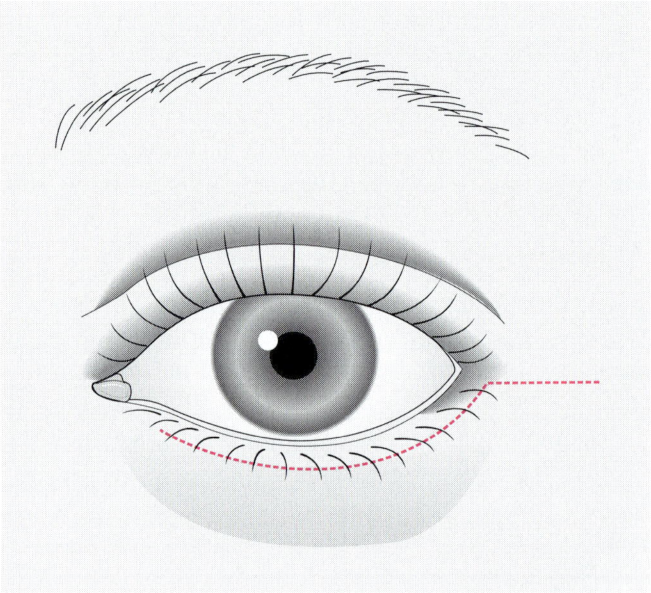

FIG. 20-30
Transcutaneous lower blepharoplasty. Typical skin incision.

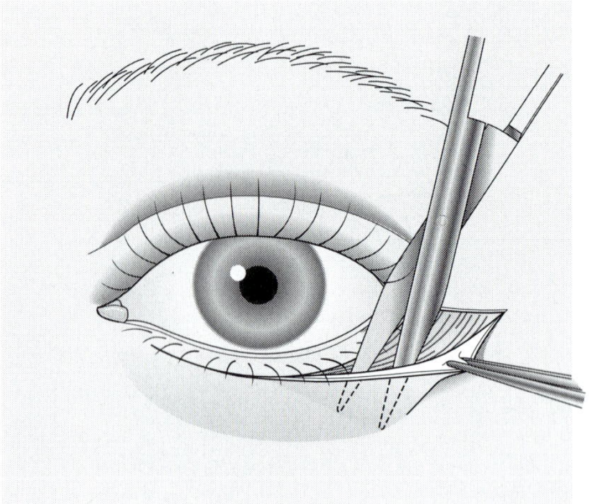

FIG. 20-31
Transcutaneous lower blepharoplasty. Some surgeons prefer to leave the pretarsal orbicularis oculi muscle intact to help decrease the risk of postoperative ectropion.

Removal of Hypertrophic Orbicularis Muscle. When orbicularis muscle hypertrophy is present, a skin flap can be dissected to expose the muscular bulge. The superior edge of prominent orbicularis mounding often begins 3 to 5 mm below the lash line and is accentuated with smiling. The muscle is reduced by partially and superficially excising muscle tissue layers along the orientation of the fibers, decreasing the anterior to posterior prominence. Bleeding is anticipated but easily controlled in this region. An alternative method uses electrosurgical modification and ablation of the orbicularis muscle to reduce the muscle prominence.[102]

Removal of Orbital Fat. In contrast to the transconjunctival approach, when the transcutaneous approach is utilized the orbital fat cannot be exposed without opening the orbital septum. The entire width of the septum may be incised at a point just above the arcus marginalis in order to expose the medial, central, and lateral fat compartments. Alternatively, three small buttonholes can be made in the septum to allow access to the fat (Fig. 20-33). Gentle pressure applied to the orbit through the lids will accentuate fat herniation. When the first lateral fat pad is removed, balloting the globe can expose a second, more posterior fat pad.[30] This fat may also need to be sculpted to avoid residual temporal lower eyelid fullness. Next the central and nasal fat pads are addressed. Fat that protrudes anterior to the rim can safely be removed using techniques described earlier. Sitting a patient upright during surgery will allow better judgment of the adequacy of liposculpting.

Fat Repositioning. Traditional blepharoplasty techniques emphasizing fat removal alone are now recognized to be too limited a strategy in rejuvenative surgery. In the presence of significant cheek fat descent, rejuvenation may additionally require a midface lift, a discussion of which is beyond the scope of this chapter.[103]

Tear trough deformities without significant malar descent can be corrected by fat preservation and repositioning. In this setting, nasal fat removal would worsen a sunken lid appearance. The inferomedial orbital rim is palpated and the septum is incised at the arcus marginalis, near the origin of the levator labii superioris alaeque nasi muscle. A periosteal elevator is used to create a subperiosteal pocket 10 mm distal to the incision spanning the length of the trough to be filled. Damage to the infraorbital foramen located 7 to 10 mm inferior to the rim at the junction of the medial third and lateral third of the eyelid is avoided.

The medial fat capsule is incised to liberate the fat lobules and allow fat to be advanced anteriorly without creating traction. The fat is fashioned into a mallet-shaped fat flap with a 5 to 7 mm diameter pedicle and positioned into the subperiosteal pocket. If properly performed, there should be no tendency for the fat to recoil posteriorly and extraocular motility should not be restricted. The fat can be secured using a 6-0 polyglactin or nylon horizontal mattress stitch that

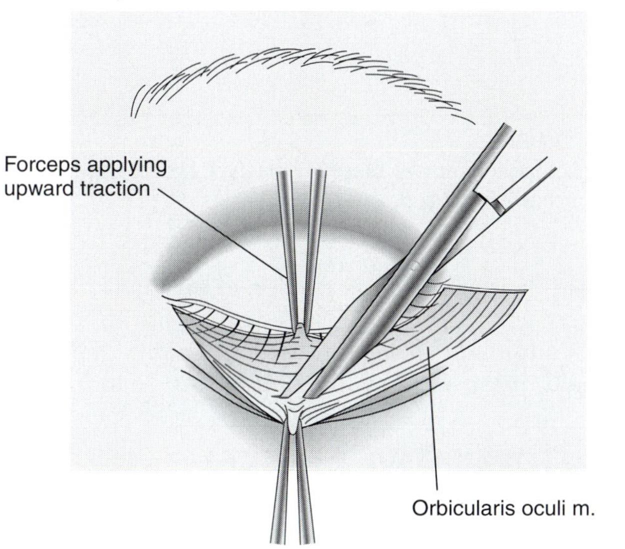

FIG. 20-32
Transcutaneous lower blepharoplasty. The preseptal orbicularis oculi muscle is opened with traction superiorly on the eyelid margin and on the inferior border of the wound.

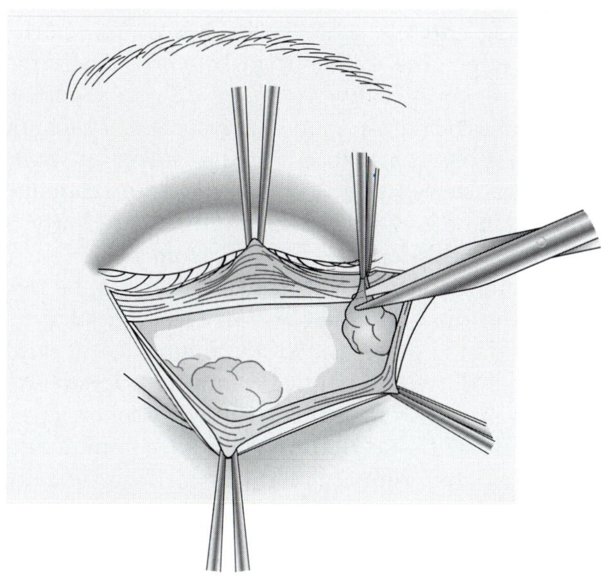

FIG. 20-33
Transcutaneous lower blepharoplasty. The skin-muscle flap is retracted, and the orbital septum has been opened to expose the central and anterior temporal fat pads. The posterior-lateral or second lateral fat pad is not pictured.

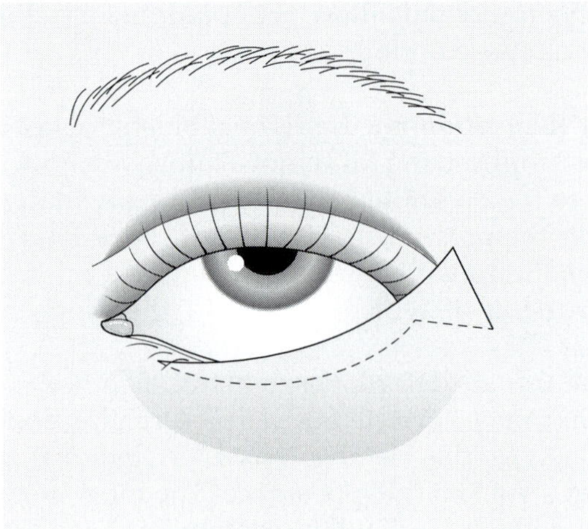

FIG. 20-34
Transcutaneous lower blepharoplasty. The skin-muscle flap is draped without traction over the incision while the patient gazes superiorly and opens the mouth, placing the lower eyelid on maximum stretch. The dashes indicate the proposed line of skin excision.

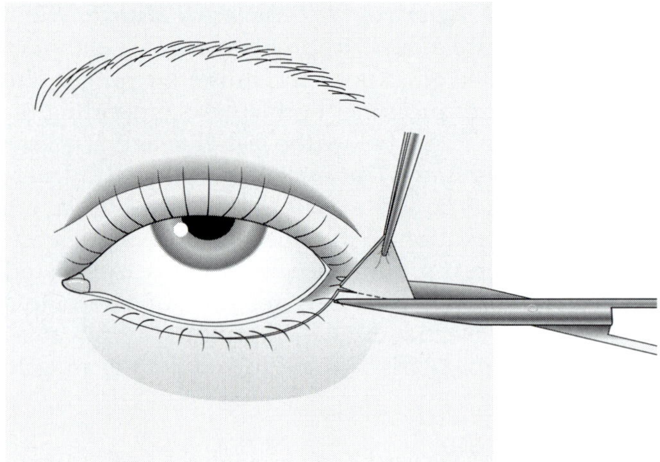

FIG. 20-35
Transcutaneous lower blepharoplasty. A "dog ear" of tissue should be excised laterally to reduce skin redundancy.

loosely engages the anterior edge of periosteum and part of the fat pedicle.

Skin Excision. The skin-muscle flap is draped without traction over the subciliary incision (Fig. 20-34). The amount of skin to be removed is determined with the patient gazing upward and opening the mouth. Excess skin extending above the subciliary incision is excised with sharp Wescott scissors. The primary lid skin tightening effect is achieved by horizontal shortening at the laugh line, rather than by vertical shortening. Therefore, conservative amounts of skin are removed from the subciliary region. Aggressive *vertical* shortening is almost guaranteed to cause lower lid malposition. The excised subciliary skin is a horizontally oriented triangle with apex pointing medially with maximal widths usually ranging from 1 to 4 mm.

As mentioned, skin tightening should be accomplished in the horizontal vector. The edge of the skin-muscle flap is draped laterally along the curvature of the lower lid with a gentle amount of traction and the overlap is excised to reduce skin redundancy. The extra "dog ear" of tissue is eliminated by a combination of extending the original laugh line incision (usually not more than 15 mm) and excising a triangle of the skin-muscle flap with apex at the inferior extent of the lateral incision (Fig. 20-35).

Skin Closure. The subciliary portion of the wound should not be under tension and can be closed using 7-0 chromic gut, silk, or nylon sutures in a running fashion from medially to laterally. The lateral wound extent is

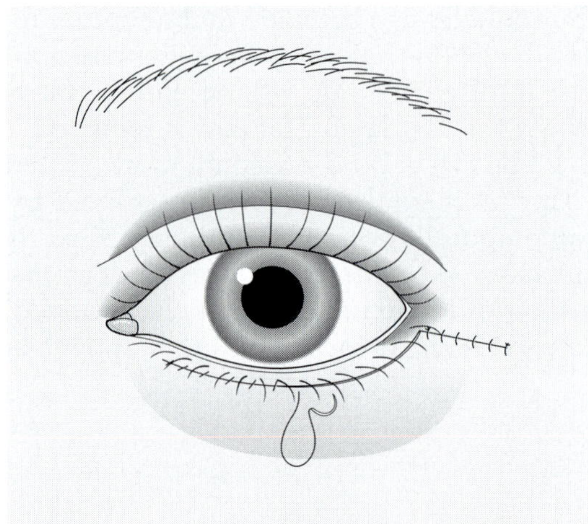

FIG. 20-36
Transcutaneous lower blepharoplasty. Correct appearance of wound as it is closed.

closed in an interrupted fashion to maximally align the closure and distribute tension. Sutures are removed in 5 days, although in laser-assisted incisions, the sutures should remain for 7 to 10 days (Figs. 20-36 to 20-38).

POSTOPERATIVE CLINICAL CONSIDERATIONS

Written postoperative instructions should include information on activity restrictions, wound care, and expected wound appearance. It is difficult to list every specific restriction or contraindication, so an explanation of why the limitations are recommended will allow the patient to extrapolate and employ good judg-

A B

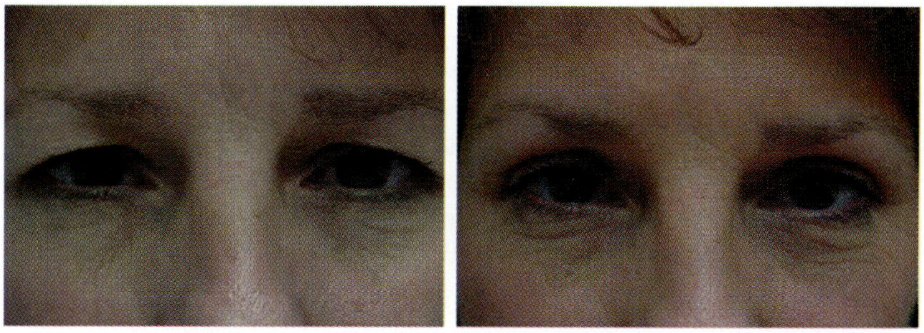

FIG. 20-37
Clinical photographs before **(A)** and 1 month after **(B)** upper blepharoplasty.

A 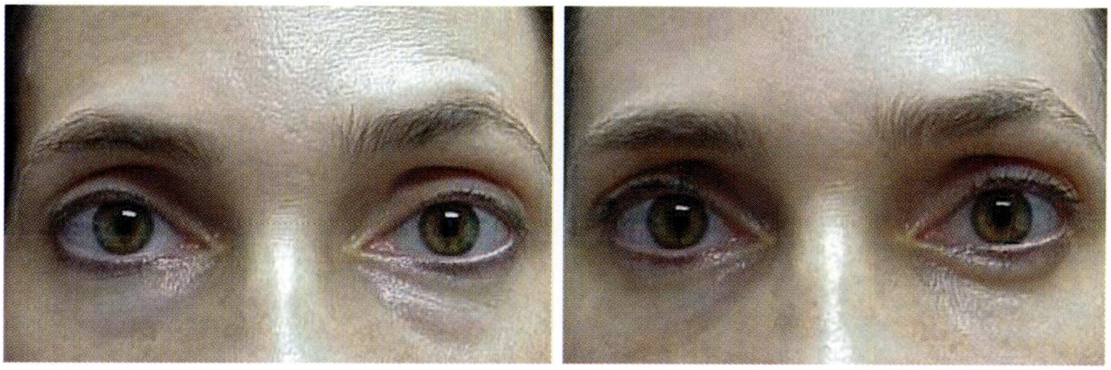 B

FIG. 20-38
Clinical photographs before **(A)** and 1 month after **(B)** transconjunctival lower blepharoplasty.

ment. The patient should be informed of signs or symptoms that warrant medical attention and then urged to maintain a low threshold for seeking your medical advice. It is important to indicate whom to contact in the event of an ocular emergency.

Wound Care and Appearance

Patients are instructed to apply ice compresses as often as possible for the first 48 to 72 hours in order to reduce eyelid swelling and improve comfort level. Crushed ice or frozen peas can be placed in resealable plastic bags. Direct application of compresses to the skin has been known to cause frostbite, which can be avoided by placing a moistened gauze or towel on the lids to buffer the intense cold of the ice pack. On the day of surgery, initial applications of 30 minutes duration each hour are suggested, with decreasing intensity over the subsequent 2 days after surgery. Beyond this, ice has limited efficacy and warm compresses are recommended for improved subjective comfort. The patient is instructed to keep the head and neck elevated 30 to 45 degrees with 2 or 3 stacked pillows during sleep to further reduce periocular accumulation of dependent edema for at least the first 3 days. A combination antibiotic-steroid ointment is applied to the suture line three to four times per day to reduce tissue reaction to sutures.

Patients should be prepared to expect eyelid swelling and bruising beginning on the first postoperative day. The edema is expected to diminish 2 to 3 weeks after surgery. Consumption of salty foods or a systemic state of fluid retention may aggravate eyelid swelling. Darkening of the skin in the early postoperative period may represent deposition of hemosiderin and resolves spontaneously. Persistent pigmentation may occur as a result of sun exposure while lids are ecchymotic. Patients are thus instructed to avoid such exposure by wearing sunglasses or a hat.

Activity Restrictions

To avoid bleeding induced by positive pressure to the orbital or eyelid vasculature during the first postoperative week, patients should refrain from heavy lifting or exertion, lowering the head beneath the heart, or other activities that result in Valsalva maneuver. If patients live a significant distance from a medical facility, they should arrange to stay nearby for the first night after surgery. Patients should be contacted by telephone on the evening of surgery and the following day. If a patient reports persistent bleeding, swelling, significant pain, decreased vision, erythema, or discharge from the wound, prompt examination is required. If there are no unanticipated concerns, the patients are then seen again on postoperative day 5 to 10 for suture removal.

Analgesia

Satisfactory postoperative analgesia is usually achieved with acetaminophen alone, although some patients require narcotics. Nonsteroidal anti-inflammatory agents and aspirin must be avoided for at least 3 to 4 days after surgery to diminish bleeding risks. Application of ice compresses often provides additional comfort.

Anticipated Recovery

Low-exertion exercise may be resumed after 1 week, and more vigorous activities after 2 weeks.

Contact lens wear may be resumed 1 to 2 weeks after surgery, but the patient must be reminded to limit lid manipulation. This anticipated postoperative contact lens wear abstinence should be discussed with patients preoperatively so they may be prepared to wear glasses during the early postoperative period. Patients are told to expect 80% of the swelling to resolve over 2 weeks, while the remaining 20% may take 3 months or longer to completely resolve. Makeup may be applied to the upper eyelids 1 to 2 days after the sutures have been removed. Concealer may be applied to the eyelids remote from incision lines to cover ecchymosis soon after surgery, but patients must exercise caution in removing the cosmetics to avoid excessive periocular manipulation.

Blepharoplasty Revision

It is normal for patients to experience a phase of self-image adjustment following cosmetic eyelid surgery. Some individuals will become acutely aware of findings that may or may not have been present before surgery. Patients should be counseled that it may take 3 to 12 months before the results of surgery may be fully judged. The surgeon should resist any surgical modification before 6 months in order to allow completion and stabilization of the cicatricial properties of the surgical wound. If a patient is dissatisfied, the surgeon should acknowledge the patient's concerns and recommend a course of action rather than defensively deny the merit of the issues.

It is advisable to proceed cautiously when considering revisions in patients whose surgery was performed by another surgeon. The patient should be encouraged to discuss concerns with the original surgeon before transferring care to a new surgeon. Only after the relationship between the patient and initial surgeon has ended should one become involved in the care of a dissatisfied blepharoplasty patient. Before any additional surgery is performed, the goals and limitations of the planned procedure should be clearly defined and understood. Some surgeons ask patients to sign a waiver stating that the operating surgeon is released from responsibility for the results of the original surgery and that the results of subsequent procedures are not guaranteed. Clear communication and accessibility remain the best means of managing these challenging situations.

REFERENCES

1. Celsus AC. De Medicina. With an English translation by WG Spencer, Vol. 3, Book VII, Section 9. Cambridge: Harvard University Press, 1935:338-343.
2. Reifler DM. The American Society of Ophthalmic Plastic & Reconstructive Surgery (ASOPRS). The First 25 Years: 1969-1994; History of Ophthalmic Plastic Surgery: 2500 BC-AD 1994. San Francisco: Norman Publishing, 1994:4-6.
3. Katzen LB. The history of cosmetic oculoplastic surgery. In: Putterman AM. Cosmetic Oculoplastic Surgery: Eyelid, Forehead, and Facial Techniques. 3rd ed. Philadelphia: WB Saunders, 1999:3-10.
4. von Graefe CF. De Rhinoplastice. Berlin: Reime, 1818:13.
5. Albert DM. Ophthalmic plastic surgery. In: Albert DM, Edwards D, eds. The History of Ophthalmology. Cambridge: Blackwell Science, 1996:235-253.
6. Garrison FH. An Introduction to the History of Medicine. 4th ed. Philadelphia: WB Saunders, 1929:1-35.
7. Miller CC. Cosmetic Surgery: The Correction of Featural Imperfections. 2nd ed. Chicago: Oak Printing, 1908:40-42.
8. Miller CC. Cosmetic Surgery: The Correction of Featural Imperfections. Philadelphia: FA Davis, 1924:30-32.
9. Sayoc BT. Plastic reconstruction of the superior palpebral fold. Am J Ophthalmol 1954; 54:424-431.
10. Pang RG. Surgical formation of upper lid fold. Arch Ophthalmol 1961; 65:783-784.
11. Baker SS, Muenzler WS, Small RG, Leonard JE. Carbon dioxide laser blepharoplasty. Ophthalmology 1984; 91:238-243.
12. Wesley RE, Bond JB. Carbon dioxide laser in ophthalmic plastic and orbital surgery. Ophthalmic Surg 1985; 16:631-633.
13. Goldberg RA, Edelstein C, Balch K, Shorr N. Fat repositioning in lower eyelid blepharoplasty. Semin Ophthalmol 1998; 13:103-106.
14. Hamra ST. The role of orbital fat preservation in facial aesthetic surgery: a new concept. Clin Plast Surg 1996; 23:17-28.
15. Weinstein C. Ultrapulse carbon dioxide laser removal of periocular wrinkles in association with laser blepharoplasty. J Clin Laser Med Surg 1994; 12:205.
16. Wiess JS, Swanson NA, Baker S. Anatomy and physiology of aging skin. In: Krause CJ, Pastorek N, Mangat DS, eds. Aesthetic Facial Surgery. Philadelphia: Lippincott, 1991:461-467.
17. Tolleth H. Concepts for the plastic surgeon from art and sculpture. Clin Plast Surg 1987; 14:585-586.
18. Farkas LG, Kilar JC. Anthropometric guidelines in cranio-orbital surgery. Clin Plast Surg 1987; 14:1.
19. Gonzalez-Ulloa M, Flores ES. Senility of the face: basic study to understand its causes and effects. Plast Reconstr Surg 1965; 36: 239-246.
20. Daniel RK, Tirkanits B. Endoscopic forehead lift: aesthetics and analysis. Clin Plast Surg 1990; 22:605-618.
21. Callahan M, Beard C, eds. Beard's Ptosis. 4th ed. Birmingham: Aesculapius Publishing, 1990:1-50.
22. Doxanas MT, Anderson RL. Oriental eyelids: an anatomic study. Arch Ophthalmol 1984; 102:1232-1235.

23. Chen WPD. Comparative anatomy of the eyelids. In: Chen WPD, ed. Asian Blepharoplasty: A Surgical Atlas. Boston: Butterworth-Heinemann, 1995:1-19.
24. Whitnall SE. The Anatomy of the Human Orbit and Accessory Organs of Vision. 2nd ed. London: Oxford Medical Publishers, 1932:57-65.
25. Shore JW. Changes in lower eyelid resting position, movement, and tone with age. Am J Ophthalmol 1985; 99:415-423.
26. Lemke BN, Lucarelli MJ. Anatomy of the ocular adnexa, orbit, and related facial structures. In: Nesi FA, Lisman RD, Levine MR, eds. Smith's Ophthalmic Plastic and Reconstructive Surgery. 2nd ed. St. Louis: Mosby, 1997:1-75.
27. Barker DE. Dye injection studies of intraorbital fat components. Plast Reconstr Surg 1977; 59:82-85.
28. Yousif NJ, Sonderman P, Dzwierzynski. Anatomic considerations in transconjunctival blepharoplasty. Plast Reconstr Surg 1995; 96:1271-1278.
29. Lowe NJ, Wieder JM, Shorr N, et al. Infraorbital pigmented skin: preliminary observations of laser therapy. Dermatol Surg 1995; 21:767-770.
30. Putterman AM. Simultaneous treatment of lower eyelid dermatochalasis and abnormal-appearing skin. Am J Ophthalmol 1983; 96:6-9.
31. Manuskiatti W, Fitzpatrick RE, Goldman MP. Treatment of facial skin using combinations of CO_2, Q-switched alexandrite, flashlamp-pumped pulsed dye, and Er:YAG lasers in the same treatment session. Dermatol Surg 2000; 26:114-120.
32. Lemke BN, Stasior OG. Eyebrow incision making. Adv Ophthal Plast Reconstr Surg 1983; 2:19-23.
33. Lemke BN, Stasior OG. The anatomy of eyebrow ptosis. Arch Ophthalmol 1982; 100:981-986.
34. Doxanas MT, Anderson RL. Eyebrows, eyelids, and anterior orbit. In: Clinical Orbital Anatomy. Baltimore: Williams & Wilkins, 1984:57-88.
35. Meyer DR, Linberg JV, Wobig JL, McCormick SA. Anatomy of the orbital septum and associated eyelid connective tissues. Ophthal Plast Reconstr Surg 1991; 7:104-113.
36. Hisatomi C, Fujino T. Anatomical considerations concerning blepharoplasty in the Oriental patient. Adv Ophthal Plast Reconstr Surg 1983; 2:151-165.
37. Liu D, Hsu WM. Oriental eyelids: anatomic difference and surgical consideration. Ophthal Plast Reconstr Surg 1986; 2:59-64.
38. Putterman AM. The mysterious second temporal fat pad. Ophthal Plast Reconstr Surg 1985; 1:83-86.
39. Hoenig JA, Shorr N, Shorr J. The suborbicularis oculi fat in aesthetic and reconstructive surgery. Int Ophthalmol Clin 1997; 37: 179-191.
40. Kikkawa DO, Lemke BN, Dortzbach RK. Relations of the superficial musculoaponeurotic system to the orbit and characterization of the orbitomalar ligament. Ophthal Plast Reconstr Surg 1996; 12:77-88.
41. Mitz V, Peyronie M. The superficial musculoaponeurotic system (SMAS) in the parotid and cheek area. Plast Reconstr Surg 1986; 58:80-88.
42. Reuss W, Owsley JQ. The anatomy of the skin and fascial layers of the face in aesthetic surgery. Clin Plast Surg 1987; 14:677-682.
43. Hargiss JL. Surgical anatomy of the eyelids. Trans Pac Coast Otolaryngol Ophthalmol Soc 1963; 44:193-202.
44. Lucarelli MJ, Khwarg SI, Lemke BN, et al. The anatomy of midfacial ptosis. Ophthal Plast Reconstr Surg 2000; 16:7-22.
45. Owsley JQ. Lifting the malar fat pad for correction of prominent nasolabial folds. Plast Reconstr Surg 1993; 91:463-474.
46. Furnas DW. Festoons, mounds, and bags of the eyelids and cheek. Clin Plast Surg 1993; 20:367-385.
47. Owsley JQ. Anatomy of the head and neck for aesthetic surgery. In: Owsley JQ, ed. Aesthetic Facial Surgery. Philadelphia: WB Saunders, 1994:7-24.
48. Aiache AE, Ramirez OH. The suborbicularis oculi fat pads: an anatomic and clinical study. Plast Reconstr Surg 1995; 95: 37-42.
49. Hamra ST. Repositioning the orbicularis oculi muscle in composite rhytidectomy. Plast Reconstr Surg 1992; 90:14-22.
50. Tucker SM, Linberg JV. Vascular anatomy of the eyelids. Ophthalmology 1994; 101:1118-1121.
51. Doxanas MT, Anderson RL. Clinical Orbital Anatomy. Baltimore: Williams & Wilkins, 1984:153-170.
52. Stuzin JM, Wagstrom L, Kawamoto HK, Wolfe SA. Anatomy of the frontal branch of the facial nerve: the significance of the temporal fat pad. Plast Reconstr Surg 1989; 83:265-271.
53. Ben-Bassat M, Ben-Bassat J, Kaplan I. An ultrastructural study of the cut edges of skin and mucous membrane specimens excised by carbon dioxide laser. In: Kaplan I, ed. Laser Surgery II. Jerusalem: Academic Press, 1976:95-100.
54. Schroder T, Hukki J, Castren M. Comparison of surgical and conventional methods in skin incisions. Scand J Plast Reconstr Surg 1989; 23:187-190.
55. Biesman BS, Wesley RE, Klippenstein KA. The Er:YAG laser in soft tissue incisional surgery: an update. Lasers Surg Med Suppl 2000; 12:55.
56. Biesman BS, Bernstein E. The Er:YAG laser as a soft tissue incisional device. Lasers Surg Med Suppl 1999; 11:64.
57. David LM, Sanders G. CO_2 blepharoplasty: a comparison to cold steel and electrocautery. J Dermatol Surg Oncol 1987; 13: 110-118.
58. Morrow DM, Morrow LB. CO_2 laser blepharoplasty: a comparison with cold-steel surgery. J Dermatol Surg Oncol 1992; 18:307-313.
59. Apfelberg DP, Maser MR, Lash H, et al. Sapphire tip technology for the YAG laser excisions in plastic surgery. Plast Reconstr Surg 1989; 84:273-279.
60. Putterman A. Scalpel neodymium:YAG laser in oculoplastic surgery. Am J Ophthalmol 1990; 109:581-584.
61. Mittelman H, Apfelberg DB. Carbon dioxide laser blepharoplasty—advantages and disadvantages. Ann Plast Surg 1990; 24:1-6.
62. Glassberg E, Babapour R, Lask G. Current trends in laser blepharoplasty: results of a survey. Dermatol Surg 1995; 2:1060-1063.
63. Lowry JC, Bartley GB. Complications of blepharoplasty. Surv Ophthalmol 1994; 38:327-350.
64. DeMere M, Wood T, Austin W. Eye complications with blepharoplasty or other eyelid surgery: a national survey. Plast Reconstr Surg 1974; 53:634-637.
65. Koorneef L. The architecture of the musculo-fibrous apparatus in the human orbit. Acta Morphol Neerl Scand 1977; 15:35-64.
66. Neuhaus RW. Complications of blepharoplasty. American Academy of Ophthalmology Focal Points 1990; 8(3):1-12.
67. Mahaffey PJ, Wallace AF. Blindness following cosmetic blepharoplasty—a review. Br J Plast Surg 1986; 39:213-221.
68. Schechter RJ. Management of inadvertent intraocular injections. Ann Ophthalmol 1985; 17:771-775.
69. Nelson CC, Passyk KA, Dootz GL. Eye shield for patients undergoing laser treatment. Am J Ophthalmol 1990; 110:39-43.
70. Hayworth RS, Lisman RD, Muchnick RS, Smith B. Diplopia following blepharoplasty. Ann Ophthalmol 1984; 16:448-451.
71. Rainin EA, Carlson BM. Postoperative diplopia and ptosis: a clinical hypothesis base on the myotoxicity of local anesthetics. Arch Ophthalmol 1985; 103:1337-1339.
72. Perlman JP, Conn H. Transient internal ophthalmoplegia during blepharoplasty: a report of three cases. Ophthal Plast Reconstr Surg 1991; 7:141-143.
73. Harley RD, Nelson LB, Flanagan JC, Calhoun JH. Ocular motility disturbances following cosmetic blepharoplasty. Arch Ophthalmol 1986; 104:542-544.

74. Jordan DR, Anderson RL, Thiese SM. Avoiding inferior oblique injury during lower blepharoplasty. Arch Ophthalmol 1989; 107: 1382-1383.
75. Levine MR, Boynton J, Tenzel RR, Miller GR. Complications of blepharoplasty. Ophthalmic Surg 1975; 6:53-57.
76. Wesley RE, Pollard ZF, McCord CD Jr. Superior oblique paresis after blepharoplasty. Plast Reconstr Surg 1980; 66:283-286.
77. Alfonso E, Levada AJ, Flynn JT. Inferior rectus paresis after secondary blepharoplasty. Br J Ophthalmol 1984; 68:535-537.
78. Baylis HI, Sutcliffe T, Fett DR. Levator injury during blepharoplasty. Arch Ophthalmol 1984; 102:570-571.
79. Carraway JH, Mellow CG. The prevention and treatment of lower lid ectropion following blepharoplasty. Plast Reconstr Surg 1990; 85:830.
80. Edgerton MT Jr. Causes and prevention of lower lid ectropion following blepharoplasty. Plast Reconstr Surg 1972; 49:42-52.
81. Kamer FM, Mikaelian AJ. Preexcision blepharoplasty. Arch Otolaryngol Head Neck Surg 1991; 117:995-999.
82. Mandel MA. Closure of blepharoplasty incisions with autologous fibrin glue. Arch Ophthalmol 1990; 108:842-844.
83. Kosko PI. Upper lid blepharoplasty: skin closure achieved with butyl-2-cyanoacrylate. Ophthalmic Surg 1981; 12:424-425.
84. Baylis HI, Goldberg RA, Wilson MC. Complications of upper blepharoplasty. In: Putterman AM. Cosmetic Oculoplastic Surgery: Eyelid, Forehead, and Facial Techniques. 3rd ed. Philadelphia: WB Saunders, 1999:411-428.
85. Smith B, Lisman RD. Dacryoadenopexy as recognized factor in upper lid blepharoplasty. Plast Reconstr Surg 1983; 71:629-632.
86. Collin JRO. Blepharochalasis: a review of 30 cases. Ophthal Plast Reconstr Surg 1991; 7:153-157.
87. Jelks GW, Jelks EB. Preoperative evaluation of the blepharoplasty patient: bypassing the pitfalls. Clin Plast Surg 1993; 20: 213-223.
88. Frankel AS, Kamer FM. The effect of blepharoplasty on eyebrow position. Arch Otolaryngol Head Neck Surg 1997; 123:393-396.
89. Shagets FW, Shore JW. The management of eyelid laxity during lower eyelid blepharoplasty. Arch Otolaryngol Head Neck Surg 1986; 112:729-732.
90. Hill JC. An analysis of senile changes in the palpebral fissure. Can J Ophthalmol 1975; 10:32-35.
91. Hill JC. The role of the lateral canthal tendon in lower eyelid laxity (commentary). Plast Reconstr Surg 1982; 69:623.
92. Neuhaus RW. Anatomic basis of "senile" ectropion. Ophthalmic Plast Surg 1985; 1:87-89.
93. Ousterhout DK, Weil RB. The role of the lateral canthal tendon in lower eyelid laxity. Plast Reconstr Surg 1982; 69:620-622.
94. Smith B, Nesi FA. The complications of cosmetic blepharoplasty. Ophthalmology 1978; 85:726-729.
95. Tenzel RR. Treatment of lagophthalmos of the lower lid. Arch Ophthalmol 1969; 81:366-368.
96. Wolfley DE. Blepharoplasty: the ophthalmologist's view. Otolaryngol Clin North Am 1980; 13:327-363.
97. Ullmann Y, Levi Y, Ben-Izhak O, et al. The surgical anatomy of the fat in the upper eyelid medial compartment. Plast Reconstr Surg 1997; 99:658-661.
98. Baker SS. Carbon dioxide laser upper lid blepharoplasty. Am J Cosmet Surg 1992; 9:141-145.
99. Biesman BS. Precautions in the use of the laser for blepharoplasty. Plast Reconstr Surg 1997; 99:275-277.
100. Ries WR, Clymer MA, Reinisch L. Laser safety features of eye shields. Laser Safety Surg Med 1996; 18:309-315.
101. David LM, Baker SS. David-Baker eyelid retractor. Am J Cosmet Surg 1992; 9:147-148.
102. Weber PJ, Wulc AE, Moody BR, et al. Electrosurgical modification of orbicularis oculi hypertrophy. Ophthal Plast Reconstr Surg 2000; 16:407-416.
103. Putterman AM. Cheek and midface lift combined with full-thickness temporal lower eyelid resection. In: Putterman AM. Cosmetic Oculoplastic Surgery: Eyelid, Forehead, and Facial Techniques. 3rd ed. Philadelphia: WB Saunders, 1999:235-247.

CHAPTER 21

Surgical Rhytidectomy: Face Lifts and the Endoscopic Forehead Lift*

STEVEN H. DAYAN
STEPHEN W. PERKINS

SECTION ONE

History and Scientific Review

BACKGROUND AND HISTORY

The majority of cosmetic surgical procedures have developed out of procedures designed to gain functional improvement. Therefore, written records, debates, and publications date back many years. In contrast, surgery for the aging face and rhytidectomy in particular originated as procedures intended to enhance self-image. Early on, aesthetic surgery was negatively perceived in the medical community. Many physicians and surgeons did not believe in the benefits of enhancing self-esteem through elective cosmetic surgery and forced this practice into shameful hiding. Others, recognizing the merit of self-improvement, felt that elective surgery with its inherent risks was an inappropriate method by which to achieve this betterment.

German and French surgeons are credited with pioneering face-lift surgery. Lexer is thought to have performed surgery in 1906 to treat wrinkles, but it was Hollander in 1912 who was the first to report a case.[1] Other European physicians including Joseph (1921) and Passot (1919) developed their own techniques to treat the aging face. Yet, for whatever reasons, these founding fathers were often guarded when it came to sharing their wisdom. Following the Great War, the practice of reconstructive plastic surgery blossomed. Along with the explosion of new ideas and techniques came the inevitable increased interest in cosmetic surgery. Although still shrouded in secrecy, its existence was recognized by even the most prominent physicians of the time. Many of these well-respected leaders were rumored to perform cosmetic surgery in their own private clinics or offices. Gilles in 1935 stated, "The operations for removal of eyelid wrinkles, cheek folds and fat in the neck are justifiable if the patients are chosen with honest discrimination."[1]

Following World War II, with the advent of newer medications and improved anesthesia methods, elective surgery became more of a reality. Additionally, a progressive affluent society expressed interest in equating appearance with a youthful outlook on life. However, the occult field of cosmetic surgery, surrounded by shameful secrecy, jealousy, and greed, had not allowed for the fostering of ideas and advancement that was common to the other surgical specialties of the time. Therefore, the results achieved by face-lift surgery were marginal and not long lasting. Sam Fomon, a pioneer in facial cosmetic surgery and also a founding father of what was to become the American Academy of Facial Plastic and Reconstructive Surgery (AAFPRS), was instrumental in teaching cosmetic surgery to all those interested. He recognized the limits of face-lift surgery when he stated, "The average duration of the beneficial effects, even with the best technical skill, cannot be expected to exceed three or four years."[1] At the time, face-lift surgery techniques consisted of a limited subcutaneous dissection and skin elevation resulting in a tightening of the preauricular skin and often an obvious "operated look." Unfortunately, these methods did not change significantly until the 1970s. The social renaissance of the 1960s and 1970s brought a new openness and acceptance to cosmetic surgery. This fueled scientific advances and dialogue leading to better surgical techniques and results.

The first major contribution in a half century was provided by Skoog, who touted the benefits of dissecting in a subfascial plane.[2] This allowed for a significant improvement in the lower third of the face. The validity of this new fascial plane was solidified by Mitz and Peyronie's landmark article in 1976, defining this fascia as the superficial musculoaponeurotic system (SMAS).[3] In order to achieve a more natural look, numerous modifications have since been made in the sub-SMAS rhytidectomy. Early sub-SMAS dissections mostly pro-

*From Perkins SW, Dayan SH. Rhytidectomy. In: Papel ID, Sykes JM, Toriumi DM, et al, eds. Facial Plastic and Reconstructive Surgery. 2nd ed. New York: Thieme, 2002.

vided for an improved jaw line. However, today's surgeons, recognizing the importance of facial harmony, have concentrated efforts on improving the mid face and nasolabial fold region. Hamra, the pioneer of the deep plane and composite rhytidectomy, continues to present the beneficial effects that can be achieved in the middle third of the face.[4,5] Others have concurred with the improved results possible with deep plane rhytidectomy.[6,7] Still, there are those who design different methods to achieve facial balance, including venturing into a subperiosteal plane.[8-10] There are even those who are revisiting the subcutaneous dissection, considering it their method of choice in select situations.

The variety of anatomically sound rhytidectomy techniques offers the surgeon options in challenging the effects of aging. However, in addition to the recent advances in surgical techniques, emphasis today has been placed on recognizing the importance of the individualized patient. Each surgical technique has its place; the key is the prudent surgeon who appropriately evaluates the patients, both physically and emotionally, and then utilizes the correct treatment for the proper diagnosis.

CONSULTATION ANALYSIS AND PREOPERATIVE PREPARATION OF THE RHYTIDECTOMY PATIENT

During the one-on-one initial consultation, it is important to develop an immediate rapport with the patient. It is important to understand the motivating forces behind the patient's request for improvement in facial appearance. Is the main concern truly correctable by standard facial rhytidectomy procedure? Often, the main concern may be true rhytides of the superficial surface of the face, more appropriately treated by means other than a face-lift procedure. If deep cheek-lip grooves are the primary motivation and the patient is less concerned about jowling or submental skin and fat ptosis, a rhytidectomy (better described as a face lift) may not be the appropriate procedure.

It is the surgeon's responsibility to determine, with the patient's assistance, what the true motivation for the surgery is. Being in the middle of a life-changing situation, such as divorce, is not in itself a contraindication for proceeding with face-lift surgery. However, the patient who expects that the cosmetic surgical procedure or procedures will solve the situational dilemma may not be a proper candidate for the procedure. The patient who truly believes the surgery is for his or her own self-esteem and not for anyone else's benefit is likely to have a successful psychological benefit. The patient must be realistic about what can and cannot be achieved by surgery, and this is a critical part of the surgeon's responsibility to impart during the consultation.

It is important to evaluate the patient's family history to determine the likely speed at which the loss of elasticity of the tissues and the overall aging process is occurring. One must determine lifestyle and social habits, taking into account issues such as solar exposure and smoking, which speed the overall aging process.

One must ask for or have the patient complete a detailed history questionnaire. It is important to identify whether the patient has had previous cosmetic surgery or any other surgery, including his or her experience and any difficulties with particular medications or anesthetic techniques. This often weighs heavily on the patient's mind. Preparing the patient for an appropriate positive mental experience is crucial. If the patient is terrified of anesthetics or the idea of surgery, one must get past this to proceed with the positive expectations of what can be achieved by surgery.

It is important to take a complete medical history to ascertain the existence of any medical conditions that would preclude face-lift surgery. Cardiovascular disease, in itself, is not a contraindication to surgery, but a complete clearance by the cardiologist is imperative prior to scheduling surgery. Certainly, an unstable cardiac history precludes any kind of anesthetic or surgical intervention. Liver and renal functions are important in determining the patient's sensitivity to anesthetics. Allergies to any medications that are required for the surgery should be taken into consideration.

There are a few diseases that would preclude face-lift surgery. The history of advanced autoimmune diseases relating to the skin of the face itself may be a contraindication for facial surgery. Scleroderma or systemic lupus erythematosus are not a contraindication to surgery, unless the patient has the disease manifested in the face itself. Some of the other autoimmune diseases may be looked at with suspicion, particularly depending upon the type of medication the patient is taking to suppress the autoimmune response. These medicines may suppress the patient's immune response or inhibit the healing process. Unstable cardiovascular disease is a contraindication to elective facial surgery. Diabetes mellitus, in itself, is not a contraindication to surgery, nor is taking chronic steroids, particularly in the lower dose ranges. Sjögren's syndrome may be a relative contraindication depending upon the involvement of the parotid glands and stasis of salivary tissues. The autoimmune diseases that relate to perivasculitis are of most concern.

A history of full course radiation treatment to the preauricular regions or infra-auricular neck would preclude surgical intervention. The long-term chronic vascular compromise to the skin's microvasculature would make skin flap elevation too risky. Accutane, although unusual in the face-lift age group population, is only a relative contraindication to any surgical intervention. There is little evidence of delayed healing of incisions specifically due to Accutane treatment. The current standard of care is to wait 6 to 12 months after finishing a course of Accutane therapy before proceeding with elective face-lift surgery. Medications that would preclude the surgeon from using epinephrine in a local anesthetic or true allergies to any of the local anesthetic classes of medication would prevent performing face-lift surgery with necessary, proper hemostasis.

Obesity, in itself, is not a contraindication to face-lift surgery if you take into consideration that the results of the procedure may be less than satisfactory. Certainly a patient who is overweight and plans dramatic weight loss in the ensuing 3 to 6 months should be counseled to appropriately lose the weight prior to contemplating the face-lift surgery. Generally, a loss or gain of 10 to 15 pounds postoperatively will not affect the overall results of the procedure. Conversely, any patient who is in the midst of dieting that may diminish vitamin and other nutritional intake should be advised against any kind of surgery. Not only should one be healthy at the time of surgery, but a proper diet is imperative for proper healing as well as electrolyte balance during the surgery. There truly are patients who are significantly overweight and should be advised against face-lift surgery because of the inherent limitations of the procedure, even if a large amount of suction-assisted lipectomy is included. The face lift itself is not a weight reduction procedure, and thinning the midfacial tissues is inappropriate and fraught with complications.

During the physical examination of the patient, part of the consultation, the surgeon should be able to advise the patient as to his or her expected outcome from the rhytidectomy itself. The physical examination is absolutely necessary for the surgeon to perform before showing the patient what the likely neckline and jawline result will be. A good candidate for face-lift surgery is a patient who has moderately thick skin and minimum sun damage and who has retained some hereditary elasticity to the skin, particularly appropriate for chronologic age. Patients with premature loss of elasticity to the skin, although it is smooth and not photodamaged, may have a less-than-satisfactory length of improvement in terms of the expectations of the surgeon and the patient.

Thick-skinned and overweight patients should not expect too much from the rhytidectomy procedure. The initial result is limited, and the length of time in which soft tissues will remain firm and in an upward position may be shorter than the average, as well as shorter than the patient expects, because of the heavier than normal weight of the tissues and gravity.

The visible loss of elasticity in the jowl tissues, as well as laxity in the skin, platysma, and fat of the submental and submandibular regions, are obvious reasons to entertain the idea of a face lift as an appropriate procedure for the patient. Certainly, benefits have to be significant to warrant the surgical intervention and the potential risks involved. Patients who have a minor degree of ptosis of these tissues or of the signs that a face lift corrects should be counseled either to consider other procedures or to return at a later date when the signs of aging have progressed and the procedure may be more indicated. Today's patient population may be slightly more anxious than they should be as to the appropriate time to begin the face-lift process to turn back the early signs of aging. It is incumbent upon the surgeon not to be too eager to recommend, or the patient too eager to undergo, this procedure for marginal benefits.

Patients who are good candidates for face-lift surgery may have a forward chin and strong bony structures, particularly prominent cheek bones. Patients with heavy cheeks and jowls and minimum malar prominences may be disappointed in the outcomes of soft tissue lifting alone. Malar augmentation may enhance the overall angulation of the face that they desire. Additionally, midfacial hypoplasia or loss of midfacial subcutaneous soft tissue due to the hereditary and aging processes often necessitates submalar augmentation to achieve appropriate rejuvenation with a standard face-lift procedure. The alternatives to these two augmentation procedures may involve a different approach to face lifting, such as midfacial lift or a composite face lift. Equally, patients with class II malocclusion, hypoplasia of the mentum, or microgenia may be poor candidates for an improved neckline result. Orthognathic consultation or, at the minimum, alloplastic augmentation of the mentum at the time of the face lift is indicated to truly achieve a satisfactory aesthetic result. It is important for the surgeon to evaluate the cervicomental angle with respect to the underlying muscular tissues and position of the hyoid bone. Many patients are poor candidates for an improved neck angle because of a low-positioned hyoid, and this needs to be carefully shown to them. It is ethically necessary to show patients the true possible results of a face lift on them. This may determine whether patients are satisfied or dissatisfied postoperatively with what they perceive the surgeon has done for them. Repositioning the hyoid itself or sculpting the digastric musculature has been described, but it is not recommended in the routine or standard neck portion of the rhytidectomy procedure. One must understand that sculpting lipectomy and platysmaplasty can accomplish remarkable results at times but have their inherent limitations.

Before leaving the consultation room, the surgeon must adequately answer all the patient's questions and then proceed to discuss the entire procedure, its alternatives, risks, and limitations. A fully informed patient understands the risks and the benefits of the procedure, as well as alternative forms of management that might be appropriate. Patients must understand the surgical procedure and the maneuvers involved, even if they do not understand or need to know the exact surgical steps. They must be adequately informed of complication possibilities, their occurrences, and their relative rates of incidence. The risks of anesthesia should be covered in terms of the choices and alternatives in a general sense. It is appropriate, however, that the risks of any particular anesthetic type should be covered by the administering physician.

FURTHER OFFICE PROTOCOL FOLLOWING CONSULTATION

At the end of the initial consultation with the patient, adequate medical photodocumentation of the current condition of the patient's aging face, neck, and jowls must be performed. Adequate preoperative photographic documentation and analysis is state of the art and the standard of care in terms of preoperative chart documentation, as well as long-term evaluation of results. Professional self-evaluation and improvement can be achieved only with adequate preoperative and postoperative photographic documentation.

Standard preoperative photographic views for face-lift surgery include the full face frontal view, as well as full face left and right oblique views and left and right lateral views. One may choose a close-up perioral photograph, as well as a photograph showing a closer detailed condition of the submental neck tissues. A close-up view of each auricle with hair pulled behind the ears, earrings removed, and all photographs taken in a Frankfort horizontal line is imperative.

It is up to the surgeon whether to show the patient, at his or her request, preoperative and postoperative photographs of other face-lift patients or merely to use computer video imaging to show the expected results in that person's case. Adequate disclaimers as to guaranteed final result must be understood by the patient. Video imaging consents are appropriate and should be signed by the patient before he or she undergoes this portion of the evaluation. Any patient viewing preoperative and postoperative photos of previous face-lift patients must understand that the confidentiality of those patients has been maintained and their permission for use in this setting was given. Furthermore, results may not be comparable from one patient to the next. Once the full evaluation is undertaken by the physician and proper photographs have been taken, the patient must be presented with the financial implications of the potential face-lift surgery. At this time patients need to be well informed as to whether this procedure will be performed in an ambulatory surgical suite or in a hospital environment. Some patients may choose extended overnight stays for their own convenience, but this is not required. Appropriate arrangements for someone to drive them to the surgical suite and to take them home is, however, critical. Most patients remain sedated postoperatively for 12 to 24 hours and should not be responsible for themselves without assistance.

If the patient chooses to schedule surgery, a date should be selected and the appropriate informed consent needs to be signed. The informed consent reiterates what was covered in the consultation, and the patient's signature reaffirms that he or she has been fully informed by the doctor of the risks and benefits of the procedure, as well as its alternatives. Further, it must state that all questions were appropriately answered. Consent for use of any kind of photography for purposes other than medical record documentation must be obtained from the patient prior to using the photos. The patient is then asked to obtain appropriate preoperative laboratory and other physical assessment measures. Any reservations about the patient's ability to undergo anesthesia may dictate further physical examination and consultation with the appropriate medical specialist.

Finally, at all times the entire confidentiality of the consultation and plans for surgery must be assured. Patients must give permission for any contact with outside laboratories, physicians, or insurance companies. Any patient reservations on whom to contact at his or her business must be documented in the chart and complied with.

ANATOMIC CONSIDERATIONS AND TYPE OF FACE LIFT PERFORMED

The fundamental decision as to type of face lift required for each individual patient is based primarily upon the preexisting condition of the patient as outlined and observed in the physical examination portion of the consultation. Not every patient requires the same degree of surgical intervention to achieve a satisfactory result. Generally there are three types of face-lift procedures based on the general categories of surgical intervention required to achieve a satisfactory surgical result. This discussion will cover each procedure, whether it involves a minimum degree of skin undermining, plication or imbrication of the underlying SMAS, treatment of the platysma muscles, or extensions into the deeper layers of the face, including the subperiosteal approach. Most of the decisions are based on the preexisting condition of the patient, the underlying philosophy of the surgeon, and what the surgeon believes the long-term results of the surgical maneuvers may be (Boxes 21-1 and 21-2).

First, the fundamental concept of face lifting is based on certain anatomic relationships of the tissues. The elasticity and condition of the overlying skin, including its degree of photodamage and rhytide formation, is important. The relationship with the underlying subcutaneous adipose tissue, including the loss of position with gravity, true ptosis, or abnormal accumulation and distribution, must be noted. The underlying fascial arrangement of face, neck, and mid face is such that the facial musculature is enveloped by a continuous fascia that extends to the preparotid region. This fascia, which is contiguous with the platysma muscle of the neck, is called the SMAS and was first described as a dynamic contractile and fibromuscular web by Mitz and Peyronie. They termed this the superficial musculoaponeurotic system (SMAS). The fascia deep to this is the superficial layer of the deep cervical fascia that envelops and covers the sternocleidomastoid muscle, as well as the parotid tissues. It is superficial to the superficial layer of the temporalis muscular fascia, as well as superficial to the periosteum of the forehead. The SMAS is contiguous with the galea of the scalp. In the neck anteriorly, the platysma muscle may or may not be interdigitated to form a connected sling. Often, there is a laxity and dehiscence of the anterior borders of the platysma muscle, creating banding in the neck. It is the very nature and existence of this SMAS layer that allows for a deeper plane of face-lifting surgery than was performed in the original rhytidectomy procedure. Only skin was lifted, elevated, excised, and resutured in a more cephalic and posterior position. Skin, because of its inherent creep phenomenon and rebound stretch characteristics, would often not hold for any length of time. Therefore, the effects of the face-lift surgery were brief when this was the only layer approached. Skin, particularly in the mid and more central portion of the face, is directly connected to the SMAS layer by firm dermal fibrous filaments. Accompanying these dermal filaments often is some penetrating vascularity from the deeper vascular systems to the superficial dermal plexus. It is easily demonstrable that lifting and pulling the SMAS layer with its integral attachment to the platysma muscle and midfacial muscles lifts and repositions the skin in the same fashion (Fig. 21-1). A superior and posterior vector of the pull of this fascia repositions the facial tissues in a more youthful position. The effect of gravity on these anatomic tissues is directly affected and improved by the face-lifting procedures.

It is equally important to understand the anatomic relationships of the neurosensory and neuromotor branches of the face that supply sensation to the overlying skin as well as function to the mimetic muscles of the face. These relate directly to the expected sequela of face-lifting surgery for all patients: loss of sensation and paresthesias. Most often this is temporary but can be permanent. The fifth cranial nerve supplies sensation to the cutaneous surfaces of the face, head, and neck. The fact that to perform any type of face-lifting surgery requires elevation and a certain degree of preauricular and postauricular skin necessitates interruption of the immediate innervation of this portion of the face. Typically, unless any major branch of the greater auricular nerve is interrupted, sensation returns to the skin in a relatively short period of time. The patient can expect return of sensation in the first 6 to 8 weeks, but occasionally it may require 6 months to a year for full return. Rarely, the patient may report a decreased overall postoperative sensation to the skin, even beyond 1 year.

BOX 21-1 Ideal Characteristics for Face Lift

- Good skin tone with minimal photoaging and few wrinkles
- Strong facial bony structures
- Strong forward chin
- Prominent cheek bones
- Fuller mid face
- Shallow cheek-lip grooves
- Sharp cervicomental sulcus
- Nonsmoker

BOX 21-2 Poor Characteristics for Face Lift

- A low hyoid producing an obtuse cervicomental angle
- Receded or weak chin
- Low-slung submandibular glands
- Deep oral commissure cheek-chin grooves
- Deep nasolabial grooves and prominent cheek mounds or folds

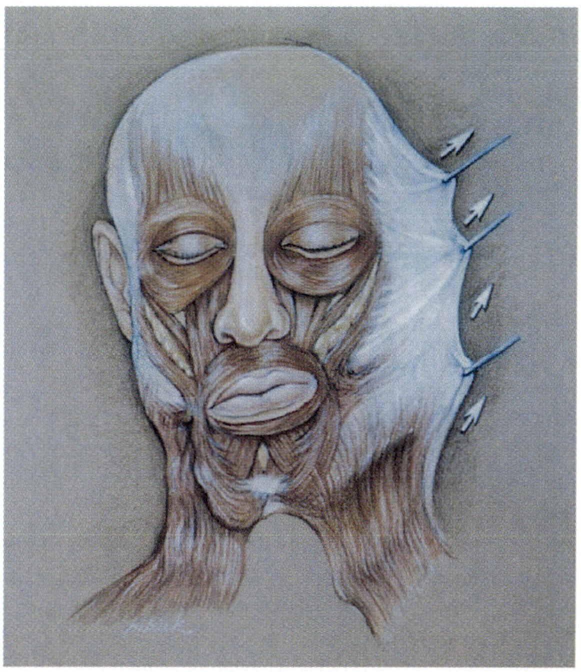

FIG. 21-1
SMAS connected with platysma and facial musculature.

Sympathetic and parasympathetic reinnervation of the skin proceeds more rapidly in the postoperative period. Although the most common major nerve branch injured in face-lifting surgery is the greater auricular nerve as it crosses over the sternocleidomastoid, even this rarely causes permanent loss of sensation of the auricle or the preauricular skin. As one is dissecting skin and its dermal attachments away from the superficial layer of the sternocleidomastoid muscular fascia, interruption of this fascia may cause direct injury to this large, visible nerve branch. When injury is recognized at the time of surgery, direct suture reanastomosis is indicated and return of nerve function within 1 to 2 years is expected. Motor branches to the facial mimetic musculature are potentially in danger during face-lifting surgery. Branches of the facial nerve become superficial as they extend past the parotid masseteric fascia. The marginal mandibular branch is at some risk as it crosses the mandibular margin, deep to the platysma muscle, and deep to the superficial layer of the deep cervical fascia. Techniques requiring deep plane elevation underneath the SMAS layer into the mid face endanger branches to the orbicularis, zygomatic, and buccinator muscles. Innervation to these muscles is still to the under surface of the muscles, and deep plane technique at this point would be superficial to those muscles. Direct visualization of the nerve is part of this procedure and will be discussed further in this chapter.

A branch of the facial nerve potentially injured in face-lifting surgery, with or without temporal forehead lifting, is the frontal (temporal) branch of the facial nerve. This branch becomes superficial at the level of the zygomatic arch and extends just beneath the subcutaneous tissues underlying the thin SMAS layer of the temporal region before its innervation of the deeper surface of the frontalis muscle. As it traverses this area, approximately 1.5 to 2 cm preauricular and halfway between the lateral orbital rim and the temporal tuft of hair, the nerve is at most risk. It is imperative that the surgeon understand the anatomic relationships of the layers of the face and temporal region in order to prevent injury to the nerve. One can elevate the skin all the way to the lateral canthal region, the preauricular area overlying the zygomatic arch, up to the orbicularis muscle, as long as dissection is in the immediate subcutaneous layer. Additionally, the surgeon can dissect freely underneath the frontalis fascia beneath the galeal layer superficial to the periosteum and the overlying superficial fascia of the temporalis muscle without injury to the frontal branch of the facial nerve, which is external to this avascular layer. However, at the level of the zygomatic arch, one needs to make the transition to beneath the periosteum, or the facial nerve may be transected as one follows the same plane overlying the zygomatic arch. Reinnervation of the frontalis muscle may not be possible after injury to the nerve in this area.

SECTION TWO
Atlas of Surgical Procedures
The Face-lift Procedure

Planning incisions and marking the appropriate locations for the incisions is crucial to the patient's long-term happiness and successful outcome. Changes in hairline or scars that are placed in visible locations may cause the patient's total dissatisfaction with an otherwise good lift result. The natural look to the patient's hairline, the freedom with which hair can be styled, and the invisibility of the scar lines separate the good face-lift surgeon from the one sought after by patients as the best in any given community. The face-lift surgeon who pays attention to the details of incision placement and planning can often be the one known and referred to by hairdressers and other cosmeticians who see the results from this portion of the face lift.

There are three critical points that must be taken into consideration in planning the face-lift incisions:

1. How to manage and maintain the preauricular tuft of hair, including the sideburn, must be decided. Each patient is different, as can be the location of the lower portion of the sideburn and the width at which it extends anteriorly from the insertion of the helical curvature. If the preauricular sideburn hairline is 1 or 2 cm below the insertion of the superior portion of the helical insertion, it can be appropriate to design an incision that curves up into the temporal hair and allows some posterior superior lifting of the hairline. The curved hairline incision—not a straight vertical incision—is required to interrupt the forces of contracture, maintain a minimally wide scar, and prevent alopecia (Fig. 21-2). As long as the hairline is not lifted higher than the insertion of the

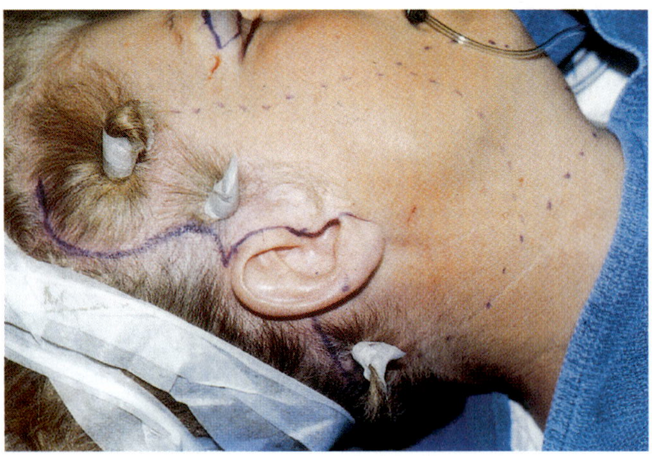

FIG. 21-2
Typical face-lift incision for patient with low sideburn tuft of hair.

superior helical insertion, the patient will have no cosmetic disturbance of this area. If the sideburn is at the helical insertion preoperatively, an inferior sideburn incision is required and this will, therefore, usually be associated with a separate temporal incision if a lift is required in this region. At no time should the incision be carried anteriorly around the sideburn tuft and along the pre-temporal hairline. All scars in this area will be visible and cannot be camouflaged with the fine, severely sloped hair as it exits the skin naturally in a posterior direction.

2. Preauricularly, the incision must at least follow the apparent curvatures of the auricle itself. There is a strong preference by the patient population for an incision hidden behind the posterior edge of the tragus so that the incision appears "inside the ear." No preauricular incision will be seen, as it otherwise follows the normal curvature of the helic insertion and goes behind the tragus about 1 to 2 mm, then exits at the junction of the earlobe with the face. As an alternative to this, for patients with hearing aids or deep pretragal depressions and tall tragi, a curved incision extending into the incisura and then out around the curve in the helix may be acceptable. However, loss of pigmentation in the scar, no matter how thin, will leave a visible line forever and may require a hairstyle modification to hide this in the future.
3. Postauricularly, the incision must be directed up onto the posterior aspect of the auricle above the sulcus, so when the ear settles posteriorly and the scar heals with some contracture of the scar, it falls into the postauricular sulcus and not out on the postauricular skin. The incision should make a gentle curve across the junction of the auricle with the postauricular skin, not crossing the non-hair-bearing skin at the level where the auricle meets the hairline. For most cases the incision should be gently sloped back into the postauricular hair. When advancing the postauricular skin posteriorly and superiorly, the posterior hairline can then be approximated with no step off or other deformity. However, when a patient has a significant amount of neck skin that needs to be repositioned posteriorly, it is often imperative that the incision be designed to run down along the postauricular hairline before being swung posteriorly into the hair. That way, a large amount of skin can be moved posteriorly and superiorly without stepping off the postauricular hairline. At no time should the incision be left visible at the base of the hairline toward the anterior neck.

Additionally, a small 1 to 3 cm incision is required in the submental area, just anterior to the preexisting deep submental crease in order to perform the portion of the operation required in the anterior neck. Prior to the infiltration of the anesthetic, a dotted line is often used to determine the area to be anesthetized and the area that will be subsequently undermined. Some surgeons prefer to mark the area of the zygomatic arch, McGregor's patch, and the angle of the mandible.

Further outlining of the jowl itself and any platysma banding may be of benefit to highlight areas that need correction during the operation.

One variation in the male face-lift patient and the woman who has a fair amount of hirsute preauricular skin is an incision that is gently curved in the preauricular area in what is often a preexisting preauricular crease. This incision should not be entirely straight but needs to be a distance away from the incisura and in front of the tragus. One must leave a non-hair-bearing portion of skin when moving the bearded skin or hair-bearing skin posteriorly and superiorly (Fig. 21-3). (An important part of the consultation is to outline exactly where you plan to make the incisions and to note this in the chart graphically, as well as in written form.)

Anesthesia for face-lift surgery requires an appropriate amount of local infiltration anesthetic combined with epinephrine to control cutaneous bleeding with a comfortable, well-sedated patient. Although many surgeons prefer inhalation anesthetics for a complete general anesthetic, this is not usually required. What is required is a patient who is intravenously sedated and fully monitored with continuous cardiac blood pressure and oxygen saturation monitors. A person is designated to monitor the patient, whether this be an anesthesiologist, certified nurse anesthetist, or an RN under the direction of the operating surgeon. A well-assured patient preoperatively is critical to the success of a conscious sedation anesthesia. The patient who is comforted knowing that he or she will not experience pain or discomfort or otherwise be mistreated during the operation will be mentally prepared for the appropri-

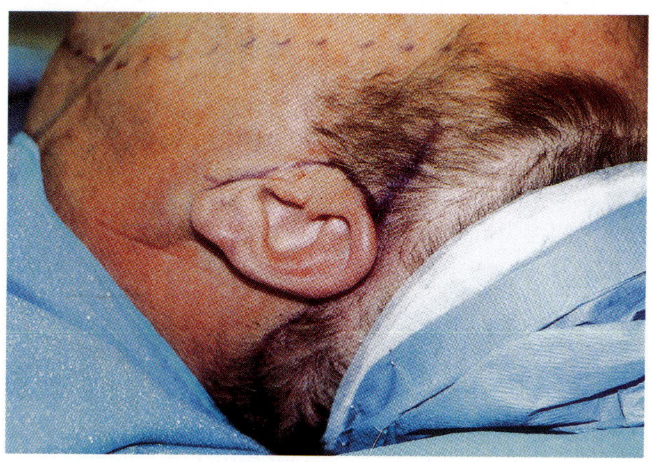

FIG. 21-3
Typical incision for a male with beard, preserving non-hair-bearing preauricular skin.

ate effects of the sedation medicine. It is generally a good idea to provide the patient some oral medication for relaxation prior to administering intravenous sedation. Current medications include a significant amount of amnestic effect as well as proper sedation and analgesia. Any anesthetic administered should have some prolonged effect so that the patient remains comfortable for several hours in the immediate postoperative period. Infiltration of the incision lines is best accomplished with 1% lidocaine with 1:50,000 epinephrine. This will provide not only good anesthesia but also the maximum possible hemostasis for vasoconstriction. Infiltration of the areas to be undermined should be done with 0.5% lidocaine with 1:100,000 or 1:200,000 epinephrine. Some hemostasis is still required. The total volume of lidocaine must be carefully monitored. At no time should more than 500 mg of lidocaine with epinephrine be infiltrated at one time or within a 1- to 2-hour period. Overdosage of lidocaine with resultant lidocaine toxicity can result from injudicious volume infiltration of this local anesthetic. It may be advisable to infiltrate one side of the face and complete this portion of the operation before infiltrating the other side of the face. This sequential infiltration, as long as it is performed 10 to 15 minutes before the incision on that side is made, is quite safe and effective.

The patient must then be prepared for the surgical operation by twisting and securing small bundles of hair to keep them out of the incision lines and the operative field. This may require taping these bundles in a secure fashion prior to prepping. Once the patient is prepped and draped with a head drape in the usual sterile manner, the operation may commence. No shaving of the hair is required. Preoperative antibiotic prophylaxis is given to all patients, using a cephalosporin 1 day preoperatively and continuing for 4 days postoperatively.

Treatment of the Submentum, Jowl, and Neck

Initial treatment of the neck involves correction of the jowl, submandibular, and submental lipoptosis. In type I face lifts, there is generally very little or no need for any intervention in the neck. Posterior tightening of the skin-SMAS-platysma is all that is required for that particular patient. However, in the majority of patients, some attention to the submandibular, submental, and jowl lipoptosis is required. If only debulking and reduction of this lipoptosis is required, a small 1 cm incision is made in the submental crease in order to admit a liposuction cannula. If one has determined by examination that no platysma redundancy is present and there is some elasticity to the skin remaining, liposuction is carried out as the only neck procedure.

The initial 1 cm dissection is performed just beneath the skin in the middle of the fat layer or subcutaneous

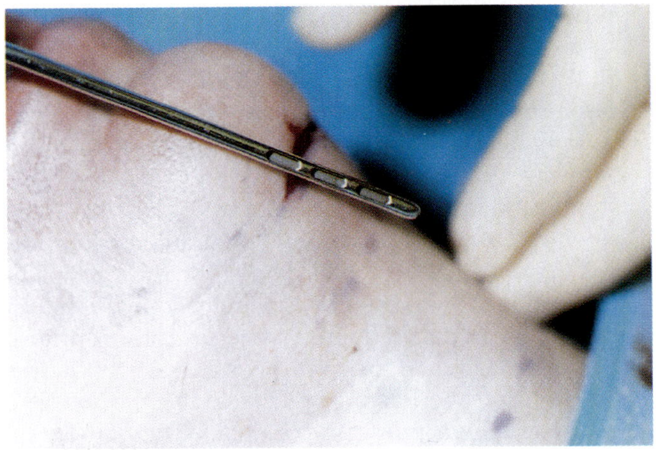

FIG. 21-4
A 3 mm three-opening liposuction cannula.

tissues. Small 1 cm tunnels are started and then completed with a 2 or 3 mm liposuction cannula. No suction is applied initially, creating the tunnels all the way from the submental area across the mandibular margin into the jowl region, to the anterior border of the sternocleidomastoid and down and across the cervicomental angle to the area of the thyroid cartilage. This is done in a fanlike fashion from one jowl across the neck to the opposite jowl. A circular liposuction cannula with three openings on one side is then used to perform this liposuction maneuver (Fig. 21-4). Very careful and judicious liposuction in the jowl areas is performed so as to hold the tissues away from the mandibular margin and not create blunt trauma to the marginal mandibular nerve. Very minimum liposuction is performed in an even fashion in order to prevent the creation of any furrows, tunnels, or dimpling. This can happen easily in the jowl areas, so care is taken to underperform this maneuver in this region. Depending upon the amount of liposuction required in the submental and submandibular neck, a larger liposuction cannula may be required, advancing to a 4 mm and sometimes a 6 mm flat cannula with one opening on the inferior surface of the cannula. Good bimanual palpation is required to determine the symmetry and equality of the removal of the fat. Leaving a degree of subcutaneous fat is required to give supple skin contour. Do not perform overly aggressive liposuction across the cervicomental angle, as this has the potential for creating dermal injury and subdermal scarring with late development of banding. Often, this is all that is required in a type II face lift. However, in advanced type III face lifts with a tremendous amount of fat and some platysma ptosis, as well as type III face lifts with significant collections of fat, laxity of skin, and platysma

A 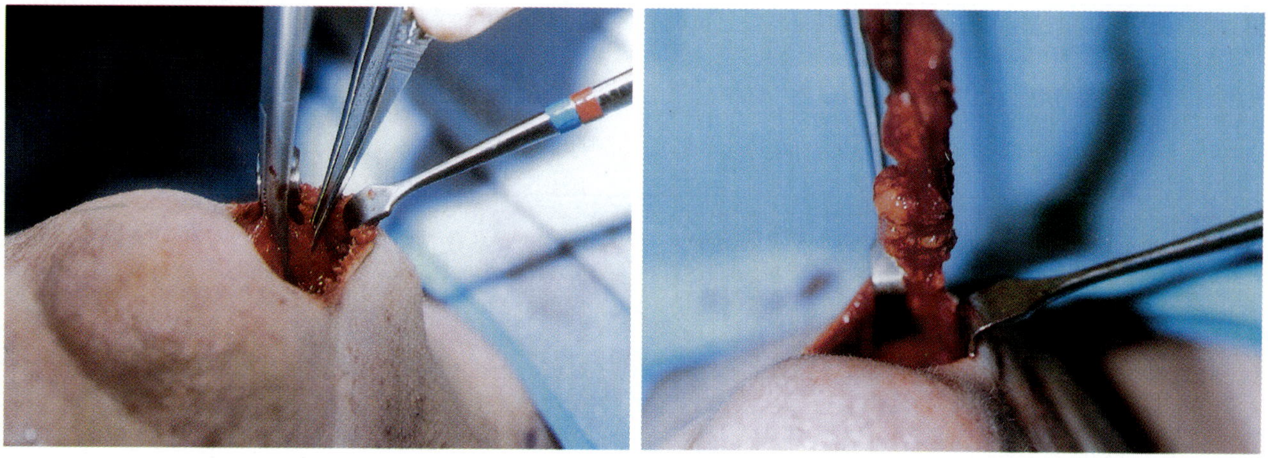 B

FIG. 21-5
A, Use of Kelly clamp to tighten anterior platysma and anterior submental fat for incremental excision. **B,** Sequential removal of redundant submental muscle and fat past cervicomental angle.

sagging, further work is required. The incision may be extended to at least 2.5 to 3 cm. Direct subcutaneous elevation is then performed after the liposuction to elevate the skin from the platysma muscle. This is performed in a wide fashion, usually extending to the anterior border of the sternocleidomastoid and past the cervicomental angle. This then allows the surgeon to directly view the remaining lipoptosis beneath the platysma muscle and view the redundancy and laxity of the anterior platysma bands. Their dehiscence is easily visible.

The laxity and redundancy of these tissues is determined and, using a grasping forceps and a long curved Kelly clamp, these tissues are tightened in the midline. Their redundancy is progressively excised, taking care to maintain adequate hemostasis, suturing the anterior transected borders of the platysma together into a midline corset. The excess fat and muscle are removed all the way down past the cervicomental angle (Fig. 21-5). Several mattressing sutures using a 3-0 Vicryl suture are done. Once a firm muscular corset is created and a sharper cervicomental angle is achieved, the remainder of the face-lift skin undermining will be accomplished from the posterior position. Redundancy of skin in the submental area will be determined at the end of the operation after tightening the bilateral preauricular and postauricular skin in a superior posterior direction.

To further define the cervicomental angle, on occasion it has been found helpful to tunnel under the neck flap an interlocking midline platysmal suspending suture. A midline mattress suture is passed from the left platysmal border out under the right postauricular flap. A second mattress suture from the right platysmal border is interlocked with the previous suture and brought out under the left postauricular flap. These sutures are then secured to the mastoid periosteum. A permanent suture is preferable, although long-lasting success has been achieved with a 3-0 nonpermanent suture. Modest tension is key, as excess pull on the suture may lead to a skeletonized neck.

Skin Elevation and Undermining

The extent of undermining is dependent on the amount of redundancy of skin in the neck and to some degree on the facial tissues. With the use of SMAS lifting, the degree of undermining is much less than in older classic rhytidectomies. A large degree of undermining increases the risk of vascular compromise as well as the development of small seromas, hematomas, and irregularities. However, when a large degree of skin and platysma redundancy is present in the neck, it is often necessary to separate the skin from the underlying lateral platysma muscle in order to redrape each in a sequential fashion and achieve the maximum improvement. Generally, lifting the SMAS and the deep facial tissues is as effective and much safer than separating the skin all the way out to the melolabial crease. Although some surgeons still prefer this older technique, today this large amount of undermining has not been shown to be more effective than the SMAS techniques in improving the jowl or deep melolabial fold.

Undermining the skin begins in the postauricular area and can be done with a beveled face-lift scissors in an advance-spreading technique (Fig. 21-6). Direct knife elevation is an alternative. It is important to begin deep to the level of the hair follicles in this region so as not to injure the hair follicles and create permanent alopecia. However, once the dissection is continued anterior to the postauricular hairline, it should be quite superficial in the immediate subcutaneous layer. This subcutaneous layer is minimal in the postauricular region, and the skin closely adheres to the overlying fascia of the sternocleidomastoid muscle. This layer must be carefully separated until the dissection is anterior to the sternocleidomastoid. Injury to the greater auricular nerve, as mentioned previously, is somewhat common due to the lack of a thicker subcutaneous layer and adherent dermal attachments in this region. Elevation is then continued to the subcutaneous plane superficial to the platysma muscle and anteriorly as far as the amount of neck surgery dictates (Fig. 21-7*A*). Often, the undermining is completed and meets the undermining that was previously done in the submental area. Although the undermining may extend up slightly above the mandibular margin, it is generally confined to the neck region.

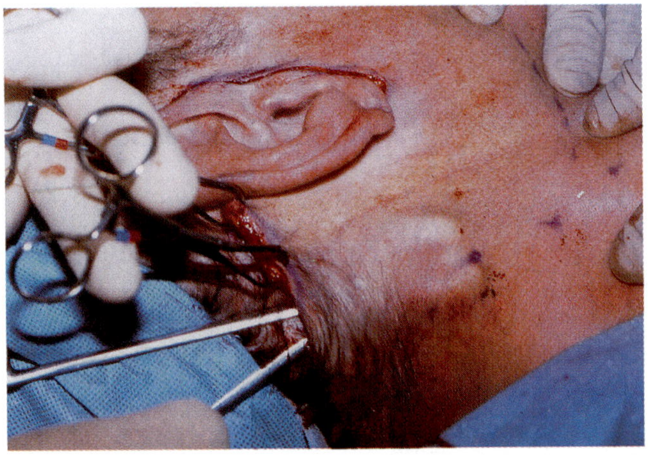

FIG. 21-6
Undermining with beveled face-lift scissors with advance and spread technique.

Once the undermining of the neck has been achieved, undermining begins in the temporal area. Temporal lifting is required to achieve smoothing of the lateral canthotemporal skin and lateral brow. Incisions are made down through the scalp tissues through the superficial galea and the superficial layer of the temporalis fascia is identified. Undermining can be performed in this layer all the way down to the lateral brow and the superior edge of the zygomatic arch. Elevation of the temporal unit is not required in all face lifts and is usually not required in type I face lifts. It is usually required when there is laxity of tissues in the lateral brow and lateral orbital region that need to be redraped so as not to create bunching when the cheek tissues are brought up superiorly. The temporal lift may or may not be connected with other means of lifting the brow-forehead complex. Elevation is then begun in the preauricular area at the level of the temporal tuft in the immediate subcutaneous layer. This is a layer distinctly different from the layer for the temporal elevation, and a noninterrupted bridge of SMAS and neurovascular bundles should be left intact extending superiorly toward the frontalis muscle. By maintaining this nonconnected bridge of tissue, one will not injure the frontal branch of the facial nerve (Fig. 21-7*B*). Undermining can then proceed to the malar area, extending in the preauricular region anywhere from 4 to 6 cm depending on the elasticity of the

A

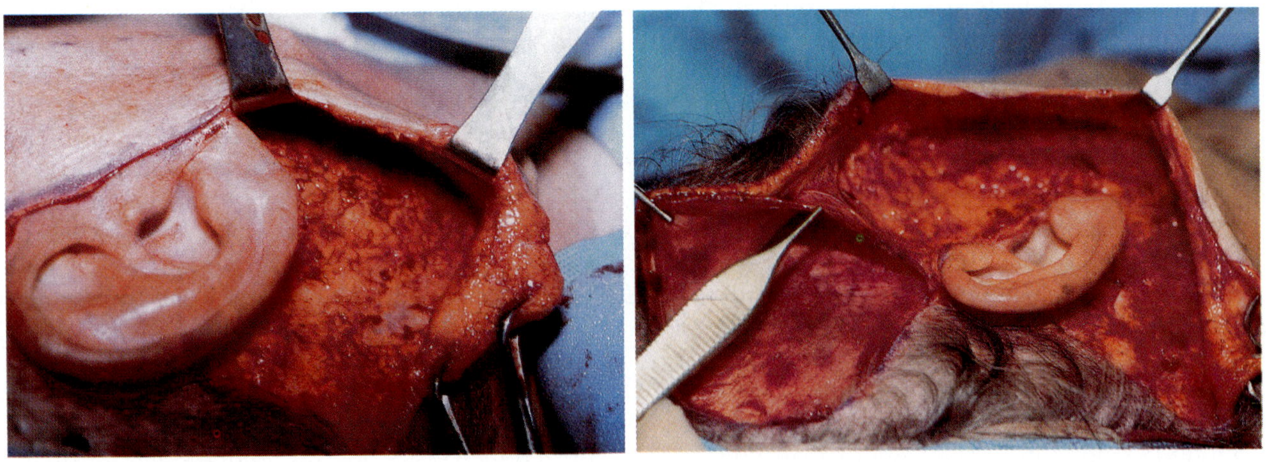

B

FIG. 21-7
A, Postauricular and neck flap elevated within subcutaneous fat layer over the sternocleidomastoid muscle. **B,** Maintaining a noninterrupted bridge of tissue in the temporal region to avoid injury to the frontal branch of the facial nerve.

skin. This undermining is continued in this intra-adipose layer, easily separating the subcutaneous dermal fat, leaving it with the skin flap, from the underlying fat overlying the SMAS. This preauricular space is connected to the same layer of elevation overlying the platysma muscle in the neck. Hemostasis is then assured under direct vision.

Depending on the nature of the face lift, one must determine the degree of intervention and manipulation of the SMAS layer. Even type I face lifts may require imbrication or deep plane maneuvers, depending on the need for elevation of the midfacial tissues. If only a small amount of jowl repositioning and posterior repositioning of the platysma muscle is required, plication of the SMAS may be the only maneuver (Fig. 21-8). However, one must remove the adipose tissue that is still on top of the SMAS in a semilunar fashion in the preauricular area so as to pull the SMAS over upon SMAS while suturing. Otherwise, there will be no fibrous adherence of the SMAS and the lift may fail when the sutures give way. Some surgeons prefer a permanent suture for this plication or folding of the SMAS because it needs to be maintained in this position over time.

Generally, face lifts do require some undermining of the SMAS layer and platysma so that it can be advanced superiorly and posteriorly (Fig. 21-9*A*). The degree of this undermining will be dictated by the need to lift the jowl, platysma muscle, and midfacial tissues. This is imbrication of the SMAS, whereby the SMAS will be lifted, advanced, trimmed, and sutured end to end. This can be done with a long-lasting, but not permanent, suture.

For those patients requiring midfacial lift of the subcutaneous soft tissues, as a minimum a modification of the deep plane face lift is performed. This requires elevation of the SMAS layer at the level of the zygomatic arch over the malar eminence and superficial to the zygomaticus muscle. Complete deep plane face-lift techniques necessitate undermining the SMAS layer all the way anterior to the anterior border of the masseteric muscle and connecting this to the elevation of the full neck tissues superficial to the platysma muscle. Transition must be made, however, in the mid cheek to the superficial layer overlying the zygomaticus muscle or injury will occur to the nerve to this muscle, or the buccinator. Once the appropriate elevation of the midfacial tissues has been accomplished with the corresponding SMAS and platysma, this layer is advanced in an appropriate posterior superior direction (Fig. 21-9*B*). Direct vision allows one to see the movement of the melolabial tissues and the jowl back and upward into a more youthful position. Often, a slip of this SMAS fascia is brought up to the firm preauricular tissues and used as a sling suspension. Similarly, the SMAS is divided at the level of the earlobe and an inferior slip of SMAS platysma is sutured with a 0-Vicryl suture as a supporting sling to the mastoid fascia and periosteum (Fig. 21-9*C* and *D*). This provides crisp, sharp delineation of the cervicomental angle. Redundancies of platysma and SMAS are trimmed and a few sutures placed to the posterior postauricular fascial tissues. Anteriorly, the SMAS is trimmed, the excess is discarded, and the SMAS is sutured end to end with a long-lasting, temporary monofilament suture such as 3-0 PDS.

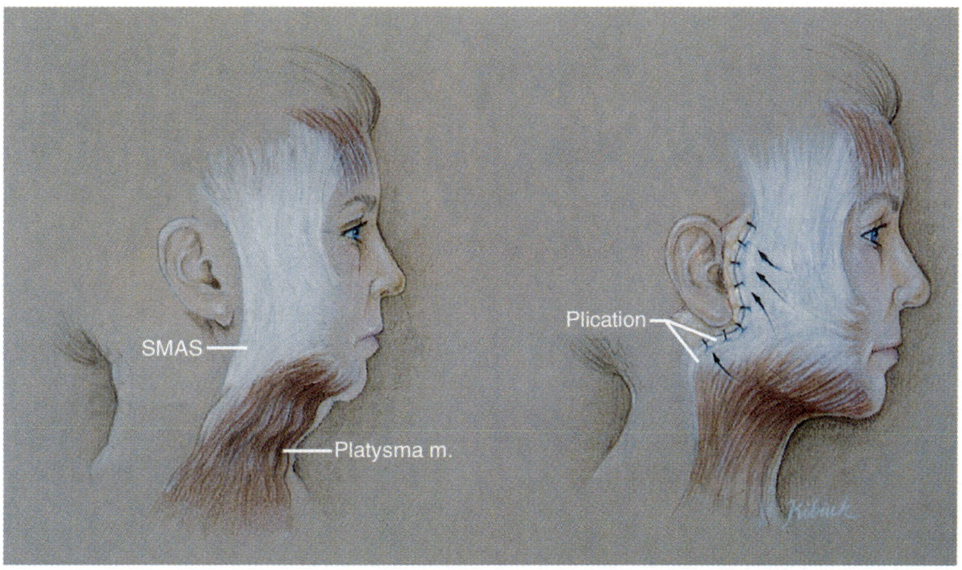

FIG. 21-8
Plication of the SMAS and platysma with posterior suspension.

A B C D

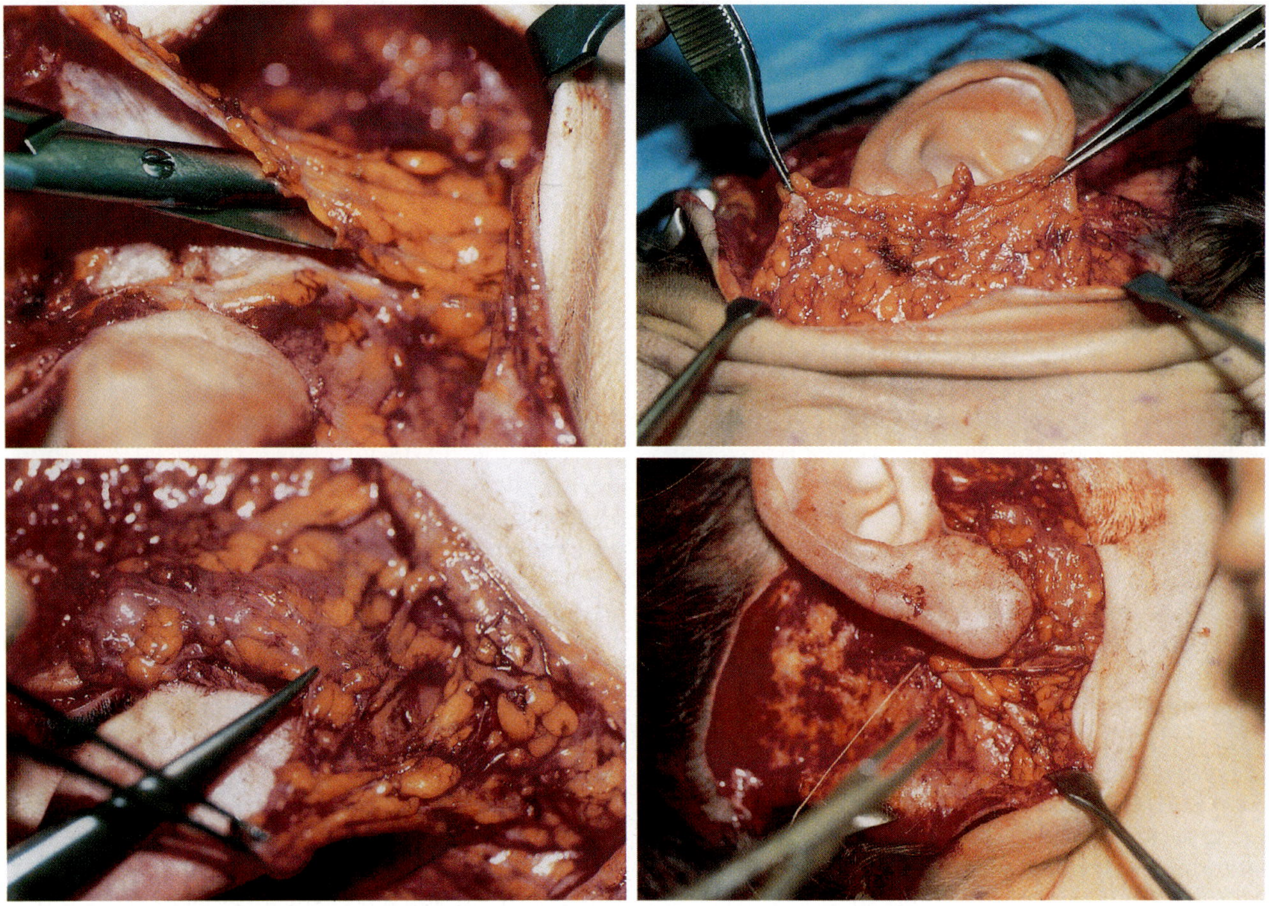

FIG. 21-9
A, Metzenbaum scissors elevation of the preauricular SMAS. **B,** Advancement of the undermined SMAS prior to imbrication. **C,** Splitting the SMAS-platysma flap at the earlobe for suspension of sling of platysma. **D,** Suspension of posterior slip of platysma-SMAS with 0-Vicryl suture to the mastoid periosteum.

Skin Flap Advancement

After adequate deep fascial lift has been completed for the long-term foundation of the face lift, the skin flap can be repositioned and modified as necessary. One can see, with minimum tension, the redundancy of skin that is draped over the ear in a posterior superior vector. The preauricular skin is moved mostly posteriorly and slightly superiorly, taking care not to let the sideburn tuft of hair be pulled too high. The neck skin is lifted in the postauricular area in a posterior but mostly superior fashion so as not to create a large step off deformity of the postauricular hairline. Once the skin has been secured in the high preauricular and postauricular regions, an incremental cut is made and a staple placed (Fig. 21-10*A*). The skin along the postauricular occipital hair is incised in a beveled fashion, and surgical staples are used to approximate these scalp tissues. The skin in the non-hair-bearing postauricular areas are sutured in a running interlocking fashion with a 5-0 plain gut type suture. As there is no tension, no deep sutures are required. The earlobe is positioned with a deep 5-0 Vicryl suture and the skin is trimmed so that the earlobe is tucked in a superior position. It is often important to exaggerate the upward lift to the earlobe so that when the tissues heal and drift inferiorly, the earlobe is not pulled down. An inferiorly distracted earlobe looks like a satyr's ear and is an obvious postoperative face-lift deformity. The preauricular tissues are trimmed appropriately according to the planned preoperative incision. A tragal flap is left significantly redundant so that when it is closed there is absolutely no tension in the earlobe and the tragal flap is bunched together in a pie-shaped fashion exaggerating the new tragus. When this heals, it will contract and look extremely close to a normal tragus and not be pulled anteriorly by overly tightened scar contracture from injudicious trimming of the flap. The preauricular skin is closed with a running interlocking 5-0 plain gut suture.

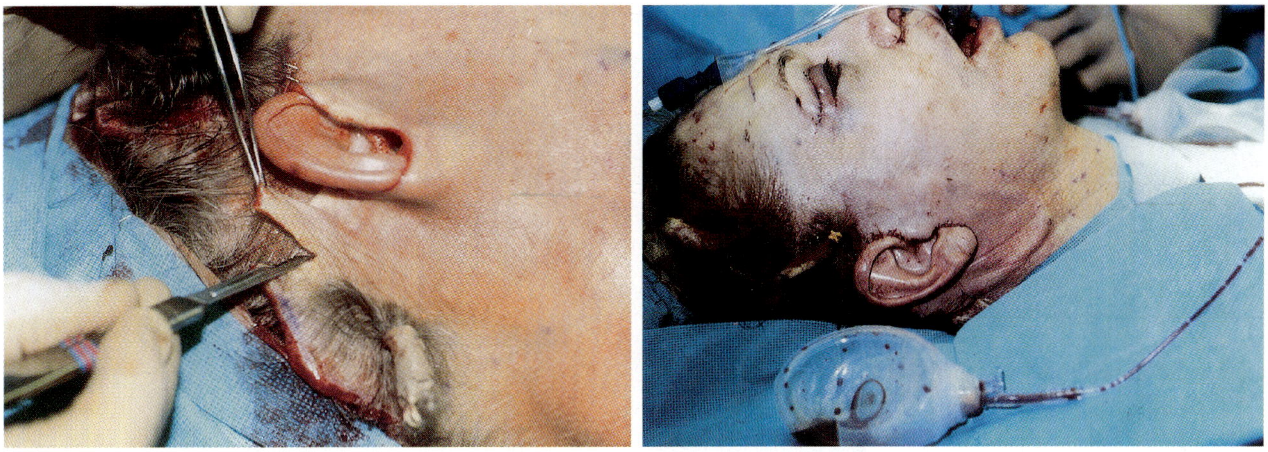

A B

FIG. 21-10
A, Posterior draping of the skin flap requires alignment of the occipital hairline. **B,** A closed suction drain is used to prevent serohematomas.

The temporal incision is closed, as was the occipital scalp, with interrupted surgical staples. Prior to complete closure, a flat 4 mm closed suction drain is placed with an exit wound hidden in the postoccipital hair (Fig. 21-10*B*). The drain is brought just to the level of the anterior angle of the mandible. The submental skin is then trimmed, if there is excess, in a semilunar fashion with care being taken not to create dog-ears laterally or skin redundancies.

Prior to the placement of the dressing in the operating room, the patient's hair twirls are removed, the hair is washed, and any blood is rinsed. An antibiotic ointment is applied to a nonadherent dressing, which is placed in the preauricular and postauricular areas. A few 4 × 4s are placed over the undermined areas, and a cotton batting is then loosely applied under the chin and over the top of the head. This is held in place with a minimally constrictive elastic type chin strap. Care is taken not to put pressure on the undermined skin flaps (Fig. 21-11).

The patient is discharged from the operating room to the recovery area and stays until he or she is able to be assisted to the car and driven home. The patient needs to be ambulatory with assistance before discharge and must be with someone through the entire night. It is important to maintain phone contact with the patient for that evening. The patient is required to stay within a 15- or 20-minute drive from the operative facility in the event immediate postoperative care would be required. The patient is requested to return the following morning, 12 to 18 hours postoperatively. At that time, the dressing is removed, the drains are generally removed, and a light chin strap is applied for 24 more hours. Throughout the week the patient is asked to shower once a day and to keep the wounds clean and moist with peroxide and antibiotic ointment.

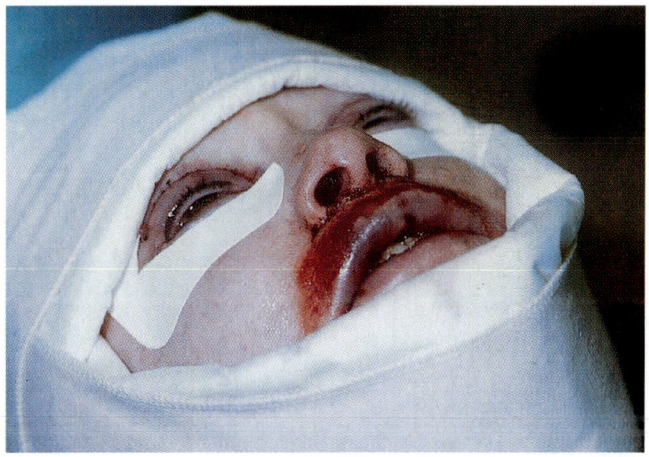

FIG. 21-11
Postoperative face-lift dressing for mild compression.

One week postoperatively, the patient returns for staple and suture removal.

The patient is then asked to return 10 to 14 days postoperatively for reexamination and the opportunity to meet with the makeup artist consultant. The meeting includes an introduction to appropriate makeup coverage for any residual ecchymoses as well as a full skin care lesson. The makeup artist introduces appropriate moisturizers, makeup, and sun screens and teaches future appropriate skin care to maintain the face-lift results.

It is imperative to see patients at 1 month, 3 months, 6 months, and 1 year postoperatively to follow their results (Figs. 21-12 to 21-15). In the second to the fourth week, patients often require emotional support, as they are still adjusting to their new appearance and reassimilating to work or social activities. Many of the post-

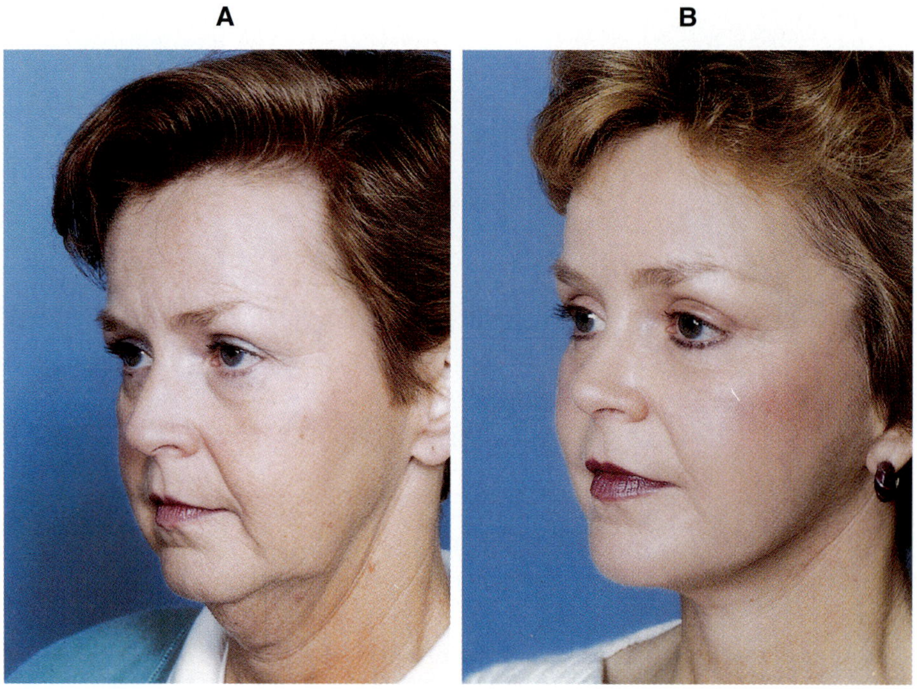

FIG. 21-12
A, Before face lift, oblique view. **B,** Six months after face lift, oblique view.

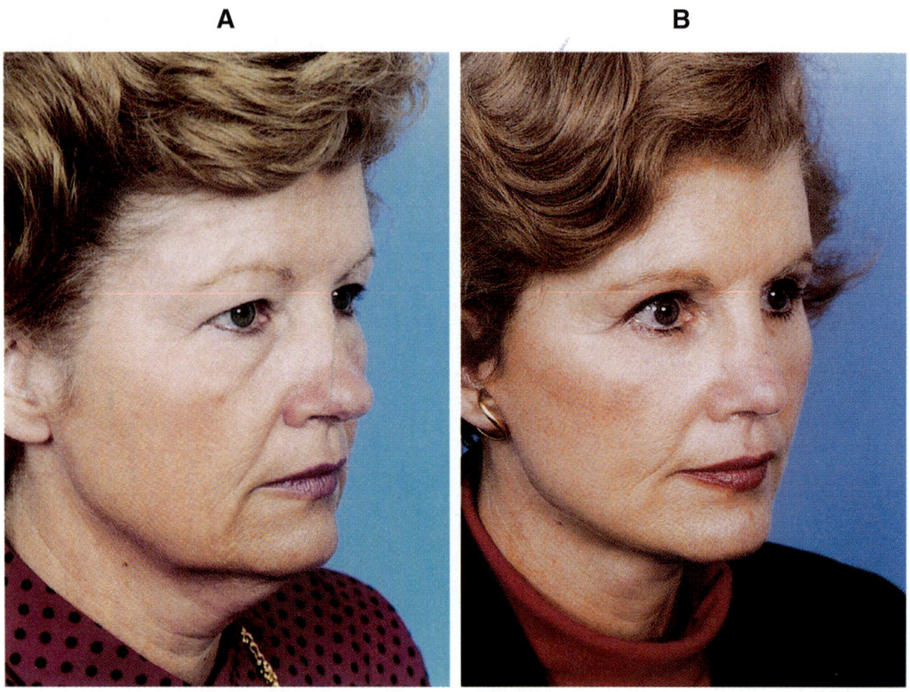

FIG. 21-13
A, Before face lift, oblique view. **B,** Two years after face lift, oblique view.

operative sensations they will be experiencing, as well as minor healing variabilities that they were told will occur, have been forgotten, and they require reassurance that everything is progressing as expected. Continuous reaffirmation of postoperative instructions and expectations is critical to the happiness of these cosmetic surgical patients. Your office needs to be a place they feel comfortable calling as well as returning to in this immediate postoperative time. The patients must feel that you are there for them, to answer their questions and to reassure them. This is critical to their long-term happiness. For longer-term follow-up, it is important for you to intervene if there is any tendency toward hypertrophic healing in the postauricular areas. Intralesional steroids may occasionally be required to settle down a slightly thickening postauricular scar.

A B

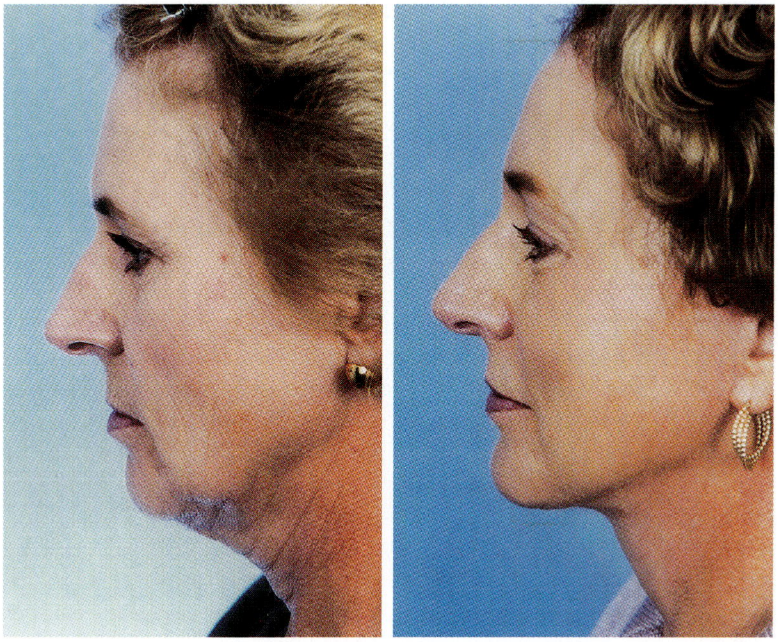

FIG. 21-14
A, Before face lift, lateral view. **B,** Eighteen months after face lift, lateral view.

A B

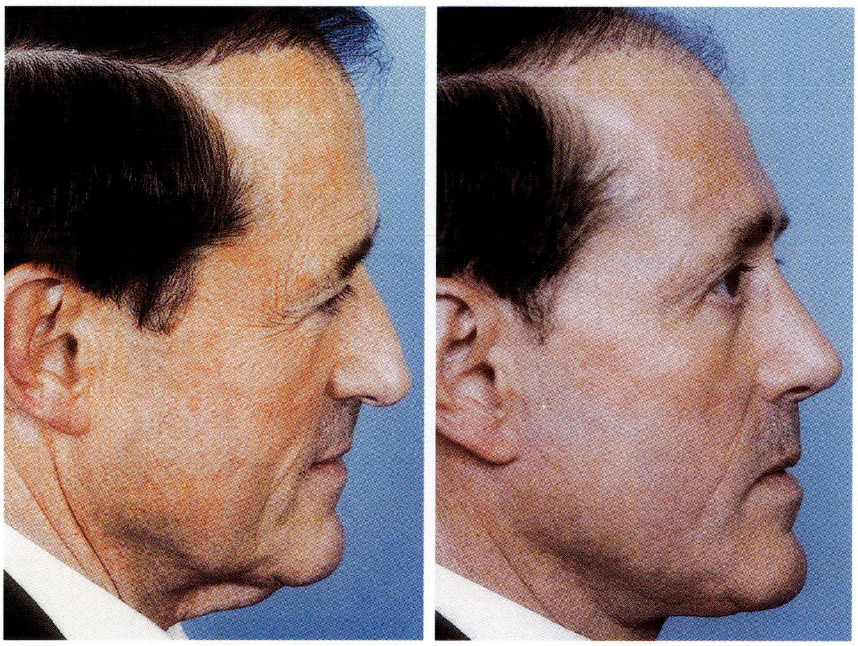

FIG. 21-15
A, Before male face lift, lateral view. **B,** Ten months after male face lift, lateral view.

Additionally, at the 4- to 6-week postoperative period, if patients are going to experience some temporary surgical alopecia in the hair-bearing areas, they need complete reassurance that these hair follicles will regenerate hair shafts and that within 4 to 6 months all of the hair will regrow. Patients further need reassurance throughout the first 3 to 6 months that the strange hypersensitivities and neuresthesias they are experiencing are completely normal and part of the normal healing process.

Tuck-ups and Secondary Rhytidectomy

As you follow your patients in the 6-month to 1-year postoperative period, it is inevitable that they will experience a certain degree of rebound relaxation in the superficial tissues of the face and neck. This is despite excellent and maximum efforts on your part to give them a long-term tightened jawline and neckline. This is very much a function of their inherent hereditary elasticity, which occasionally requires a small procedure to improve the overall results. Submental tuck-up procedures to take care of small residual submental band or fullness can be required in 5% to 10% of patients, depending on their preoperative condition and elasticity of the skin. This should be offered to them as part of the overall face-lift experience. It has nothing to do with the overall technique that you provided for them. Rarely, the jowl, because of its fullness and preexisting condition, will recur enough to require a cheek tuck-up to improve this area and obtain some lasting improvements. This is the area most likely to leave the patient less than satisfied with the overall result. The patient must understand that the melolabial fold and groove is minimally helped with a standard face lift, but it can be quite disconcerting when the jowl does settle somewhat because of this rebound relaxation. A cheek-only portion and an SMAS plication may be helpful in selected patients to give them the long-term results they had expected.

Despite all good efforts, however, in the first year there are patients whose face-lift results do not last as long as they had desired. This is often related to the age of the patient, the condition of the facial skin, and heredity. Patients must understand that a secondary face lift is never required and that they will continue to age and look normal but will always look better than if they had never had the face lift. They will always look more youthful than their chronological age. A repeat face lift can be done in the future but is not usually necessary for 5 to 8 years postoperatively. Techniques similar to the original face lift may be required, depending on the advancement of the aging process in all layers of tissues involved.

RHYTIDECTOMY COMPLICATIONS

Hematoma

The most common complication following rhytidectomy is hematoma formation, occurring in 2% to 15% of patients.[11-13] A major hematoma requiring reoperation and exploration usually presents within the first 12 hours postoperatively (Fig. 21-16). Hematoma formation is heralded by pain and increasing facial edema. Interestingly, there is no correlation between the volume of intraoperative blood loss and hematoma occurrence. Conversely, hypertension predisposes to hematoma formation, increasing its incidence 2.6 times.[14] The importance of blood pressure control cannot be overstated; it must be closely monitored both intraoperatively and throughout the postoperative period. Particular attention should be paid to assuring a smooth emergence from anesthesia and avoidance of postoperative nausea, vomiting, and anxiety. Other predisposing factors associated with hematoma formation include ingestion of aspirin-containing products, nonsteroidal anti-inflammatory drugs, high doses of vitamin E, and the dominantly inherited Ehlers-Danlos syndrome.[15] A detailed list of aspirin-containing products should be distributed, since many of these medications are not obvious. All of these products need to be stopped at least 2 weeks preoperatively and discontinued for at least 1 week postoperatively. Certainly, those taking anticoagulants need to be managed in

A

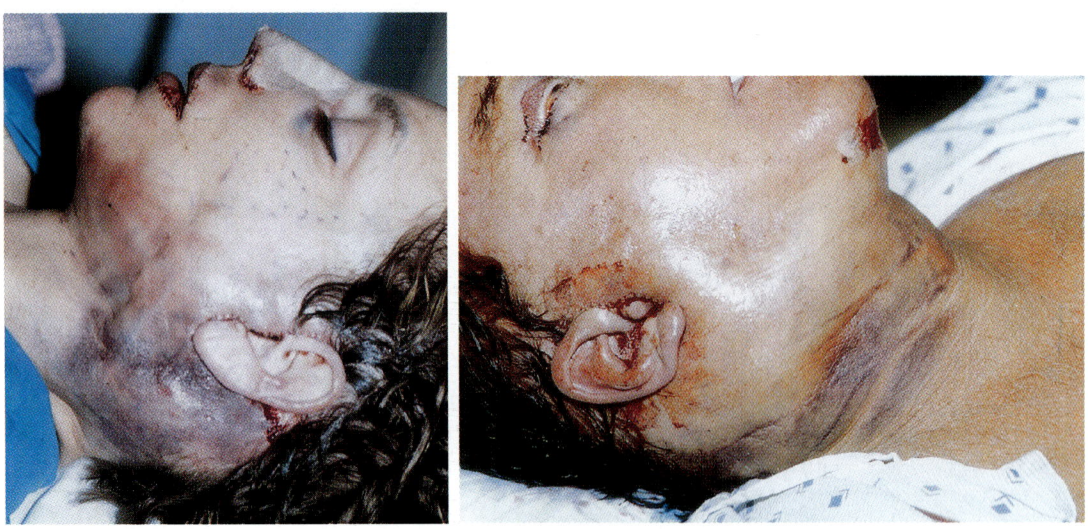

B

FIG. 21-16
A, Acute hematoma 1 hour after face lift. **B,** Acute expanding hematoma 3 hours after face lift.

conjunction with the prescribing physician. We routinely screen all patients with prothrombin time, partial thromboplastin time, and platelet counts, referring them for further workup if abnormal values are noted twice.

Special precaution needs to be afforded to males because the consensus among most facial plastic surgeons is that they are more susceptible to hematoma. Although not proven, it is felt to be secondary to an increased blood supply to the skin and beard follicles.

Delay in treatment may lead to skin flap necrosis, especially in those with a malignant, rapidly expanding hematoma. Additionally, the fluid accumulation may become an ideal culture media, increasing the chances of infection. At the time of evacuation it is often difficult to identify a single vessel at fault; rather, the norm is a diffuse oozing. Treatment should consist of clot evacuation, irrigation, exploration, and cautery of suspicious bleeding vessels. Suction drains and pressure dressing should be reapplied.

Minor hematomas are commonly encountered and probably account for the large range of hematoma percentages reported. Minor hematomas are usually identified in the first week postoperatively and consist of small pockets of fluid usually in the postauricular area. Once liquefied, these fluid collections can be evacuated by 18-gauge needle aspiration under sterile conditions. If the hematoma is not yet liquefied, a small opening in the incision line may be necessary to remove the clot. These patients are refitted with a pressure dressing, and an extended course of antibiotics is prescribed. Undetected hematomas lead to fibrosis, skin puckering, and discoloration, which can take months to resolve (Fig. 21-17). If such a course is encountered, serial steroid injections of triamcinolone 10 mg/ml or triamcinolone 40 mg/ml may be helpful.

Flap Necrosis

Skin flap necrosis occurs when blood supply to the distal ends of the random skin flap is compromised. Predisposing conditions include poor flap design, extended subcutaneous flap elevation, injury to the subdermal plexus, extensive closing tension, certain systemic medical conditions, and smoking. The postauricular area followed by the preauricular area are at greatest risk for necrosis. Deep plane and SMAS rhytidectomy benefit from a decrease in necrosis by allowing for a more robust vascular flap and decreased closing tensions. The toxic effects of nicotine and smoking have long been identified as the most preventable jeopardy to blood supply in random skin flaps. The risk for flap necrosis is increased 12.6 times in smokers.[16] It is imperative that patients abstain from smoking for at least 2 weeks before and after surgery. Systemic diseases like diabetes mellitus, peripheral vascular disease, and multiple connective tissue disorders may predispose patients to vascular compromise and warrant strong consideration preoperatively (Fig. 21-18).

Flap necrosis is preceded by venous congestion and flap discoloration. Frequent massaging of the area and an extended antibiotic course is instituted. Necrosis is usually accompanied by eschar formation. The compromised area should be treated conservatively with daily peroxide cleaning, limited débridement, and topical antibiotic ointment. Fortunately, most affected areas will heal nicely by secondary intention, but fre-

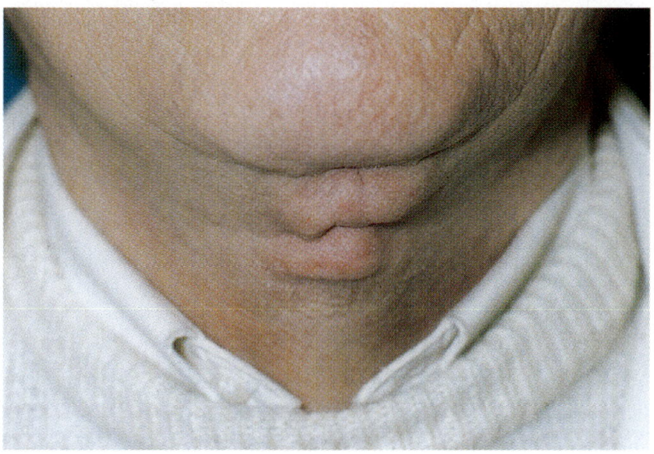

FIG. 21-17
Fibrosis and skin irregularities 2 months after hematoma and seroma in submental neck.

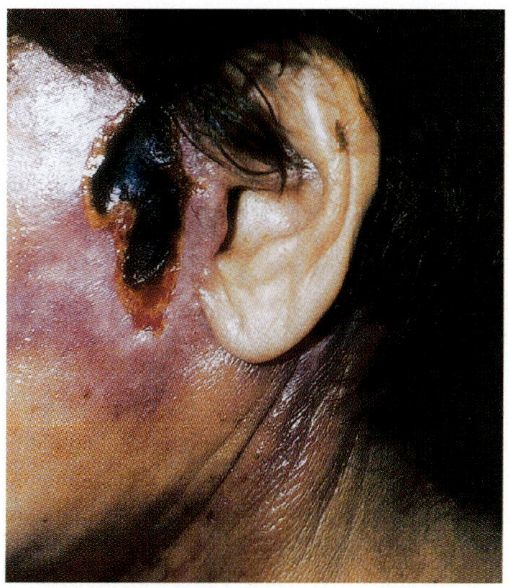

FIG. 21-18
Partial face-lift flap necrosis in a patient taking immunosuppressive drug for severe arthritis.

quent postoperative visits and patient reassurance are necessary.

Nerve Damage

A cervical sensory branch, the great auricular nerve, is the most commonly injured nerve in face-lift surgery, occurring in 1% to 7% of patients.[13,17] This nerve can be found at the anterior border of the sternocleidomastoid muscle. The skin flap tends to get thinner approaching the postauricular and mastoid area. Care must be taken not to violate the muscle and the nerve during this dissection. Increased bleeding is often a sign of muscle injury. Great auricular nerve injury is often noted at the time of surgery, in which case the ends should be anastomosed with epineural repair using 9-0 nylon suture. Failure to repair the injury will lead to regional hypoesthesias and possibly painful neuroma formation.

Motor branch injury fortunately is much less common, occurring in 0.53% to 2.6% of face-lift patients.[11,18] The two most commonly injured nerves are the temporal branch and the marginal mandibular branch of the facial nerve. The more commonly injured of the two branches depends on the method of surgery performed and the report cited. However, both of these injuries can lead to devastating outcomes for the patient and the physician. Mastery of facial nerve anatomy is mandatory to all those planning to perform face-lift surgery. The temporal branch of the facial nerve assumes a superficial course at the level of the zygomatic arch. Dissection in this area needs to be immediately subcutaneous or subperiosteal to avoid injury. Rather than the single branch that is often depicted in textbooks, the temporal branch of the facial nerve consists of multiple rami. Anatomic studies have identified the rami crossing the middle portion of the inferior arch. Dissection in the immediate preauricular 10 mm of the arch and the distal 19 mm of the arch is safe. Unfortunately, injury to the facial nerve is usually not recognized at the time of surgery, but if it is, attempts should be made for direct anastomosis. Microscopic assistance may be helpful. When immediate postoperative facial paralysis or paresis presents, do not panic. Initially, allow at least a 4- to 8-hour time period for the effects of local anesthesia to dissipate. In the unfortunate event that a motor branch injury has occurred, surgical exploration and attempt for anastomosis of these small distal branches is not practical. However, be reassured that clinical evidence has shown a majority of these injuries (85%) will resolve with time.[6] The high incidence of recovery may be because injury was due to a temporary neuropraxia from local insult. Others theorize that in the case of the temporal nerve, multiple branches may allow for reinnervation even in the case of the neurotmesis.[19] However, if recovery is not evident by at least 1 year, then reconstructive options must be considered, including brow lift, contralateral frontal branch neurolysis, and eyelid reanimation procedures.

Subplatysmal dissection places the marginal mandibular branch of the facial nerve at risk. Staying in the immediate subplatysmal plane and dissecting using a blunt scissors with the blades moved vertically will protect the nerve from injury. The nerve initially runs posterior and inferior to the mandible; it enters a superficial plane over the mandible 2 cm lateral to the modiolus.[18] Dissection in the subcutaneous plane in this area is without benefit and may be disastrous. Zygomaticus and buccal branch nerves surface at the anterior end of the parotid gland and are rarely identified in standard face-lift techniques. However, in deep plane dissections, the branches are often encountered. Injury in this area may be obscured by the multiple branches and anastomosis.

Bell's palsy recurrence has been reported following face-lift surgery, and patients with a history of Bell's palsy should be counseled on the possibility.[20] Total facial paralysis should be referred to the appropriate colleague for consultation. Electrical nerve testing may be of prognostic benefit in these patients, as well as in those with isolated motor branch injuries.

Hypertrophic Scarring

Hypertrophic scarring can occur if excessive tension is placed on flap closure, and is more commonly associated with the isolated subcutaneous flap dissection (Fig. 21-19). Hypertrophic scarring can rear itself as early as 2 weeks postoperatively and usually occurs within the first 12 weeks. Interval intralesional injections with steroids have been helpful. Excision and primary closure of the hypertrophic scarring should be delayed for at least 6 months.

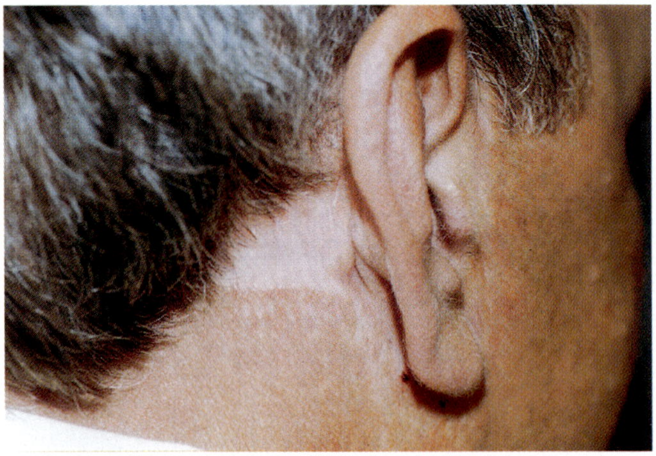

FIG. 21-19
Postauricular hypertrophic scar with widening due to excess tension on closure.

Incision Line Irregularities

Poor planning of incision lines may lead to loss of the temporal tuft of hair, alopecia, excessive dog-ear formation, and hairline stair-stepping pattern. The temporal tuft of hair can be recreated with micrograft placement or through creative local flap designs. Hair loss is usually secondary to follicular shock (telogen effluvium), and reassurance can be given. However, if follicles were transected or tension on closure is excessive, hair loss may be permanent (Fig. 21-20). After a waiting period of 3 to 6 months, if there has been no hair recovery, alopecia areas may be excised and closed primarily. Micrografting can also help to camouflage the area.

Failure to advance and rotate the postauricular flap can lead to a stair-stepping of the hairline. Fortunately, for most patients this area is easily hidden. However, if it is a problem for those interested in wearing their hair back, flap revision may be necessary.

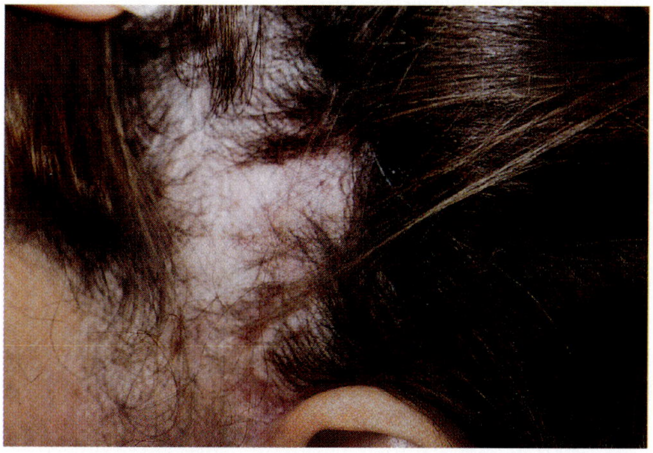

FIG. 21-20
Temporal alopecia secondary to excess tension and damage to hair follicles.

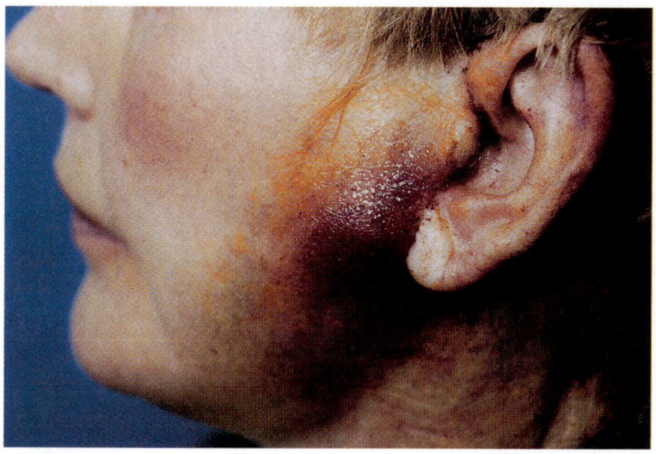

FIG. 21-21
Postoperative abscess and infection 1 week after face lift.

Infection

Infection is rare in rhytidectomy patients. Mild cases of cellulitis will respond well to an extended antibiotic course covering the common variants of staphylococcus and streptococcus. These patients generally heal without sequelae. In the rare event of abscess formation, incision, drainage, and wound culturing is necessary (Fig. 21-21). Intravenous antibiotics should be considered.

Earlobe Deformity

Satyr ear (devil's ear) can occur if the earlobe is not tucked up properly. During the healing period, the earlobe is drawn inferiorly (Fig. 21-22). Poor placement of the earlobe can lead to the telltale signs of face-lift surgery. Repairing the unnatural earlobe can be difficult. The best method to create the inferior lobe sulcus is by V-Y plasty, but this should be delayed for at least 6 months after surgery.

Parotid Injury

Parotid parenchyma injury leading to sialocele or fistula formation is rare. Intraoperative injury should be

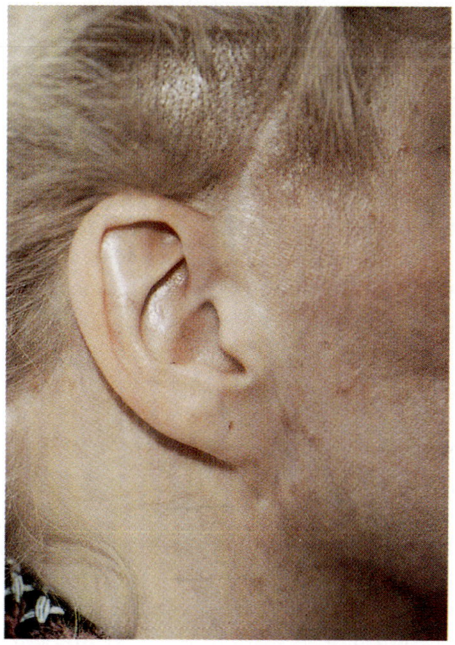

FIG. 21-22
Satyr ear (devil's ear) with poor scar placement.

oversewn with available SMAS. Postoperative fluid accumulation may be treated with needle aspiration and pressure dressing. Persistent fluid accumulation may require a drainage procedure.

Sequelae of telangiectasia, hypertrichosis, and temporary hypoesthesia over the elevated flap tend to improve with time. However, persistent vascular lesions and problematic excessive hair can be effectively ameliorated with appropriate laser treatments.

ENDOSCOPIC RHYTIDECTOMY

Endoscopic face lifting has been described as a method for achieving excellent results in the mid face and a complete harmony of the upper and middle one third of the face. It allows for small incisions and extended access to deep planes of the mid face. Many surgeons who began with this technique are using the endoscope less as they become more familiar with the tissue planes. The additional experience affords the confidence to carry out a majority of the surgery blindly, with the endoscope reserved for areas of particular concerns. Despite reports of excellent results, this method is yet to be widely practiced. Perhaps as this technique becomes more standardized it will become the treatment of choice. However, for now, more experience and research are needed to find the best methods of operation.[21] The failure of this technique to be universally adopted may be due to the steep learning curve, the potential for nerve injury, and the relevant satisfaction with SMAS techniques.

ENDOSCOPIC FOREHEAD LIFTING

To achieve a natural result in facial rejuvenation surgery, attention to the upper one third of the face is indicated. Surgeons who limit lifting procedures to the lower face achieve a youthful neckline but one that is not in balance with heavy brows. Additionally, there is a risk of accentuating rhytides at the temporal border of the face lift. In the evolution of cosmetic treatments of the face, techniques developed for treating the forehead have lagged behind those developed for the lower one third of the face. Neglecting the forehead in patients undergoing face-lift surgery often results in an "operated look." Additionally, in the patient inquiring about eyelid surgery the contribution of brow ptosis is often overlooked. The novice cosmetic surgeon must be cognizant of brow position in all blepharoplasty candidates. At times a crowded upper eyelid is secondary to brow ptosis, and a blepharoplasty procedure would be the incorrect treatment and might even predispose to a complication such as lagophthalmos. Frequently the calculated combination of brow elevation plus excision of redundant eyelid skin allows for an opening of the eyes and a more attractive look.

Treatment options for the redundant sagging forehead, heavy brow, and deep glabellar creases are many, and successful correction has been achieved with a variety of approaches. The gold standard for forehead rejuvenation has been the coronal lift, but the expected sequelae and possible complications may be unacceptable to many patients. Additionally, those patients with a high hairline or the male experiencing male pattern baldness are not appropriate candidates for this approach. The solution to many of these problems appeared to be answered with the advent of endoscopic techniques. Initial enthusiasm was tempered with reports of early relaxation and brow position rebound. This has led to the development of a variety of surgical and fixation techniques to suspend the elevated brows into a natural position. Many now claim results from endoscopic forehead lift that are equal or superior to the results from a coronal lift.[22-24]

After a decision to treat the brows has been made, the approach selected must be targeted to the individual patient. In 1939, Fomon felt the best method for lasting eradication of forehead wrinkles was through a suprabrow incision bluntly elevating tissues of the forehead and then advancing the redundancy inferior over the brow with excision of the excess. Everting interrupted sutures were then placed in horizontal wrinkles for 24 to 36 hours.[1] Early coronal approaches to forehead wrinkles did not include release of the arcus marginalis or treatment of the corrugators, and these procedures were predestined to create only temporary improvement. As surgeons gained experience and began to treat the forehead more completely, improvements were seen in the long-term result of the coronal forehead lift. This approach then became the standard for forehead and brow rejuvenation. However, if the patient's hairline is naturally high (5 cm above the brow or greater), then an incision placement modification is recommended. A trichophytic or pretrichial incision affords a similar dissection without elevating the hairline. A well-camouflaged healing line is expected if standard plastic surgery principles are adhered to upon closure. These three approaches will allow excellent visualization of the depressor brow muscles. Myotomies of the corrugators, procerus, and depressor supercilii can be performed accurately under direct vision. After this release, elevation of the brow is dependent on scalp excision. It is generally thought that there is a ratio of 2.5:1 or 3:1 for coronal scalp excision to brow elevation, although for trichophytic and pretrichial incisions this ratio may be slightly less. Unfortunately, this method of fixation tends to increase tension at the closing site, predisposing to the possibility of alopecia. Additionally, patients may mention annoying scalp numbness or occasionally pain.

In the late 1980s endoscopic techniques excited all fields of surgery, and facial cosmetic surgery was no exception. Minimal incision, extended access surgery has allowed for a quicker recovery time, less morbidity, and greater patient acceptance.[22] Endoscopic forehead lifting also added a new philosophy to elevating the brow. As in the open approach, sectioning of the antagonistic brow depressor is necessary, but the difference is in releasing the posterior scalp so as to allow the whole forehead complex room to shift back. Brow elevation no longer depended on excising scalp and the resultant increased tension at the closure site, therefore decreasing the risk for alopecia. Small interrupted incisions strategically placed in the scalp avoid damaging the deep branch of the supraorbital nerve and avoid the hypoesthesias of an open approach.[25] The endoscopic method also enlarged the pool of potential patients for forehead lift. Small incisions heal well and can be hidden in thin and receding hairlines. Initial enthusiasm for the endoscopic forehead lift was lessened by the inconsistent outcomes. Many early disappointing results may have been due to inexperience, as a learning curve certainly exists. This has led to debate on the ideal dissection plane (subgaleal or subperiosteal) and fixation method. We have found the subperiosteal plane to be the optimal choice affording a clean optical dissection. The key to achieving elevation is releasing the periosteum at the arcus marginalis. The transposed forehead flap repositions superiorly and anchors to the cranium at an elevated position. A temporary fixation method is necessary until the periosteum fixes to the skull. Many methods exist, but we have found drilling a precise bone tunnel into the outer cortex, facilitated by a handheld instrument (marketed by Xomed), allows for suture fixation and is a superior technique. Recent advancement with autologous and homologous tissue adhesives are promising and may become standard. A preference for each of the multiple methods of dissection and fixation can be argued well, but conclusive scientific evidence objectively determining the ideal technique is still pending.

Patient Preparation

Patients shampoo their hair on the morning of surgery with Septisol. Following mark placement, obstructing hair is twisted on itself and secured with rubber band and paper tape. Local anesthesia and vasoconstriction are achieved with injection of 1% lidocaine with 1:50,000 epinephrine into incision lines. Field blocks are completed with 1% lidocaine with 1:100,000 epinephrine to the forehead and scalp area.

Technique

Endoscopic surgery is facilitated with a 5 mm, 30-degree endoscope. Approach to the forehead is through two temporal incisions placed 2 to 3 cm behind the hairline and either two vertically placed paramedian incisions 1 to 3 cm behind the frontal hairline or a 3 to 4 cm midline trichophytic incision in those with a high hairline. A firm sweep with a blunt elevator in the loose areolar tissue of the subgaleal plane allows for release and mobilization of the parietal and occipital scalp. Anterior dissection is performed bluntly and blindly in a subperiosteal plane to 2 cm above the orbital rims. This technique safeguards the supraorbital bundle from inadvertent injury. Lateral dissection is begun on the superficial layer of the deep temporalis fascia and directed anteriorly and medially. Care is taken not to violate this plane, as the frontal branch of the seventh nerve runs in the adjacent superficial musculoaponeurotic fascia. To mobilize the lateral brow, ligamentous periosteal-cutaneous attachments of the lateral brow are released, which can be done blindly. It is important to keep the index finger of the nondissection hand on the orbital rim to prevent injury to the globe following a sudden release of the ligament. Under endoscopic assistance, transitional zone fibers separating the temporal dissection from the frontal dissection are sharply transected and periosteum is released off the superior and orbital rims. The periosteum is incised at the arcus mariginalis, allowing for release of the brows. Care is taken not to extend into orbital fat. Corrugator muscle resection and procerus muscle transections are performed under endoscopic vision with care to preserve branches of the supraorbital and supratrochlear neurovascular structures. A cauterizing hook is helpful to isolate and transect these fibers. The frontalis muscle may be incised in the midline if prominent horizontal creases exist. Forehead skin, galea, and periosteal tissues are repositioned posterior and anchored to the outer table of the cranium with 2-0 Vicryl sutures threaded through bone tunnels. Scalp incisions are closed with a tension-reducing deep 3-0 Vicryl suture. Everted hair-bearing skin edges are stapled together. If a trichophytic incision was made, it is closed precisely. The epidermis and superficial dermis of the posterior flap, which is at the frontal hairline, is sharply excised in a beveled fashion, leaving intact hair follicles at the base. Following excision of a calculated amount of forehead skin, the anterior flap of skin is sutured to the posterior flap skin line with the distal portion of the anterior flap overriding the hair follicles of the posterior flap. This allows for hair growth through the scar and camouflage of the incision line. Drains are not necessary, and a compression dressing is removed the next day.

Complications

Alopecia has not been a problem with judicious cauterization and a tension-free closure. Assuming the supraorbital nerve bundle isn't injured, regional scalp hypoesthesia is temporary, and rarely has a patient expressed concern. Facial nerve injury is avoided with meticulous dissection and respect for tissue planes. Temporary temporal (frontal) branch paresis is rare, although it may occur. If the nerve was not directly injured, full recovery is expected and usually occurs within 6 months. An area where the facial nerve is at particular risk is the transitional zone separating the medial from the lateral compartment. Dissecting from lateral to medial prevents inadvertent injury, as does staying immediately on the superficial layer of the deep temporal fascia or just below it. Additionally, a more obscure area is approximately 1 cm lateral to the orbital rim, where the frontal branch runs in close proximity to a sentinel vessel (medial temporozygomatic vein). Control of vessel bleeding in this area should be done with caution to avoid inadvertent nerve injury.

Conclusion

The endoscopic forehead lift is a proven, minimally invasive low-morbidity procedure for achieving symmetric and lasting brow elevation. The coronal forehead lift is still our preferred method in the patient with severe brow ptosis and deep forehead creases. However, the benefits of this open approach must be weighed against the potential sequelae of scalp hypoesthesias, elevated hairline, and possible alopecia. For those patients with less severe ptosis, and interested in a more rapid recovery, the endoscopic approach is a well-accepted option for achieving the desired results.

REFERENCES

1. Fomon S. The Surgery of Injury and Plastic Repair. Baltimore: Williams & Wilkins, 1939.
2. Skoog T. Plastic surgery: the aging face. In: Plastic Surgery: New Methods and Refinements. Philadelphia: WB Saunders, 1974:300-330.
3. Mitz V, Peyronie M. The superficial musculo-aponeurotic system (SMAS) in the parotid and cheek area. Plast Reconstr Surg 1976; 58:80-88.
4. Hamra ST. The deep plane rhytidectomy. Plast Reconstr Surg 1990; 86:53.
5. Hamra S. Composite rhytidectomy. Plast Reconstr Surg 1992; 90: 1-13.
6. Kamer FM. One hundred consecutive deep plane face lifts. Arch Otolaryngol Head Neck Surg 1996; 122:17-22.
7. Godin MS, Johnson CM. Deep plane/composite rhytidectomy. Facial Plast Surg 1996; 12:231-239.
8. Ramirez OM. The subperiosteal rhytidectomy: the third generation face lift. Ann Plast Surg 1992; 28:218-232.
9. Psillakis JF, Rumley TO, Camargos A. Subperiosteal approach as an improved concept for correction of the aging face. Plast Reconstr Surg 1988; 82:383-392.
10. Baker SR. Tri-plane rhytidectomy. Arch Otolaryngol Head Neck Surg 1997; 123:1167-1172.
11. Rees A. Complications of rhytidectomy. Clin Plast Surg 1978; 5: 109-119.
12. Lawson N. Male face lift. Arch Otolaryngol Head Neck Surg 1993; 119:539.
13. Perkins SW. Personal experience of 89 consecutive facelifts. July 1998-July 1999. Unpublished.
14. Straith RE, Raju DR, Hipps CJ. The study of hematomas in 500 consecutive face lifts. Plast Reconstr Surg 1977; 59:694-698.
15. Muenker R. Problems and variation in cervicofacial rhytidectomy. Facial Plast Surg 1992; 8:33-51.
16. Adamson P, Moran ML. Complications of cervicofacial rhytidectomy. Facial Plast Surg Clin N Am 1993; 112:257-270.
17. McKinney P, Katrana DJ. Prevention of injury to the great auricular nerve during rhytidectomy. Plast Reconstr Surg 1977; 59:525-529.
18. Liebman E, Webster R, Gaul J, Griffin T. The marginal mandibular nerve in rhytidectomy and liposuction surgery. Arch Otolaryngol Head Neck Surg 1988; 114:179-181.
19. Gosain A, Sewall S, Yousif NJ. The temporal branch of the facial nerve: how reliably can we predict its path? Plast Reconstr Surg 1997; 99:1224-1236.
20. Castanares S. Facial nerve paralyses coincident with or subsequent to rhytidectomy. Plast Reconstr Surg 1974; 54:637-643.
21. Celik M, Tuncer S, Buyukcayir I. Modifications in endoscopic facelifts. Ann Plast Surg 1999; 42:638-643.
22. Ramirez OM. Why I prefer the endoscopic forehead lift. Plast Reconstr Surg 1997; 100:1033-1039.
23. Hutcherson R, Keller GS. Endoscopic techniques in facial rejuvenation surgery. Facial Plast Surg 1996; 12:303-310.
24. Steinsapir KD, Shorr N, Hoening J, et al. The endoscopic forehead lift. Ophthal Plast Reconstr Surg 1998; 14:107-118.
25. Knize DM. Reassessment of the coronal incision and subgaleal dissection for foreheadplasty. Plast Reconstr Surg 1998; 102:478-492.

CHAPTER 22

Leg Vein Management: Sclerotherapy, Ambulatory Phlebectomy, and Laser Surgery

ROBERT A. WEISS
JEFFREY S. DOVER

SECTION ONE

History and Scientific Review

BASIC SCIENCE

Unsightly or symptomatic venulectasia or telangiectasia on the legs occurs in 29% to 41% of women and 6% to 15% of men in the United States.[1] These smaller vessels are most often directly or indirectly connected to larger reticular or varicose "feeding" veins. Even though up to 53% of patients with leg telangiectases have associated symptoms, the most common reason patients seek consultation is cosmetic.[2] The ideal treatment for unwanted leg veins would be painless and clear 100% of vessels in one treatment with no associated side effects. The variation in vessel size, flow, depth, and type preclude the possibility of a single effective treatment modality. Vessel types include varicosities, reticular or feeder veins, and superficial spider veins. Despite the fact that sclerotherapy has a long list of potential side effects, including pain, swelling, urticaria, systemic allergic reaction, hyperpigmentation, telangiectatic matting, skin necrosis, and phlebitis, it remains the treatment of choice for most leg veins less than 4 mm in diameter.[3-5]

Telangiectases, although readily visible on the skin surface of the leg, are often manifestations of abnormal physiology of its venous system. When accompanied by larger varicose veins, associated telangiectases cannot be successfully treated without addressing the problems induced by hydrostatic pressure. Hydrostatic pressure leads to sequestration and stagnation in the venous system as blood backs up into veins with malfunctioning valves. This process may cause even smaller surface veins such as reticular veins and associated telangiectatic webs to expand with pressure, producing symptoms.

Ambulatory phlebectomy allows treatment of virtually all large truncal varicose veins; compression sclerotherapy can be used to treat large varicose veins and reticular varicose veins. Once venous pressure is addressed, telangiectases may be treated either with sclerotherapy or with intense pulsed light devices. In patients with isolated telangiectases without pressure problems, sclerotherapy or laser/light therapy may be instituted primarily. In cases where an incompetent valve occurs at the main valve of the greater saphenous vein (GSV) at the junction of the femoral vein, other surgical techniques or the new radio frequency occlusion techniques may be required. All these approaches may be performed in the office setting. Each of these approaches and the role of lasers and light sources in the treatment of leg veins will be addressed in this chapter.

DIAGNOSIS

Physicians must acquire the knowledge to diagnose origins of reverse flow, which causes varicose or reticular veins and ultimately associated telangiectases. Reverse flow through incompetent valves frequently leads to abnormal veins on the leg. Diagnostic instruments include Doppler ultrasound (analogous to a stethoscope), digital photoplethysmography (analogous to an electrocardiogram), and duplex ultrasound (analogous to an echocardiogram).

Knowledge of basic superficial venous anatomy is essential. Three important superficial venous systems include the greater saphenous vein (GSV), the lesser saphenous vein (LSV), and the lateral subdermic venous system (LSVS) (Figs. 22-1 and 22-2).

Physical examination is performed to determine whether telangiectatic webs or varicose veins seen on the surface originate from venous pressure in one or more of these three segments of venous anatomy. Younger patients (20s and 30s) usually present with telangiectatic webs originating from reverse flow or re-

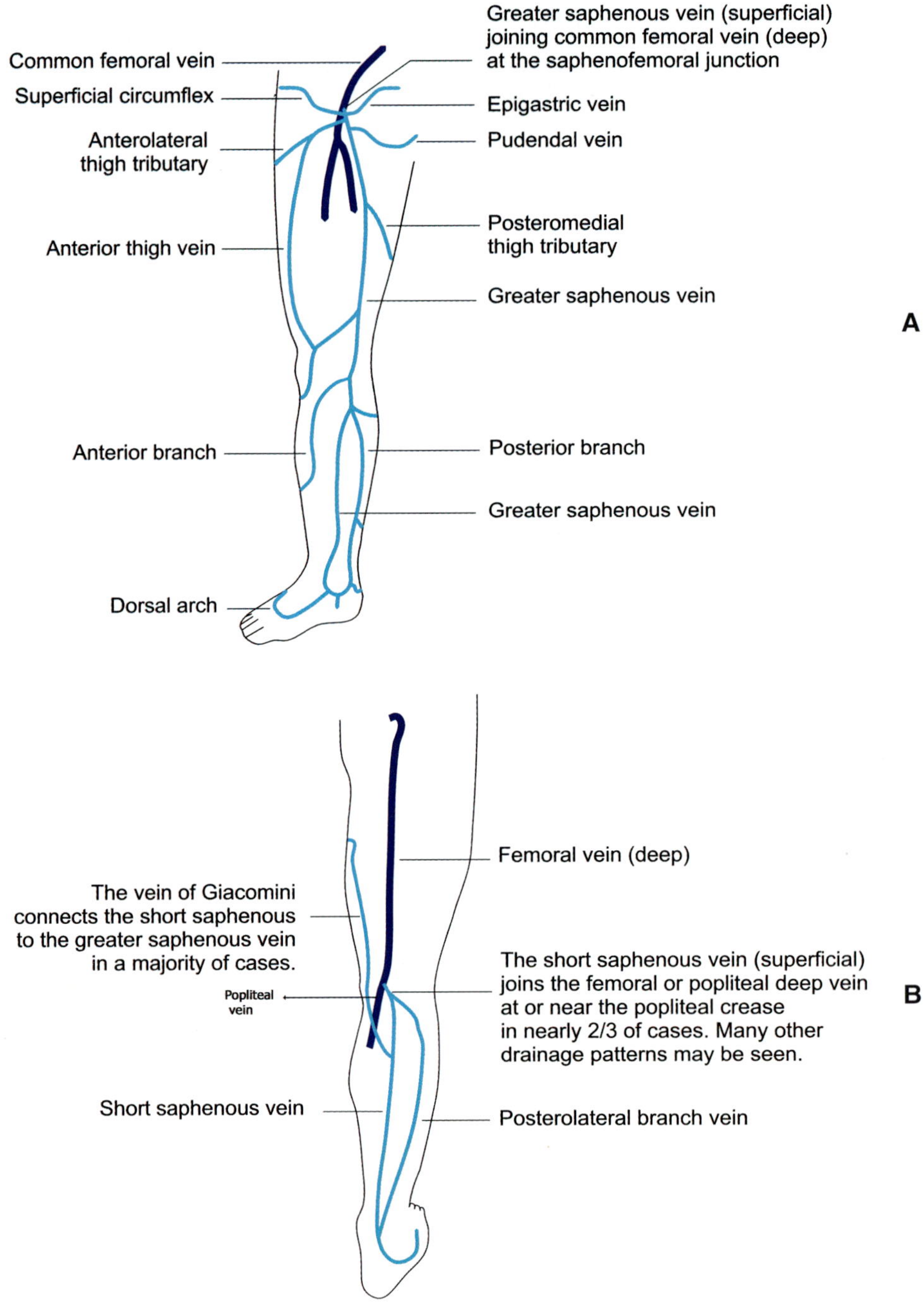

FIG. 22-1
Superficial anatomy of the venous system. **A,** Greater saphenous vein. **B,** Lesser saphenous vein. (From Weiss RA, Feied CR, Weiss MA. Vein Diagnosis and Treatment: A Comprehensive Approach. New York: McGraw-Hill, 2001.)

flux in the lateral venous system unless there is a strong family history of larger varicose veins. When there is a positive family history of large varicose veins, reflux originating from the GSV or LSV must be suspected. A duplex ultrasound study on patients presenting for treatment of "cosmetic" leg veins demonstrated a relatively high incidence of early associated axial or truncal reflux in the GSV.[6]

The microanatomy responsible for the transmission of venous hypertension into telangiectases via reticular varicosities has been documented by high-resolution duplex ultrasound.[7] A reticular vein is a thin-walled blue superficial venulectasis thought to be part of a network of subcuticular veins communicating with the venous system via direct connections to the saphenous system or by small perforating veins that can course through superficial and deep fascia. These reticular veins are commonly called "feeder" veins, since the assumption is that reflux through them causes the groups of telangiectases, although physiologically these reticular veins drain blood from, not to, the telangiectases.

Doppler ultrasound findings on thousands of patients confirm that reflux through the lateral subdermal venous system is very frequently associated with large areas of painful telangiectatic webs on the lateral and posterior thighs.[7,8] This lateral venous system may re-

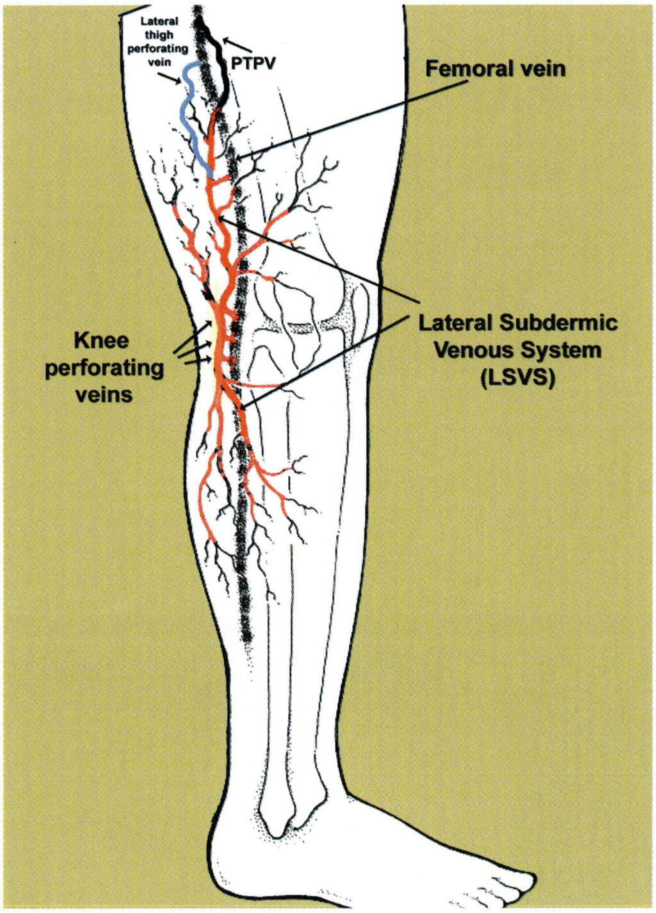

FIG. 22-2
Lateral subdermic venous system. (From Weiss RA, Feied CR, Weiss MA. Vein Diagnosis and Treatment: A Comprehensive Approach. New York: McGraw-Hill, 2001.)

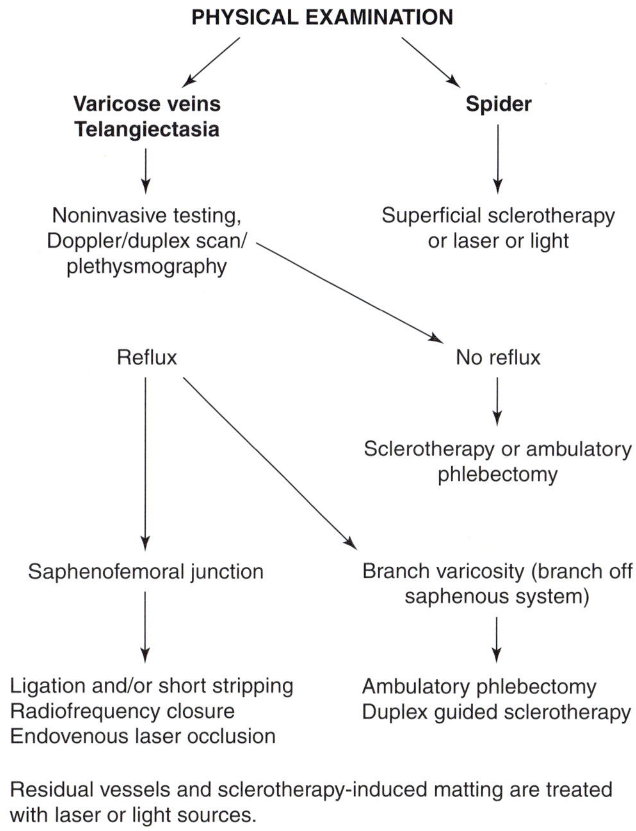

FIG. 22-3
Algorithmic approach to diagnosis and treatment of the venous system.

ceive reflux from knee perforating veins, lateral thigh perforating veins, or posterior thigh perforating veins. Perforating veins connect the deep and superficial venous systems of the leg. Figure 22-2 shows a schematic of the lateral subdermal venous system anatomy.

ALGORITHMIC APPROACH TO THE TREATMENT OF LEG VEINS

Treatment of varicose veins follows an algorithmic and logical approach[5] (Fig. 22-3). When leg veins are managed in this systematic approach, feeder vessels or larger varicose veins are first eliminated surgically or with radiofrequency (RF) occlusion, and sclerotherapy proceeds from largest to smallest vessels, with 80% to 90% of vessels responding to one or two treatments.[9] Given the high success rate of sclerotherapy, the relative low cost of ambulatory phlebectomy, compression sclerotherapy, and superficial sclerotherapy, and the relatively limited improvement demonstrated with lasers and light sources, we recommend using laser and light therapy only in certain situations.[10] Only those vessels that do not respond to sclerotherapy, that are too small to be injected, that remain after feeding vessels are treated, or that are suspected arteriolar spider malformations should be considered for laser and light treatment. By adhering to these principles, patients will receive cost-effective, efficient, and logical care.

Doppler Ultrasound

The handheld Doppler ultrasound is the main tool used to detect reverse flow or reflux in the superficial venous system. Optimal frequencies for examining superficial vessels (1 to 2 cm below the skin) are 8 to 10 MHz, while deeper vessels require a lower frequency of 4 to 5 MHz.[11,12] Blood flow is slow and intermittent; it is mainly pulsed by calf muscle contraction. To generate an audible signal of flow, a maneuver such as manual compression of the calf (simulating a muscle contraction) must be performed by the examiner. When compression is released, gravitational hydrostatic pres-

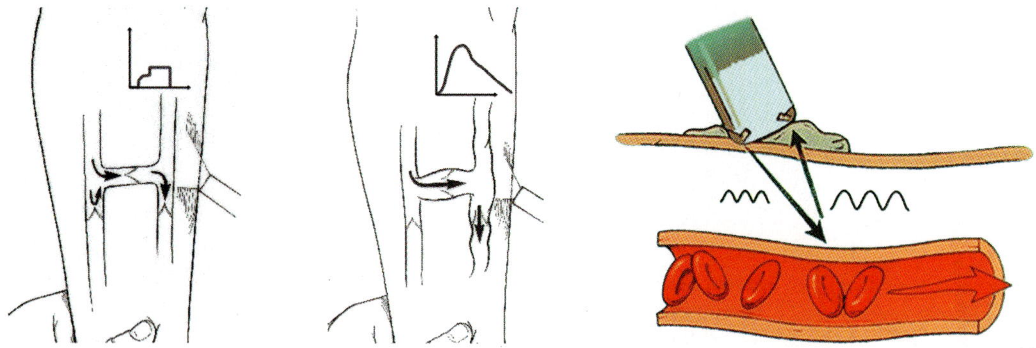

FIG. 22-4
Gravitational flow along with external muscle compression is required to hear flow sounds. **A,** Compression and release with normal valves. **B,** Compression and release with refluxing valves. **C,** Principle of Doppler transducer.

sure causes reverse flow to cease within 0.5 to 1.0 second when valves are competent, but a long flow sound is audible when valves are incompetent.

The Doppler examination is usually performed with the patient standing or sitting, because gravitational hydrostatic pressure enhances the volume and velocity of retrograde flow and makes it easier to detect. To perform this test, the nondominant hand gently squeezes the leg well below (distal compression) or above (proximal compression) the point of auscultation, while the dominant hand holds the Doppler transducer lightly against the skin. Under normal circumstances, flow should be heard only during active distal compression. Flow that is heard during proximal compression or immediately after the release of distal compression is retrograde flow—a clear sign of incompetent valves (Fig. 22-4).

Plethysmography

The term *plethysmography* describes a number of techniques used to measure pressure or volume changes directly or indirectly. A plethysmograph consists of a mechanism to sense a change within the lower leg and a modifying unit (transducer) that translates changes from a displacement-sensing device into electrical energy that is then recorded. Photoplethysmography (PPG) and the minor variant of PPG known as light reflection rheography (LRR) measure changes in light absorption within dermal capillaries.

For PPG examination, the patient sits on a chair in a relaxed position with the knees bent at a 110- to 120-degree angle. A small probe containing light-emitting and sensing diodes is taped to the medial aspect of the lower leg about 8 to 10 cm above the medial malleolus. The leg is allowed to fill for several minutes, and the patient then dorsiflexes the foot 8 to 10 times, activat-

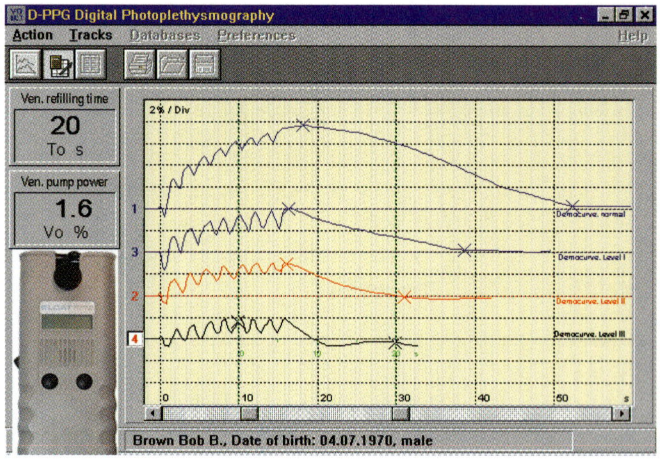

FIG. 22-5
Sample tracings of the D-PPG. Actual handheld instrument is shown at left lower corner inset. The tracings demonstrate grade I (normal) through grade IV (severe) venous insufficiency.

ing the calf muscle pump to empty the venous system. As the skin venous plexus empties, it causes increased reflectance of light because less hemoglobin remains to absorb light. A tracing is made of the changes in reflected light from the skin under the probe (Fig. 22-5).

After the calf muscle pumping ceases, blood refills the skin plexus that absorbs increasing amounts of light as blood fills venules, and the PPG tracing returns to its initial resting value. Although PPG reflects regional venous volume changes, it may be construed to represent the entire venous volume of the leg.[13]

While venous Doppler ultrasound is used to detect anatomic sites of reverse flow, PPG permits quantification of the physiologic significance of these findings.

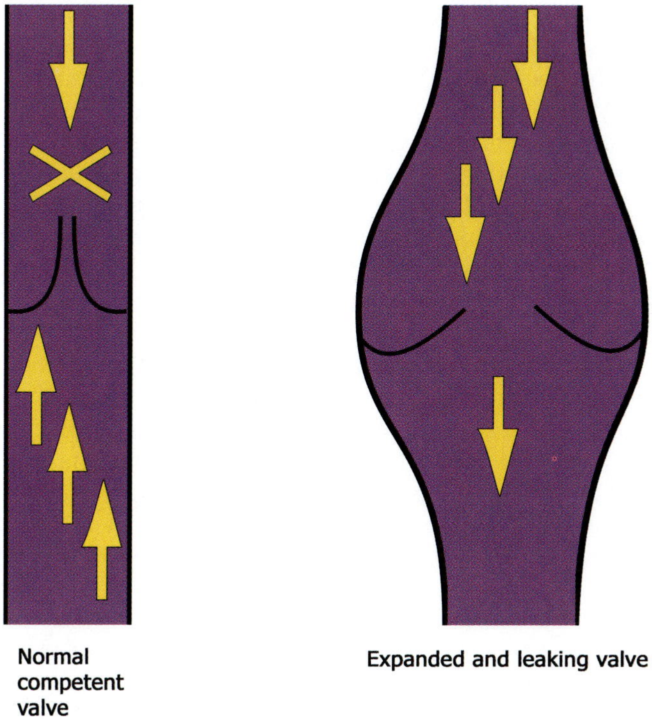

FIG. 22-6
Valve leaflets that fail to meet allow reflux.

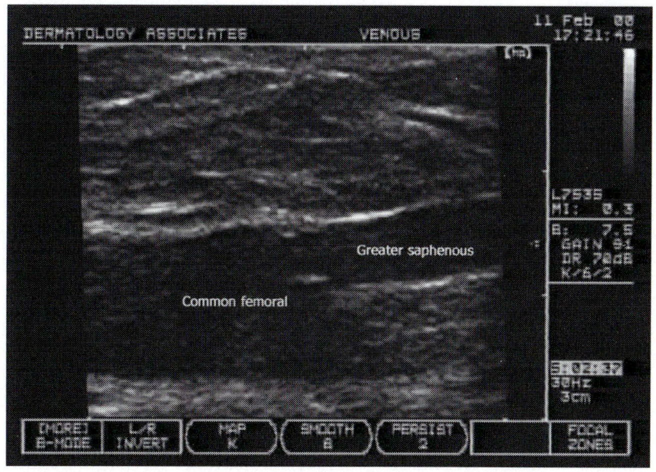

FIG. 22-7
Duplex view of the greater saphenous vein entering the femoral junction, known as the sapheno-femoral junction (SFJ).

PPG is independent of examiner experience. Recent advances have led to even greater reliability and quantitative results with digital PPG (ELCAT GmbH, Wolfratshausen, Germany) in which a dedicated microprocessor standardizes the signal so that measurements are reliable regardless of skin color or edema.[14] A refill time shorter than 25 seconds indicates significant venous valvular insufficiency. Longer refill times indicate normal venous valve function. An abnormal PPG requires further investigation by Doppler, duplex, or other means before treatment by sclerotherapy, ambulatory phlebectomy, or laser/light source is initiated.

Duplex Ultrasound

Duplex ultrasound is a dual mode diagnostic tool that allows a timed pulse echo to be superimposed with the continuous wave Doppler. This allows one to "see" the anatomy in two dimensions while superimposing the Doppler flow signal as a color marker. Reflux can then be demonstrated visually rather than purely audibly as with the handheld. The site of origin of reflux can be pinpointed. Duplex may also be used to guide treatment by direct visualization of the needle.

Structures that absorb, transmit, or scatter ultrasonic waves appear as dark areas, while structures that reflect the waves back to the transducer appear as white areas in the image. Vessel walls reflect ultrasound, while blood flowing in a vessel absorbs and scatters ultrasound in all directions; thus the normal vessel appears as a dark-filled white-walled structure. Nonflowing blood and thrombus are somewhat ultrasonically reflective, although less so than the vessel wall; thus they appear as heterogeneous areas of gray echogenicity within the vessel.

Reflux is diagnosed by placing the transducer over the vessel in a longitudinal plane and observing the Doppler signal in the vessels while (with the free hand) the distal leg is momentarily compressed and released to increase the cephalad movement of blood. Functional valves permit flow only in the antegrade direction, but normal vessels can demonstrate brief retrograde flow due to slow closing of valves (Fig. 22-6). Retrograde flow of duration greater than 0.5 second is considered pathologic reflux, and reflux that lasts more than 2 seconds is hemodynamically significant.

In the longitudinal view, the origin of the greater saphenous vein is identified as it courses off the common femoral vein (Fig. 22-7). Two valves can be visualized in the greater saphenous vein. The first is the terminal valve, which lies at the vein origin. Distal augmentation for Doppler flow reveals competence or incompetence of this valve. The second valve, the subterminal valve, is examined in the same fashion. Valsalva maneuver may also show incompetence of these valves. Major tributaries that empty into the region of the sapheno-femoral junction can be identified here. These include the circumflex, pudendal, epigastric, and others. Most commonly seen is the epigastric because of its size and position in the same plane as the termination of the greater saphenous vein.

SECTION TWO

Atlas of Surgical Procedures

TREATMENT WITH SCLEROTHERAPY

No matter how small and how localized the telangiectasia, every patient must initially be evaluated by detailed history and physical examination, with noninvasive diagnostic vascular tests performed as necessary. Once any reflux in the saphenous system has been identified and treated, then treatment of the smaller branch veins may begin. Once the patient understands the nature and risks of treatment and signs the consent form, digital images of the leg veins are recorded. These readily accessible images enable evaluation of treatment progress and allow patients to assess improvement for themselves. Many patients have great difficulty distinguishing partial resolution from no improvement, particularly when some treated areas demonstrate hyperpigmentation (Fig. 22-8). The "before" treatment images are invaluable to improve both the patient's satisfaction and the physician's satisfaction with the procedure.

The room in which sclerotherapy is performed is kept cool to minimize vasovagal reactions. The first treatment session is usually limited to a small number of sites in order to observe the patient for any allergic reactions and ability to tolerate the burning or cramping of a hypertonic solution, judge the effectiveness of a particular concentration and class of sclerosing agent, and observe any reactions to the tape or foam pads used for compression. It also serves to familiarize the patient with the treatment, treating physician, clinic surroundings, and the sensation of the fine needle. This allows more extensive treatment on the second visit, as the patient is typically more relaxed. The test site also complies with the suggestion in the package insert of sodium tetradecyl sulfate, which states that a small area should be treated initially to observe any signs of allergic reaction.

The patient returns in 4 to 6 weeks to compare the test site with pretreatment digital images. The patient is

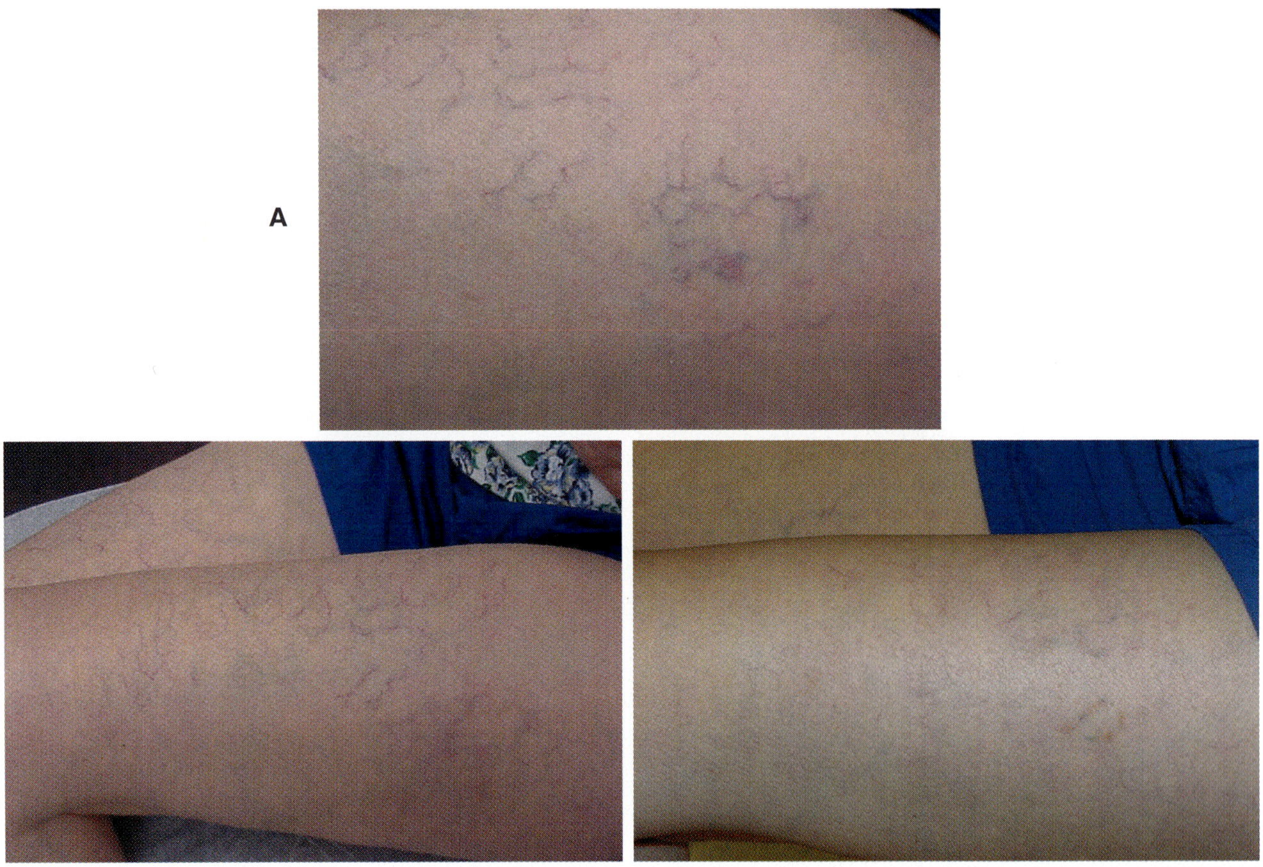

A

B

C

FIG. 22-8
Hyperpigmentation postsclerotherapy. **A,** Telangiectases before treatment. **B,** One month after treatment some matting is seen. **C,** Following a second treatment some residual pigmentation remains at 3 months, but the patient is convinced there is no improvement. Once shown the before photo **(A),** patient understands the progression.

now familiar with the procedure, a response to sclerosing solutions can be predicted, and more areas can be treated with the patient less fearful and muscles relaxed. The order of treatment is varicose veins, reticular veins, purple venulectases, telangiectatic webs or networks, and finally treatment of the smallest and most isolated telangiectases. Injection of telangiectases should not be undertaken until larger diameter reflux sources flowing back into the telangiectatic area are eliminated. Reflux from larger vessels typically originates proximally but rarely may originate distally.

Transillumination may help identify the sources of reticular veins connected to telangiectatic webs (Fig. 22-9). When no clear feeder vessel is identified by Doppler or transillumination, then the point at which the telangiectases begin to branch out is the site at which to begin injection. Whenever possible, it is best to inject telangiectases during the visit when the reticular veins are injected. We believe that concomitant injection of reticular veins in visible association with telangiectatic webs decreases the total number of treatments.[15,16] Once sclerotherapy treatment sessions are complete, many of the "stragglers," vessels too small to cannulate with a 30-gauge needle, can be treated with laser or light sources.

Injection of Telangiectases

The typical sclerotherapy tray setup includes (1) cotton balls soaked with 70% isopropyl alcohol, (2) protective gloves, (3) 3 cc disposable syringes, (4) 30-gauge disposable transparent hub needles, (5) cotton balls or STD pads for compression, (6) Transpore or paper tape, (7) nitroglycerine paste (for use in the case of prolonged blanching of an injection site). The following sclerosing solutions are used:

1. Sodium tetradecyl sulfate (STS) (concentrations 0.1% to 0.5%)
2. Hypertonic saline (11.7% to 23.4%)
3. Hypertonic saline (10%) and dextrose (25%) (mixed by local pharmacy)
4. Polidocanol (concentrations 0.25% to 1%) (pending FDA approval)

Technique. The patient is placed in either the prone or supine position. Treatment sites may be wiped with cotton balls heavily saturated with 70% isopropyl alcohol, although cooling of the skin may cause contraction of the reticular veins. It is supposed that alcohol application reduces infection risk, but it certainly helps to visualize vessels by increasing light transmission through otherwise reflective white scale on the epidermal surface. Following complete evaporation of the alcohol, a 30-gauge needle, bent to an angle of 10 to 30 degrees with the bevel up, is placed on the skin so that the needle is parallel to the skin surface. A 3 cc syringe filled with 1.5 to 2 ml of solution is held between the index and middle fingers while the fourth and fifth fingers support the syringe against the leg in a fixed position facilitating accurate penetration of the vessel (Fig. 22-10). The nondominant hand is used to stretch the skin around the needle and may offer additional support for the syringe.

The firmly supported needle is then moved slowly 1 to 2 mm forward, piercing the vein just sufficiently to allow infusion of solution with the most minimal pressure on the plunger. Magnifying lenses on the order of ×1.5 to ×3 are often helpful to visualize cannulation of the smallest telangiectases.

A very sharp needle is critical to cannulate but not shear small telangiectases. The 30-gauge needle is changed as often as every three to four punctures. Use of 32- to 33-gauge needles is not advised, as they veer off course easily. Injection of a tiny bolus of air (<0.05 ml) may be helpful to establish that the needle is within the vein, as slight clearing 1 to 3 mm ahead of the bevel

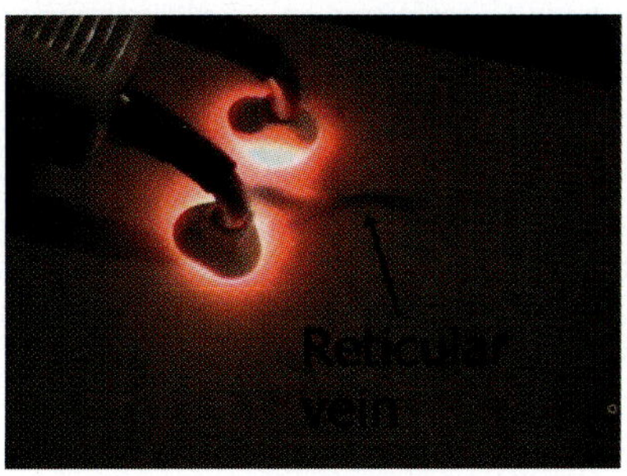

FIG. 22-9
Transillumination of a reticular vein leading to a group of telangiectases.

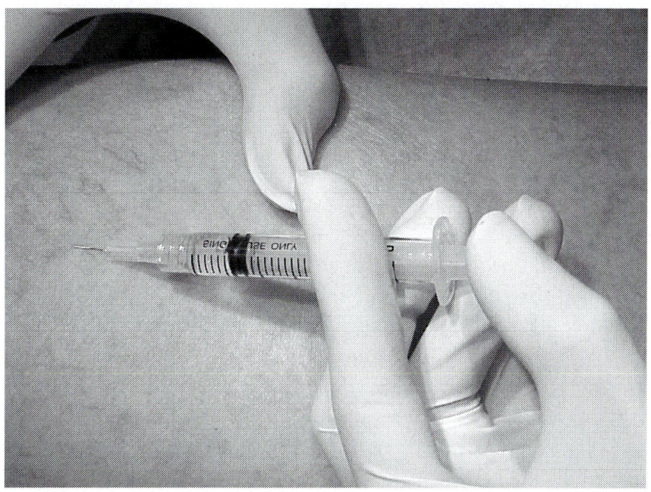

FIG. 22-10
Proper hand positioning during sclerotherapy.

can be seen. A larger air bolus theoretically allows the arborizing vessels to clear instantly, allowing greater spread of the sclerosing solution,[17,18] but we and others have found this to occur infrequently and generally find a larger air bolus not necessary.[2,9,19]

Concentrations of sclerosants used for telangiectases are less than those needed for reticular veins. We recommend 0.1% to 0.2% STS, 0.25% to 0.5% polidocanol (not approved by the U.S. FDA), 11.7% to 23.4% hypertonic saline, or hypertonic saline and dextrose (not FDA approved). The initial concentration is typically the lowest concentration listed above, termed the minimal effective sclerosant concentration.[20] Higher concentrations increase the risks for matting and pigmentation. The concentration may always be increased at subsequent treatments if ineffective sclerosis occurs. Increase of sclerosant concentration is more effective than an increased volume per injection. STS dissolves some of the rubber of the syringe plunger, making it difficult to move the plunger and contaminating the sclerosing solution with rubber breakdown products (personal communication, Wyeth-Ayerst Laboratories). For this reason, we strongly recommend the use of latex-free syringes (Terumo Medical Corp., Somerset, NJ) to avoid allergic reactions due to latex contamination of the sclerosant. In the experience of one of the authors (R.A.W.), using latex-free syringes in 10,000 patients reduced the incidence of allergic reaction to STS to zero.

Reticular Veins

This procedure is similar to the injection of telangiectases except that a much greater volume of solution is injected. A 3 cc syringe with a 27- to 30-gauge needle bent to an angle of 10 to 30 degrees is inserted into the reticular vein, which is usually superficial and visibly blue. When the sensation of piercing the vein is felt, the plunger is gently pulled back with the thumb of the dominant hand until blood is seen beginning to back up into the transparent plastic hub. If the wall of the reticular vein is thin, the suction created by pulling back on the syringe may cause the wall to adhere to the needle bevel and prevent aspiration of blood. In this case one can move the needle gently forward and backward, and if no resistance is felt, the vein has probably been cannulated and the injection may proceed cautiously.

Reticular veins undergo contraction following a cannulation attempt or when the skin temperature is cool. If this occurs, another injection site along the reticular vein must be sought. The cannulation of a reticular vein can be more difficult than protuberant venulectases or telangiectases. Usually the volume per injection site is no more than 0.5 ml, but the capacity of long reticular veins may easily exceed 1 ml. The progress of solution may be followed visually and the injection stopped when the entire reticular vein has cleared of blood.

The strength of sclerosants for treatment of reticular veins are 0.2% to 0.5% sodium tetradecyl sulfate (STS, Sotradecol), 0.5% to 1% polidocanol (Aethoxysklerol) (not FDA approved), 23.4% hypertonic saline, or hypertonic saline and dextrose (Sclerodex) (not FDA approved).[9,21] See Table 22-1 for a summary of sclerosing solutions.

Until experience is gained in cannulating reticular veins, cautious injection is the rule. Resistance to injection will be felt when the reticular vein has not been properly cannulated and then will be followed by a small hematoma. Necrosis is rare with extravascular injection at this depth. After injection, all sites treated are noted in anatomic diagrams in the patient's record. Concentration and volumes of all sclerosing solutions are recorded.

Varicose Veins

Treatment of varicose veins is performed by cannulation with a straight 27- or 30-gauge needle in a recumbent patient. The patient's veins are typically marked with the patient standing prior to beginning treatment. One must be absolutely positive of the intravascular positioning of the needle, since higher volumes of higher-concentration sclerosants are used.

The patient is typically placed in a supine or prone position as necessary, and a syringe and needle are used to inject a small volume of sclerosant at each one of the previously marked points along the veins to be treated. A 27- to 30-gauge needle on a 3 cc syringe is often employed for this technique. The needle is advanced while aspirating the syringe until dark venous blood indicates penetration of the lumen. At this point 0.5 to 1.5 ml of concentrated sclerosant is injected at the site. The needle is withdrawn and redirected to the next site. At the conclusion of treatment the vein should visually appear contracted. This is a rapid and efficacious technique that is used by the majority of phlebologists treating large veins in the United States today.

When this technique is used, it must be recognized that the vessels being injected are not fully empty of blood, thus the sclerosant being injected must be more concentrated to allow for dilution by the blood remaining in the vessel. The largest vessels contain more blood and therefore require higher concentrations of sclerosant and possibly higher volumes to produce effective sclerosis after dilution. Sclerosing solutions used are 0.5% to 3% STS and 1% to 3% polidocanol. Volumes per injection site should not exceed 1 ml. Volume per session should not exceed the equivalent of 10 ml of 3% STS.

Starting Sclerotherapy

A substantial investment of time and effort is required to develop expertise in sclerotherapy of any sized veins. Prior experience with venipuncture helps little with treatment of larger veins and is completely irrele-

Table 22-1 Sclerosing Solutions Commonly Used in the United States

Solution: Chemical Name	Brand Names	Category	Advantages	Disadvantages
Sodium tetradecyl sulfate	Sotradecol Fibro-Vein Thrombovar	Detergent (emulsifier): rapid dissolution of endothelium	■ Painless intravascular ■ Painful extravascular ■ Strong for varicose veins ■ Effective at low concentration	■ Skin necrosis with extravasation of concentrations >0.25% ■ Expensive ■ Pigmentation: postsclerosis ■ Dissolves rubber: must use latex-free syringes to avoid latex allergic response
Polidocanol	Aethoxysklerol Sclero-Vein	Detergent (emulsifier)	■ Always painless ■ Cutaneous necrosis low ■ Effective at low concentration	■ Urticaria (immediate) at injection site ■ Skin necrosis from painless arteriolar injection ■ Not FDA approved*
Hypertonic saline (23.4%)	None	Hyperosmolar: slow crenation of endothelium	■ Low allergic risk ■ Readily available ■ Rapid action	■ Painful stinging and cramping ■ Highly ulcerogenic: high risk for skin necrosis
Saline and dextrose	Sclerodex	Hyperosmolar	■ High viscosity: remains in treated veins ■ Low allergic risk ■ Low risk of necrosis	■ Too weak for larger varicosities ■ Slight stinging ■ One concentration only ■ Not FDA approved*

*Under FDA review.

vant in the treatment of the smallest veins. Successful treatment requires the correct technique, the correct diagnosis, and the correct treatment plan for the type and size of vein to be treated. The procedure is mastered by reading written descriptions of proper technique and by observing and emulating the fastidious technique of skilled physicians. Many different techniques have been used in the treatment of small veins, but certain basic principles are universal.

The basic principle of treatment from the largest to the smallest varicosities holds true no matter what the size being treated (Box 22-1). Sclerotherapy of telangiectases begins with injection of the feeding reticular veins, then venulectases, then telangiectatic webs or networks and finally the smallest and most isolated telangiectases. For the inexperienced practitioner, beginning with reticular veins and associated telangiectases should be understood and practiced first before embarking on the treatment of larger varicosities of the saphenous system. Skills for larger veins are best learned at intensive hands-on workshops.

BOX 22-1 Principles of Varicose Vein Sclerotherapy

- Larger veins treated prior to smaller veins
- Reflux at the SFJ is eliminated surgically
- Reflux points determined initially and treated specifically
- Vein must be emptied of blood by various maneuvers before injection (or use foamed sclerosant)
- Direct finger pressure in a spreading and compressing motion following injection
- Immediate and adequate compression until sustained vein contraction is observed

Minimizing Complications of Sclerotherapy

Compression. After massaging the injection site to distribute the sclerosant more evenly, cotton balls are secured over the injection sites by paper tape or Transpore tape. Graduated 20 to 30 mm Hg or 30 to 40 mm Hg support hose are then applied, particularly in patients with protuberant telangiectases or telangiectases in association with reticular veins.[22] Some physicians prefer to skip the cotton balls and have the patients wear compression stockings. These are best applied while the patient is still supine immediately after the procedure has been completed. Having the patient stand before putting on the stockings increases blood flow in the sclerosed vessels and is believed to decrease the effectiveness of the treatment session.

The duration of compression needed after sclerotherapy is still a matter of debate, although most recommend 2 to 3 weeks. The classic descriptions of sclerosis of varicose veins described by Fegan, Hobbs, and Doran recommend compression for 6 weeks.[23-25] A few small randomized studies have suggested that most of the value of compression may come in the early phase and that results may be comparable no matter whether compression is maintained for 6 weeks, for 3 weeks, or for only 3 days.[26,27] A recent well-controlled study concluded that 3 weeks of compression may be ideal, but 1 week or 3 days of compression is sufficient to improve results.[28] In the United States, few patients can tolerate 6 weeks of uninterrupted compression, but most are able to comply with 2 weeks of compression stockings, and nearly all can tolerate a protocol that uses relatively uninterrupted compression for the first 3 days, then continues compression interrupted only for showering for the next 2 weeks.

Patients are encouraged to walk, and not restrict their activities, with the exception of any exercise such as weightlifting with sustained muscle contraction that results in a sharp rise in venous pressure. Treatment intervals vary, but allowing 4 to 8 weeks between treatments helps to minimize the number of necessary sessions. In the case of laser and pulsed light treatment, waiting 8 to 12 weeks between treatments yields optimal results. Often telangiectases will ultimately improve with at least partial clearing after exhibiting no initial response within the first 2 weeks. A typical patient undergoes three to five treatments spaced 4 to 8 weeks apart. After the initial series of treatments, a "rest" period of 4 to 6 months allows pigmentation and matting to clear and allows remaining reticular veins to establish "new" routes of drainage. Approximately 80% of vessels treated clear satisfactorily during the first course of treatment. The physician may then judge and reevaluate any remaining telangiectatic webs or new telangiectases for the best approach for another round of sclerotherapy.

Hyperpigmentation. The incidence of hyperpigmentation depends on the sclerosing agent, the concentration, and the technique used. In general, the incidence of hyperpigmentation is higher when a stronger agent is used and higher when stronger concentrations of an agent are used. Larger veins also have a higher incidence of pigmentation, since more trapping of red blood cells occurs. The cause of pigmentation is most likely a combination of postinflammatory hyperpigmentation and direct hemosiderin deposition. Hyperpigmentation is rare in vessels less than 1 mm in diameter.[29]

The rate of hyperpigmentation after sclerotherapy varies from 10% to 80%. An incidence of 10% to 30% has been reported for hypertonic saline and polidocanol[4] but up to 80% with 0.5% STS.[9] The occurrence of pigmentation can be reduced by using minimal concentrations of sclerosing solutions, applying compression, and avoiding injection into sites receiving reflux from larger associated varicosities. There is no highly effective method for treating hemosiderin hyperpigmentation. Treatments that may have some value include exfoliation, chelation, and short-pulsed pigment specific laser therapy. Most patients will have spontaneous resolution of hyperpigmentation within 1 year, and watchful waiting with periodic photographic documentation of the pigmentation is satisfactory in most cases. It is important to remind patients to return for drainage if they notice any hyperpigmented firm or nodular areas after treatment, as the duration of hyperpigmentation is lessened by prompt drainage of coagula (preferably within 6 weeks).

Matting. Telangiectatic matting refers to appearance of tiny new red (occasionally violaceous) telangiectases that appear in patients after sclerotherapy or surgical removal of varicose veins or venulectasia. Telangiectatic matting presents as "blush type" regions containing large numbers of "new" blood vessels less than 0.2 mm in diameter, located in and around the site of treatment.

The incidence of telangiectatic matting is between 15% and 24%.[30,31] It is predominantly seen in women but can also occur in men.[4] Telangiectatic matting may occasionally be associated with intolerable burning pain and with leg edema[32]; it usually resolves spontaneously in 3 to 12 months.[29,30] Occasionally telangiectatic matting can be permanent, and pretreatment patient information should make this clear in an explicit manner.[33]

It is widely believed, though unproven, that telangiectatic matting is more common when higher infusion pressures, larger volumes, and higher concentrations of sclerosant are used. We have observed that when infusion pressure is increased, resulting in blanching of the entire capillary network of the skin, telangiectatic matting is more likely to occur. Patient factors associated with an increased risk of telangiectatic matting include excessive body weight, a family history of telangiectases, and longer duration of spider veins.[30]

The most important first step in treating this complication is to repeat the clinical evaluation of the patient, looking for any previously unrecognized sources of hydrostatic pressure. Transillumination may help locate a previously unseen reticular vein. At the minimum, Doppler examination of the problem areas should be done to listen for unresolved reflux. Much more information can be gained from a duplex ultrasound examination. The duplex study should be performed with the patient in the standing position, because previously unrecognized high-pressure reflux from an intermittently incompetent (clinically inapparent) saphenous vein may be the culprit.

The patient is given a mild anti-inflammatory cream to apply to the area, and photographs of the area are

Table 22-2 Common Side Effects and Prevention

Side Effect	Incidence	Prevention
Telangiectatic matting	10%-50%	■ Use minimal sclerosant concentrations ■ Limit blanching per injection to an area 1 to 2 cm in diameter ■ Use low injection pressures to avoid backup of solution into capillaries ■ Encourage weight loss prior to institution of therapy ■ Consider recommendation to discontinue oral contraceptives
Hyperpigmentation	11%-80%	■ Eliminate high-pressure reflux before treating smaller vessels ■ Minimize risks of vessel rupture ■ Avoid excessive syringe pressure ■ Minimize intravascular pressure by elevating leg during treatment ■ Select a sclerosant with the least inflammatory effects ■ Use a sclerosant concentration appropriate for vessel size ■ Apply compression immediately posttreatment ■ Remove postsclerotherapy coagula as early as possible ■ Avoid concomitant use of minocycline ■ Direct treatment at the deepest site in a telangiectatic cluster ■ Avoid treating patients with known defects in iron transport
Necrosis	1%-5%	■ Use meticulous technique to avoid extravasation ■ Avoid prolonged blanching ■ Treat arteriolar spasm with vigorous local massage ■ Arteriolar spasm may be treated with 2% nitroglycerine ointment ■ If a small bleb of low concentration of solution is extravasated, massage for 1 minute ■ Use right-size compression garment and the right amount of compression

taken at 6- to 8-week intervals until resolution occurs. Patients can be reassured that even the worst matting can resolve completely over time and are much more tolerant of this waiting period when they have been suitably informed before start of treatment that telangiectatic matting may occur.

Necrosis. To minimize skin necrosis, extravasation must be avoided. If resistance to the easy injection of sclerosant or the beginning of any "bleb" at the injection site is noted, stop injecting immediately. The physician needs to keep an eye on the injection site at all times in order to notice the "bleb" at the moment of its occurrence. Some physicians keep a syringe containing 5 to 10 ml of normal saline nearby to flush and dilute any areas of extravasation that may develop. If sclerosant extravasates, it may also be diluted with 0.5% to 1% lidocaine without epinephrine. The benefit of dilution has not been proven but is based on the theory that further dilution of a sclerosing solution will minimize the capacity for further tissue destruction. A prolonged period of blanching following injection indicates possible arteriolar compromise, and for this, immediate application of topical nitroglycerine paste is recommended. Application is made in small "dabs" rubbed into the skin until a faint blush replaces the blanch.

Sclerosing solutions vary in the degree of cellular necrosis they produce. Hypertonic saline at 23.4% is a caustic sclerosing agent, and when an inexperienced practitioner uses this agent, small spots of superficial epidermal damage often are seen at points of injection where a small bleb of the solution has escaped from the vein.[34] The incidence of significant necrosis following sclerotherapy in experienced hands is estimated at less than 1%.

Fortunately, when ulcerations do occur they are usually fairly small, averaging 4 mm in diameter. At this size, primary healing usually leaves an acceptable scar but will often result in pigmentation changes on the skin lasting from months to years. Occlusive or hydrocolloid dressings apparently decrease wound healing time. More importantly, occlusive dressings decrease the pain associated with an open ulcer. Left alone, ulcers may take 4 to 6 weeks to completely heal. If this is unacceptable, excision and primary closure is a reasonable alternative, depending on the anatomic location. Excision of the ulcer with split- or full-thickness grafting usually leads to a worse cosmetic result than healing by secondary intention. A summary of complications, incidence, and means of prevention is shown in Table 22-2.

AMBULATORY PHLEBECTOMY (AP)

Indications

In younger patients with varicose veins, the walls may be thicker, more muscular, and thus less susceptible to penetration and injury by sclerosing solutions. These thicker veins, particularly in athletic individuals, diminish the likelihood that sclerotherapy will be effective. Other situations more amenable to ambulatory phlebectomy include areas of high flow such as large truncal or branch veins of the greater and lesser saphenous system. Phlebectomy leads to good results except when significant reflux at the saphenofemoral and saphenopopliteal junctions is present. In the case where reflux at these junctions is present, we recommend ligation and short stripping or the new endovenous RF occlusion technique called Closure.

The decision to treat by ambulatory phlebectomy vs. sclerotherapy usually is determined by anatomic location, patient preference, and estimated thickness of vein wall. When a "blue" vein is observed, this indicates a wall so thin that blood may easily be visualized within it. Full-thickness damage by sclerosing solutions is more likely, and these blue veins easily shred when trying to hook them by ambulatory phlebectomy. Therefore visibly flesh-colored veins are better treated by ambulatory phlebectomy.

Once the origin point of reflux is diagnosed in truncal (axial) varicose veins, ambulatory phlebectomy may be preferred over traditional surgery, since little or no scar occurs compared with ligation incisions. Ambulatory phlebectomy also avoids possible complications of sclerotherapy for larger subcutaneous varicose veins including intra-arterial injection, superficial thrombophlebitis, skin necrosis, and months of hyperpigmentation.[35,36] The recurrence rate of large varicose veins is also reduced, but only when the major source of reflux (if present) at the saphenofemoral or saphenopopliteal junctions is eliminated as well.

History

Ambulatory phlebectomy is a surgical procedure attributed to Swiss dermatologist Robert Muller.[37,38] He first performed the technique in an office setting in Neuchâtel, Switzerland, in the late 1950s as an alternative to hospital-based surgery and sclerotherapy. Acceptance of this technique was very slow. It became popular in the 1990s when reduced time to resolution and longer-lasting resolution was realized. Importantly, new instruments became more widely available.[39]

Procedure

Instrumentation requirements are quite basic; the hooks are shown in Figure 22-11. The Muller hook, available in four sizes, with a blunt tip, resembles a crochet hook that elevates the vein from below. Oesch's hook, available in three sizes, is characterized by a massive squared off grip and is designed with a small barb at the tip to pierce the vein from the lateral aspect and elevate. Ramelet's hook, available in two sizes, is a smaller, fine, sharp hook, elevating the vein from above by lifting from adventitia. The cylindrical shape of the grip permits a gentle rolling of the hook between the fingers, diminishing wrist and hand stress during the procedure.

Other necessary equipment includes a No. 11 scalpel or 18-gauge needle to perform the incisions or punctures (Box 22-2). A half dozen or more mosquito clamps or curved clamps should be on the tray with the phlebectomy hooks. An operating table allowing rotation in the Trendelenburg position and good overhead lighting is necessary. The presence of an assistant to provide compression at sites of oozing is essential.

Sedation, if required, consists usually of an oral benzodiazepine. Varicose vein bulges are carefully delineated with a skin marker pen on the standing patient.

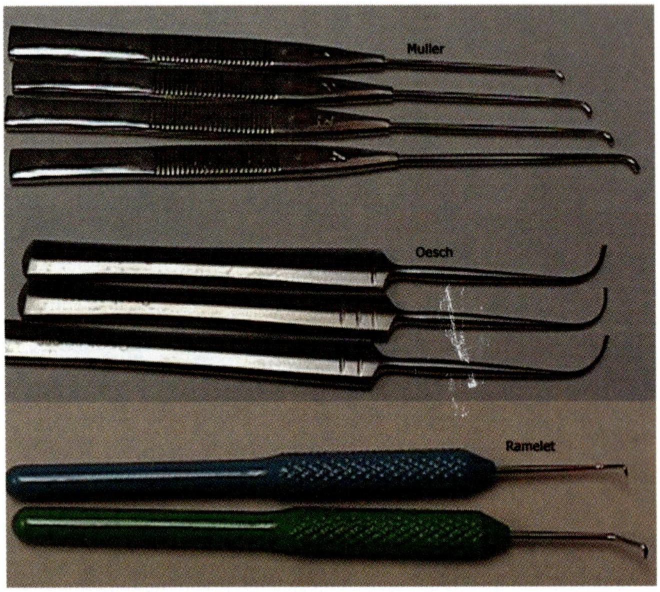

FIG. 22-11
Hooks for ambulatory phlebectomy.

BOX 22-2 Phlebectomy Supplies

1. Skin marking pen
2. Iodine prepping solution
3. Disposable face mask, sterile gloves
4. Local anesthetic, syringes, needles
5. Ambulatory phlebectomy hooks: Muller, Oesch, Ramelet, Varady
6. Clamps, sterile 4 × 4 gauze pads
7. Needle 18 gauge, scalpel No. 11
8. Mosquito forceps (one dozen)
9. Hydrogen peroxide for postoperative washing of the leg
10. Absorbent dressings
11. Inelastic compression wrap
12. Elastic graduated compression stockings

The patient is then placed supine and the vein position is reexamined using a transilluminator. Areas that are deeper and will be more difficult to hook are noted and marked. Local anesthesia using a tumescent anesthesia technique requires a higher concentration than tumescent anesthesia for liposuction. Typically 0.2% lidocaine with 1:500,000 epinephrine in normal saline is prepared. Injection is with a 22-gauge spinal needle that dissects the tissue just under the varicose vein to be avulsed. Usually no more than 200 ml is required for fairly long segments. Anesthesia of the leg often persists for 10 hours. Only with work in the popliteal fossa may patients experience a temporary foot drop from anesthesia of the peroneal nerve and require assistance for ambulating and driving home.

Cutaneous incisions performed with No. 11 scalpel blade or 18-gauge needle should be vertical along the thigh and lower leg and follow the skin lines at the knee or the ankle. The distance between the incisions varies from 2 to 15 cm, but is typically 3 to 4 cm. Once the ambulatory phlebectomy hook is inserted into the puncture site, the targeted vein is gently dissected by undermining with the shaft of the phlebectomy hook. Attempts to pull vein through the puncture site may initially result in shreds of adventitial fibroadipose attachments. Sometimes it is not until the third or fourth attempt at lifting that a loosened vein segment can then be elevated with the sharp tip of the hook. As the vein loop is exposed and pulled through the small incision, mosquito forceps are then used to clamp the vein loop. Traction is maintained by pulling as far as the vein slides easily. Too much tension will result in breakage. A gentle rolling motion accompanied by massage can be helpful.

Novices are warned to avoid the popliteal fossa, dorsum of the foot, peripatellar or pretibial region, and recurrent varicose veins after phlebitis or sclerotherapy. Hemostasis is achieved with intraoperative and postoperative local compression and by Trendelenburg positioning of at least 10 degrees. Venous ligation is not necessary, as stretching of the vein causes rapid hemostasis most likely due to more exposed endothelial sites for platelet aggregation. Avoiding ligation eliminates all the additional complications of foreign material left just below the skin.

A typical session lasts 30 to 60 minutes with the major portion of a varicose vein extending from thigh to mid calf. Occasionally incision sites in the mid thigh may stretch with removal of large truncal veins and may require one 5-0 suture. Postoperative pain seldom occurs because of long action of the tumescent anesthesia, but some patients have reported a slight burning at the site of incisions during the first postsurgical night. Analgesia is easily achieved by acetaminophen. Immediate ambulation reduces risks of deep venous thrombosis to a negligible rate.

Postoperative Course

Hematoma and bleeding are the most likely complications of ambulatory phlebectomy (Box 22-3). Therefore meticulous postoperative compression bandaging is required. The entire course of the removed varicose vein is covered with four layers of gauze pads or a single layer of the most absorbent sanitary napkins. These are secured with a low-stretch bandage (such as Comprilan, Beiersdorf-Jobst, Charlotte, NC) stretched to 80% of maximal stretch to obtain a low resting pressure dressing. Hematomas are minimized by placing compression at least 4 cm beyond the most proximal incision. An elastic graduated compression stocking is also worn to obtain high resting pressure. The patient walks for 10 minutes in the office and the dressing is observed for any signs of bleeding. If the dressing remains dry, the patient may drive home without assistance as long as local anesthesia has not compromised motor function.

Dressings are changed after 24 hours, and the incision sites are visually inspected. A less bulky dressing of gauze and inelastic compression is applied, and the compression stocking is placed over this again. The inner dressing may be removed at 48 hours, but daytime elastic graduated compression stockings are mandatory for 7 to 14 days. Hematomas are barely visible at 24 hours but become more prominent by 7 days.

Short showers are allowed 2 to 3 days postoperatively. Surgical puncture sites are usually totally invisible after 3 to 6 months but may persist much longer in younger patients with tighter skin. Hematomas rapidly disappear and pigmentation usually fades within 2 to 3 weeks. Long-term results are excellent as long as the source of venous reflux has been correctly eliminated (Fig. 22-12). Since susceptibility to varicose veins is genetic, patients need to be warned about recurrences or

BOX 22-3 Complications of Ambulatory Phlebectomy

Frequent

Skin: transient pigmentation, vesicles from pressure dressing

Vascular: hematoma

Uncommon

Skin: contact dermatitis, infection, scar, tattoo from marking pen, silicon (foreign body) granuloma

Vascular: postoperative bleeding, telangiectatic matting

Neurologic: postoperative pain, transitory sensory defect, neuroma

Rare

Superficial thrombophlebitis

Lymphatic pseudocyst

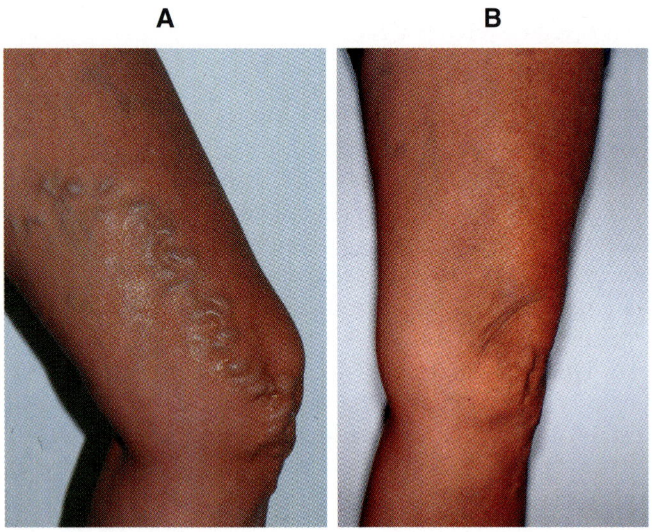

FIG. 22-12
Before and after ambulatory phlebectomy. **A,** Large primary branch varicosity of the greater saphenous vein. **B,** Six weeks after ambulatory phlebectomy.

new varicosities in the future even with definitive eradication by ambulatory phlebectomy.

LASERS AND LIGHT SOURCES

Theoretical Considerations

Sclerotherapy remains the gold standard for treatment of leg veins and telangiectases. Public interest in laser and light treatment of leg veins is high, and under the right circumstances they can produce excellent results. As with all the other treatment techniques, reverse pressure from associated reticular or varicose veins must be recognized or treatment will be doomed to failure. In many patients, a combination of treatments is necessary, as lasers and light sources do not effectively treat associated reticular and varicose veins.

Lasers have been used to treat leg telangiectases since the early 1970s. While it was not until the development of the pulsed dye lasers in the late 1980s that the first reasonable results were achieved, recent development of longer wavelength, longer pulse duration, pulsed lasers, and light sources has improved outcomes significantly. Basic requirements for a laser or light source to treat leg veins are (1) a wavelength that is proportionately better absorbed by the target (hemoglobin) than surrounding chromophores, (2) penetration to the full depth of the target blood vessel, (3) sufficient energy to damage the vessel without damaging the overlying skin, and (4) an exposure duration long enough to slowly coagulate the vessel and its lining without damaging the surrounding tissue.

Ideal parameters, therefore, depend on wavelength, pulse duration, and beam diameter. In general, longer-wavelength visible light penetrates deeper into skin and should be chosen to target deeper vessels. The larger the vessel diameter, the longer the required pulse duration in order to slowly heat the entire vessel. Larger spot sizes penetrate deeper into tissue and optimize fluence delivery to the target (Table 22-3).

The choice of wavelength(s) and pulse duration is related to the type and size of target vessel treated. Deeper vessels require a longer wavelength to allow penetration to their depth. While pulse duration must be matched to vessel size, the larger the vessel diameter, the longer the pulse duration required to effectively damage the vessel thermally. The relative importance of the hemoglobulin absorption peaks in green (541 nm) and red to infrared (800 to 1000 nm) shifts as the depth and size of blood vessel changes (Fig. 22-13). Absorption by hemoglobin in the long visible to near infrared range appears to become more important for vessels over 0.5 mm in diameter and at least 0.5 mm below the skin surface.[40]

Table 22-3 Ideal Laser/Light Parameters for Treatment of Vascular Lesions

	Wavelength (nm)	Pulse Duration (ms)	Beam Diameter (mm)
Diameter of Vessels			
100 μm	580	1	—
300 μm	590	10	—
600 μm to 1 mm	600	20-100	—
Vessel Depth			
Less than 1 mm	>500	—	Small
Greater than 1 mm	>600	—	Larger

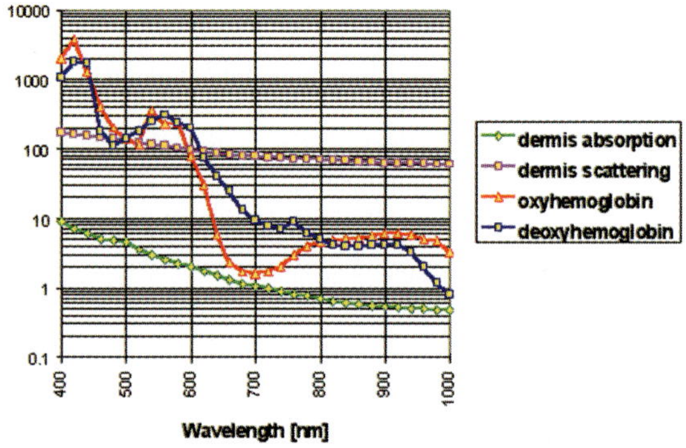

FIG. 22-13
The relative importance of the hemoglobulin absorption peaks in green (541 nm) and red to infrared (800 to 1000 nm) shifts as the depth and size of blood vessel change. (Courtesy Lumenis, Santa Clara, CA.)

Successful treatment by lasers and light sources is also hindered by the fact that leg telangiectases course at different depths with greatly varying diameters in each segment. Large-diameter segments require a longer pulse duration to allow sufficient time for diffusion of heat evenly throughout the cylindrical vessel lumen.[41]

Various devices have been utilized in an effort to enhance clinical efficacy and minimize the adverse sequelae of telangiectasia treatment (Table 22-4). Unfortunately, most have also been associated with adverse responses in excess of and response rate far lower than those associated with sclerotherapy. This is related both to insufficient vessel destruction and to competition from overlying melanin and the lack of treatment of hydrostatic pressure from the "feeding" venous system.

Table 22-4 Lasers and Light Sources for Vascular Lesions in Order of Increasing Wavelength

Laser/Light Source (Manufacturer)	Wavelength (nm)	Pulse Duration (ms)
Pulsed KTP	532	1-200
VersaPulse (Lumenis)		
Illustra (Cynosure)		
Diolite (Iriderm)		
Aura/Orion (Laserscope)		
Pulsed dye	585	0.450
SPTL-1b (Candela)		
LV (Cynosure)		
Long-pulsed dye		
Vbeam (Candela)	585, 590, 595, 600	0.5-40
PhotoGenica V-Star (Cynosure)	595	0.5-40
Long-pulsed alexandrite	755	3-20
GentleLASE (Candela)		
LPIR (Cynosure)		
EpiTouch Alex (Lumenis)		
Diodes	800, 810, 930	1-250
Diomed (LaserLite)		
LightSheer (Lumenis)		
Long-pulsed Nd:YAG	1064	
Vasculight (Lumenis)		2-16
CoolGlide (Altus)		10-100
CoolTouch Varia		0.3-100
Lyra (Laserscope)		50
VeinLase (HGM)		1-50
Intense pulsed light source	515-1200	0.5-20
Vasculight (Lumenis)		

Continuous Wave Lasers

Carbon Dioxide Laser. Carbon dioxide lasers were used early on in an effort to obliterate telangiectatic vessels by means of precise vaporization without significant damage to adjacent tissue.[42-44] However, because carbon dioxide laser light is so well absorbed by water in the epidermis and dermis overlying the blood vessel, nonspecific thermal injury is guaranteed regardless of whether pulsed or continuous wave sources are used.[43] All reported studies demonstrate unsatisfactory cosmetic results.[42-44] Treated areas show multiple hypopigmented punctate scars with either minimal resolution of the treated vessel or neovascularization adjacent to the treatment site. Because of its nonselective action, the carbon dioxide laser has no advantage over the electrodessication needle in treating leg telangiectasia.

Argon and Continuous Wave Dye Lasers. Argon (488 and 514 nm) and continuous wave dye lasers (515 to 590 nm) are well absorbed by hemoglobin and penetrate to the depth of middermal vessels, over 1 mm into skin. Because of unwanted, nonspecific thermal damage that occurs because of the continuous nature of the beam, results of treatment of leg veins have been discouraging (Dover JS and Arndt KA, unpublished observations, November 1987). In a report of 38 patients treated by Apfelberg et al.[44] 49% had poor or no results from treatment and only 16% had what were considered acceptable results. In addition, almost half of the patients had hemosiderin bruising. In another series, Dixon et al.[45] noted significant improvement in just under half of their patients. They speculated that after initial improvement, incomplete thrombosis, recanalization, or new vein formation produced reappearance of the vessels after 6 to 12 months.

In an effort to enhance therapeutic success with leg vein sclerotherapy, the argon laser has been used to interrupt the telangiectasis every 2 to 3 cm prior to injection of a sclerosing agent.[46] In 11 of 16 patients who completed treatment, 2 developed punctate depigmented scars and 3 developed hyperpigmentation. However, 93.7% of patients were reported to have "satisfactory" results. Cooling the skin simultaneously with argon or argon dye (577 nm, 585 nm) laser treatment has been demonstrated to produce improvement in 67% of leg telangiectases 1 mm in diameter or less.[47] This may, however, have been due to temperature related vasomotor changes in blood flow.[48]

Continuous Wave Neodymium:Yttrium Aluminum Garnet (Nd:YAG) Laser. The Nd:YAG laser at 1064 nm has also been used to treat leg telangiectasia.[49] Because absorption in blood is relatively poor at this wavelength, the penetration depth is so great (up to 3.7 mm), and so much nonspecific damage is produced, there is no role for the continuous wave Nd:YAG laser in the treatment of leg vessels.

Pulsed Lasers and Light Sources

KTP Lasers. Early unsuccessful attempts were made to treat leg vessels with the CW potassium titanyl phosphate (KTP) crystal laser. A group of pulsed KTP lasers have recently been introduced for treatment of vascular lesions (see Table 22-4). The 532 nm KTP light was chosen for a variety of reasons, including the fact that 532 nm light is absorbed by hemoglobin as well as 585 nm light, and the penetration depth is almost the same. KTP crystals are highly reliable, convenient to work with, and easily available to laser manufacturers. While these devices use various mechanisms, each produces millisecond domain pulses at 532 nm.

The VersaPulse (Lumenis, Santa Clara, CA) produces a true millisecond domain pulse while other lasers in this category group nanosecond domain Q-switched pulses into millisecond laser pulses, resulting in slightly lower energy output.

Results of treatment of facial vessels have been excellent.[50] Early results in the treatment of leg veins using small spots and pulse durations of 10 ms or less were disappointing.[51] Recent results with the VersaPulse KTP laser have been more promising using larger spot sizes (3 to 5 mm) and longer pulse durations of 10 to 50 ms at fluences of 14 to 20 J/cm². Utilizing fluences between 12 and 20 J/cm² delivered with a 3 to 5 mm diameter spot size, a train of pulses is delivered over the vessel until spasm or thrombosis occurs. For leg vessels less than 1 mm in diameter that are not directly connected to a feeding reticular vein, and with use of a 4°C chilled tip to protect the epidermis, this method can be quite effective. We found that two to three treatments were necessary for maximal vessel improvement, although some have reported 100% resolution of the treated leg vein with one treatment.[52] Patients with darker or tanned skin have a relatively high risk of temporary hypopigmentation in my experience (R.A.W.). Cooling appears to be of significant benefit in protecting the epidermis, thus allowing use of higher, more effective fluences.[52]

Flashlamp Pumped-Pulsed Dye Laser. The traditional pulsed dye laser (PDL) (585 nm, 450 μs pulse duration) is highly effective in treating a variety of cutaneous vascular lesions, including port wine stains and facial telangiectases (Table 22-5). It is less effective, however, in the treatment of leg veins. The original PDL was developed for the treatment of port wine stains in children, where the average vessel is superficial and has a diameter of 100 μm and an average depth of 0.46 mm. While 585 nm light can penetrate 1.2 mm to reach the typical depth of leg telangiectasia,[53] the pulse duration is inadequate to effectively damage all but superficial fine vessels, approximately 0.1 mm or smaller in diameter. In general, telangiectases of the lower extremities treated with the PDL are less responsive and more prone to posttherapy hyperpigmentation than when treated with sclerotherapy.

Table 22-5 600 nm Flashlamp-Excited Pulsed Dye Lasers

	Candela Vbeam	Cynosure PhotoGenica V-Star
Pulse duration	1.5 to 40 ms	0.500 to 40 ms (LV) (pulse train of 0.500 pulses)
Pulse rate	Single or 1 Hz	Single or 1 Hz or 2 Hz
Spot sizes	3 × 10, 7, 10 mm	7, 10 mm
Maximum fluence	22 J/cm²	22 J/cm²

Advantages: Clearance of vessels 1.0 mm in diameter, but most effective for vessels 0.5 mm in diameter. Cynosure PhotoGenica V-Star combines characteristics of short-pulsed and long-pulsed lasers.

Disadvantages: Postoperative erythema, purpura, and postoperative pigmentation.

Polla et al.[54] treated 35 superficial leg telangiectases with the traditional PDL. The only parameters revealed in the report were that vessels were treated an average of 2.1 times with a maximum of four separate treatments. Red-purple raised, and blue flat vessels were treated without regard for the existence of reticular or feeder vessels. Fifteen percent of treated vessels had greater than 75% clearing, but 73% of treated vessels showed little or no response to treatment. The only lesions that responded at all were red-pink tiny telangiectases. Almost 50% of the treated patients developed persistent hypopigmentation or hyperpigmentation.

In preliminary animal studies in the rabbit ear vein, approximately 50% of vessels treated with an effective concentration of sclerosant demonstrated extravasated red blood cells (RBCs), while after PDL treatment extravasated RBCs were apparent in only 30% of vessels treated.[55] Rabbit ear vein treatment with the PDL resulted in a relative decrease in perivascular inflammation, compared with vessels treated with sclerotherapy alone.

Goldman and Fitzpatrick systematically examined the clinical effects of various fluence of the PDL in specific leg telangiectases.[56] They chose red superficial telangiectases less than 0.2 mm in diameter and telangiectatic matts induced by prior sclerotherapy. Thirty women with telangiectatic leg veins were treated. Telangiectases were superficial, red, and less than 0.2 mm in diameter. Thirteen of 101 telangiectatic areas were noted to have an associated reticular "feeding" vein between 2 and 3 mm in diameter that was not treated. Thirty-nine telangiectatic areas, chosen randomly, and seven patients with 25 areas of telangiectatic matting after previous sclerotherapy were treated with the traditional PDL (Candela, Wayland, MA) using a 5 mm spot with fluences of 6.5 to 8 J/cm^2 without concomitant cooling. At the conclusion of treatment, compression stockings were continuously worn over a foam dressing for approximately 72 hours. Sixty-seven percent of linear telangiectatic areas had cleared completely within 4 months of a single treatment. The best results were seen in vessels in which there was no identifiable feeder vessel. Hyperpigmentation, which developed in less than 10%, resolved completely within 6 months. There were no episodes of cutaneous ulceration, thrombophlebitis, or posttelangiectatic matting, perhaps because the PDL produces less inflammation than sclerotherapy. Hypopigmentation developed in all patients who were tanned at the time.

Long-Pulsed Dye Lasers. Based on the theory of selective photothermolysis, the predicted pulse duration ideally suited for thermal destruction of vessels the size of leg telangiectases (0.1 to several mm in diameter) is in the 1 to 50 ms domain.[41] Four "long-pulsed" dye lasers, two with 1.5 ms pulse durations (ScleroPLUS, Candela, Wayland, MA, and PhotoGenica VLS, Cynosure, Chelmsford, MA) and two with variable pulse durations as long as 40 ms (Vbeam, Candela, and PhotoGenica V-Star, Cynosure) are now available (see Table 22-5). Each device uses a rhodamine dye to produce wavelengths of 585, 590, 595, or 600 nm. These longer pulse durations and wavelengths theoretically improve our ability to treat deeper, larger-caliber vessels.

Six studies have assessed the effectiveness of these long-pulsed dye lasers in the treatment of leg veins. Results have been variable. In 18 patients with vessels ranging in diameter from 0.6 to 1 mm (in whom feeding vessels were previously treated successfully with sclerotherapy), a single treatment was performed with a 2 × 7 mm elliptical handpiece through a transparent hydrogel dressing. At a fluence of 15 J/cm^2, 50% of vessels cleared, while at 18 J/cm^2, 67% of vessels cleared.[57] Side effects included crusting, hyperpigmentation, and hypopigmentation. In a similar study that demonstrated that 595 nm was the more effective wavelength, results and side effects were similar.[58]

In a single treatment of vessels less than 0.4 mm in diameter using the 595 nm, 1.5 ms pulsed dye laser (Cynosure) and an experimental 595 nm, 4 ms pulsed dye laser, clearing rates were not clinically significant with either device, and the rates of both hypopigmentation and hyperpigmentation were significant.[59]

In a multiple treatment study, three treatments were performed 6 weeks apart using the 595 nm, 1.5 ms PDL (Candela) through a transparent hydrogel dressing with a 2 × 7 mm elliptical spot at 20 J/cm^2. All patients (100%) had at least 50% clearing, but 50% of treated areas became hyperpigmented and 20% hypopigmented.[60]

Lee and Lask treated 25 women with leg telangiectases less than 1 mm in diameter with the long-pulsed PDL (Candela).[61] Each patient had four areas treated; two at a wavelength of 595 nm with energies of 15 or 20 J/cm^2 and two additional areas treated with a 600 nm wavelength at 15 or 20 J/cm^2 respectively. A maximum of three treatments were performed at 6-week intervals. All patients noted improvement. The best results were achieved at 595 nm and 20 J/cm^2. Treatment response was variable and unpredictable, with some patients having complete resolution and some having only slight improvement. Three patients had superficial scabbing that resolved without apparent scarring. Hyperpigmentation occurred in over half of the treated sites but resolved completely within several months.

Reichert treated 250 sites of leg telangiectases ranging in size from 0.1 to 1.0 mm in diameter in 80 patients with the 1.5 ms pulsed dye laser (Candela) at wavelengths of 585 to 600 nm.[62] Patients were selected in whom refluxing reticular veins either were not present or had been previously treated. Ice packs were used to cool the skin before treatment. Total clearing was achieved after one or two treatments 6 weeks apart in all vessels with diameters up to 0.5 mm, while vessels 0.5 to 1 mm in diameter faded in approximately 80% of the cases after up to four separate treatments. Scarring, thrombophlebitis, and telangiectatic matting never occurred, but there was transient hyperpigmentation in 50% of cases and hypopigmentation in 50% of cases.

No studies have yet been published using dye lasers with pulse durations longer than 1.5 ms to treat leg veins, but if the results of long-pulsed Nd:YAG lasers are any indication, longer-pulsed dye lasers will be more effective than short-pulsed dye lasers in the treatment of leg vessels.

Other Pulsed Lasers

On the basis of deep penetration of long-wavelength visible and near infrared light and a small peak of hemoglobin absorption in the 700 to 900 nm range, long-pulsed alexandrite and Nd:YAG lasers have been developed to treat moderately deep, larger-caliber spider and feeding reticular veins. Characteristics of the available alexandrite lasers are wavelength of 755 nm and pulse durations of 3 to 20 ms; of the Nd:YAG lasers, wavelength 1064 nm, pulse durations up to 100 ms; and of the diode lasers, wavelengths 800, 810, and 930 nm and pulse durations of 10 to 250 ms.

Table 22-6 Long-Pulsed Solid State Alexandrite Lasers 755 nm

	EpiTouch Alex	GentleLASE	LPIR/Apogee
Pulse duration	2, 10, 20, or 40 ms	3 ms	5, 10, or 20 ms
Pulse rate	5-10 Hz	1 Hz	Single and 1 Hz
Spot sizes	5, 7, and 10 mm	8, 10, 12, 15 mm	7, 10, 12.5 and 6 × 10 mm (optional)
Maximum fluence	1-50 J/cm^2	8 mm, 100 J/cm^2; 10 mm, 60 J/cm^2; 12 mm, 45 J/cm^2; 15 mm, 30 J/cm^2	7 mm, 50 J/cm^2; 10 mm, 35 J/cm^2; 6 × 10 mm, 50 J/cm^2
Other features	Rapid repetition rate, integrated scanner 10 × 10 cm	Cryogen spray cooling	Cooling tip
Manufacturer	Lumenis, Santa Clara, CA	Candela, Wayland, MA	Cynosure, Chelmsford, MA

Advantages: Deeper penetration, less melanin absorption, effective for reticular veins, no postoperative purpura.

Disadvantages: Less effective for vessels less than 0.5 mm.

Long-Pulsed Alexandrite Laser. To penetrate more deeply to treat larger vessels and to allow for greater thermal diffusion time, the alexandrite laser (Table 22-6) has been modified to allow pulse durations of up to 20 ms. This wavelength theoretically penetrates 2 to 3 mm deep. In two excellent clinical trials, this wavelength at long pulse duration has been effective in the treatment of midsized leg veins. Optimal treatment parameters for long-pulsed alexandrite lasers appear to be 20 J/cm^2, double pulsed at a repetition rate of 1 Hz. In one study, after three treatments at 4-week intervals, subjective grading indicated a 63% reduction in leg telangiectases.[63] Medium-diameter vessels (0.4 to 1 mm) responded best; small vessel diameters responded poorly. This would match the theory that larger vessels have a larger thermal relaxation time, while smaller vessels absorb shorter pulses more readily. The best response in this study of the long-pulsed alexandrite laser was seen with sclerotherapy performed as a supplemental technique, confirming the importance of sclerotherapy for leg veins. In a separate study, patients with skin types I to III and leg veins 0.3 to 2 mm in diameter were treated using an 8 mm spot and fluences of 60 to 80 J/cm^2 with concomitant cryogen cooling. A total of 48 treated sites were available for evaluation 4 weeks after a single treatment; 35% of these sites had cleared by more than 75%, and another 33% had cleared by more than 50%. By week 12, almost two thirds of treated sites were more than 75% clear, and an additional 22% of sites had cleared by more than 50%. The treatment was uncomfortable, and in a third of the treated sites, temporary hyperpigmentation developed. The elliptical spots in the latest pulse lasers have been designed to limit laser damage to the targeted vessel, but even more valuable is the use of cooling to protect the epidermis when high fluences are in use.[64]

Table 22-7 Diode Lasers 800 nm

	FeatherLite	LightSheer
Laser type	Gallium arsenide	AlGaAs semiconductor diode
Pulse duration	50-250 ms	5-30 ms
Pulse rate	5 Hz	0.5 Hz
Spot sizes	2, 5, 2 × 4 mm	Spot 9 × 9 mm
Maximum fluence	60 watts	10-40 J/cm^2
Other features		Chill tip
Manufacturer	LaserLite, Boston, MA	Star Medical Tech, Pleasanton, CA

Advantages: Deeper penetration, less melanin absorption, effective for reticular veins, no postoperative purpura.

Disadvantages: Less effective for vessels ≤0.5 mm.

Diode Lasers. A group of 800 nm diode lasers (5 to 250 ms pulse duration) have been used in the treatment of superficial and deep small- to medium-size leg telangiectases with encouraging results (Table 22-7). The concept behind using near infrared wavelengths lies not only in the deeper penetration of this wavelength and in decreased melanin absorption, but most importantly because there is a tertiary hemoglobin absorption peak at 915 nm. By choosing these longer wavelengths, even moderately deep vessels such as feeder reticular veins can be treated, and by varying the pulse width from a few ms to several hundred ms a variety of different sized vessels can also be targeted.

Diode lasers generate coherent monochromatic light through excitation of small diodes. Two methods of delivery for diode lasers are available. These include fiber-

Table 22-8 Long-Pulsed Nd:YAG (1064 nm) Lasers

	CoolGlide	CoolTouch Varia	Lyra	Vasculight	VeinLase
Laser type	Nd:YAG	Nd:YAG	Nd:YAG	Flashlamp pumped Nd:YAG	Nd:YAG
Pulse duration	10 to 100 ms	300 μs-100 ms	1-50 ms	16 ms	50 ms
Pulse rate	Up to 2 Hz	1 Hz	1-50 Hz	2 Hz	1-25 Hz
Spot sizes	7 and 10 mm	4, 6, and 8 mm	1.5, 3.5, and 10 mm	6 mm	2 mm
Maximum fluence	Up to 200 J/cm^2	Up to 150 J/cm^2	1-400 J/cm^2	150 J/cm^2	100 J/cm^2
Other features	Integrated contact cooling	Integrated cryogen spray cooling before or after laser pulse	Contact cooling, photon recycling, ergonomic handpieces	Synchronized double or triple pulses; total duration up to 50 ms	Fluence not variable
Manufacturer	Altus	CoolTouch Corp.	Laserscope	Lumenis	HGM Medical

Advantages: Poor absorption in skin permits penetration to target relatively deep vessels. Long pulse durations ideally suited for large-caliber vessels. Some devices allow shorter pulse durations to treat smaller vessels.

Disadvantages: Insufficient data to make conclusions on effectiveness.

optic transmission of an 810 nm (gallium-arsenide) beam (LaserLite, Boston, MA) or an overlapping 800 nm diode array with a fixed spot size of 9 × 9 mm (Star Medical, a division of Lumenis). These devices are therefore lightweight, reliable, and portable with a relatively small desktop footprint. Dierickx et al. evaluated an 800 nm diode array laser (Star Medical) on eight areas of leg veins.[65] The laser was utilized at 15 to 40 J/cm^2 given in 5 to 30 ms pulses as double or triple pulses separated by a 2 second delay time. Veins were treated every 4 weeks for three sessions and evaluated 2 months after the last treatment; 100% clearing occurred in 22%, 75% clearing in 42%, and 50% clearing in 32%.

Garden et al.[66] used an 810 nm diode laser with a 750 μm spot size at 40 watts and 50 ms pulses for a total of 453 J/cm^2 of fluence delivered. Twelve patients with 58 vessels 0.2 to 0.5 mm in diameter were treated with three to four passes until vessel spasm occurred. Patients were retreated every 2 to 4 weeks. There was a mean clearance of 60% after 2.2 treatments. Eighteen vessels had more than 70% clearance after three treatments.

Early results of leg vein treatment using a 930 nm pulsed diode laser nearer the 915 nm hemoglobin absorption peak have also been encouraging. The single significant side effect of pain may limit use of this wavelength.

Long-Pulsed Nd:YAG 1064 nm Laser. Long-pulsed 1064 nm lasers have recently been developed in an effort to target deep, relatively large caliber cutaneous vessels (Table 22-8). The primary benefit of this wavelength is deep penetration and the absence of absorption in melanin, thus allowing treatment even in deeply pigmented individuals. However, high energies must be utilized for adequate penetration. Only with sufficient fluence and facilitation of heat dissipation can the posterior wall of a larger diameter (1 to 2 mm) vessel filled with deoxygenated hemoglobin be reached and heated.

The newer pulsed 1064 nm lasers have pulse durations between 1 and 200 ms (Vasculight, Lumenis, Santa Clara, CA; CoolTouch Varia, Laser Aesthetics, Auburn, CA; Lyra, Laserscope, San Jose, CA; CoolGlide, Altus, Burlingame, CA). In general, treatment with long-pulsed 1064 nm laser light is relatively painful, requiring cooling and topical anesthesia. Large-caliber vessels greater than 0.5 mm in diameter respond best. Recent data suggest that by using smaller spots and even higher fluences, even small vessels respond. In our initial studies with the Vasculight, optimal settings were fluences of 80 to 120 J/cm^2 and single pulse durations of 10 to 30 ms.[67] Our most recent data indicate an approximately 75% resolution of leg telangiectases at 3 months using 16 ms pulse durations with fluences of 130 to 140 J/cm^2 [67] (Fig. 22-14). Similar earlier results in fewer patients have been reported at meetings of the ASLMS using the CoolGlide with a 10 mm spot, 100 J/cm^2 at 50 ms; the Lyra at 3 mm spot, 150 J/cm^2 at 50 ms; and the CoolTouch Varia with a 5.5 mm spot, 120 to 130 J/cm^2 at 25 to 50 ms, but none have yet been published.

For patient comfort, epidermal cooling is provided with the CoolGlide and the Lyra using contact cooling provided with the system. The CoolTouch Varia supplies a cryogen spray that can be programmed both before and after the laser pulse. The concept behind ap-

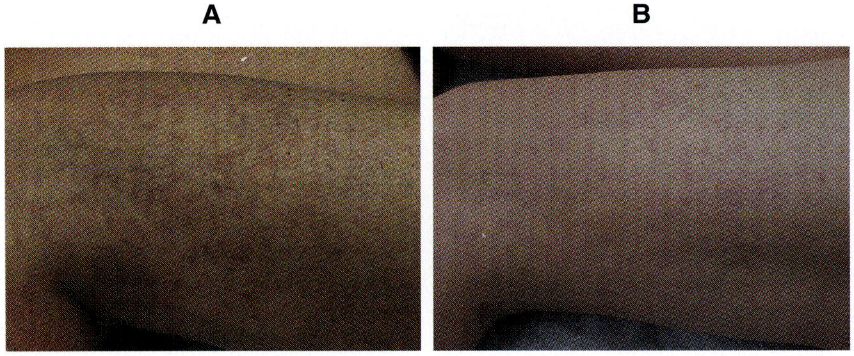

FIG. 22-14
Clinical results with 1064 nm laser. Before **(A)** and 3 months after **(B)** one treatment.

plying the spray after the cooling pulse is for thermal quenching of the heat released from larger vessels following the laser heating. For the Vasculight, cooling may be provided through cold gel or a contact skin chilling device at 1° to 4°C.

Vessels up to 3 mm can be treated with long-pulsed Nd:YAG lasers. Some of the effects of hydrostatic pressure may be addressed by treating these larger vessels, although the pain experienced by patients significantly increases beyond a 2 mm vessel.

Intense Pulsed Light Source

The high intensity pulsed light (IPL) source was developed as a device to treat ectatic blood vessels using noncoherent light emanating from a filtered flashlamp (Photoderm VL, Lumenis, Santa Clara, CA) (Table 22-9). Although Lumenis, Santa Clara, California, is the largest and best known manufacturer of the IPL device, others include Energis Technology, Swansea, United Kingdom, marketing an Energis Elite IPL system for hair removal only, and Danish Dermatologic Development, Hoersholm, Denmark, which markets the Elipse system for hair and vascular indications. The Energis system is a low-output device, with 5 to 19 J/cm^2 output, spot size of 10 × 50 mm, pulse train length of 15 to 40 ms and 4 to 5 pulses per train. There is a fixed delay between pulses of 1.5 ms. By comparison, the Lumenis device is a high-output device with up to 90 J/cm^2 output, spot size of 8 × 35 mm, variable pulse lengths of 2 to 40 ms and infinitely variable delay between pulses of 1 to 1000 ms. Parameters of the DDD system are not published.

Selectivity for IPL is obtained primarily by manipulating pulse durations to match thermal relaxation times of vessels larger than 0.2 mm and use of filters to remove lower wavelengths of visible light. Fluences can be high, with the unit delivering up to 90 J/cm^2. Sequential pulsing of 1 to 12 ms duration separated and synchronized with 1 to 100 ms rest intervals delivers wavelengths of 515 to 1000 nm. It is most commonly used with the 550 and 570 nm filters to deliver primarily the yellow and red wavelengths with some infrared.

Table 22-9 Noncoherent Intense Pulsed Light Source

Name	Photoderm VL, Multilight, Vasculight IPL, Quantum SR
Light source	Flashlamp
Wavelength	515-1200 nm (filtered to cut off lower wavelengths)
Pulse duration	2-25 ms
Pulse rate	Single, double, or triple pulses; variable delay between pulses
Spot sizes	8 × 35 mm and 8 × 15 mm
Energy range	3-90 J/cm^2
Manufacturer	Lumenis, Santa Clara, CA

Advantages: Treats vessels up to 2 mm in diameter. Parameters can be individualized for skin type and vessel size. No postoperative purpura.

Disadvantages: Long, slow learning curve; potential for pigmentary change if used with shorter wavelength filters in darker skin. Slow repetition rate (8 seconds between pulses) only for Multilight and Vasculight IPL. Newer Quantum has recycle time of 1 Hz. Newest Vasculight SR has recycle time of 0.5 Hz.

The therapeutic potential of IPL is explained by the optical properties of hemoglobin as the size and depth of its container (blood vessel) and state of oxygenation are changed (Fig. 22-15). As the size of the vessel increases to 1 mm diameter, it absorbs more than 67% of light even at wavelengths longer than 600 nm. This absorption band is even more significant for blood vessels 2 mm in diameter. Thus a light source above 600 nm should result in deeper penetration of thermal energy, thereby allowing much absorption by deoxyhemoglobin. This is because the absorption coefficient in blood is higher than that of surrounding tissue for wavelengths between 600 and 1000 nm.

A device that produces a noncoherent light as a continuous spectrum longer than 550 nm was thought to have multiple advantages over a single-wavelength laser system. These include absorption by both oxygenated and deoxygenated hemoglobin and by larger blood vessels located deeper in the dermis being affected. In reality, the primary advantage has been

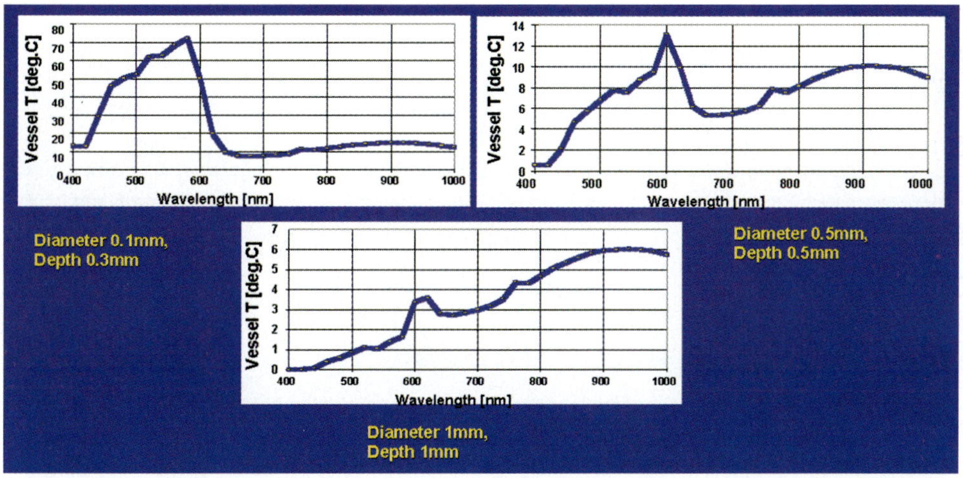

FIG. 22-15 Optical properties of hemoglobin as the size and depth of its container (blood vessel) and state of oxygenation are changed. (Courtesy Lumenis, Santa Clara, CA.)

larger spot size and relatively low incidence of purpura on facial telangiectasia.

Utilizing these theoretical considerations, IPL emitting in the 515 to 1000 nm range was used at varying energy fluences (5 to 90 J/cm^2) and various pulse durations (2 to 12 ms) to treat venulectasia 0.4 to 2 mm in diameter. Clinical trials using various parameters with the IPL, including multiple pulses of variable duration, demonstrated efficacy ranging up to 90% clearance in vessels less than 0.2 mm in diameter, 80% in vessels from 0.2 to 0.5 mm, and 80% in vessels 0.5 to 1 mm in diameter.[68] Others have reported good results, but few have confirmed the 90% clearance initially reported,[69,70] although Schroeter reported that in 73.6% of patients there was an immediate clearing, and in 84.3% a clearing after 1 month in leg telangiectases up to 1 mm in diameter.[71]

The incidence of adverse sequelae was minimal, with hypopigmentation occurring in 1% to 3% of patients, resolving within 4 to 6 months. Tanned or darkly pigmented Fitzpatrick type III patients were likely to develop hypopigmentation and hyperpigmentation in addition to blistering and superficial erosions. These all cleared over a few months. Treatment parameters that were found to be most successful ranged from a single pulse of 22 J/cm^2 in 3 ms for vessels less than 0.2 mm or a double pulse of 35 to 40 J/cm^2 given in 2.4 and 4 ms with a 10 ms delay. Vessels between 0.2 and 0.5 mm were treated with the same double pulse parameters or with a 3 to 6 ms pulse at 35 to 45 J/cm^2 with a 20 ms delay time.

More recently, increased efficacy has been reported by increasing the pulse durations to a maximum of 12 ms in two consecutive pulses separated by a 20 to 30 ms delay with a 570 to 590 nm cutoff filter and fluences of 70 J/cm^2. The development of the short pulse/long pulse protocol utilizing 2.4 to 3 ms and 7 ms pulses separated by a 10 to 20 ms delay employing the 570 nm filter has yielded the best results for leg veins using the IPL device. Response rates of 74% in two treatments with an 8% incidence of temporary hypopigmentation or hyperpigmentation has been reported.[72] By combining a shorter pulse (2.4 to 3 ms) with a longer pulse (7 to 10 ms), it is theoretically possible to ablate smaller and larger vessels overlying one another in the dermis. The shorter pulses theoretically are absorbed more selectively by smaller, more superficial vessels, while the longer pulses are absorbed by the larger-diameter vessels. Additionally, new contact epidermal cooling devices improve treatment results by allowing larger fluences with less risk to the epidermis (Fig. 22-16).

The Role of Cooling

The concept of cooling the skin in an effort to protect the epidermis during laser treatment of dermal targets was first studied by Gilchrest[73] with the use of ice prior to argon laser treatment of port wine stains. There has been a recent resurgence of interest in skin cooling during skin laser therapy in an effort not only to cool and protect the epidermis and to prevent other collateral dermal damage but also to reduce the discomfort associated with treatment. Because high fluences are required to adequately damage leg veins, cooling appears to be especially important in their treatment in an effort to limit unwanted collateral injury. Several approaches have been taken, including water-cooled chambers applied directly to the skin, through which the laser beam is directed (e.g., Chess Chamber, VersaPulse chill tip, Lumenis; Photoderm chiller, Lumenis), cooling coupling gels, and refrigerated spray cooling devices (e.g., Dynamic cooling device, Candela; cryogen spray, CoolTouch). Preliminary results suggest that cooling helps to spare epidermal damage, allowing use of higher fluences, thus yielding more damage of the targeted vessels, with a greater degree of clearing per treatment.[47,74]

A B

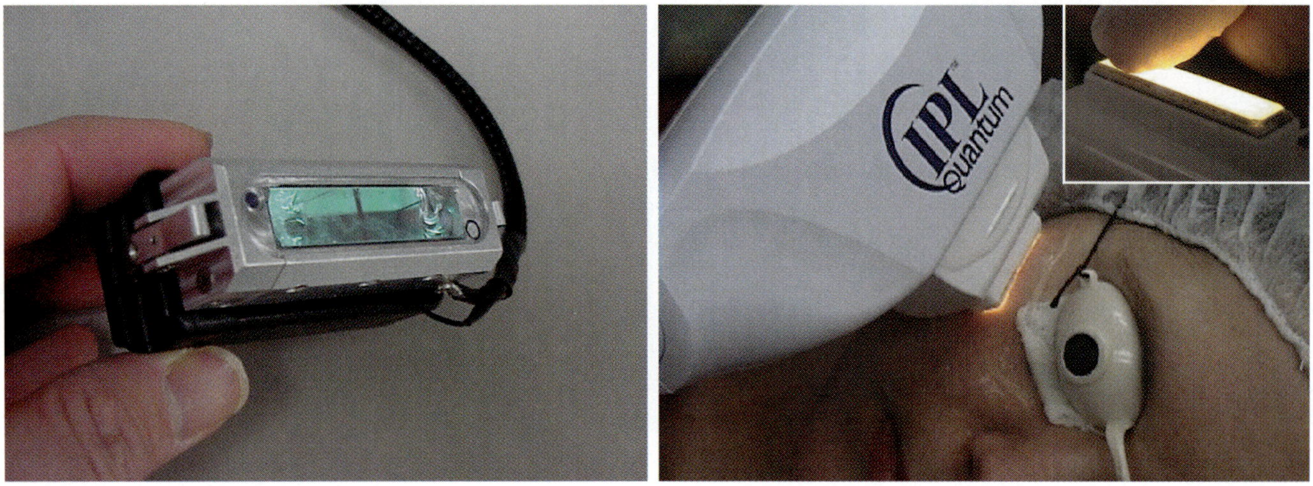

FIG. 22-16
A, Epidermal contact cooling device used with intense pulsed light source (IPL) surrounds the crystal. **B,** New lightweight IPL head with integrated cooling; ice forming on crystal shown in the inset.

Technique: Laser Treatment of Leg Veins

Technique for Laser (1064 nm) Direct Contact Method. It is critical to wear protective glasses when using the 1064 nm wavelength, as it is one of the most penetrating and damaging to the eyes. Treatment with long-pulsed 1064 nm lasers is quite painful. Cooling and either topical anesthesia or local anesthesia are necessary when treating all but the smallest veins. Many of the long-pulsed 1064 nm devices available are based on a fiber delivery system with contact or dynamic cooling. The Vasculight (Lumenis, Santa Clara, CA) may be used without a cooling device and its crystal can be placed directly on the skin (Fig. 22-17). For the contact cooling devices, water-based gel is placed directly on the skin and the crystal or spacing device is held directly against the skin. The CoolGlide (Altus, Burlingame, CA) has a small chamber of cooled water that recirculates in the tip of the handpiece, cooling the skin to just above freezing. The Lyra (Laserscope, San Jose, CA) uses ergonomically designed handpiece attachments that cool the skin to 1.5°C.

Minimal pressure is placed against the skin, since the target may be compressed with excessive hand pressure. In some cases in which a larger reticular vein is targeted for 1064 nm laser, slight pressure may be used to minimize the total diameter of the vein to allow greater penetration and less total heat accumulation by virtue of less hemoglobin heated. This may make the treatment slightly less painful. During treatment of small-caliber vessels, immediate disappearance is often

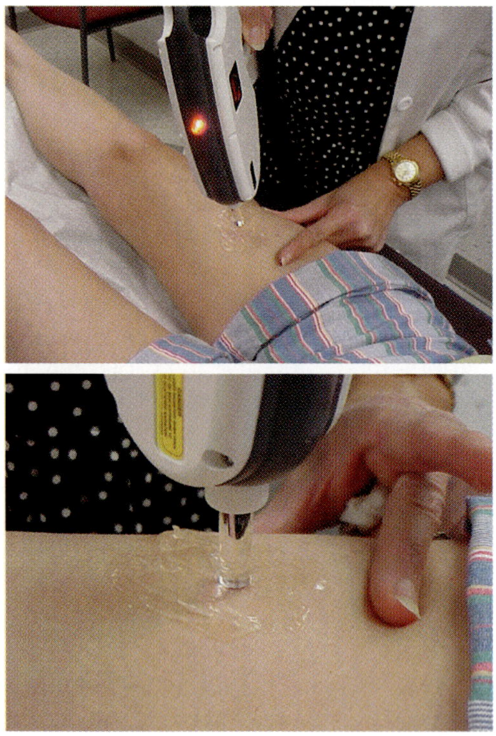

A

B

FIG. 22-17
A, Use of Vasculight with gel directly on the skin. **B,** Close up.

A

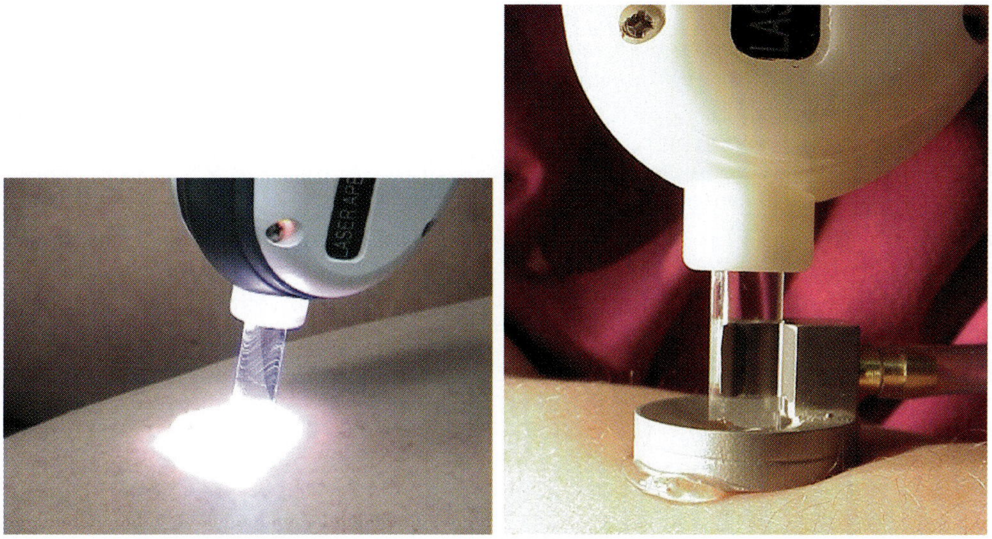

B

FIG. 22-18
A, Off skin technique of Vasculight. Tip is kept 1 to 2 cm away from skin, but gel on skin surface acts as a heat sink. **B,** Cooling collar may be used around Vasculight crystal.

seen, but during treatment of larger-caliber vessels, there is often no visible change in the treated vessel.

Off Skin Technique. Some of the devices allow a defocused beam or divergent collimated beam to be used. A small layer of gel is placed on the skin and the crystal or fiber delivering the laser energy is held 1 to 3 cm off the skin (Fig. 22-18). This causes a sudden change in interface from air to water, permits a larger spot size, causes more lateral spread of thermal energy, and causes some of the smaller vessels (0.3 to 0.5 mm) to visibly contract. Increased visualization of the treatment area is the primary advantage; greater heat accumulation toward the skin surface, the main disadvantage.

Dynamic Cooling Technique. Some devices allow an integrated cryogen spray to be timed and synchronized with the laser pulse. For smaller vessels, the cryogen is typically sprayed before the laser pulse, but for larger leg veins, CoolTouch, Auburn, California, introduced the concept of Thermal Quenching. By synchronizing the cryogen spray immediately after the laser pulse, damage from dissipated heat from larger vessels is reduced. It is thus possible to have a dynamic cooling spray both before and after the laser pulse for increased patient comfort and increased safety of the epidermis. Higher fluences can thus be delivered. The main advantage of the dynamic cooling lasers for leg veins is excellent visibility during treatment; the main disadvantage is accumulated cold injury should too many pulses be delivered in the identical spot (Fig. 22-19). The key to safety and increased patient comfort is to allow each pulse to be separated by at least 2 to 3 mm and to keep the cumulative cryogen time to less than 60 ms.

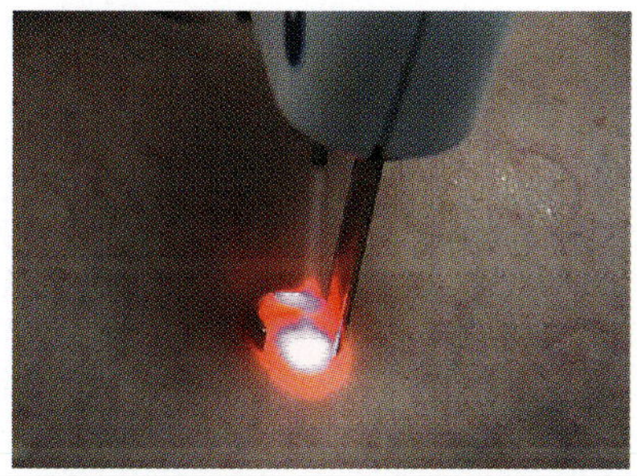

FIG. 22-19
Dynamic spray cooling with the CoolTouch Varia using 6 mm spot size. No gel is required.

IPL Technique. A thick layer of gel must be placed onto the crystal and absolutely no pressure applied as the crystal is placed over the target area, floating the crystal in gel. Compressing this 2 to 3 mm layer of gel against the skin will result in crystal placement too close to the skin, thus greatly increasing the risks of epidermal injury. Plastic spacers are available to increase the uniformity of distance of crystal and thickness of gel, although most users simply float the crystal, holding the weight of the IPL head in their hands. Newer head designs have taken this into account; they have become much more lightweight and have incorporated integral Peltier cooling devices to keep the crystals at 1°C (Quantum SR, Quantum HR, Lumenis, Santa

Clara, CA) (see Fig. 22-16*B*). For skin types I to untanned III with very fine red telangiectases, acceptable results can usually be obtained; when large areas are involved, the large spot size of the IPL allows rapid treatment. To minimize rectangular footprinting, a 10% overlap of pulse placement is used, or alternatively a second pass oriented 90 degrees from the original direction may be made.

Attaching a cooling device that surrounds the crystal has been shown to produce better results with fewer side effects.[75] Cooling is maintained by circulating water at 1°C through the metal collar around the crystal. When this contact-cooling device is utilized, only a small layer of water-based gel is placed on the cooling collar of the treatment crystal. This remains in contact for at least 10 seconds to chill down to the temperature of the circulating water set at 1° to 4°C. With absolutely minimal pressure, the cooling device with the crystal is placed directly onto the skin overlying the targeted area. No pressure is applied, as the target vessels may shut with compression. No EMLA cream is used before treatment, as there is a high incidence of vasoconstriction produced by the prilocaine component of EMLA. ELA-Max 4% lidocaine (Ferndale Labs, Ferndale, MI) is a better choice but is usually not necessary with cooling.

Indications for Laser and Leg Vein Treatment

While sclerotherapy and ambulatory phlebectomy remain the mainstay of treatment for varicose veins, reticular veins, and telangiectases, lasers certainly play a role. In general, treatment with lasers and light sources is more expensive, less predictable, and associated with more variable responses, and the risk of side effects is at least as high as with sclerotherapy. Candidates suitable for laser or light source treatment are needle phobic, have failed sclerotherapy, or have developed untoward side effects from sclerotherapy. Others suited for laser treatment are fair skinned individuals who either have vessels smaller than the caliber of a 30-gauge needle or have foot and ankle vessels, which are notoriously difficult to treat with sclerotherapy.

Clearing rates with sclerotherapy approximate 90%.[2,21] Experience gained over time greatly enhances results. Every patient should be approached with knowledge of venous anatomy and principles of reflux, thorough informed consent, photographic documentation, and familiarity with different sclerosing solution volumes and concentrations, office surgical techniques, and when laser or light therapy may be warranted. Treatment based on this foundation is highly likely to be successful.

Since sclerotherapy treatment is highly effective and inexpensive, do lasers and light sources have a role in the treatment of leg telangiectasia? A rational approach to the treatment of leg vein follows. Varicosities, incompetent perforators, and reticular veins must first be treated using appropriate surgical means or sclerotherapy where indicated. This should be followed by superficial vessel sclerotherapy until only vessels smaller than the diameter of a 30-gauge needle and vessels resistant to sclerotherapy remain. It is these vessels that respond best to pulsed lasers and light sources, along with telangiectatic matting caused by sclerotherapy. There are instances where laser and light source treatments should be considered prior to superficial sclerotherapy; patients who are fearful of needles or who do not tolerate sclerotherapy, patients whose vessels fail to respond to sclerotherapy, or who are prone to telangiectatic matting. Further carefully monitored, controlled studies are essential to better define the role of each of the available lasers and light sources in the treatment of leg telangiectasia.

REFERENCES

1. Engel A, Johnson ML, Haynes SG. Health effects of sunlight exposure in the United States: results from the first national health and nutrition examination survey, 1971-1974. Arch Dermatol 1988; 124:72-79.
2. Weiss RA, Weiss MA. Resolution of pain associated with varicose and telangiectatic leg veins after compression sclerotherapy. J Dermatol Surg Oncol 1990; 16:333-336.
3. Goldman MP, Bennett RG. Treatment of telangiectasia: a review. J Am Acad Dermatol 1987; 17:167-182.
4. Duffy DM. Small vessel sclerotherapy: an overview. Adv Dermatol 1988; 3:221-242.
5. Weiss RA, Feied CF, Weiss MA. Vein Diagnosis and Treatment: A Comprehensive Approach. New York: McGraw-Hill, 2001.
6. Thibault P, Bray A, Wlodarczyk J, Lewis W. Cosmetic leg veins: evaluation using duplex venous imaging. J Dermatol Surg Oncol 1990; 16:612-618.
7. Somjen GM, Ziegenbein R, Johnston AH, Royle JP. Anatomical examination of leg telangiectases with duplex scanning [see comments]. J Dermatol Surg Oncol 1993; 19:940-945.
8. Weiss RA, Weiss MA. Doppler ultrasound findings in reticular veins of the thigh: subdermic lateral venous system and implications for sclerotherapy. J Dermatol Surg Oncol 1993; 19:947-951.
9. Weiss RA, Goldman MP. Advances in sclerotherapy. Dermatol Clin 1995; 13:431-445.
10. Goldman MP, Weiss RA, Bergan JJ. Diagnosis and treatment of varicose veins—a review [review]. J Am Acad Dermatol 1994; 31(3:Part 1):393-413.
11. Partsch H. Primary Varikose der Vena Saphena Magna und Parva. In: Kriessman A, Bollinger A, Keller H, eds. Praxis der Doppler Sonographie. Stuttgart: Thieme, 1982:101-103.
12. Weiss RA. Evaluation of the venous system by Doppler ultrasound and photoplethysmography or light reflection rheography before sclerotherapy. Semin Dermatol 1993; 12:78-87.
13. Rosfors S. Venous photoplethysmography: relationship between transducer position and regional distribution of venous insufficiency. J Vasc Surg 1990; 11:436-440.
14. Blazek V, Schmitt HJ, Schultz-Ehrenburg U, Kerner J. Digitale Photoplethysmographie (D-PPG) für die Beinvenendiagnostik: medizinisch-technische Grundlagen. Phlebol Proktol 1989; 18: 91-97.
15. Weiss RA, Weiss MA. Sclerotherapy. In: Wheeland RG, ed. Cutaneous Surgery. Philadelphia: WB Saunders, 1994:951-981.

16. Weiss RA, Weiss MA. Painful telangiectasias: diagnosis and treatment. In: Bergan JJ, Weiss RA, Goldman MP, eds. Varicose Veins and Telangiectasias: Diagnosis and Treatment. 2nd ed. St. Louis: Quality Medical Publishing, 1999:389-406.
17. Bodian EL. Sclerotherapy: a personal appraisal. J Dermatol Surg Oncol 1989; 15:156-161.
18. Bodian EL. Techniques of sclerotherapy for sunburst venous blemishes. J Dermatol Surg Oncol 1985; 11:696-704.
19. Goldman PM. Sclerotherapy for superficial venules and telangiectasias of the lower extremities. Dermatol Clin 1987; 5:369-379.
20. Sadick NS. Sclerotherapy of varicose and telangiectatic leg veins. Minimal sclerosant concentration of hypertonic saline and its relationship to vessel diameter [see comments]. J Dermatol Surg Oncol 1991; 17:65-70.
21. Goldman PM. Polidocanol (aethoxysklerol) for sclerotherapy of superficial venules and telangiectasias. J Dermatol Surg Oncol 1989; 15:204-209.
22. Struckmann J, et al. Venous muscle pump improvement by low compression elastic stockings. Phlebologie 1986; 1:97-103.
23. Fegan WG. Continuous compression technique of injecting varicose veins. Lancet 1963; 2:109-112.
24. Hobbs JT. Surgery and sclerotherapy in the treatment of varicose veins: a random trial. Arch Surg 1974; 109:793-796.
25. Doran FSA, White M. A clinical trial designed to discover if the primary treatment of varicose veins should be by Fegan's method or by operation. Br J Surg 1975; 62:72-76.
26. Batch AJ, Wickremesinghe SS, Gannon ME, Dormandy JA. Randomised trial of bandaging after sclerotherapy for varicose veins. Br Med J 1980; 281:423-426.
27. Fraser IA, Perry EP, Hatton M, Watkin DF. Prolonged bandaging is not required following sclerotherapy of varicose veins. Br J Surg 1985; 72:488-490.
28. Weiss RA, Sadick NS, Goldman MP, Weiss MA. Post-sclerotherapy compression: controlled comparative study of duration of compression and its effects on clinical outcome. Dermatol Surg 1999; 25:105-108.
29. Weiss RA, Weiss MA. Incidence of side effects in the treatment of telangiectasias by compression sclerotherapy: hypertonic saline vs. polidocanol. J Dermatol Surg Oncol 1990; 16:800-804.
30. Davis LT, Duffy DM. Determination of incidence and risk factors for postsclerotherapy telangiectatic matting of the lower extremity: a retrospective analysis. J Dermatol Surg Oncol 1990; 16:327-330.
31. Norris MJ, Carlin MC, Ratz JL. Treatment of essential telangiectasia: effects of increasing concentrations of polidocanol. J Am Acad Dermatol 1989; 20:683-689.
32. Ouvry P, Davy A. Le traitement sclerosant des telangiectasies des membres inferieurs. Phlebologie 1982; 35:349-355.
33. Puissegur Lupo ML. Sclerotherapy: review of results and complications in 200 patients. J Dermatol Surg Oncol 1989; 15:214-219.
34. Eaglstein W. Inadvertent intracutaneous injection with hypertonic saline (23.4%) in two patients without complication. J Dermatol Surg Oncol 1990; 16:878-879.
35. Ramelet AA. La phlebectomie ambulatoire selon Mueller: technique, avantages, desavantages. J Mal Vasc 1991; 16:119-122.
36. Ramelet AA. Le traitement des telangiectasies: indications de la phlebectomie selon Muller. Phlebologie 1995; 47:377-381.
37. Muller R. Ambulatory phlebectomy. Ther Umsch 1992; 49:447-450.
38. Muller R. Traitement des varices par la phlebectomie ambulatoire. Bull Soc Franc Phlebologie 1966; 19:277-279.
39. Ramelet AA. Muller phlebectomy: a new phlebectomy hook. J Dermatol Surg Oncol 1991; 17:814-816.
40. Smithies DJ, Butler PH. Modelling the distribution of laser light in port-wine stains with the Monte Carlo method. Phys Med Biol 1995; 40:701-731.
41. Dierickx CC, Casparian JM, Venugopalan V, et al. Thermal relaxation of port-wine stain vessels probed in vivo: the need for 1-10 millisecond laser pulse treatment. J Invest Dermatol 1995; 105: 709-714.
42. Apfelberg DB, Smith T, Maser MR, et al. Study of three laser systems for treatment of superficial varicosities of the lower extremity. Lasers Surg Med 1987; 7:219-223.
43. Landthaler M, Haina D, Waidelich W, Braun-Falco O. Laser therapy of venous lakes (Bean-Walsh) and telangiectasias. Plast Reconstr Surg 1984; 73:78-83.
44. Apfelberg DB, Maser MR, Lash H, et al. Use of the argon and carbon dioxide lasers for treatment of superficial venous varicosities of the lower extremity. Lasers Surg Med 1984; 4:221-231.
45. Dixon JA, Rotering RH, Huether SE. Patient's evaluation of argon laser therapy of port-wine stain, decorative tattoos, and essential telangiectasia. Lasers Surg Med 1984; 4:181-184.
46. Corcos L, Longo L. Classification and treatment of telangiectases of the lower limbs. Laser 1988; 1:22-27.
47. Chess C, Chess Q. Cool laser optics treatment of large telangiectasia of the lower extremities. J Dermatol Surg Oncol 1993; 19:74-80.
48. Tan OT, Kerschmann R, Parrish JA. Effect of skin temperature on selective vascular injury caused by pulsed laser irradiation. J Invest Dermatol 1985; 85:441-444.
49. Apfelberg DB, Smith T, Maser MR, et al. Study of three laser systems for treatment of superficial varicosities of the lower extremity. Lasers Surg Med 1987; 7:219.
50. Keller GS. KTP laser offers advances in minimally invasive plastic surgery. Clin Laser Mon 1992; 10:141-144.
51. West TB, Alster TS. Comparison of the long-pulse dye (590-595 nm) and KTP (532 nm) lasers in the treatment of facial and leg telangiectasias. Dermatol Surg 1998; 24:221-226.
52. Adrian RM. Treatment of leg telangiectasias using a long-pulse frequency-doubled neodymium:YAG laser at 532 nm. Dermatol Surg 1998; 24:19-23.
53. Garden JM, Tan OT, Kerschmann R, et al. Effect of dye laser pulse duration on selective cutaneous vascular injury. J Invest Dermatol 1986; 87:653-657.
54. Polla LL, Tan OT, Garden JM, Parrish JA. Tunable pulsed dye laser for the treatment of benign cutaneous vascular ectasia. Dermatologica 1987; 174:11-17.
55. Goldman MP, Martin DE, Fitzpatrick RE, Ruiz-Esparza J. Pulsed dye laser treatment of telangiectases with and without subtherapeutic sclerotherapy: clinical and histologic examination in the rabbit ear vein model. J Am Acad Dermatol 1990; 23:23-30.
56. Goldman MP, Fitzpatrick RE. Pulsed-dye laser treatment of leg telangiectasia: with and without simultaneous sclerotherapy. J Dermatol Surg Oncol 1990; 16:338-344.
57. Hsia J, Lowery JA, Zelickson B. Treatment of leg telangiectasia using a long-pulse dye laser at 595 nm. Lasers Surg Med 1997; 20:1-5.
58. Garden JM, Backus AD. Treatment of leg veins with high energy pulsed dye laser. Lasers Surg Med 1996; 8:34.
59. Alora MB, Herd RH, Szabo E. Comparison of the 595 nm long pulse (1.5 ms) and the ultra-long pulse (4 ms) lasers in the treatment of leg veins. [Abstract]. Lasers Surg Med Suppl 1998; 10:38.
60. Grossman MC, Bernstein LJ, Kauvar AB, et al. Treatment of leg veins with a long pulse tunable dye laser. Lasers Surg Med Suppl 1996; 8:35.
61. Lee PK, Lask G. Treatment of leg veins by long pulsed dye laser (sclerolaser). Lasers Surg Med Suppl 1997; 9:40.
62. Reichert D. Evaluation of the long-pulse dye laser for the treatment of leg telangiectasias. Dermatol Surg 1998; 24:737-740.
63. McDaniel DH, Ash K, Lord J, et al. Laser therapy of spider leg veins: clinical evaluation of a new long pulsed alexandrite laser. Dermatol Surg 1999; 25:52-58.
64. Kauvar AN, Lou WW. Pulsed alexandrite laser for the treatment of leg telangiectasia and reticular veins. Arch Dermatol 2000; 136:1371-1375.

65. Dierickx CC, Duque V, Anderson RR. Treatment of leg telangiectasia by a pulsed, infrared laser system. Lasers Surg Med Suppl 1998; 10:40.
66. Garden JM, Bakus AD, Miller ID. Diode laser treatment of leg veins. Lasers Surg Med Suppl 1998; 10:38.
67. Weiss RA, Weiss MA. Early clinical results with a multiple synchronized pulse 1064 nm laser for leg telangiectasias and reticular veins. Dermatol Surg 1999; 25:399-402.
68. Goldman MP, Eckhouse S. Photothermal sclerosis of leg veins. ESC Medical Systems, LTD Photoderm VL Cooperative Study Group [see comments]. Dermatol Surg 1996; 22:323-330.
69. Schroeter C, Wilder D, Reineke T, et al. Clinical significance of an intense, pulsed light source on leg telangiectasias of up to 1 mm diameter. Eur J Dermatol 1997; 7:38-42.
70. Raulin C, Weiss RA, Schonermark MP. Treatment of essential telangiectasias with an intense pulsed light source (Photoderm VL). Dermatol Surg 1997; 23:941-945.
71. Schroeter CA, Neumann HA. An intense light source: the Photoderm VL-flashlamp as a new treatment possibility for vascular skin lesions. Dermatol Surg 1998; 24:743-748.
72. Weiss RA, Weiss MA, Marwaha S, Harrington AC. Non-coherent filtered flashlamp intense pulsed light source for leg telangiectasias: long pulse durations for improved results. Lasers Surg Med Suppl 1998; 10:40.
73. Gilchrest BA, Rosen S, Noe JM. Chilling port wine stains improves the response to argon laser therapy. Plast Reconstr Surg 1982; 69:278-283.
74. Waldorf HA, Alster TS, McMillan K, et al. Effect of dynamic cooling on 585-nm pulsed dye laser treatment of port-wine stain birthmarks [see comments]. Dermatol Surg 1997; 23:657-662.
75. Weiss RA, Sadick NS. Epidermal cooling crystal collar device for improved results and reduced side effects on leg telangiectasias using intense pulsed light. Dermatol Surg 2000; 26:1015-1018.

CHAPTER 23

Scar Management: Keloid, Hypertrophic, Atrophic, and Acne Scars

SANDY S. TSAO
JEFFREY S. DOVER
KENNETH A. ARNDT
MICHAEL S. KAMINER

SECTION ONE

History and Scientific Review

The wound reparative process results in a spectrum of scar formation ranging from nearly scarless healing to excessive fibrosis or atrophy. Scars can be divided into two basic categories: (1) keloidal and hypertrophic scars and (2) atrophic scars. A third scar type—a flat scar—is characterized by what is considered the normal healing process. The options for treating flat scars are numerous, frequently involving surgical revision. This is often not sought, as the flat scar in most cases becomes imperceptible with time. However, when the wound healing process produces a raised or atrophic scar, management can be modified and improvements made to the appearance of the scar through a variety of techniques. Treatment of these scars is driven in large part by the underlying anatomy and the cause of the defect.

Keloids and hypertrophic scars represent examples of exuberant scarring. Hypertrophic scars are confined to the original injury and increase in size by pushing outward and not by invasion.[1] Keloids are characterized by scar tissue that extends beyond the confines of the original wound. Acne scars and pox scars represent examples of localized, exaggerated dermal and subcutaneous atrophic scarring.

KELOIDS AND HYPERTROPHIC SCARS

Background and History

The earliest recognized description of keloids was written around 1700 BC in the Smith Papyrus.[2] As early as the tenth century the Yorubas, a West Nigerian tribe, performed ritual facial markings and earlobe perforations early in childhood to avoid what had been observed as an increased tendency to form keloids during adolescence. They also recorded the tendency of keloid formation to occur within families. Jean Louis Alibert is credited as being the first to describe cicatricial tumors in 1802. He coined the term *cheloides* to describe a keloid's tendency toward lateral growth as well as their claw-like extension into normal tissue. He observed keloids arising both spontaneously and after trauma. He noted a distinction between keloids and scars that remained within the confines of the initial trauma, currently referred to as hypertrophic scars.[3] Keloids are unique to humans. Despite an increased understanding of wound healing, the exact cause, clinical behavior, and optimal treatment of keloids and hypertrophic scars remain a challenge (Box 23-1).

The incidence of hypertrophic scars and keloids varies with age, race, sex, anatomic location, and the inciting trauma. Keloids are uncommon at the extremes of life (childhood and late adulthood). Patients with the highest incidence of keloid development are between the ages of 10 and 30 years.[4] The exact prevalence of hypertrophic scars and keloids is unknown; the male-to-female ratio is approximately 1:1. Studies that report a higher female incidence may reflect a greater cosmetic concern and more frequent earlobe piercing. Blacks and Asians are affected more often than Caucasians, with comparable incidence ratios between 5:1 and 15:1.[4] An incidence of between 4.5% and 16% in a predominantly black and Hispanic population has been reported.[5]

Keloids demonstrate a regional predilection.[6] The most susceptible regions of the body include the presternal area, anterior chest, back, shoulder, and posterior neck. The ears, abdomen and beard area are moderately susceptible to keloid formation. Keloids rarely develop on the palms, soles, mucous membranes, scalp, or genitalia. Hypertrophic scars do not appear to have a regional predisposition.

The appearance of a keloid or hypertrophic scar is often cosmetically unappealing to the affected individual. The time lag between injury and scar formation is variable, though they tend to form within the first year after the inciting skin wound.[7] They range from firm papules, nodules or plaques with telangiectases and a pearly atrophic surface to soft, doughy, pendulous nodules. Their color is variable, ranging from mildly erythematous to vivid purple. Older lesions may become hypopigmented. Keloids tend to have a thick, ropelike surface, whereas hypertrophic scars tend to have a smoother surface. Hypertrophic scars remain within the original boundaries of the injury, whereas keloids extend beyond the original site of trauma. Associated pruritus, dysesthesia, and pain, as well as restricted range of motion and contracture formation may be observed with both keloids and hypertrophic scars but tend to be more prevalent with keloids.

Hypertrophic scars differ from keloids in their tendency to regress over time. Within 6 to 12 months of scar onset the erythema begins to subside, with incremental softening and bulk reduction occurring later.[8] Keloids tend to persist over time and may continue to enlarge.

Keloids are characterized histologically by the haphazard deposition of thick, hyalinized eosinophilic collagen bundles within the dermis, forming nodules that contain an abundance of eosinophils, mast cells, plasma cells, and lymphocytes.[9,10] These nodules are encircled by numerous small vessels. Partial to full occlusion of these microvessels as a result of excessive endothelial cell proliferation is observed.[11] There are few vessels found within the nodules.

Hypertrophic scars also demonstrate increased collagen bundles histologically. The collagen still lies parallel to the epithelial surface, as observed with normal skin, but is flatter and less clearly demarcated. In hypertrophic scars, nodules are not present and the collagen lacks the hyalinized appearance noted with keloids.[9] More fibroblasts are present and microvasculature occlusion is noted. Foreign body reactions are frequently detected.

BOX 23-1 Clinical Features Distinguishing Hypertrophic Scars and Keloids

Hypertrophic Scars
- Confined to original wound
- Spontaneous regression
- Onset within 3 months of injury
- Occur at any anatomic site
- Unclear familial association
- Improved with surgery

Keloids
- Extend beyond original wound
- Persistent over time
- Onset months to years after injury
- High-risk anatomic sites
- Familial tendency observed
- May worsen after surgery

Basic Science

Hypertrophic scars and keloids may develop even after the most minor of skin wounds such as insect bites, lacerations, tattoos, vaccinations, burns, and blunt trauma. Diseases inciting inflammation (e.g., folliculitis, viral infections such as varicella zoster or herpes simplex) or follicular occlusion (e.g., hidradenitis suppurativa, acne cyst formation) may also lead to scar formation (Box 23-2). Although some individuals report spontaneous keloid formation, it may be that the affected individual has forgotten the initial skin injury that incited the keloid development. The spontaneous development of multiple keloids has been recognized in syndromes such as Rubenstein-Taybi,[12] progeria, Ehlers-Danlos, pachydermoperiostosis, osteogenesis imperfecta, and trichorhinophalangeal syndrome.

A family history of keloids is frequently elicited.[13] Both autosomal recessive[14] and autosomal dominant[15] patterns of inheritance have been reported. A predisposition for keloid formation has been noted in individuals with human leukocyte antigens (HLA) B14, BW16,[16-18] and blood type A.[19]

Other factors such as local tissue and wound tension also influence healing. A decreased incidence of keloid formation has been noted when wounds are oriented along lines of relaxed skin tension. If a keloid is removed and grafted into an area with minimal tension, the scar may undergo spontaneous flattening.

A predisposition to keloid formation has been associated with abnormal function of the hypothalamus, thyroid, and parathyroid glands. One unifying feature is thought to be an increase in melanin-synthesizing hormone (MSH). This is supported by the higher incidence of keloids in darker-skinned individuals, a greater distribution of melanocytes present in the anatomic sites of the body predisposed to keloid formation, and the increased incidence of keloid formation at puberty and during pregnancy, when levels of MSH are elevated.

BOX 23-2 Etiologic Factors in Keloid and Hypertrophic Scar Formation

- Trauma
- Follicular occlusion
- Infection
- Anatomic location
- Genetic predisposition
- Wound tension
- Endocrine factors
- Foreign body reaction

The basis for keloid and hypertrophic scar formation is not fully understood (Box 23-3). Heterogeneous fibroblast populations with different growth potentials exist within all wounds at the same time.[20] Keloid-derived fibroblasts may be self-selected by the hypoxic environment known to exist.[21] Increased levels of histamine[22] and lactate, decreased pH, and decreased nitric oxide synthase and nitric oxide production[23] contribute to the stressed environment. Keloid-derived fibroblasts produce increased amounts of collagen per cell in comparison to normal fibroblasts and appear to function autonomously.[24] Normal[25] and elevated levels of types I[26] and III collagen synthesis have been reported. Collagen synthesis is approximately 20 times greater in keloids than in normal skin.[27] This rate approaches normal scar levels within 2 to 3 years after the initial injury. Despite this increased activity, the growth characteristics of keloid fibroblasts are similar to normal fibroblasts.[28] Elevated levels of chondroitin 4-sulfate,[29] which acts to make collagen fibers resistant to collagenase degradation, have been detected within keloids. Elevated levels of collagenase inhibitors such as α_1-antitrypsin and α_2-macroglobulin[30] are also present.

Hypertrophic scar-derived fibroblasts display a similar, albeit less exuberant, elevation in collagen production in vitro. However, their response to metabolic modulators is similar to normal fibroblasts.[31]

Although both an increased collagen synthesis and turnover are observed within keloids[32] and hypertrophic scars, ultimately a disproportionate deposition of collagen is noted. A tenfold increase in collagenase production has been detected.

An immunological basis for keloid and hypertrophic scar formation has also been addressed. Elevated levels of IgG,[33] IgM, and C3[34] have been measured and fibroblast antinuclear antibodies have been detected.[35] The significance of these findings is not understood. The incidence of keloids has been directly correlated with elevated serum IgE levels. IgE mediates the release of histamine from mast cells and histamine levels are also elevated in keloids. As histamine enhances collagen synthesis[36] and inhibits lysyl oxidase, which is responsible for collagen cross-linking, this contributes to the increased amount of soluble collagen in keloids.[37]

Growth factor levels are also altered in keloid and hypertrophic scar formation. Increased transforming growth factor (TGF)-β gene expression has been detected. TGF-β induces collagen, fibronectin, and proteoglycan synthesis[38] while reducing collagenase production and increasing collagenase inhibitor production.[39] Keloid and hypertrophic scar fibroblasts demonstrate an enhanced sensitivity to TGF-β.[40] Interleukin-1, insulin-like growth factor-1,[41] platelet-derived growth factor,[42] and tumor necrosis factor (TNF), all of which increase fibroblast collagen synthesis, are also elevated in keloids.

BOX 23-3 Biochemical Alterations Detected in Hypertrophic Scar and Keloid Formation

- Increased collagen synthesis
  - Increased histamine levels
  - Increased lactate levels
  - Decreased nitric oxide and nitric oxide synthetase
  - Increased type I and III collagen
  - Increased chondroitin 4-sulfate
  - Increased proline hydroxylase
  - Increased α_1-antitrypsin and β_2-macroglobulin
- Increased collagenase production
- Altered growth factor production
  - Increased transforming growth factor-β
  - Increased interleukin-1
  - Increased platelet-derived growth factor, insulin-like growth factor
  - Increased tumor necrosis factor

Clinical Studies

The management of keloids and hypertrophic scars has proven challenging. Numerous treatment modalities have been employed with varying degrees of success. The failure to distinguish between keloids and hypertrophic scars has complicated assessments of treatment success in clinical studies. Moreover, standardized criteria that define treatment response or failure have not been established. Using our current understanding of keloid and hypertrophic scar formation, three distinctly different therapeutic approaches can be taken: (1) manipulation of the mechanical properties of wound repair; (2) correction of the abnormal balance of collagen synthesis and degradation; and (3) alteration of the immune/inflammatory response. Multiple modalities are often utilized concurrently or sequentially to successfully manage these lesions.

Surgery. Surgical excision is one of the first reported treatments for keloids, with the first description of this technique by Druit[43] noted in 1844. The futility of surgical excision alone soon became apparent, as noted by DeCosta[44] in 1903. Recurrence rates for simple surgical excision of keloids alone vary from 50% to 80%.[45] Therefore, if an excision is performed, at least one other treatment modality should be utilized to minimize recurrence. Certain keloids display a greater tendency to recur, even with adjuvant therapy. These scars are in areas of high skin tension, such as the presternal area. These scars are generally dumbbell shaped with claw-like lateral extensions. Surgical revision is not recommended for these scars.

Radiation. The rationale for the use of radiation therapy in the treatment of keloids is in the destruction of fibroblasts and neovascular buds by the ionizing radiation.[46] Once the fibroblasts are destroyed, the treated areas do not become repopulated by new fibroblasts from surrounding tissues. Fibroblasts demonstrate great heterogeneity in their response to radiation.[47] If a sufficient number of fibroblasts are eliminated, a balance is reached between collagen synthesis and degradation with resultant scar flattening. DeBeurman and Gougerot[48] were first to report the treatment of keloids with radiation in 1906. Cosman et al.[49] introduced the early postoperative use of x-ray therapy following keloid excision. He noted no advantage in combined preoperative and postoperative radiation over postoperative radiation alone. Conflicting data exist regarding this observation.[50] Numerous reports have since described the use of various combinations of radiation therapy, including external vs. interstitial radiotherapy, superficial x-ray therapy, beta-ray therapy, and electron beam treatment. All have been variably effective in the treatment of keloids.

Studies have shown that radiotherapy alone is minimally effective in the treatment of keloids, with a recurrence rate of between 50% and 100%.[51] However, postoperative radiation has proven successful in preventing keloid recurrence. The timing, administration, and dosage of postoperative radiation remains controversial. Data from several studies suggest that keloid recurrence correlates best with the total dose of radiation administered, with efficacy seen at total doses ranging between 1500 and 2000 rads.[52] Typically, treatment is initiated immediately after surgery, with several repeat doses administered over the next few days. Levy et al.[53] achieved an 88% success rate in keloid resolution, with follow-up ranging from 6 to 24 months. Studies by Ollstein et al.[54] and Enhamre and Hammer[55] revealed similar results. Postoperative interstitial radiotherapy with iridium 192 has been employed in multiple studies with keloid recurrence rates ranging from 20% to 36.8%.[56] Advantages to this treatment include ease of usage and limited irradiation exposure with efficacy comparable to external radiotherapy. Side effects include telangiectasia formation, skin atrophy, pruritus, and hyperpigmentation (Box 23-4). There is uncertainty regarding the long-term carcinogenic effects of x-rays, even at low dose exposure, thus making the use of radiotherapy in the treatment of keloids controversial. A case of medullary thyroid carcinoma in an 11-year-old boy 8 years following excision and postoperative radiation of a chin keloid has been described.[57] Many clinicians reserve radiotherapy for keloids resistant to other treatment modalities.

BOX 23-4 Side Effects of Radiation Therapy

- Hyperpigmentation
- Telangiectasia formation
- Skin atrophy
- Pruritus
- Paresthesia
- Pain
- Carcinogenic risk

Pressure. The use of mechanical pressure to treat keloids was first reported in 1835. Pressure therapy is useful for therapy of established keloids and hypertrophic scars as well as for prophylactic prevention. The use of pressure in the prevention and treatment of keloids after burn injury became standard in the late 1960s.[58] No study has been able to fully elucidate the mechanism by which pressure alters scars. Proposed explanations include (1) a decrease in blood flow with resultant decrease in α_2-macroglobulin and subsequent increase in collagenase-mediated collagen breakdown[59]; (2) decreased levels of chondroitin 4-sulfate, with resultant increase in collagen degradation; (3) decreased scar hydration resulting in mast cell stabilization and subsequent decrease in neovascularization and extracellular matrix production[60]; and (4) localized hypoxia resulting in fibroblast and collagen degradation. Pressure results in histologically looser collagen bundles, increased interstitial space, and a decreased number of inflammatory cells.[61]

Silicone Gel Sheeting. Silicone gel sheeting has recently been used for its scar hydrating effects. The sheeting—3.5 mm thick—is a soft, adherent, semiocclusive covering that is fabricated from medical-grade, cross-linked silicone polymers. Silicone gel sheeting is thought to act through scar hydration, with one half the evaporative water loss compared with normal skin. It is theorized that this hydration results in decreased capillary flow, with a reduction in collagen deposition due to decreased circulating proinflammatory cytokines. No effects with regard to pressure, change in scar temperature, and oxygen tension have been detected to date.[62] These sheets were initially used with success in the treatment of burn wounds to accelerate wound healing.[63] Various investigators have since demonstrated significant keloid and hypertrophic scar improvement following silicone gel sheeting application.[64] Katz demonstrated that 79% of revised keloid scars treated immediately with silicone gel sheeting after reepithelialization showed no evidence of recurrence after 6 months.[65]

A study by Ricketts and colleagues[66] evaluating the treatment of hypertrophic scars with silicone vs. nonsilicone gel dressings demonstrated comparable clinical improvement of the scars with both dressings. It may, therefore, be the occlusive effects of the dressing that account for the improvement observed. Thus silicone may not be a necessary component. Side effects of silicone gel application are limited to localized irritation. No release of silicone material into skin has been documented to date.

Laser Surgery. The carbon dioxide 10,600 nm laser was one of the first lasers to be employed in the treatment of keloids and hypertrophic scars. Its advantages were attributed to its atraumatic and anti-inflammatory properties.[67] Studies evaluating the effectiveness of the continuous wave carbon dioxide laser demonstrate that laser excision of keloids with healing by secondary intention alone fails to suppress keloid growth and recurrence.[68-70] At present, carbon dioxide laser keloid excision is limited to special situations such as the debulking of large keloids prior to initiation of another treatment modality.

More recent advances in laser technology have generated two new categories of char-free carbon dioxide lasers. The first are high-energy, short-pulsed carbon dioxide lasers that produce high-energy pulses with pulse durations of less than 900 μs. The second are continuous wave, scanned carbon dioxide lasers that utilize a scanner to direct a focused, continuous wave laser beam in a spiral pattern, resulting in less than 1 ms tissue exposure time. These lasers produce tissue vaporization with minimal coagulation, as they exceed the vaporization threshold of tissue, 5 J/cm^2, while also limiting the tissue exposure time (pulse duration) to less than 1 ms, which is the thermal relaxation time of the skin. Bernstein and colleagues[71] evaluated the use of the high-energy, short-pulsed carbon dioxide laser and the scanned carbon dioxide laser in the treatment of 24 postsurgical hypertrophic and keloidal scars and 6 traumatic, acne, and varicella scars. All 30 patients showed improvement of surface contour after treatment. Temporary side effects included erythema in all scars lasting 7 to 24 weeks and slight hypopigmentation in 3 scars. Long-term follow-up regarding keloid recurrence has not been reported. The short-pulsed and scanned carbon dioxide lasers offer an alternative treatment modality in the surgical ablation of keloids.

Argon Laser. The 488 nm to 514 nm argon laser was first described as a treatment for hypertrophic scars and keloids in 1978.[72] The proposed mechanism of action has been debated. It is thought to act via a coagulative effect on capillaries, leading to localized ischemia, release of lactic acid, and a subsequent decrease in pH. This pH alteration is thought to lead to decreased α_2-macroglobulin and a subsequent increase in collagen degradation. Others have proposed that the laser's effect is due to heat conduction with resultant dermal tissue shrinkage.[73] Although symptomatic improvement has been noted in keloids treated with the argon laser,[69] this effect is temporary, with symptoms returning after 6 months. At present, the argon laser is not recommended in the management of scars.

Nd:YAG Laser. A photobiological effect on collagen metabolism using the neodymium:yttrium-aluminum-garnet (Nd:YAG) 1064 nm continuous wave laser was first demonstrated by Abergel and colleagues.[74] The laser's effect is thought to be due to its hemostatic effect. Collagen production is selectively inhibited without effect on fibroblast viability or DNA replication. Once treated, the keloid demonstrates surface infarction with subsequent sloughing of the eschar and resultant keloid debulking. Use of this laser in keloid scar treatment is not recommended at present. The 1064 nm laser light is poorly absorbed by chromophores in the skin. As a result it penetrates deeply into tissue and produces diffuse heating of tissue. This results in nonspecific skin damage and a high risk of unwanted cutaneous necrosis.

Pulsed Dye Laser. In 1993, Alster and colleagues first described an improvement in atrophic and hypertrophic scars[75] with the use of a 585 nm pulsed dye laser. Ten argon laser–induced scars within port wine stains received five laser treatments over a 10-month period. It was observed that by targeting treatment to the vascular component of the scars, the pulsed dye laser induced a reduction or elimination of the erythema in these scars. In addition, normal skin markings returned and a flattening of the elevated portions of the scars was observed. No recurrence of the scars was noted at 4-year follow-up. A subsequent uncontrolled, prospective study of 14 hypertrophic and erythematous scars by Alster[76] demonstrated a 57% to 83% improvement of these scars after one or two treatments with the 585 nm flashlamp pulsed dye laser, respectively. Dierickx and associates observed similar results in their uncontrolled evaluation of hypertrophic and erythematous scars.[77] Goldman and Fitzpatrick[78] treated 48 hypertrophic and erythematous scars with either pulsed dye laser alone (n = 37) or pulsed dye laser followed by the injection of intralesional corticosteroids (n = 11). Concomitant administration of intralesional corticosteroids (triamcinolone acetonide, 5 to 10 mg/ml) and pulsed dye laser treatment achieved greater resolution of the scars than laser treatment alone at 4- to 8-week follow-up.

Improvement of keloid scars after 585 nm pulsed dye laser treatments has also been observed. Alster and Williams[79] treated median sternotomy hypertrophic scar and keloid halves and compared the clinical, textural, histologic, and symptomatic responses of the treated scar halves with the untreated control halves using photography and skin profilometry. Significant improvement was observed in all laser-treated keloids in all clinical parameters in comparison with the untreated controls.

The pulsed dye laser's mechanism of action on scar improvement is likely multifactorial. The laser's vascular specificity may lead to direct microvasculature damage, with resultant ischemia and subsequent collagen degradation. Thermal damage to collagen fibers may also result in direct dissolution of disulfide bonds. These hypotheses are supported by studies conducted by Reiken et al. on hypertrophic scar implants in athymic mice treated with the pulsed dye laser.[80] The extent of scar growth inhibition was proportional to the pulsed dye laser energy utilized, which ranged from 6 to 10 J/cm^2, and was maximal at the lowest wavelength within the range tested (585 to 600 nm). Histologic examination of the laser-treated hypertrophic scar implants suggested the primary target was the microvasculature; significant vessel wall necrosis was noted.

The optimal time for the initiation of pulsed dye laser treatment of hypertrophic scars and keloids has not yet been determined. Scars may show incremental improvement, in the absence of treatment, over 6 to 12 months after onset. Wound dehiscence may occur if treatment is initiated too soon during early scar remodeling. Fibroblasts in evolving keloids do not deviate from their normal growth pattern for at least 3 weeks after surgery.[81] Therefore, treatment initiated within this first 2- to 3-week postoperative period may serve as preventative management.

Intralesional Corticosteroid and 5-Fluorouracil Injections. Intralesional corticosteroid injections are a first-line treatment for hypertrophic scars and keloids. Corticosteroids appear to act by inhibiting fibroblast growth and inhibiting α_2-macroglobulin,[82] resulting in collagen degradation. The corticosteroid suspensions are injected directly into the scar. Corticosteroid injections alone will improve but may not eliminate a keloid. Enhanced results may be achieved when intralesional corticosteroid injections are combined with other treatment modalities (i.e., laser or cryosurgery) or initiated after surgical excision. The mechanism of action of 5-fluorouracil (5-FU) in improving hypertrophic scars and keloids has yet to be fully elucidated. In a fashion similar to that for intralesional corticosteroid injections, the 5-FU suspension is injected directly into the scars after being diluted in a suspension of corticosteroid and may be combined with other treatment modalities (i.e., laser or cryosurgery) to enhance results.

Cryosurgery. Cryosurgery utilizes a cryogenic agent or cryoprobe to cause direct cell and microcirculatory damage. The resulting stasis, thrombus formation, and subsequent anoxia leads to tissue necrosis and sloughing, followed by tissue flattening.[83] Cell destruction is selective, leaving fibroblasts intact for reepithelialization of the wound. Cryotherapy alone has resulted in complete keloid flattening in 51% to 74% of patients treated. When used in combination with intralesional steroids, an 84% response rate was seen.[84] A comparison study of intralesional triamcinolone alone vs. cryosurgery alone in the treatment of acne keloids by Layton and colleagues showed a beneficial response to both modalities, but a preferential response to cryosurgery was observed.[85]

Interferon. The use of interferons in the treatment of keloids and hypertrophic scars has been investigated because of their effects on collagen synthesis. Interferons alpha (IFN-α), beta (IFN-β), and gamma (IFN-γ) inhibit types I and III collagen synthesis by dermal and synovial fibroblasts and type II collagen synthesis by chondrocytes in a dose-dependent fashion. This inhibition occurs through a reduction in cellular messenger ribonucleic acid.[86] A double-blind controlled study of intralesional IFN-γ on the treatment of keloids[87] demonstrated a clinically significant reduction in keloid size with histologic reduction or elimination of collagen nodules and more orderly, parallel deposition of fine collagen fibers. A decrease in mast cells was also noted. Recurrences were minimal after 1 year. Larrabee et al.[88] and Pittet et al.[89] confirmed these results.

A similar reduction in keloid size has been observed after intradermal interferon alpha-2b injections.[90] A retrospective analysis of the recurrence rate of 124 excised keloids conducted by Berman and Flores[91] revealed a significantly lower rate of recurrence in keloids treated with postoperative interferon alpha-2b (18.7% recurrence), in comparison with keloids treated with excision alone (51.1%) or with postoperative triamcinolone acetonide (58.4%). Conejo-Mir and colleagues[92] observed similar findings in the evaluation of 16 earlobe keloids and 14 trunk keloids after treatment with a carbon dioxide laser followed by weekly injections of interferon alpha-2b. No recurrence was noted in 66% of these lesions after 3 years. Al-Khawajah[93] and Wong et al.[94] were unable to reproduce these findings. These conflicting results may be due to differences in dosage, manufacture, or delivery of interferon alpha-2b, location of keloids treated, or a combination of these factors. Further studies utilizing interferon alpha-2b in the treatment of keloids and hypertrophic scars are necessary to determine if this treatment is indeed effective and to standardize dosages and administration.

Pharmacologic Therapies. Novel approaches to treating keloids and hypertrophic scars are being utilized as knowledge of the underlying factors leading to their formation is revealed. Many treatments are anecdotal to date. The efficacy of the treatments listed below will require further confirmation via controlled studies.

Topical retinoic acid is thought to act via an inhibitory effect on fibroblast DNA synthesis to reduce the size of keloids. Application of 0.05% retinoic acid solution in the treatment of 28 keloids and hypertrophic scars produced improved coloration, symptomatic relief, and some flattening of the lesions.[95] The irritating nature of retinoic acid may limit its long-term use in certain anatomic areas. Studies comparing the various strengths of topical retinoic acids over time will aid in defining the most effective strength with the fewest side effects.

Colchicine has been administered to alter collagen metabolism through collagen synthesis inhibition, microtubular disruption, and collagenase stimulation.[96]

Lathyrogens, such as β-aminopropionitrile and D-penicillamine,[97] as well as other agents such as topical putrescine,[98] have been used in the treatment of hypertrophic scars and keloids to prevent collagen cross-linking. These agents increase susceptibility to collagen degradation.

Collagenase stimulation and lysyl oxidase inhibition has been achieved with the application of topical zinc tape.[99] Inhibition of collagen synthesis, decreased fibroblast proliferation, and a decrease in inflammation have been observed with the application of topical vitamins A and E.[100] Madecassol has been utilized in the treatment of keloids and is hypothesized to work via a reduction in fibroblast collagen synthesis.[101]

Intralesional verapamil and other calcium-channel antagonists have been employed in the management of keloids due to their ability to inhibit extracellular matrix proline incorporation.[102] A study evaluating the treatment response of 45 earlobe keloids to excision followed by injections of intralesional verapamil (0.5 to 2 ml, 2.5 mg/ml) for 1 month and pressure earrings for a minimum of 6 months revealed a 45% recurrence rate.[103] There were no significant differences in recurrence rates related to sex, age, keloid size, keloid age, or number of verapamil injections received.

Antihistamines have been utilized in keloid treatment to stabilize mast cells and reduce histamine levels.[104] To date, keloid response to these medications has been modest at best. Topical cyclosporine has been utilized in keloid management to alter T-cell function.[105] Other chemotherapeutic agents such as methotrexate have also been employed for their immunosuppressive effects without noted benefit.[106]

Numerous physical forms of treatment have been implemented in the treatment of hypertrophic scars and keloids. These include ultrasound,[107] static-electric field induction,[108] and iontophoretic transdermal delivery of transilast.[109] Intralesional injections of formalin,[110] hydrochloric acid, pepsin,[111] and oil of creosote have been used as digestive agents in the management of these scars with variable degrees of success.

ATROPHIC AND ACNE SCARS

Background and History

Atrophic scarring is a well-recognized consequence of acne vulgaris and varicella infection. It is the result of an inflammatory response to an initial lesion, which terminates in fibrosis. Trauma, infection, and long-standing epithelial cyst formation are processes that can also lead to atrophic scarring.

Atrophic scarring is caused by fibrotic scar tissue formation. The dermal nature of the scar produces a bound-down, often angular scar with an indented or inverted center. Although the shape of the final defect may vary, the underlying etiology is similar: fibrosis. It is unclear why certain individuals will heal with atrophic scars, while others with a similar appearing clinical lesion will heal without any evidence of scarring.

Acne affects over 80% of the population at some point in their lives, yet not all people with acne develop scarring.[112] The desire to prevent scarring is often a reason for treating acne, yet even in the presence of adequate intervention, some patients will scar from acne. Many of these patients also exhibit a poor healing response to conventional cold steel surgery, especially on the face (personal observation). Therefore, the management of atrophic and acne scars is complicated by the potentially poor response the patient will have to surgical revision.

Basic Science

In 1994, Layton et al. studied the pathogenesis of acne scarring. The authors evaluated 185 patients with a history of acne for the presence and extent of acne scarring. Facial scarring was noted to affect both sexes equally and occurred to some degree in 95% of the patients evaluated.[112] Scarring developed as a consequence of all types of acne, including pustules, papules, and nodules. The incidence of facial scarring was greater than that of truncal scarring due to site-specific responses to inflammatory stimuli.[112] Skin type and previous history of scarring did not appear to correlate with postacne scarring. A delay of 3 years between acne onset and adequate treatment correlated with the greatest degree of scarring observed in both sexes.

The gamut of acne scarring includes both contour irregularities and surface discoloration. A reddish-brown macular hue may develop at the site of a resolved acneiform lesion. This represents postinflammatory hyperpigmentation and erythema. This change is usually temporary but may persist for up to 8 to 12 months.

There are three basic types of textural acne scars: boxcar, ice pick, and rolling scars (Fig. 23-1). Perhaps the most common acne scar is the depressed, crateriform *boxcar* scar. It generally measures 3 to 4 mm or less in diameter and is similar in appearance to a varicella scar. A fibrotic lesion is present, with extension of the fibrosis into the dermis and subcutaneous fat resulting in a firm, semirigid scar. The deeper the scar, the more visible the scar becomes due to its exaggerated demarcated edges (shoulders) and resultant shadow forma-

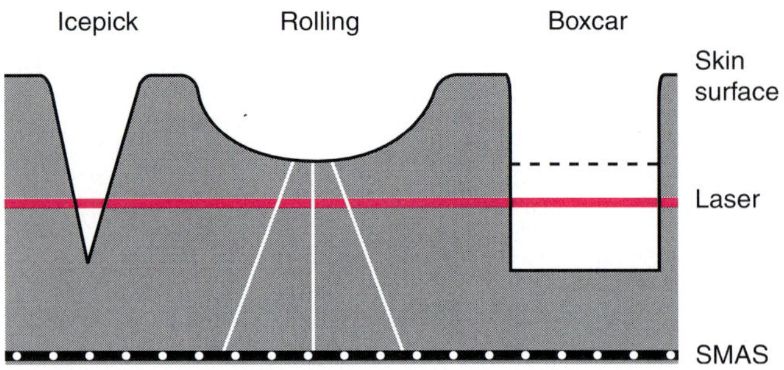

FIG. 23-1
Acne scar subtypes. The three main acne scar subtypes—ice pick, rolling, and boxcar—are depicted in schematic cross-section. White lines represent fibrous tethers that produce rolling scar bound-down appearance. Pink line indicates depth achievable with laser resurfacing. Dashed line indicates level of SMAS.

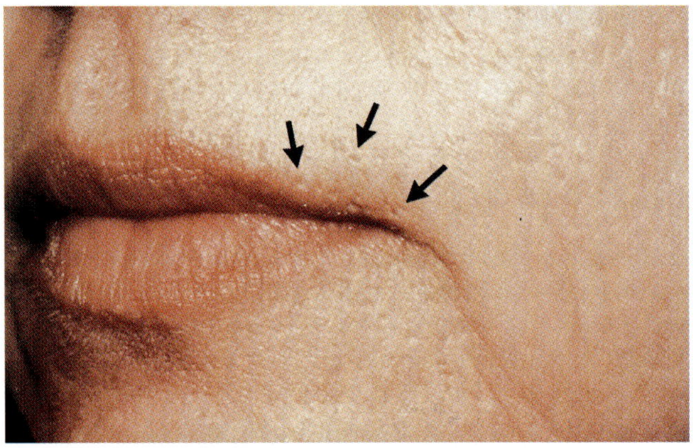

FIG. 23-2
Perioral ice pick scars. Arrows indicate individual scars.

tion. *Ice pick* scars (Fig. 23-2), or deep pitted scars, exhibit a narrow opening with a 0.5 mm or greater extension into the dermis, resembling a small hole. *Rolling* scars (Fig. 23-3) are soft, distensible, depressed scars, with a slightly wrinkled superficial base. These scars present as shallow undulations and may be subtle, but often become more noticeable with lighting changes or as the patient moves his or her head. Rolling scars can be small (less than 1 cm) or large (greater than 1 cm). Often, patients will have several individual rolling scars that coalesce to form a larger area of scarring. An individual may present with one type of scar or a combination of scar types (Box 23-5). Treatment must be tailored to the type of scarring present.

Clinical Studies

Development of acne scarring is multifactorial, including a genetic predisposition, delay in treatment administration, and a tendency toward scarring. When evaluating a patient with acne scarring, one must assess multiple aspects of the patient's acne background prior to developing a treatment plan. Key elements to evaluate in the patient with acne scarring include:

- The patient's acne history, including age of onset, duration of acne, and current acne activity.
- Patient's medical history, including endocrine/hormonal abnormalities and treatments received for these abnormalities as well as menses history (including age of onset, regular vs. sporadic cycles, correlation with acne outbreaks).
- Patient medications, including oral contraceptive use.
- Patient's acne treatment history, including past and current medications used. If isotretinoin (Accutane, Roche Pharmaceuticals, Nutley, NJ) has been taken, it is important to record the number of courses, length of each course, and the month and year of the last dose taken. A surgical procedure should not be performed within 1 year of the last dose of Accutane, as Accutane has been shown to lead to delayed postprocedural wound healing and risk of hypertrophic scarring.[113] Prior surgical procedures performed to treat the acne scarring should be documented.
- Patient's goals and expectations in the management of the acne scarring. It may not be possible to meet a patient's expectations given the extent and type of scarring present. A lengthy discussion regarding realistic treatment goals is critical in the management plan.

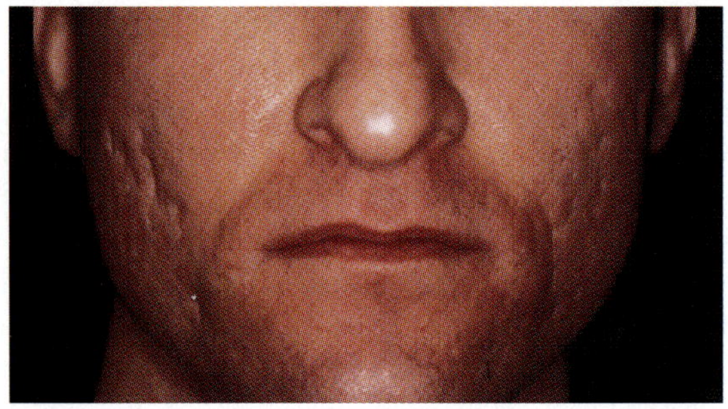

FIG. 23-3
Young man with rolling scars on bilateral cheeks.

BOX 23-5 Types of Acne Scarring

- Postinflammatory hyperpigmentation
- Crateriform "boxcar" scars
- Ice pick scars
- Shallow "rolling" scars
- Hypertrophic scars and keloids

BOX 23-6 Side Effects of Carbon Dioxide Laser Resurfacing

- Persistent erythema (temporary erythema lasting 2 to 4 months is expected)
- Hypertrophic scarring
- Infection (bacterial, viral, fungal)
- Pigmentary alteration (hyperpigmentation or hypopigmentation)
- Demarcation lines or patches
- Milia development
- Acne flare
- Ectropion formation
- Scar recurrence
- Incomplete removal
- Treatment failure

BOX 23-7 Side Effects of Pulsed Dye Laser Treatment

- Transient purpura, lasting up to 2 weeks (This discoloration is deep purple and difficult to camouflage with cosmetics.)
- Short-lived sharp, stinging pain, compared to the snap of a rubber band, followed by a sensation of heat
- Pigmentary alteration, including temporary postinflammatory hyperpigmentation and permanent hypopigmentation
- Blistering and partial-thickness burns
- Infection
- Scar formation

Procedure. The treatment area is first draped with fire-resistant materials (i.e., moistened towels). The treatment area is anesthetized locally with 1% lidocaine with or without epinephrine (1:100,000) or via a regional nerve block to eliminate patient discomfort during treatment. Protective eyewear, masks, and continuous suction are employed during the entire procedure to minimize exposure to the continuous plume of smoke and debris that is emitted during treatment.

Scar ablative treatment may be initiated with the carbon dioxide laser set in a continuous wave mode utilizing a power of 10 watts and with a 1-, 2-, or 3-mm spot handpiece. With the parameters set, aim the laser beam at a tongue depressor and test for laser function and alignment. Beam target distance greatly affects the power delivered to the skin. The laser should be aimed at the scar to deliver an impact spot of 3 to 4 mm. A single-pulse setting or repeat-pulse setting can be utilized to ensure precise treatment of the affected areas. The perimeter of the scar is traced in a continuous burst to define the treatment area, then the remainder of the tissue surface is vaporized. Once an entire pass has been completed, the char is gently removed with saline-moistened gauze. This cycle is repeated until the scar has been ablated. As the lesion is debulked, a lower power and increased target distance should be used to avoid excessive treatment.

Postprocedural Care. Immediately after treatment the area should be covered with antibiotic ointment. Wound care consists of cleansing the treatment areas with moist compresses two to three times a day to remove any formed crust, followed by the application of an emollient such as Vaseline or Aquaphor healing ointment (Biersdorf, Wilton, CT). This should be continued until complete reepithelialization has occurred.

Postoperative pain is generally limited. Analgesic use should be titrated both to the extent of the surgery and the patient's subjective experience. In general, use of acetaminophen is generally sufficient for pain relief.

Pulsed Dye Laser

Preprocedural Management. The patient's informed consent should be obtained prior to treatment. The patient should be made aware of the side effects associated with treatment (Box 23-7).

Procedure

Safety. Laser-specific protective eyewear with side shields must be worn by all persons involved in treatment, including the patient. If an area of the eyelid is to be treated, nonreflective stainless steel corneal eye shields are used to protect the patient's eyes. The inner surface of these shields is coated with an ophthalmic antibiotic ointment to decrease risk of corneal abrasion. An ophthalmologic anesthetic is used before placement for patient comfort.

The treatment site is cleaned with a noninflammatory cleanser to remove any makeup and debris present. A water-based lubricant is applied to moisten any potentially combustible materials that will fall within the laser treatment field, including patient hair.

Anesthesia. The need for anesthesia depends on the size and location of the lesion to be treated, as well as the age and pain tolerance of the patient. In general, treatment discomfort is short-lived and is tolerated without the need for pretreatment anesthesia. Topical anesthetic cream (EMLA, Astra USA, Westborough, MA) may be applied under occlusion to the scar(s) 2 hours before treatment. Also, 1% lidocaine with or without epinephrine (1:100,000) intralesionally or via a regional nerve block may be used.

Treatment. Treatment parameters are determined by the location and appearance of the lesion. Lesions of the face can tolerate higher fluences than the neck and chest. The Fitzpatrick skin type of the patient must also be considered, as melanin interferes with absorption of the pulsed dye laser energy. Skin types III and greater are treated with lower energy fluences in order to decrease the risk of epidermal blistering, pigmentary change, and scarring. Recommended pulsed dye laser treatment parameters for hypertrophic scars and keloids include energy fluences of 6 to 7.5 J/cm^2 utilizing a 5 to 7 mm spot size (Candela Corp., Wayland, MA) at treatment intervals of 4 to 8 weeks. If a larger spot size is used, treatment is performed using a lower fluence.

Postprocedural Care. A cool hydrogel or compress is applied immediately after treatment to decrease patient discomfort. Aquaphor healing ointment (Biersdorf, Wilton, CT) or equivalent emollient is applied over the subsequent 2 to 3 days following treatment to minimize epidermal crusting.

Corticosteroid and Other Intralesional Therapy

Procedure. Varied intralesional corticosteroid preparations have been utilized in the treatment of hypertrophic scars and keloids. We routinely use triamcinolone acetonide, 10 mg/ml, to initiate treatment of keloids and hypertrophic scars. If no improvement is noticed after one or two treatments, the concentration should be doubled with each treatment to a maximum concentration of 40 mg/ml. An alternate therapy is the use of triamcinolone diacetate, 25 mg/ml.

Steroid preparations may be diluted with 1% lidocaine with or without epinephrine (1:100,000). The use of lidocaine reduces the pain of multiple injections, as well as the pain incurred immediately post treatment. The vasoconstrictive properties of epinephrine may allow for prolonged presence of the steroid at the treatment site. An alternate diluent is buffered sterile saline. Regardless of which diluent is used, the contents within the syringe must be mixed continuously throughout the treatment in order to ensure an even concentration of the mixture throughout the syringe. For scars, we routinely use a 1 or 3 ml Luer-Lok syringe with a 1-inch 27- or 30-gauge needle. Alternate injection devices include a dental syringe or a mechanical injector. Mechanical injectors are thought to be less painful but may not provide the accuracy of injection necessary for optimal treatment.

The corticosteroid preparation is injected directly into the bulk of the keloid or hypertrophic scar. It is vital to ensure that the needle is within the body of the scar and not above or below it in order to decrease the risk of side effects.[142] If correctly placed, a whitening of the scar will be observed as the preparation is injected. Injection into the scar is often difficult because of the fibrotic nature of the scar. If the injection appears easy to perform and there is little resistance to the injection, the needle may be placed too low in the subcutaneous tissue. With improper placement, subcutaneous atrophy may result. To facilitate injection, the needle should be advanced to create a tract, and the corticosteroid should be injected while the needle is withdrawn. An alternative method is to treat the scar with cryosurgery for 15 to 30 seconds prior to the injection. This allows for tissue edema and subsequent softening of the scar prior to intralesional corticosteroid injection.[84] Intralesional corticosteroids have an approximately 30- to 40-day duration of action. Injections are therefore administered at intervals of 4 to 6 weeks to limit side effects (Box 23-8). Therapy may require repeated treatments over several months.[106]

Intralesional 5-fluorouracil (5-FU) has been successfully utilized at a concentration of 50 mg/ml in the management of hypertrophic scars[143] and keloids. Frequent initial injections (one to three times weekly) are employed, with a reduction in frequency to weekly or monthly injections as improvement is noted. The addition of triamcinolone acetonide at a final concentration of 5 mg/ml 5-FU (i.e., dilution of nine parts 50 mg/ml 5-FU to one part 10 mg/ml triamcinolone acetonide) increases the efficacy of this treatment when employed on a monthly basis. A major disadvantage to the use of intralesional injections of 5-FU or corticosteroids is the pain experienced by patients during injections, which may lead to noncompliance.

Cryosurgery

Preprocedural Management. A complete medical history must be obtained before treatment to exclude patients with preexisting conditions that may preclude this treatment (Box 23-9).

BOX 23-8 Side Effects of Intralesional Corticosteroid Injections

- Skin atrophy
- Hypopigmentation or hyperpigmentation
- Telangiectasia formation
- Necrosis or ulceration
- Subepidermal white deposits that resolve slowly over time
- Systemic response to corticosteroids (rare)

BOX 23-9 Contraindications to Cryosurgery Treatment

- Autoimmune and collagen disorders
- Raynaud's disease
- Cryoglobulinemia or cryofibrinogenemia
- Intolerance to cold
- Blood dyscrasias or platelet deficiency disease
- Myeloma or lymphoma
- Concurrent treatment with immunosuppressive drugs
- History of pyoderma gangrenosum
- History of cold anaphylaxis

Procedure. Cryosurgery can be performed in an outpatient facility or office setting. Agents that are available include nitrous oxide, chlorodifluoromethane (Verruca Freeze), propane (Histofreezer), dimethyl ether, carbon dioxide, and liquid nitrogen (Box 23-10). Liquid nitrogen is the coldest cryogen available. It is the preferred method for cryotherapy.

Liquid nitrogen storage requires an insulated aluminum tank in order to avoid evaporation. The liquid nitrogen can then be transferred to a thermos or handheld cryogen delivery system. A thermos must be able to allow evaporating gas to escape. The cryogun is available in various sizes, with special applicator tips that have different size apertures that can be interchanged according to lesion size.

It is not possible to see the depth of freezing that occurs below the surface of a treated area once the cryogenic agent is applied. A thermocouple device may be inserted into the skin to detect the depth of freeze, but few physicians employ this technique. For keloids and hypertrophic scars, treatment is gauged by the freezing time, determined by the time it takes for the treatment site to become frozen white. With these scars, the physician must limit the amount of lateral spread of whitening in order to avoid surrounding tissue damage (Box 23-11).

A dipstick method of applying liquid nitrogen to the scars may be performed via a cotton-tipped applicator dipped frequently into liquid nitrogen in a Styrofoam cup and applied to the lesion. The major disadvantages of this method are different reproducibility and variable depth of freeze depending on the amount of pressure applied during treatment.

The cryogun operates via a trigger mechanism to deliver a continuous spray, allowing for controlled delivery. Treatment usually involves one freeze-thaw cycle lasting from 10 to 30 seconds at each treatment session to achieve keloid flattening. Generally 2 to 10 sessions, separated by 20 to 30 days, are required. Lack of efficacy of cryosurgery may be due to inadequate freeze times or the failure to continue treatment when initial results are not impressive.

BOX 23-10 Boiling Points of Various Cryogens

Cryogen	Boiling Point (°C)
Dimethyl ether	–24
Chlorodifluoromethane	–41
Propane	–42
Carbon dioxide	–79
Nitrous oxide	–90
Liquid nitrogen	–196

BOX 23-11 Side Effects of Cryosurgery

- Permanent pigmentary alteration (hypopigmentation, hyperpigmentation)
- Blistering
- Intradermal hemorrhage
- Postoperative infection
- Postoperative pain
- Scar formation
- Neuropathy

Postprocedural Care. Postoperative care may include application of bacitracin ointment followed by the placement of a bandage on the treated area.

Interferon Gamma

Procedure. Intralesional injections of 10 to 200 μg of interferon gamma are made into the keloid twice weekly for 4 weeks.

Postprocedural Care. Overall, intralesional injections of interferon gamma are well tolerated. However, injections tend to be painful, which may require regional anesthesia prior to treatment. A flulike syndrome, characterized by myalgia, headaches, and low-grade fever (37.5°C), has been observed. These symptoms may persist for 6 to 48 hours after the intralesional injection. The use of acetaminophen may be useful in managing these symptoms. No significant biochemical, hematologic, or renal abnormalities have been reported.

ATROPHIC AND ACNE SCARS

Preoperative Clinical Considerations

Proper selection of surgical techniques is paramount to treatment success. Many patients present with a variety of atrophic scar subtypes, each requiring an individualized approach to produce the best treatment results (Table 23-1). It is essential that the physician take the proper time to diagnose the patient's scarring subtypes. Therapeutic decision making hinges on making the proper diagnosis in these patients. Once the pa-

Table 23-1 Therapy of Acne Scars

Scar Type	Excision	Punch Elevation	Subcision	CO_2/Er:YAG Laser
Ice pick	+++	–	–	–
Superficial boxcar	+	+	–	+++
Deep boxcar	+++	++	–	+
Rolling	–	+	+++	+

tient's scar subtypes have been identified, a treatment plan and timeline can be implemented.

Ice pick scars, given their depth of fibrotic scarring, respond well to punch excision, which allows for full removal of the deep aspects of the scar. Ice pick scars do not improve with punch elevation or subcision and have minimal if any response to laser skin resurfacing or dermabrasion.

Boxcar scars respond to a variety of treatments. Shallow boxcar scars can be effectively treated with laser skin resurfacing but may obtain additional improvement with prelaser punch elevation. Deep boxcar scars require surgical treatment. Punch excision works well for narrow (less than 3 mm) deep boxcar scars, whereas punch elevation is preferred for wider deep boxcar scars.

Rolling scars are best treated by subcision. The skin overlying the lesion usually appears normal to slightly wrinkled and therefore does not need to be removed to produce good results. Rather, scar elevation alone will often produce substantial improvement due to the elimination of shadowing. Many rolling scars are too wide (greater than 3 mm) to be treated with excision due to the visible nature of the incision scar.

Most scar types will respond best to a combination of therapies. The addition of laser skin resurfacing 6 to 12 weeks after surgical treatment of atrophic scars tends to improve final contours. This occurs through two mechanisms. Scars that are too small to treat with surgical techniques are often improved with laser skin resurfacing, and this tends to improve the final appearance of the skin. In addition, recently created surgical scars from excision, punch elevation or excision, or subcision can undergo remodeling and improvement with the addition of laser resurfacing.

Patients are asked to stop all medications that can cause bleeding 2 weeks prior to surgery (i.e., NSAIDs, vitamin E). Preoperative and perioperative antibiotics (penicillins or cephalosporins) are routinely prescribed for excision or punch elevation of multiple lesions. Oral antibiotics are also prescribed for large subcision cases (greater than 5 cm^2).

Procedural Techniques

Surgical Excision. Various excisional techniques are available for the effective treatment of atrophic scars. Each technique utilizes similar equipment to perform the procedure.

Procedure. The scars are outlined with a marking pen. The treatment areas are sterilely prepped and draped. The areas are then infiltrated with 1% lidocaine with epinephrine (1:100,000) and the patient is allowed to sit for 10 to 20 minutes prior to the procedure to allow for the vasoconstrictive effects of the epinephrine.

Punch excision. Ice pick scars and deep boxcar scars may be excised with a 1.5, 2, 2.5, or 3 mm punch tool (Fig. 23-5). By placing outward traction on the punch site at the time of excision, the circular wound is changed into an ellipse. To ensure that the ellipse runs parallel to the skin lines, the outward traction should be applied perpendicular to the skin lines (Fig. 23-6). The scar tissue is removed and the wound sutured with one to three interrupted sutures using 6-0 nylon or Prolene (Ethicon, Somerville, NJ). If the punch excision is 2.5 mm or greater, a 6-0 Vicryl (Ethicon, Somerville, NJ) subcutaneous suture can be placed prior to epidermal closure. We have found that this absorbable deep su-

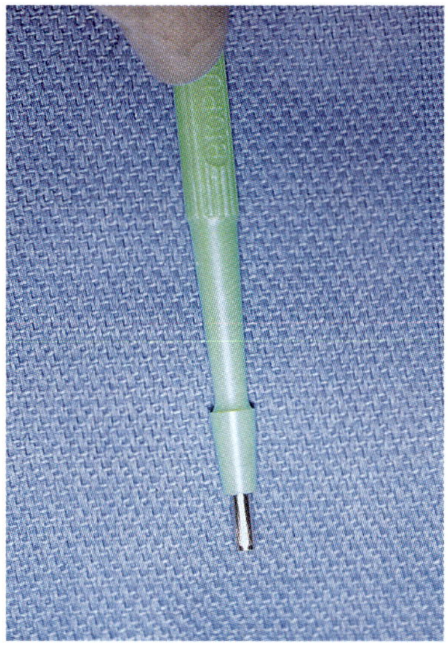

FIG. 23-5
A 2 mm punch tool.

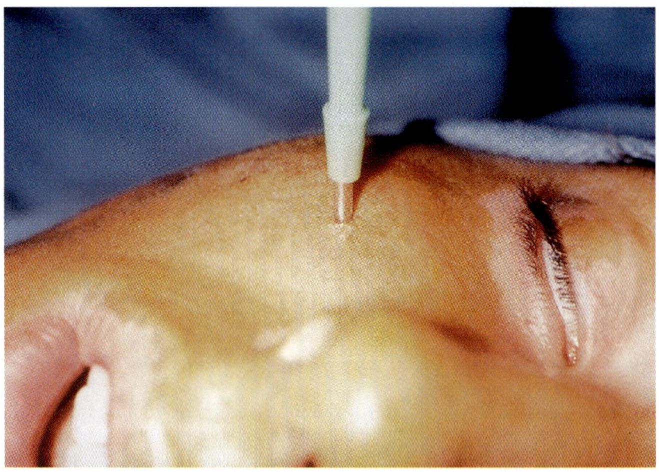

FIG. 23-6
Technique for punch excision.

ture helps to promote wound edge eversion and facilitates proper healing.

Punch elevation. Wide boxcar scars (greater than 3 mm) are the type of scars most amenable to this treatment. A punch that is exactly sized to match the inner diameter of the crateriform scar is selected for treatment. The punch is performed using a quick, rotating motion. This releases the bound-down scar. The plug is elevated with forceps and carefully freed from the underlying tissue. The plug is then elevated and positioned to lie slightly higher than the surrounding skin.

The coagulum that forms is responsible for holding the graft in place temporarily. Dermabond skin adhesive (Ethicon, Somerville, NJ) may be applied to assist in graft placement and stabilization. Dermabond is a fast-setting, 2-octyl cyanoacrylate tissue adhesive used to hold approximated, noninfected wound skin edges together. It is utilized solely for the closure of epidermal edges, as entrance into the wound itself may impede wound healing or result in foreign body reaction due to polymerization of the adhesive polymers. Its use is also limited to dry areas of low skin tension to provide maximal adhesion. Dermabond adhesive use is contraindicated in patients with known hypersensitivities to formaldehyde or cyanoacrylate. It should also not be applied to mucosal surfaces or to any wound with evidence of active infection. Steri-Strips are applied to the treatment sites whether Dermabond is applied or not. These are left in place for 4 to 5 days. An advantage to this procedure is that one avoids the issue of color or texture mismatch, which may occur with punch grafting. A disadvantage is that the punch is scar tissue and therefore may demonstrate persistent textural irregularities once healed. These textural irregularities may be further improved with subsequent treatment with carbon dioxide or erbium laser resurfacing performed 6-8 weeks after the excision is performed.

Punch grafting. This procedure is utilized for deep, irregular pits and tethered boxcar scars.[144] The technique is similar to that of a punch elevation. The plug is removed and a graft plug of tissue obtained from the postauricular area transferred to the plug site. The punch graft should be 0.5 mm larger than the punch used to excise the scar. Smaller grafts can be secured into place with liquid adhesive or Dermabond glue (Ethicon, Somerville, NJ) and Steri-Strips. Larger grafts may require suturing. This technique is more successful for scars located on less mobile regions of the face such as the malar area and the forehead, and less successful in perioral sites.

Complications that may be observed include poor graft take, graft extrusion, and graft visibility. Poor color and textural mismatch are also frequently observed. Given these postoperative sequelae, the authors do not recommend this procedure as first-line treatment for boxcar or ice pick scars.

Excision. Deep, sharply demarcated scars larger than 4 mm may be best managed with elliptical excision. A concern regarding this technique revolves around the increased sebaceous gland activity and prominence often present in the treatment area of patients with acne scars, which may lead to an increased risk of wound depression and widening. To minimize this risk, as much subcutaneous tissue as possible must be preserved to serve as an anchoring base for the overlying wound tissue. For small scars, a simple fusiform excision along relaxed skin lines may be performed (Fig. 23-7). Use of a curvilinear or lazy S incision adds an increased element of concealment in some areas. Larger scars may be excised in a staged fashion, with 4 to 6 weeks allowed between serial excisions.

A

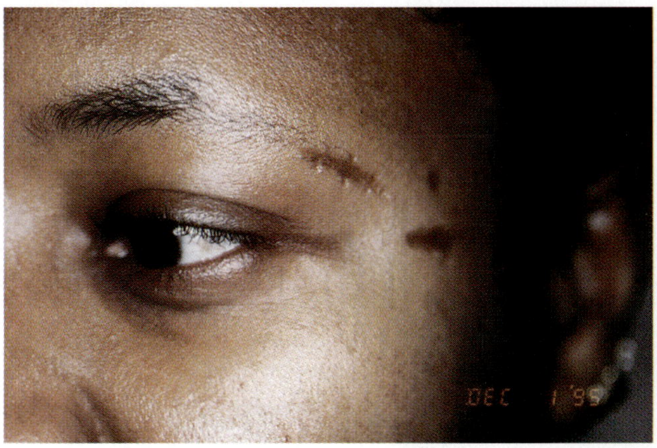

B

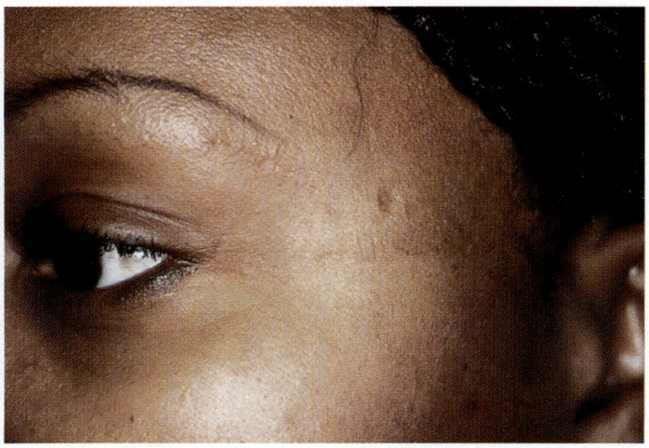

FIG. 23-7
Woman with left temple traumatic scars. **A,** Preoperative appearance. **B,** At 6 months after excisional surgery.

All these techniques may benefit from the addition of carbon dioxide or erbium laser resurfacing, as well as dermabrasion (Figs. 23-8 and 23-9). These procedures may be performed 6 to 8 weeks after the excisional procedures have been completed. By carefully elevating or removing long-standing scar tissue, the surgeon is able to create new scars that are less noticeable than the originals. However, subtle textural irregularities can persist despite meticulous technique. Resurfacing the skin as the surgical wound remodels allows the surgeon to improve the final skin surface contours.

Postprocedural Care. Wound care is performed with twice daily cleansing with soap and water, followed by the application of bacitracin ointment. The sutures are removed in 1 week.

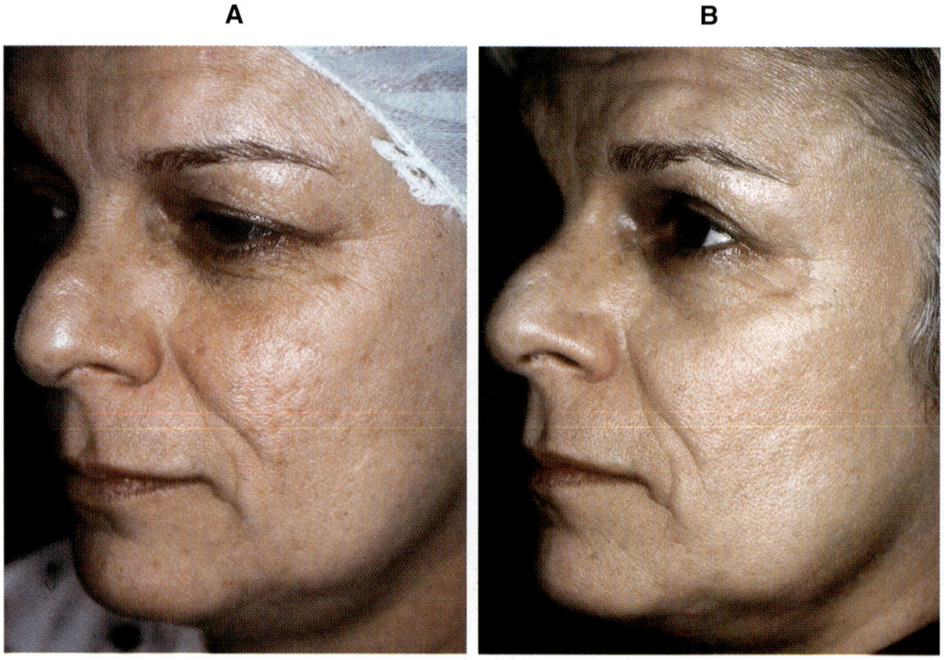

FIG. 23-8
Woman with boxcar acne scarring on cheeks. **A,** Preoperative appearance. **B,** At 6 months after punch excisions followed by carbon dioxide full face resurfacing.

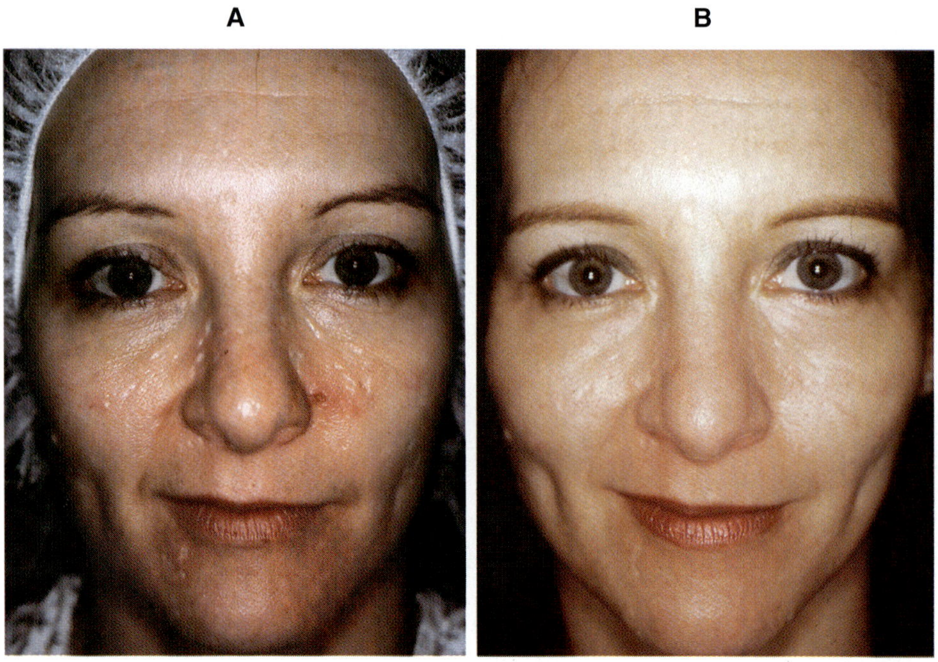

FIG. 23-9
Woman with severe boxcar scarring on face. **A,** Preoperative appearance. **B,** At 1 year after treatment with punch and linear excisions, followed by erbium and carbon dioxide full face resurfacing.

Subcision

Procedure. Following marking of the rolling scars to be treated (with the patient in the sitting position), anesthesia is obtained with injectable 1% lidocaine with 1:100,000 epinephrine. It is advisable to wait 15 to 30 minutes to allow maximal hemostasis. The patient is prepped and draped in the usual sterile fashion.

A sterile, NoKor (Becton Dickinson, Franklin Lakes, NJ) hypodermic 18-gauge needle is inserted through a needle puncture into the skin (Fig. 23-10). The needle is inserted at an acute angle, with the blade oriented parallel to the skin surface (Fig. 23-11). The free, nondominant hand is used to stretch and stabilize the treatment site. Various maneuvers are used to release the subcutaneous fibrotic strands (Fig. 23-12). *Lancing* is a technique involving a linear inserting-withdrawing needle motion similar to pistonlike liposuction cannula movement to subcise very fibrotic scars. *Fanning* involves needle movement, in side-to-side and back-and-forth motions, while withdrawing the needle in a fanlike motion, similar to cutting the bands. A combination of these techniques may be applied, approaching the scar via multiple puncture sites to maximize release of the fibrotic strands. During treatment of bound-down scars, the needle is inserted into the superficial subcutaneous plane and, in some cases, the deep dermis. The final result should be a scar that appears smooth and is elevated from its preoperative bound-down appearance (Fig. 23-13).

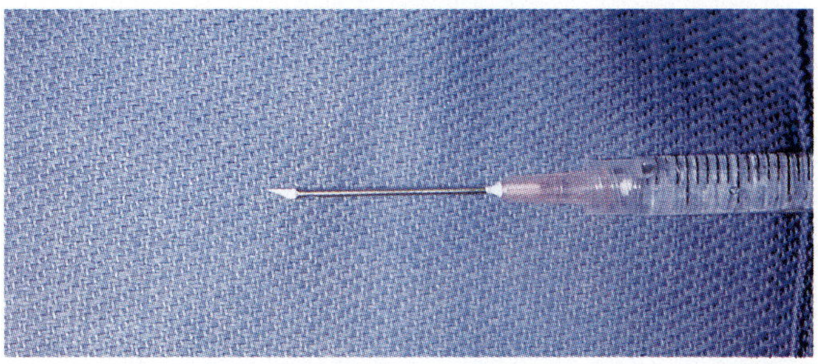

FIG. 23-10
NoKor hypodermic 18-gauge needle.

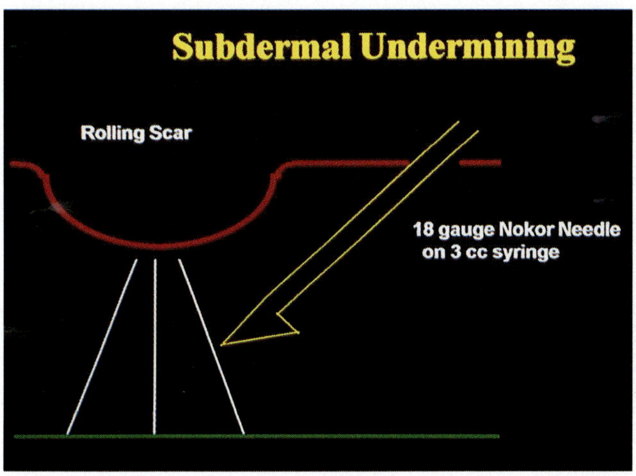

FIG. 23-11
Schematic diagram of subcision technique.

Postprocedural Care. Firm, direct pressure is applied to the treated sites for several minutes after the procedure to obtain hemostasis. The patient is instructed to wash the treatment sites twice daily with soap and water, followed by bacitracin ointment until the needle entrance sites are healed. Camouflage makeup may be applied to cover the bruised areas. Side effects include localized bruising, hypertrophic scarring, and scar recurrence (Box 23-12). If hypertrophic scarring is noted during healing, the affected sites may be treated with monthly injections of intralesional triamcinolone acetonide, 3.3 to 10 mg/ml until flattening occurs.

Carbon Dioxide Laser

Preprocedural Management. The patient's informed consent must be obtained prior to treatment. The patient should be aware of the potential side effects (see Box 23-6). Patients are given prophylactic antiviral medications (500 mg valacyclovir PO bid or 400 mg acyclovir tid) initiated 2 days prior to the procedure and continued for 10 to 14 days until complete reepithelialization has occurred. Antibiotics (500 mg cephalexin PO bid) are administered 1 day prior to the procedure and are continued for 7 to 10 days postoperatively. The patient is made aware that approximately 2 weeks at home will be needed for full recovery.

Procedure. For full face resurfacing, a combination of topical, local, regional nerve blocks, and intravenous (IV) anesthesia are employed to achieve an adequate level of comfort during the procedure. For resurfacing of localized areas, local anesthesia is administered intralesionally or via a nerve block. When intravenous therapy is administered, an anesthesiologist or nurse anesthetist should be present. Typically, IV anesthesia is achieved with propofol, fentanyl, midazolam, or ketamine. Appropriate monitoring equipment, including

BOX 23-12 Side Effects of Subcision

- Bruising
- Hypertrophic scarring
- Scar recurrence
- Discoloration

a blood pressure monitor, electrocardiogram, and oxygen saturation monitor are required, as is an emergency cart complete with Ambu bag and resuscitation medications. Tumescent anesthesia may be utilized. If so, treatment areas should be highlighted with a marker prior to infiltration, as subtle variations in skin topography may be obscured.

A facial scrub should be performed prior to the procedure. Avoidance of all flammable materials, including alcohol swabs, is vital. Hair-bearing areas are covered with wet towels and a nonflammable lubricant. Nonreflective eye shields or protective eye goggles are worn throughout the procedure to prevent eye injury.

When using the UltraPulse laser system (Lumenis, Santa Clara, CA), the 3 mm collimated handpiece is used at energies of 350 to 500 mJ, with a power of 3 to 7 watts. One to three passes are performed over the cosmetic unit or full face without overlapping treatment spots. The treated skin is gently wiped with saline-soaked gauze between laser passes. After the

A B C

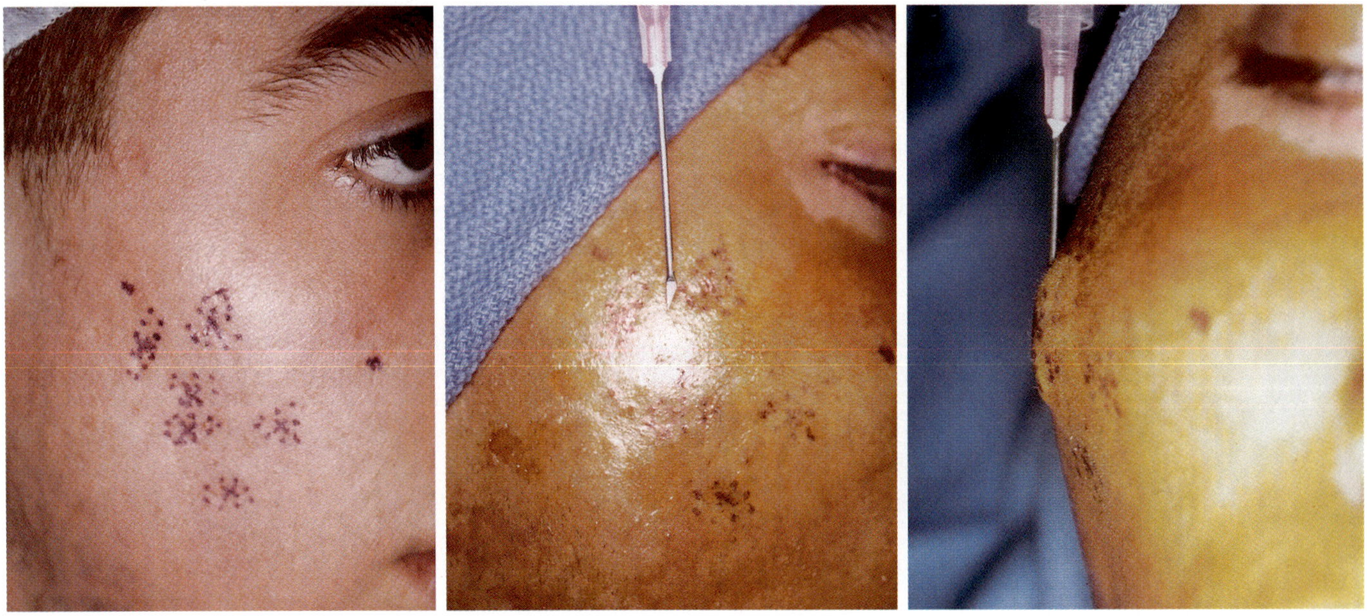

FIG. 23-12
Young man with rolling scars on cheek. **A,** Areas to be subcised marked with "X." **B,** Correct placement of NoKor needle with blade oriented to skin surface. **C,** Tenting with fanning to release fibrotic bands.

A 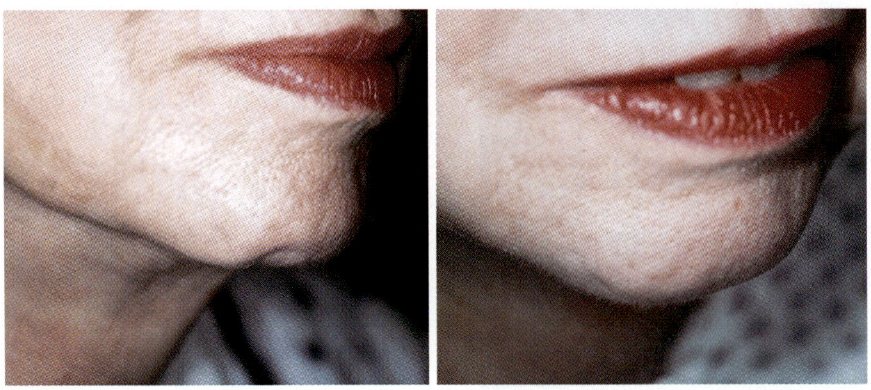 B

FIG. 23-13
Woman with depressed scar on lower chin. **A,** Preoperative appearance. **B,** At 1 year after subcision.

first laser pass, the scars will become more evident as white, slightly depressed scars. Once the face or cosmetic unit has been treated, further laser passes can be made around the scar edges first, then across the scar to even the texture. Care must be taken to avoid overtreatment of the scar, as this may result in a more visible scar once healed. The CPG handpiece may also be used at an energy of 300 mJ, power of 60 watts, a density of 4 to 6, and a size setting of 6 to 8. Generally one or two passes are first made with the CPG, and the fine tracing is performed with the 3 mm collimated handpiece.

When using the SilkTouch laser (Lumenis, Santa Clara, CA), a power of 5 to 7 watts is employed with a 0.2 second pulse duration for spot sizes 2 to 4 mm and a power of 15 watts with a 0.2 second duration for the 6 mm spot size. Treatment is performed as for the UltraPulse laser. Other carbon dioxide lasers available include the NovaPulse (Luxar, Bothell, WA) and TruPulse (Tissue Technologies, Albuquerque, NM).

The erbium:YAG laser is often employed as additional treatment following carbon dioxide resurfacing (see the following discussion).

Postprocedural Care. Immediate postoperative care includes the continuous use of ice packs or cool compresses every 1 to 2 hours. This is followed by the application of Aquaphor (Biersdorf, Wilton, CT) or similar emollient that provides hydration. We recommend the postoperative application of a biocclusive dressing such as Silon TSR (BioMed Sciences, Bethlehem, PA) over the treatment sites for the first 24 to 72 hours, as this results in more rapid reepithelialization and decreased patient discomfort. Once the dressing is removed, soaks are then initiated every 1 to 2 hours until reepithelialization is noted. Postoperative pain control is achieved by administration of oral analgesics and nighttime sedatives. Close follow-up is required for the first few weeks postoperatively to ensure that the patient is able to care for the treated areas properly and that the desired healing is evident. Camouflage makeup may be used after the crusting and oozing have subsided. Optimal results are generally observed 6 to 12 months after full face resurfacing.

Erbium:YAG Laser

Preprocedural Management. Preoperative care is similar to that for the carbon dioxide laser resurfacing patient.

Procedure. Most Er:YAG lasers generate repetition rates from 1 to 10 pulses per second and spot sizes of 3 to 7 mm. Treatment is performed by overlapping pulses by approximately 10% across the treatment area. Approximately 4 μm of tissue is affected for each joule per square centimeter of energy. Settings are adjusted according to the depth of tissue one desires to ablate with each pass. A setting of 5 J/cm^2 will ablate the epidermis in four passes. Care must be taken to limit the extent of tissue ablation for the best treatment control. In general, a range of two to six passes of the Er:YAG laser may be necessary to achieve scar effacement. If scarring is limited, spot laser resurfacing may be employed. The area around and over the scar is resurfaced first, followed by resurfacing of the scar edges until it is completely effaced. If scarring is extensive, the entire face should be resurfaced to obtain more consistent color and textural change. Frequently the Er:YAG laser will be utilized immediately following carbon dioxide laser resurfacing to remove the zone of thermal necrosis left by the carbon dioxide laser as well as to produce additional contouring. In these cases, much more conservative settings and a smaller number of passes should be performed in order to limit the risk of scarring and depigmentation.

Postprocedural Care. Postoperative care measures are similar to those described for carbon dioxide laser resurfacing. Reepithelialization generally occurs over 3 to 10 days.

Autologous Fat Transplantation

Preprocedural Care. The patient's informed consent should be obtained prior to the procedure (Box 23-13). Patients should be aware that the treatment is not permanent and that an average of 50% of the transplanted fat will be resorbed after 1 year.

Procedure. The patient is given an anxiolytic sedative (e.g., diazepam, lorazepam) approximately 15 minutes before the procedure. The selected donor site is sterilely prepped and draped. Cannula insertion sites are selected and anesthetized with a small bolus of 0.1% tumescent lidocaine anesthesia. Small incisions only large enough to allow for introduction of an infusion cannula are made with a No. 11 blade at these sites. Tumescent 0.1% anesthesia is introduced to the donor site subcutaneously via a blunt sprinkler tip infusion cannula attached to a 20 to 60 cc syringe. Anesthesia is allowed to sit for 30 to 45 minutes to obtain maximum

BOX 23-13 Side Effects of Autologous Fat Transplantation

- Minimal bruising
- Temporary edema and erythema
- Minimal pain of the donor site
- Temporary drainage of the donor site
- Infection
- Scarring (rare)
- Unilateral blindness (rare) when used in glabella, periorbital areas[145]

anesthesia and hemostatic effect. The fat is removed using a 12-gauge Klein cannula attached to 10, 20, 30, or 60 cc Luer-Lok syringes (Becton-Dickinson, Franklin Lakes, NJ). The cannula is introduced subcutaneously, and once it is in place, the syringe plunger is pulled back to create negative pressure. The cannula is then moved in a pistonlike motion, with the cannula parallel to the skin. The filled syringes are capped and placed standing in an upright position for 10 minutes to allow for separation of the infranatant from the intact adipocytes by gravitational pooling. The infranatant is discarded to leave blood-free, yellow adipose tissue. If significant blood remains, normal saline solution may be added to the adipocytes, mixed, and allow to settle. The infranatant can again be discarded. The adipocytes are transferred to 3 cc syringes using a female-to-female adapter.

The recipient area is sterilely prepped and draped. A small amount of 1% lidocaine with epinephrine is injected subdermally into the defect, with care not to substantially elevate the depressed treatment areas. A tract can be created by advancing a NoKor needle into the depressed scar. Lipoinjection is then performed with a 16- or 18-gauge needle. The needle is advanced into the depressed scar, and adipose tissue is injected while the needle is withdrawn. Control of fat deposition is obtained by applying manual pressure along the edges of the defect. Lipoinjection is continued until an overcorrection of 20% to 30% is achieved. When complete, the graft is gently molded for precise localization.

Postprocedural Care. Bacitracin and a pressure bandage are placed on the donor site, and bacitracin is applied to the graft sites. The patient is instructed not to shower for 24 hours and to limit facial motion as much as possible, including extensive chewing, over a 24-hour period to limit graft movement. Ice should be applied by the patient intermittently throughout the day. The incision sites are cleaned daily, followed by the application of bacitracin ointment to avoid scab formation and decrease infection risk. Scarring is uncommon. Repeat injections may be performed at 6- to 8-week intervals. Fat can be stored for up to 12 months at –4°C and reused for subsequent injections.

Collagen Injections

Preprocedural Management. The patient's informed consent must be obtained prior to testing and implantation are performed. Skin testing is mandatory prior to the implantation of collagen to eliminate the risk of an allergic reaction, which is seen in 3% of patients tested. Testing is administered as an intradermal injection in the forearm of 0.1 ml of collagen. This is monitored for 4 weeks for signs of sensitivity, including erythema, induration, swelling, or tenderness at the treatment site. Most reactions are noted at 72 hours but may occur at any time within the first month. A second test is administered after 4 weeks. This test will detect those 1.5% to 2% of patients who are at risk of developing a treatment site reaction but have a negative first test. This second test is observed for 2 weeks before collagen implantation.

Patients should be aware of the temporary nature to these treatments, with augmentation lasting between 3 and 6 months. They should also be made aware of the temporary discomfort incurred during treatment.

Procedure. The treatment area is cleansed with alcohol. Implantation is performed with a 30-gauge needle inserted at a 15- to 20-degree angle when Zyderm I or II is injected and at a 30- to 45-degree angle when Zyplast is injected. Injections are made with the needle bevel up. Zyderm I is injected in the superficial papillary dermis, whereas Zyplast is placed in the reticular dermis. Zyderm II should be placed in the mid dermis. White blanching should be avoided when Zyplast is used, and if it is noted, the treated area should be vigorously massaged.

Injectable collagen has proven useful in the treatment of soft, undulating, distensible scars. The more mature and supple the boxcar or rolling scar, the better the results. Ice pick scars and postvaricella scars do not respond well to this treatment. Extensively fibrotic scars are also difficult to treat, as the implant must be placed into scarred dermis under great pressure, and it is difficult to achieve the overcorrection necessary to gain the maximum benefit of the implant. Zyderm II and Zyplast afford the best results for many scars, but Zyderm I is a useful adjunct for maximal contour correction. The scar should be elevated and overcorrected by approximately 50% with Zyderm II. The scar should not be overcorrected when Zyplast is used. Layering of Zyderm I or II over Zyplast can be a particularly effective technique. The number of needlesticks should be minimized to eliminate points of bleeding. If a sudden release of pressure of the syringe is noted during injection, implantation into the subcutaneous tissue may be occurring, which should be avoided, as implantation here is ineffective. Zyplast should be used with caution in the glabella region because of the risk of blindness.

Postoperative Care. Patients are given an ice pack, which may be applied to the treatment areas intermittently throughout the day. No further care is required.

Microdermabrasion

Preprocedural Management. The patient is instructed to wash the treatment areas with a mild facial soap before the procedure to remove any makeup and facial debris present. Protective eye goggles are worn, and cotton gauze is applied to the auricular ostia of both the patient and physician to limit exposure of these areas to aerosolized crystals. No anesthesia is necessary.

Procedure. The handpiece is held against the face, and pressure is adjusted to obtain a suction pressure that results in superficial epidermal microtrauma. The handpiece is moved across the treatment areas in an even, linear motion with a foot pedal controlling the pressure. To minimize patient discomfort, care must be taken not to pull the handpiece across the treatment areas in an upward fashion. The pressure may be increased and treatment repeated to the depressed acne, pox, or trauma scars alone to increase the therapeutic response.

Postprocedural Care. The treatment areas are cleansed to remove any residual crystals present. An emollient is applied to the face, and the patient is instructed to continue applying emollients twice daily until the erythema subsides. Side effects are minimal (Box 23-14). Healing is complete in 1 to 3 days, and treatment may be repeated every 1 to 2 weeks. Multiple treatments (between 5 and 15) generally are necessary for clinical improvement.

Dermabrasion

Preprocedural Management. A prophylactic antiviral medication is initiated 2 days before the procedure, and a prophylactic antibiotic medication is initiated 1 day before the procedure. Preprocedural consent must be obtained after both expectations and side effects of treatment are discussed (Box 23-15).

Procedure. Dermabrasion is performed in an operating room setting. Patients generally require sedation and local anesthesia. Most procedures can be accomplished with low doses of preoperative meperidine (25 to 50 mg IM), hydroxyzine (25 mg IM), and diazepam (5 to 10 mg PO). Facial anesthesia is achieved with local anesthesia using 1% lidocaine with or without epinephrine (1:100,000) or regional nerve blocks. The operating room staff must be protected from airborne and aerosolized particles during the procedure. Appropriate protective measures include gloves, gowns, masks, and protective eyewear.

The area is sterilely prepped and draped. Great care is taken to avoid free gauze, hair, and towels within the surgical field in order to avoid interaction of these materials with the treatment device. Vaseline and gauze pads are used to protect the patient's eyes, ears, and nose. The treatment areas are outlined with gentian violet or surgical ink.

Refrigeration of the skin is performed with spray anesthesia prior to dermabrasion. The choice of spray anesthesia includes Frigiderm (Freon 114, Dermatology Lab and Supply, Council Bluffs, IA) and Fluro-Ethyl (Freon 114 plus ethyl chloride, Gebauer Chemical, Cleveland, OH), which cool to –40°C to –42°C in 25 seconds, and Cryosthesia (Chemtrex, Great Neck, NY) which cools to –52°C to –60°C, resulting in greater tissue necrosis. Frigiderm and Fluro-ethyl are generally recommended, given fewer side effects associated with their use. The spray anesthesia is applied by the assistant in a circular motion for 20 to 30 seconds until the skin becomes frigid and has a white frost on it. Delineation of the area to be frozen is limited to no greater than 2 or 3 cm^2. Towels are used to protect the adjacent skin. Tumescent anesthesia is an alternative method of obtaining good tissue turgor for treatment.

Several types of dermabraders are available, most of which employ a flexible-shaft instrument suggestive of a dental drill. The operative portion may be mounted on a stand or placed on a table. Speeds of 40,000 to 60,000 rpm can be achieved with these instruments, resulting in a greater depth of planing. Hand engines are also utilized, achieving speeds up to 35,000 rpm while providing maximum flexibility of use. These engines are the most popular. The cutting tools for dermabrasion include diamond fraises, wire brushes, and serrated wheels. Diamond fraises are stainless steel wheels with diamond chips bonded to the wheels in different grades of coarseness (regular, coarse, and extra-coarse). They are available in ¾ inch and 3⁄16 inch sizes. Experienced dermabraders utilize the coarser fraises. The wire brush is a stainless steel wheel with wires arranged at an angle. The wire brush is preferred by experienced operators but requires greater skill to control, as it can cut deeply and rapidly. A narrow wire brush permits point contact at its perimeter, allowing for precise control of treatment. Cutting tools are held by a mandrel held in a chuck attached to a flexible cable. A foot pedal rheostat controls speed.

BOX 23-14 Side Effects of Microdermabrasion

- Temporary erythema and desquamation
- Postinflammatory hyperpigmentation
- Granuloma formation
- Eye irritation, including photophobia, epiphora, punctate keratopathy
- Failure to improve mild to moderate scars
- Question of role of aluminum dust in lung disease, Alzheimer's disease

BOX 23-15 Side Effects of Dermabrasion

- Pigmentary alteration (hyperpigmentation or hypopigmentation)
- Hypertrophic scar or keloid
- Infection (bacterial, fungal, or viral)
- Persistent erythema
- Temporary milia

Treatment is performed by spraying and abrading one area at a time, moving from the outermost and dependent areas toward the central and upper areas of the face. The skin is placed under gentle, spreading tension between the thumb and index finger of the non-operating hand. The operator moves the brush or fraise over the frozen skin with firm, steady, back-and-forth strokes with even pressure. The plane of the rotating head is held parallel to the skin's surface while light, brushing strokes are performed. The handpiece is kept in motion at all times in order to avoid heat conduction to the underlying tissue and to produce a more uniform wound depth. At the periphery of the field the pressure and number of strokes are decreased to produce a gradual feathering between treated and non-treated areas. The dermabrasion is usually carried to the end of natural folds of the face (i.e., nasolabial fold, hairline, and under the jawline) to avoid visible demarcation lines that can occur with spot dermabrasion.

Recognition and control of the proper depth of wounding are the most important concepts of dermabrasion. Dermabrasion is normally performed to the level of the papillary (sebaceous glands visible) or superficial reticular (white collagen visible) dermis. Generally two cycles of spraying and abrading are necessary to achieve the desired effect. Undertreatment may result in persistent lines and overtreatment may result in permanent scarring. Chemical exfoliation with 30% to 50% trichloroacetic acid may be applied to adjacent unabraded areas (i.e., lower eyelids and upper lip) for additional blending. Care must be taken when combining the two procedures to prevent pigmentary alterations.

Postprocedural Care. Application of compresses saturated with 1% lidocaine with epinephrine (1:100,000) are applied to the treated areas to assist in vasoconstriction and control bleeding. Vaseline is then applied to the face and a biologic dressing such as Vigilon (Bard Home Health Division, C.R. Bard, Murray Hill, NJ) placed directly on the abraded sites, followed by a Telfa dressing (Kendall Hospital Products, Boston, MA), sterile gauze pads, and wrap. The dressing is changed at 24-hour intervals. After 2 to 4 days the dressings are discontinued and an antibiotic ointment is applied to prevent crusting. Mild soap can be introduced 5 or 6 days postoperatively. Gentle soaking and antibiotic ointment application is performed until reepithelialization occurs.

Lipocytic Dermal Augmentation

Procedure. Adipose tissue is harvested from the donor site as described for autologous fat transplantation, with a total of 10 to 15 ml of fat harvested from the abdomen or thigh. The harvested fat is allowed to stand for 5 minutes, allowing for separation of the fat from the infranatant. The fluid infranatant is decanted and the remaining fat is centrifuged at 1000 rpm for 1 minute. After centrifugation the remaining infranatant is discarded and the fat transferred into 3 cc syringes via a bi-Luer-Lok adapter. The fat is manipulated back and forth through two 3 cc syringes in a sterile fashion to disrupt the adipocytes and connective tissue septa. One milliliter of sterile, distilled water may be added before centrifugation to facilitate this separation.

The recipient site is sterilely prepped and draped. Local anesthesia using 1% lidocaine with epinephrine (1:100,000) is injected subdermally into the borders of the defects, with care to preserve the existing architecture. Lipoinjection is performed with a 16- or 18-gauge needle. The needle is advanced into the depressed scar and adipose tissue is injected while the needle is withdrawn. Control of fat deposition is obtained by applying manual pressure along the edges of the defect. Intradermal lipoinjection is continued until an overcorrection of 20% to 30% is achieved. When complete, the graft is gently molded for precise localization.

Postprocedural Care. Bacitracin and a pressure bandage are placed on the donor site, and bacitracin is applied to the graft sites. The patient is instructed not to shower for 24 hours and to limit facial motion as much as possible, including extensive chewing, over a 24-hour period to limit graft movement. Ice should be applied by the patient intermittently throughout the day. The incision sites are cleaned daily, followed by the application of bacitracin ointment to avoid scab formation and decrease infection risk. Scarring is uncommon. Repeat injections may be performed at 6- to 8-week intervals.

REFERENCES

1. Peacock EEJ, Madden JW, Trier WC. Biologic basis for the treatment of keloids and hypertrophic scars. South Med J 1970; 63: 755-760.
2. Breasted JH. The Edwin Smith Surgical Papyrus: Hieroglyphic Transaction and Commentary. Chicago: University of Chicago Press, 1970; I:403-406.
3. Addison T. On the keloid of Alibert and on true keloids. Mediocochir Trans 1835; 19:19.
4. Cohen IK, McCoy BJ. The biology and control of surface overhealing. World J Surg 1980; 4:289-295.
5. Cosman B, Crikelair GF, Ju DM. The surgical treatment of keloids. Plast Reconstr Surg 1961; 27:335-358.
6. Crockett DJ. Regional keloid susceptibility. Br J Plast Surg 1964; 17:245-253.
7. Ketchum LD, Cohen IK, Masters FW. Hypertrophic scars and keloids: a collective review. Plast Reconstr Surg 1974; 53:140-154.
8. Muir IFK. On the nature of keloids and hypertrophic scars. Br J Plast Surg 1990; 43:61-69.
9. Blackburn WR, Cosman B. Histologic basis of keloid and hypertrophic scar differentiation. Arch Pathol 1966; 82:65.
10. Kischer CW, Shetlar MR. Collagen and mucopolysaccharides in the hypertrophic scar. Connect Tissue Res 1974; 2:205.

11. Kischer CW. The microvessels in hypertrophic scars, keloidal scars and related lesions: a review. J Submicrosc Cytol Pathol 1992; 24:281-296.
12. Kurwa AR. Rubenstein-Taybi syndrome and spontaneous keloids. Clin Exp Dermatol 1979; 4:251.
13. Omo-Dave P. Genetic studies on keloids. J Natl Med Assoc 1975; 67:428.
14. Murray JC, Pollack SV, Pinnell SR. Keloids: a review. J Am Acad Dermatol 1981; 4:461-470.
15. Bloom D. Heredity of keloids: a review of the literature and report of a family with multiple keloids in five generations. NY State J Med 1956; 56:51-519.
16. Castagnoli C, Pervecci OD, Stella M. The HLA-DR beta 116 allogenotype constitutes a risk factor for hypertrophic scarring. Hum Immunol 1990; 24:229-232.
17. Castagnoli C, Stella M, Magliacani G. Anomalous expression of HLA class II molecules on keratinocytes and fibroblasts in hypertrophic scars consequent to thermal injury. Clin Exp Immunol 1990; 82:350-354.
18. Laurentaci G, Diguardi D. HLA antigens in keloids and hypertrophic scars. Arch Dermatol 1977; 113:1726.
19. Ramakrishnan KM, Thomas KP, Sundararjan CR. Study of 1,000 patients with keloids in South India. Plast Reconstr Surg 1974; 53:276-280.
20. Bordin S, Page RC, Narayanan AS. Heterogeneity of normal human diploid fibroblasts: isolation and characterization of one phenotype. Science 1984; 223:171-173.
21. Kischer CW, Theis AC, Chrapil M. Perivascular myofibroblasts and microvascular occlusion in hypertrophic scars and keloids. Hum Pathol 1982; 13:819.
22. Cohen IK, Beaven MA, Horakova Z. Histamine and collagen synthesis in keloid and hypertrophic scars. Surg Forum 1972; 23:509-510.
23. Wang R, Ghahany A, Shen YJ. Nitric oxide synthetase expression and nitric oxide production are reduced in hypertrophic scar tissue and fibroblasts. J Invest Dermatol 1997; 108:438-444.
24. Diegelmann RF, Cohen IK, McCoy B. Growth kinetics and collagen synthesis of normal skin, scar and keloid fibroblasts in vitro. J Cell Physiol 1979; 98:341-346.
25. Clove JN, Cohen IK, Diegelmann RF. Quantitative assays of types I and III collagen synthesized by keloid biopsies and fibroblasts. Acta Biochem Biophys Acad 1979; 586:384-390.
26. Uitto J, Perejda AJ, Abergel RP. Altered steady-state ratio of type I/III procollagen mRNAs correlates with selectively increased type I procollagen biosynthesis in cultured keloid fibroblasts. Proc Natl Acad Sci USA 1985; 82:5935-5939.
27. Cohen IK, Keiser HR, Sjoerdsmo A. Collagen synthesis in human keloid and hypertrophic scars. Surg Forum 1971; 22:488.
28. Russell JD, Witt WS. Cell size and growth characteristics of cultured fibroblasts isolated from normal and keloid tissue. Plast Reconstr Surg 1976; 57:207-212.
29. Linares HA, Lasron DL. Proteoglycans and collagenases in hypertrophic scar formation. Plast Reconstr Surg 1978; 62:589-593.
30. Diegelmann RF, Bryant CP, Cohen IK. Tissue alpha globulins in keloid formation. Plast Reconstr Surg 1977; 59:418-423.
31. Tuan T, Nichter LS. The molecular basis of keloid and hypertrophic scar formation. Mol Med Today 1998; 1:19-24.
32. McCoy BJ, Galdun J, Cohen IK. Effects of density and cellular aging on collagen synthesis and growth kinetics in keloid and normal skin fibroblasts. In Vitro 1982; 18:79-86.
33. Cohen IK, McCoy BJ, Mohanakuma T. Immunoglobulin complement and histocompatability antigen studies in keloid patients. Plast Reconstr Surg 1979; 63:689-695.
34. Block ER, Hall MG, Densin MJ. General immune reactivity in keloid patients. Plast Reconstr Surg 1984; 73:448-451.
35. Janssen de Limpens AM, Cormane RH. Keloids and hypertrophic scars: immunological aspects. Aesthetic Plast Surg 1982; 6:149-152.
36. Sandberg N. Accelerated collagen formation and histamine. Nature 1962; 194:183.
37. Harris EDJ, Sjoerdsma A. Collagen profile in clinical conditions. Lancet 1966; 2:707-711.
38. Ignotz RA, Massague J. Transforming growth factor-B stimulates the expression of fibronectin and collagen and their incorporation into the extracellular matrix. J Biol Chem 1986; 261: 4337-4345.
39. Overal CM, Wrane JL, Sodek J. Independent regulation of collagenase, 72-kd-progelatinase and metalloproteinase inhibitor (TIMP) expression in human fibroblasts by transforming growth factor-B. J Biol Chem 1989; 264:1860-1869.
40. Younai S, Nichter LS, Wellisz T. Modulation of collagen synthesis by transforming growth factor-B in keloid and hypertrophic scar fibroblasts. Ann Plast Surg 1994; 33:148-151.
41. Ghahany A, Shen YJ, Nedelec B. Enhanced expression of mRNA for insulin-like growth factor-1 in post-burn hypertrophic scar tissue and its fibrogenic role by dermal fibroblasts. Mol Cell Biochem 1995; 148:25.
42. Lynch SE, Colvin RR, Antoniades HN. Growth factors in wound healing: single and synergistic effects on partial thickness porcine skin wounds. J Clin Invest 1989; 84:640.
43. Druit R. Modern Surgery. Philadelphia: Lea and Blanchard, 1844.
44. DeCosta JC. Modern Surgery. Philadelphia: Saunders, 1903.
45. Darzi MA, Chowdi NA, Kaul SK. Evaluation of various methods of treating keloids and hypertrophic scars: a 10-year follow-up study. Br J Plast Surg 1992; 45:374.
46. Hintz BL. Radiotherapy for keloid treatment. J Natl Med Assoc 1973; 65:71-75.
47. Ma S, Fang RH, Chang WP. Heterogeneity in radiosensitivity of human diploid fibroblasts from keloids and normal skin. Cell Biol Int 1996; 20:289-292.
48. DeBeurman R, Gougerot H. Cheloides des muquescies. Ann Dermatol Syphilol 1906; 7:151.
49. Cosman B, Crikelair GF, Faulin TC. The surgical treatment of keloids. Plast Reconstr Surg 1961; 27:335.
50. Levitt WM, Fagillies H. Radiotherapy in the prophylaxis and treatment of keloids. Lancet 1942; 1:440.
51. Borok TL, Bray M, Sinclair I. Role of ionizing irradiation for 393 keloids. Int J Radiat Oncol Biol Phys 1988; 15:856-870.
52. Doornbos JF, Stoffel TJ, Haas AC, et al. The role of kilovoltage irradiation in the treatment of keloids. Int J Radiat Oncol Biol Phys 1990; 18:833-839.
53. Levy DS, Salter MM, Roth RE. Postoperative irradiation in the prevention of keloids. Am J Roentgenol 1976; 127:509.
54. Ollstein RN, Siegel HW, Gillooley F. Treatment of keloids by combined surgical excision and immediate postoperative x-ray therapy. Ann Plast Surg 1981; 7:281.
55. Enhamre A, Hammer H. Treatment of keloids with excision and postoperative x-ray irradiation. Dermatologica 1983; 90:167.
56. Malaker K, Ellis F, Paine CH. A new method of treatment combining surgery with interstitial radiotherapy. Clin Radiol 1976; 27:179-183.
57. Hoffman S. Radiotherapy for keloids? Ann Plast Surg 1982; 9: 205.
58. Linares HA, Larson DL, Willis-Galstaun BA. Historical notes on the use of pressure in the treatment of hypertrophic scars or keloids. Burns 1993; 19:17-21.
59. Kischer CW, Shetlar MR, Shetlar CC. Alteration of hypertrophic scars induced by mechanical pressure. Arch Dermatol 1975; 11: 60-64.
60. Baur PS, Larson DL, Stacey TR. Ultrastructural analysis of pressure-treated scars by mechanical pressure. J Trauma 1976; 10: 958-967.

61. Carr-Collins JA. Pressure techniques for the prevention of hypertrophic scars. Clin Plast Surg 1992; 19:733-743.
62. Quinn KJ. Silicone gel in scar treatment. Burns 1987; 113:533-540.
63. Perkins K, Davey RB, Walis KA. Silicone gel: a new treatment for burns and contractures. Burns 1982; 9:406-410.
64. Dockery GL, Nilson RZ. Treatment of hypertrophic and keloid scars with Silastic gel sheeting. J Foot Ankle Surg 1994; 33:110-119.
65. Katz BE. Silicone gel sheeting in scar therapy. Cutis 1995; 56:65-67.
66. Ricketts CH, Martin L, Faria DT. Cytokine mRNA changes during the treatment of hypertrophic scars with silicone and non-silicone gel dressings. Dermatol Surg 1996; 22:955-959.
67. Bailin P. Use of the CO_2 laser for non-PWS cutaneous lesions. In: Arndt KA, Noe JM, Rosen S, eds. Cutaneous Laser Therapy: Principles and Methods. New York: John Wiley, 1983:187-200.
68. Norris TE. The effect of carbon dioxide laser surgery on the recurrence of keloids. Plast Reconstr Surg 1991; 87:44-49.
69. Apfelberg DB, Maser MR, Lash H. Preliminary results of argon and carbon dioxide laser treatment of keloid scars. Lasers Surg Med 1984; 4:283-290.
70. Olbricht SM, Arndt KA. Lasers in cutaneous surgery. In: Fuller T, ed. Surgical Lasers: A Clinical Guide. New York: Macmillan, 1987.
71. Bernstein LJ, Kauvar ANB, Grossman MC. Scar resurfacing with high-energy, short-pulsed and flashscanning carbon dioxide lasers. Dermatol Surg 1998; 24:101-107.
72. Ginsbach G, Kuhnel W. The treatment of hypertrophic scars and keloids by argon laser: clinical data and morphological findings. Plast Surg Forum 1978; 1:61-67.
73. Hulsbergen-Henning JP, Roskann Y, vanGemert M. Treatment of keloids and hypertrophic scars with an argon laser. Lasers Surg Med 1986; 6:72-75.
74. Abergel RP, Merke CA, Lam TS. Control of connective tissue metabolism by lasers: recent developments and future prospects. J Am Acad Dermatol 1984; 11:1142.
75. Alster TS. Alteration of argon laser-induced scars by the pulsed dye laser. Lasers Surg Med 1993; 13:368-373.
76. Alster T. Improvement of erythematous and hypertrophic scars by the 585 nm pulsed dye laser. Ann Plast Surg 1994; 32:186-190.
77. Dierickx C, Goldman MP, Fitzpatrick RE. Laser treatment of erythematous/hypertrophic and pigmented scars in 26 patients. Plast Reconstr Surg 1993; 95:84-90.
78. Goldman M, Fitzpatrick RE. Laser treatment of scars. Dermatol Surg 1995; 21:685-687.
79. Alster TS, Williams CM. Treatment of keloid sternotomy scars with 585 nm flashlamp-pumped pulsed dye laser. Lancet 1995; 345:1198.
80. Reiken SR, Wolfort SF, Berthiaume F. Control of hypertrophic scar growth using selective photothermolysis. Lasers Surg Med 1997; 21:7-12.
81. Mancini RE, Quaife JV. Histogenesis of experimentally produced keloids. J Invest Dermatol 1962; 38:143.
82. McCoy B, Diegelmann RF, Cohen IK. In vitro inhibition of cell growth, collagen synthesis and prolyl hydroxylase activity by triamcinolone acetonide. Proc Soc Exp Biol Med 1980; 163:216-222.
83. Rusciani L, Rosse G, Bono R. Use of cryotherapy in the treatment of keloids. J Dermatol Surg Oncol 1993; 19:529-534.
84. Ceilley RI, Barin RW. The combined use of cryosurgery and intralesional injections of suspension of fluorinated adrenocorticosteroids for reducing keloids and hypertrophic scars. J Dermatol Surg Oncol 1979; 5:54.
85. Layton AM, Yip J, Cunliffe WJ. A comparison of intralesional triamcinolone and cryosurgery in the treatment of acne keloids. Br J Dermatol 1994; 130:498-501.
86. Jimenez SA, Freundlich B, Rosenbloom J. Selective inhibition of human diploid fibroblast collagen synthesis by interferons. J Clin Invest 1984; 74:1112-1116.
87. Granstein RO, Rook A, Flotte TJ. Controlled trial of intralesional recombinant interferon-gamma in the treatment of keloidal scarring. Arch Dermatol 1990; 126:1295-1302.
88. Larrabee WFJ, East CA, Jaffee AS. Intralesional interferon gamma treatment for keloids and hypertrophic scars. Arch Otolaryngol Head Neck Surg 1990; 110:1159-1162.
89. Pittet B, Rubbia-Brandt L, Desmoulieve A. Effect of gamma-interferon on the clinical and biological evolution of hypertrophic scars and Dupuytren's disease: an open pilot study. Plast Reconstr Surg 1994; 93:1224-1235.
90. Berman B, Duncan MR. Short-term keloid treatment in vivo with human interferon alpha-2b results in a selective and persistent normalization of keloidal fibroblast collagen, glycosaminoglycans and collagenase production in vivo. J Am Acad Dermatol 1989; 21:694-702.
91. Berman B, Flores F. Recurrence rates of excised keloids treated with postoperative triamcinolone acetonide injections or interferon alfa-2b injections. J Am Acad Dermatol 1997; 37:755-757.
92. Conejo-Mir JS, Corbi R, Linares M. Carbon dioxide laser ablation associated with interferon alfa-2b injections reduces the recurrence of keloids. J Am Acad Dermatol 1998; 39:1039-1040.
93. Al-Khawajah MM. Failure of interferon-alpha 2B in the treatment of mature keloids. Int J Dermatol 1996; 35:515-517.
94. Wong TW, Chiu HC, Yip KM. Intralesional interferon alfa-2b has no effect in the treatment of keloids. Br J Dermatol 1994; 130: 683-684.
95. Janssen de Limpens AMP. The local treatment of hypertrophic scars and keloids with topical retinoic acid. Br J Dermatol 1980; 103:319-323.
96. Peacock EE. Pharmacological control of surface scarring in human beings. Ann Surg 1981; 193:592-597.
97. Schorn D, Francis MJD, London M. Skin collagen biosynthesis in patients with rheumatoid arthritis treated with penicillamine. Scand J Rheumatol 1979; 8:124.
98. Dolynchuk KN, Ziesmann M, Serletti JM. Topical putrescine (fibrostat) in treatment of hypertrophic scars: phase II study. Plast Reconstr Surg 1979; 97:117-123.
99. Soderberg T, Hallmans T, Bartholson L. Treatment of keloids and hypertrophic scars with adhesive zinc tape. Scand J Plast Reconstr Surg 1982; 16:261-266.
100. Ehrlich HP, Tavier H, Hunt TK. Inhibitory effects of vitamin E on collagen synthesis and wound repair. Ann Surg 1972; 175: 235.
101. Bosse JP. Clinical study of a new anti-keloid agent. Ann Plast Surg 1972; 175:235.
102. Lee RC, Ping JA. Calcium antagonists retard extracellular matrix production in connective tissue equivalent. J Surg Res 1990; 49:463-466.
103. Lawrence WT. Treatment of earlobe keloids with surgery plus adjuvant intralesional verapamil and pressure earrings. Ann Plast Surg 1996; 37:167-169.
104. Topol BM, Lewis VL, Benveniste K. The use of antihistamines to retard the growth of fibroblasts derived from human skin, scar and keloids. Plast Reconstr Surg 1981; 68:227-232.
105. Duncan JL, Thomson AW, Muir LFK. Topical cyclosporin and T-lymphocytes in keloid scars. Br J Dermatol 1991; 124:109.
106. Pollack SV, Gosler JB. The surgical treatment of keloids. J Dermatol Surg Oncol 1982; 8:1045-1049.
107. Walker JJ. Ultrasound therapy for keloids. S Afr Med J 1983; 64:270.
108. Hirschowitz B, Lindenbaum E, Har-Shai Y. Static-electric field induction by a silicone cushion for the treatment of hypertrophic and keloid scars. Plast Reconstr Surg 1998; 10:1173-1183.
109. Shigeki S, Murakani T, Yata N. Treatment of keloid and hypertrophic scars by iontophoretic transdermal delivery of transilast. Scand J Plast Reconstr Hand Surg 1997; 31:151-158.
110. Smyth J. Treatment of keloids. Br Med J 1913; 2:811.

111. Ahlswede E. Digestion of keloids, cicatrices and buboes with pepsin and hydrochloric acid. Arch Dermatol Syphilol 1921; 142.
112. Layton KM, Henderson CA, Cunliffe WJ. A clinical evaluation of acne scarring and its incidence. Med Exp Dermatol 1994; 19: 303-308.
113. Roenigk HH Jr, Pinski JB, Robinson JK, Hanke CW. Acne, retinoids, and dermabrasion. J Dermatol Surg Oncol 1985; 11:396.
114. Orentreich DS, Orentreich N. Subcutaneous incisionless (subcision) surgery for the correction of depressed scars and wrinkles. Dermatol Surg 1995; 21:543-549.
115. Spangler AS. New treatment for pitted scars. Arch Dermatol 1957; 76:708-711.
116. Gottlieb S. GAP repair technique (Poster exhibit). December, 1977; Annual Meeting of the American Academy of Dermatology, Dallas, TX.
117. Koranda FC. Treatment modalities in facial acne scars. In: Thomas JR, Holt GR, eds. Facial Scars: Incision, Revision and Camouflage. St. Louis: Mosby, 1989:285.
118. Fitzpatrick RE, Tope WD, Goldman MP, Satur NM. Pulsed carbon dioxide laser, trichloroacetic acid, Baker-Gordon phenol, and dermabrasion: a comparative clinical and histologic study of cutaneous resurfacing in a porcine model. Arch Dermatol 1996; 132:469-471.
119. Apfelberg DB. A critical appraisal of high-energy pulsed carbon dioxide laser facial resurfacing for acne scars. Ann Plast Surg 1997; 38:95-100.
120. Alster TS, West TB. Resurfacing of atrophic facial scars with a high-energy, pulsed carbon-dioxide laser. Dermatol Surg 1996; 22:151-155.
121. Kye YC. Resurfacing of pitted facial scars with a pulsed Er:YAG laser. Dermatol Surg 1997; 23:880-883.
122. Cho SI, Kim YC. Treatment of atrophic facial scars with combined use of high-energy pulsed CO_2 laser and Er:YAG laser: a practical guide of the laser techniques for the Er:YAG laser. Dermatol Surg 1999; 25:959-964.
123. Neuber F. Fat grafting. Cuir Kongr Verh Otsum Ges Chir 1893; 20:66.
124. Peer LA. Loss of weight and volume in human fat grafts. Plast Reconstr Surg 1950; 5:217.
125. Gurney CE. Studies on the fate of free transplants of fat. Proc Staff Meet Mayo Clin 1937; 12:317.
126. Matsudo PKR, Toledo LS. Experience of injected fat grafting. Aesthetic Plast Surg 1988; 12:35.
127. Asken S. Autologous fat transplantation: micro and macrotechniques. Am J Cosmet Surg 1987; 4:111.
128. Hudson DA, Lambert EV, Bloch CE. Site selection for autotransplantation: some observations. Aesthetic Plast Surg 1990; 14:195.
129. Coleman WPI, Lawrence N, Sherman RN, et al. Autologous collagen? Lipocytic dermal augmentation: a histopathologic study. J Dermatol Surg Oncol 1993; 19:1032-1040.
130. Knapp TR, Kaplan EN, Daniels JR. Injectable collagen for soft tissue augmentation. Plast Reconstr Surg 1977; 60:398.
131. Kromayer E. Die Heilung der Akne durch ein Neves Narbrnlases Operationsverfahren: das Stanzen. Illustr Monatsscht Aerztl Polytech 1905; 27:101.
132. Kromayer E. Cosmetic Treatment of Skin Complaints. English translation of the Second German Edition. London: Oxford University Press, 1930.
133. Iverson PC. Surgical removal of traumatic tattoos of the face. Plast Reconstr Surg 1947; 2:427-432.
134. Burke JW Jr. Wire Brush Surgery. Springfield, Ill: Charles C Thomas, 1956.
135. Monteleone G. Microdermabrasion with aluminum hydroxide powder in scar camouflaging. Proceedings of the Third Meeting of the Southern Italy Plastic Surgery Association. Benevento. December 9-10, 1988.
136. Tsai R-Y, Wang C-N, Chan H-L. Aluminum oxide crystal microdermabrasion: a new technique for treating facial scarring. Dermatol Surg 1995; 21:539-542.
137. Apfelberg DB, Maser MR, Lash H. The use of epidermis over a keloid as an autograft after resection of the keloid. J Dermatol Surg Oncol 1976; 2:409.
138. Weimar VM, Ceilley RI. Treatment of keloids on earlobes. J Dermatol Surg Oncol 1979; 5:522.
139. Murray RD. Kenalog and the treatment of hypertrophied scars and keloids in negroes and whites. Plast Reconstr Surg 1963; 31: 275.
140. Davies DM. Scars, hypertrophic scars and keloids. Br Med J 1985; 19:733-743.
141. Wong T, Chiu H, Chen J. Symptomatic keloids in two children. Arch Dermatol 1995; 131:775-776.
142. Friedman SJ, Butler DR, Pittelkow MR. Perilesional linear atrophy and hypopigmentation after intralesional corticosteroid therapy. J Am Acad Dermatol 1988; 19:537-541.
143. Fitzpatrick RE. Treatment of inflamed hypertrophic scars using intralesional 5-FU. Dermatol Surg 1999; 25:224-232.
144. Johnson WC. Treatment of pitted scars: punch transplant technique. J Dermatol Surg Oncol 1986; 12:260-265.
145. Temouria B. Blindness following fat injections. Correspondence and brief communications. Plast Reconstr Surg 1988; 80:361.

Index

Note: Page numbers followed by f refer to figures; page numbers followed by t refer to tables; page numbers followed by b refer to boxes.

C

D

T

X

Y

Z